HARRY J. GRIFFITHS, M.D.
Associate Professor of Radiology and Orthopedics,
The University of Rochester School of
Medicine and Dentistry;

Senior Radiologist,
Strong Memorial Hospital,
Rochester, New York.

ROBERT C. SARNO, M.D.
Assistant Professor of Radiology,
Tufts University School of Medicine;

Assistant Radiologist,
New England Medical Center Hospital,
Boston, Massachusetts.

with a chapter on Nuclear Medicine by

WILLIAM D. KAPLAN, M.D.
Assistant Professor of Radiology,
Harvard Medical School;

Chief, Oncologic Nuclear Medicine,
Sidney Farber Cancer Institute,
Boston, Massachusetts.

CONTEMPORARY RADIOLOGY

An Introduction to Imaging

HARRY J. GRIFFITHS

and

ROBERT C. SARNO

1979

W. B. SAUNDERS COMPANY
PHILADELPHIA • LONDON • TORONTO

W. B. Saunders Company: West Washington Square
Philadelphia, PA 19105

1 St. Anne's Road
Eastbourne, East Sussex BN21 3UN, England

1 Goldthorne Avenue
Toronto, Ontario M8Z 5T9, Canada

Contemporary Radiology: An Introduction to Imaging ISBN 0-7216-4282-9

 Made in the United States of America. Press of W. B. Saunders Company. Library of Congress catalog card number 78-64711.

Last digit is the print number: 9 8 7 6 5 4 3 2 1

We would like to dedicate this book to

OUR MOTHERS

and

to two great teachers of radiology

ALICE ETTINGER and the late GEORGE SIMON

PREFACE

This book separates naturally into two parts: The first seven chapters compose a catalogue of many radiological procedures available today. We begin with plain film studies and go on to contrast media procedures, including many relatively sophisticated techniques. Discussions of nuclear medicine and ultrasound follow, which encompass the more traditional imaging procedures in these fields as well as some more advanced techniques that may not be generally available at the moment but will probably become more widely accepted soon. The seventh chapter is a look into the future, with a discussion of some other methods of imaging.

The second half of the book, consisting of six chapters, is clinically oriented. Most of the common signs and symptoms are discussed and are illustrated with short case histories. It is our intention that the reader be entertained as well as informed as to the best way to approach a given clinical situation (such as a patient with dyspnea or a headache).

It is obviously impossible to cover every clinical situation and yet have a volume of reasonable size. Such diagnostic dilemmas as severely traumatized or suicidal patients have been excluded from this work, which was written primarily for medical students in clinical years of study and for interns, and for residents just beginning their careers. We hope, however, that the book will appeal to emergency room personnel and to radiological technicians, who, although they are responsible for performing many of the studies outlined in this book, are actually kept "in the dark" with respect to interpretations and results.

"I wish thee as much pleasure in the reading as I had in the writing."

FRANCES QUARLES

ACKNOWLEDGMENTS

Many people who have helped with the planning and writing of this book deserve our thanks, particularly those friends who have provided suitable names and literary inspiration and who have helped drink the local vino. We would also like to thank Anne Sophie and Michael Grant for the use of their wonderful house, where the majority of the manuscript was put together for the first time. Among the friends who helped at that early stage were Peter Manzi, Debbie Hall, Jeffrey Rich, and Steven Hammerschlag.

We are indebted to the various people who proofread the manuscript at later stages in its production; we thank them all for their time, patience, and perseverance. Although we are unable to mention everyone in this regard, we would particularly like to mention Dr. Harry Fischer for the care he took in reading most of the manuscript and for many helpful suggestions. We would also like to thank Dr. Alice Ettinger for her advice, Dr. Steven Hammerschlag for his help with the neuroradiology section, Dr. Robert Paul for his help in general, Dr. Ray Gramiak for his advice about the ultrasound chapter, and Dr. Robert O'Mara for his assistance with the nuclear medicine section.

Although many of the illustrations and case histories have been collected by us over the years (some were collected in the last two days), we are especially indebted to Dr. Barbara Carter for the use of the teaching file at Tufts–New England Medical Center and to Dr. Jeffrey Moore for the use of material from the Temple University collection. In fact, without Dr. Carter's orderly collecting, this book would not have been possible. We would like to thank Barbara Billings and Pat Jayson, also at Tufts–New England Medical Center, for the help in rounding up ideas, cases, and material.

Dr. Stanley Rogoff gave us the use of the University of Rochester teaching collection. Thanks are extended also to Ginny Bleier and Dr. Marilyn Goske in Rochester.

Photographs for the illustrations were produced by the photographic departments of Tufts Medical School and the University of Rochester, and we thank personnel of both departments (especially Tom Moon) for their patience, assistance, and workmanship. We would like to express our gratitude to Robert Blake for his help and understanding with the earliest images.

Several people who gave us invaluable help with the collection of cases outside our own fields of interest deserve mention: Richard Weschler for the CT scans, Mully Wolpert and Eric Farber for neuroradiology, Victor Millan for angiography, and Debbie Hall for xeroradiography as well as some other cases. We also thank Curt Robison, Stuart Belkin, Marc Homer (our mentor in mammography), Roy McCauley, Jovitas Skucas, and Walter Plassche among others for help in acquiring specific cases that we needed to complete the illustrations.

The initial draft of the manuscript was typed by Mrs. Joan Foley in great good humor. Natalie Shaheen followed R.S. through countless redrafts and last-minute taxi rides to Logan airport. Thelma LaPierre and particularly Ellie Markum made the ten-finger effort to complete the final draft.

Choosing cases and radiographs from a variety of sources, especially teaching collections, makes failures of proper acknowledgment almost inevitable. We would like to apologize to anyone whose case appears in this book without acknowledgment, and we welcome notification of such oversights for correction in later editions.

In the final analysis, this book would not have been possible without the help and cooperation of H.G.'s secretary, Alyce Norder. Her help, understanding, unfailing good humor, and magnificent typing, and especially her uncanny ability to read H.G.'s writing (as well as his mind) have been of incalculable assistance throughout the production of this book.

HARRY J. GRIFFITHS
ROBERT C. SARNO

CONTENTS

CHAPTER 1

HISTORY AND PRINCIPLES OF RADIOLOGY

HISTORICAL BACKGROUND

Conrad Roentgen discovered x-radiation by accident in November 1895 while working with accelerated electrons in cathode ray tubes. He presented a paper on it before the Medico-Physical Society of Wurtzberg in January 1896. Roentgen's discovery and his rapid evaluation of the potential of the x-ray resulted in his being awarded the first Nobel Prize for physics in 1901. This new discovery swept the world, and by 1900, there were flourishing radiological societies in New York, Chicago, Vienna, Berlin, and London. As early as November 1896, experimentation was being conducted with various substances in the hope of discovering an agent that would opacify hollow organs. Air, calcium sulfate, lead, bismuth, and other heavy metals were all tried. In 1910, the first liquid angiographic medium was used (bismuth in oil), but it was found to be extremely toxic. It was not until 1923, when a 20 per cent sodium iodide solution was injected into the antecubital vein of a man, that angiography as we know it today was really launched.

Retrograde pyelography was first attempted in 1904, and the first intravenous pyelograms, using colloidal suspensions of heavy metals, were performed in 1905. In 1923, the first intravenous pyelograms using sodium iodide were performed, but this contrast agent was found to be very toxic; in 1928 the first modern non-toxic agents were in use routinely for opacification of the renal tract. By 1910, opacification of both the upper and the lower gastrointestinal tract became commonplace. Fluorescent screens were introduced in 1899, although it was not until the 1920s that effective fluoroscopy became widely available. Finally, image intensification, which produces a brighter radiographic image and is an inherent part of television fluoroscopy units, became a reality in 1941, after having been described as "distant electric vision" as early as 1911. The use of image intensification and television has revolutionized many special procedures. More recently computerized axial tomography (the CT or CAT scanner) was introduced. Initially intended to scan only the head, the process was modified in 1972 to scan the whole body.

PHYSICAL PRINCIPLES

Most people are familiar with various forms of electromagnetic radiation such as visible light, ultraviolet light, radiant heat, and that used in radio and television communication. The only difference among the various types of electromagnetic radiation is their wavelength and corresponding frequency. X-rays are electromagnetic radiations of specific wavelengths (1.0 Å to 0.1 Å) and are produced in an x-ray tube by the deceleration of fast-moving electrons. The x-ray tube consists of a glass cylinder with a vacuum inside. The electrons are produced from a tungsten coil (termed the *cathode*) which the coil is heated.

One of the variables in the production of diagnostic x-rays is the number of electrons to be accelerated; this can be controlled by selecting the milliamperage of exposure that will determine the number of electrons to be boiled off the cathode. After the electrons are produced in the tube, they are accelerated from the cathode toward the positively charged anode by a potential, which is placed across the x-ray tube between the cathode and the anode. As the electrons strike the anode, the most significant effect is the production of a large amount of heat, although a small percentage (about 1 per cent) of the accelerated electrons produce x-rays. The x-rays are produced primarily by means of a phenomenon termed *bremsstrahlung*, in which a negatively charged electron with high kinetic energy is slowed down by a positively charged nucleus from the tungsten anode. The energy lost from the fast-moving electron is expelled as x-rays. This process accounts for the majority of x-rays used in diagnostic radiology. However, small amounts of radiation are also produced in the anode by the ejection of electrons from the anode's tungsten atoms. As an electron is ejected from a shell near the nucleus of the tungsten atom, more peripherally located electrons fill the vacancy in the inner shell. As this occurs, *characteristic radiation* is produced.

A second controllable variable in the production of diagnostic x-rays is the potential across which the electrons are accelerated in the x-ray tube. The potential is measured in kilovolts. Higher kilovoltage levels cause electrons to be accelerated faster, in turn producing x-rays of higher energy.

A third variable in the amount of radiation produced is the time factor. This is simply the duration in seconds of exposure of the patient to the x-rays themselves. In diagnostic radiology, therefore, one speaks of kilovoltage, milliamperage, and time when determining the extent of patient exposure.

After they are produced, the x-rays exit in a fan-shaped beam toward the patient. Lead panels are placed to contain the lateral extent and the size of the radiation beam. The beam is directed through the patient. Behind the patient is a film, which is often contained in a metal cassette (merely a housing around the radiographic film itself). The cassette serves two purposes: it prohibits light exposure of the radiographic film, and it frequently contains a screen that fluoresces in the presence of x-rays. Fluorescence or production of light within the cassette exposes the film directly. It is important to remember that the image seen on the radiographic film is not merely the result of the direct effect of the x-rays on the film but is primarily due to the light exposure of the film inside the cassette.

RADIOLOGICAL PRINCIPLES

The x-radiation interacts with different substances in the body in different ways, depending on the degree to which the beam is attenuated by the substance. This variation in interaction results in four basic densities on a film: *air* which appears *black*, *fat* which appears *dark grey*, *soft tissue* which appears *light grey*, and *bone* which appears *white*. All radiographic images depend on the differences in these tissues and the interfaces that may be seen between them. Let us take a chest x-ray as an example (Fig. 1–1). Look for the air above the shoulders as well as in the lung fields. Look at the heart and diaphragms; the interface between these structures and the air in the lungs allows us to see their outline. However, should there be a consolidation in the medial segment of the right middle lobe, part of the right heart border would be lost; this is the *silhouette sign* (Fig. 1–2). Similarly, a pneumonia in the left lower lobe would efface the inner margin of the left hemidiaphragm. The ribs and spine are bone and can be clearly seen through the overlying soft tissues. Fat is more difficult to recognize immediately, but it can be seen separating the muscles in the shoulder or the leg. Visualization of the renal outlines

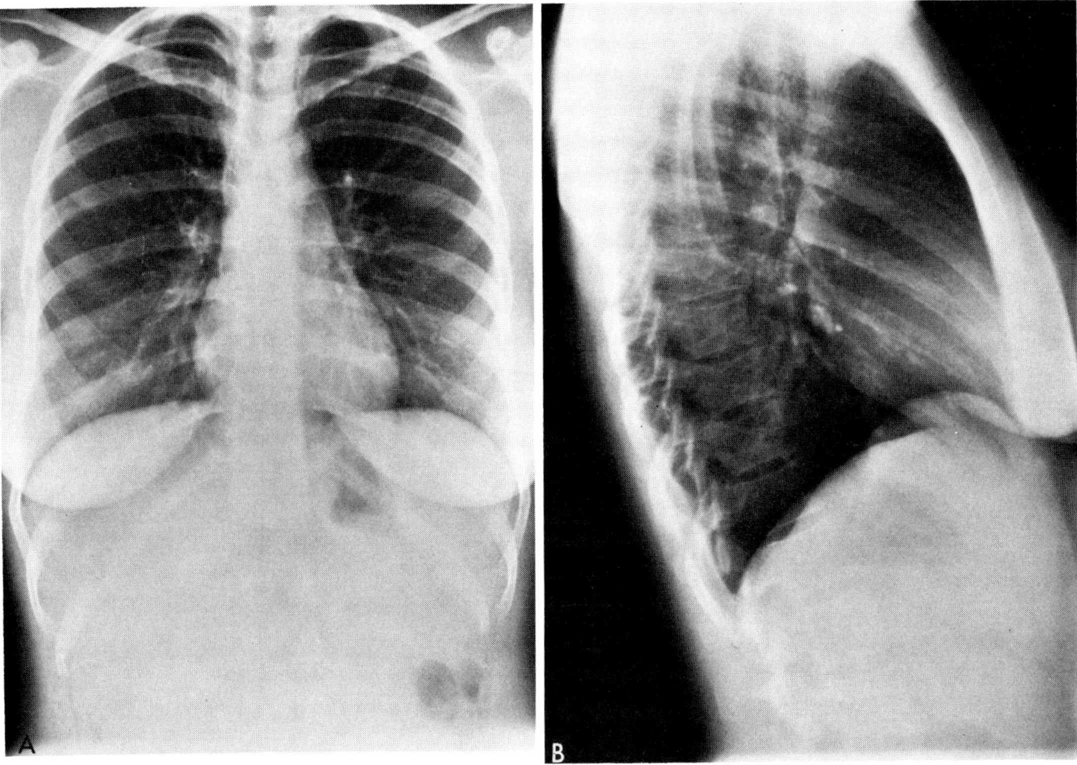

Figure 1–1. Normal chest x-ray, PA view (*A*) and lateral view (*B*). Note the different tissue densities: *air* in the lungs, outside the body and in the intestine; *fat* in the flank stripes; *soft tissues* in the breasts, the abdomen, and the blood vessels in the lungs; and *bones* in the ribs and spine.

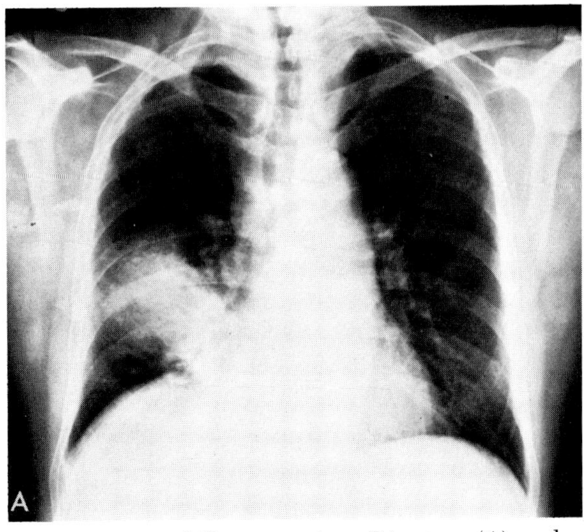

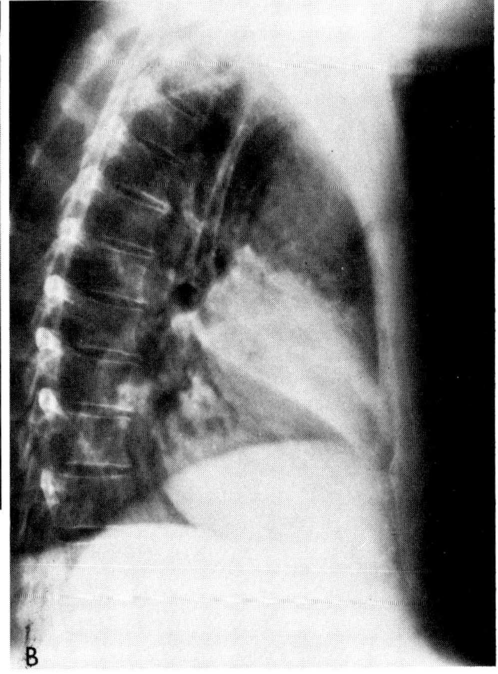

Figure 1–2. Silhouette sign, PA view (*A*) and lateral view (*B*). In this 63-year-old female patient with right middle lobe pneumonia, loss of the right heart border is apparent because of the juxtaposition of soft tissue (heart) and soft tissue (pneumonia) and hence loss of the silhouette.

depends on the presence of fat in the renal bed.

GUIDELINES FOR THE RADIOLOGIST

There are a few basic radiological premises of great importance. Although examples of each will be given in subsequent chapters, it is important to enumerate them here.

1. *Wherever possible get more than one view.* As a general rule, all parts should be x-rayed in two and possibly three planes. For example, views of the chest should be posteroanterior (PA) and lateral; for the abdomen, supine and erect; for bones anteroposterior (AP) and lateral; and for joints, anteroposterior (AP) and axial. Should the patient be too ill to be moved, a cross-table lateral view with a horizontal beam may be useful.

2. *If possible use previous radiographs for comparison.* This is particularly useful in looking at chronic obstructive pulmonary disease or tumors in the lung.

3. *Soft tissue changes may provide useful information.* For example, the *fat pad sign* in an elbow means that an effusion is present, so look for a fracture, particularly in the radial head (Fig. 1–3).

4. *X-ray the opposite side for comparison.* If there is any question of fracture or discrete pathologic condition, a picture of the other side will make diagnosis easier.

5. *Keep in mind the concept of a "ring of bone."* If there is a fracture through one side of a bony ring, look for another fracture or dislocation (an "entry point" and an "exit point"). The classic examples are: pelvis, orbit, maxillary antrum, radius and ulna, and tibia and fibula (Fig. 1–4).

6. *X-rays of long bones should include both articulations.* For example, a radiograph of the femur should include the hip and the knee.

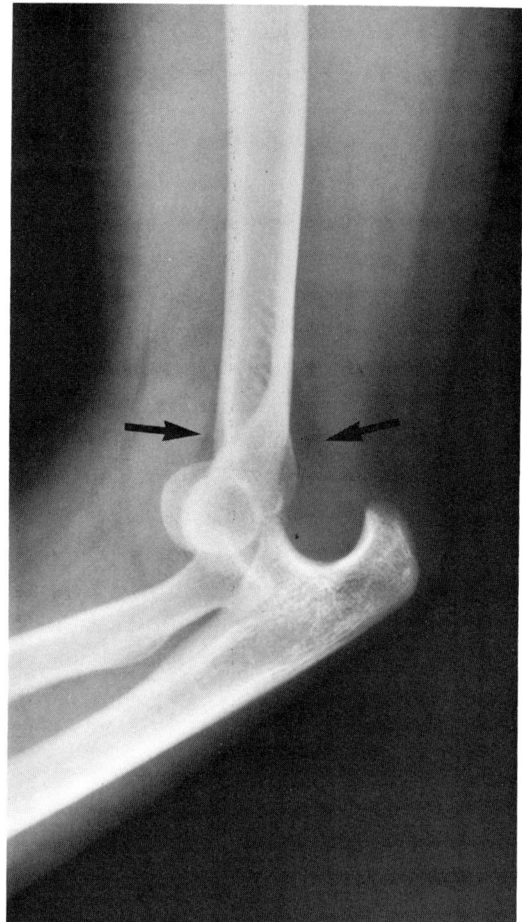

Figure 1–3. Fat pad sign in fracture of the elbow. Following a fall down the stairs, this 21-year-old male student dislocated his elbow and sustained a fracture of the radial head. The joint effusion displaces the anterior and posterior fat pads outwards *(arrows)*.

THE ROLE OF THE RADIOLOGIST

The radiologist plays a decisive role in the work-up and final diagnosis of most patients. It is important, therefore, to provide the radiologist with adequate information on the clinical signs and symptoms as well as suspicions with respect to the probable diagnosis. Too often, the radiologist is kept in the dark (literally and metaphorically), and it is the patient who ultimately suffers. With a particularly difficult clinical problem, it is often wise to consult the radiologist personally with regard to the best way to evaluate the patient radiographically. Although the radiologist may not know as much about the fecal vanadium levels as a clinician does, his or her specialty is the radiological approach to disease, and the radiologist will know not only what procedures are available at the present time but also the correct order in

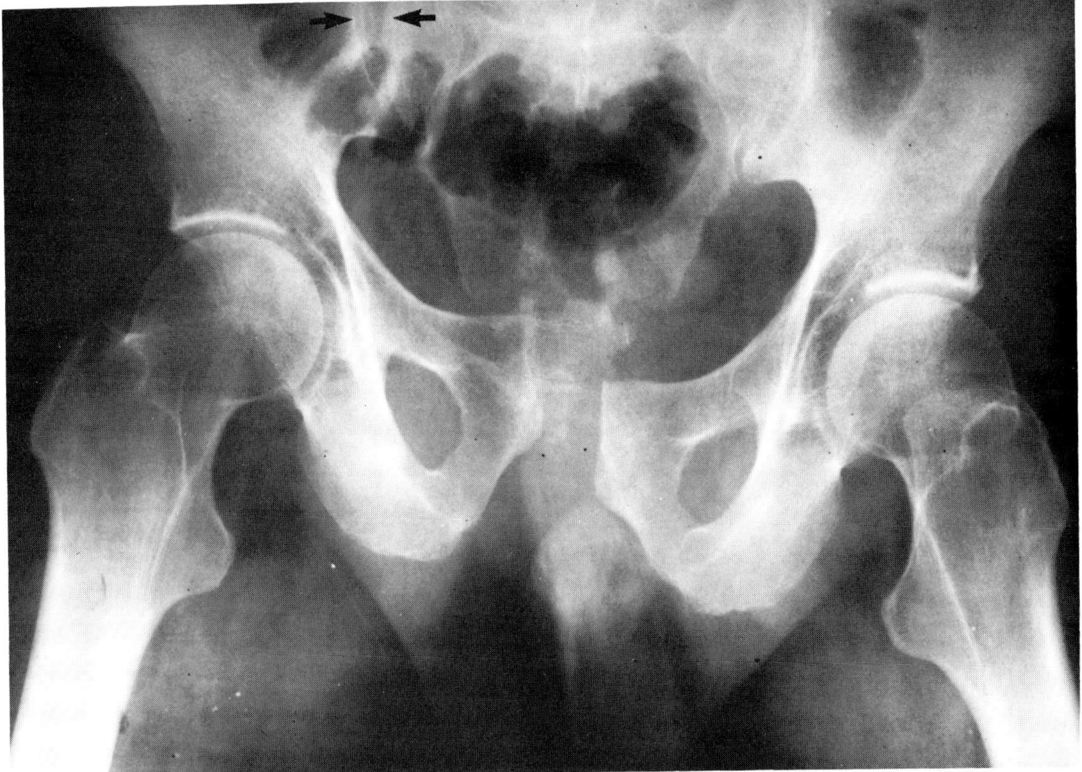

Figure 1–4. "Ring of bone" in a pelvic fracture. This man fell off a scaffold and sustained pelvic injuries as well as a ruptured urethra. The separation of the symphysis pubis is obvious. Since the pelvis is a "ring of bone," there must be another injury; where is it? Look at the sacroiliac joints—the right one is widened *(arrows)*.

which to perform them. The radiologist is a consultant, not just a film reader.

Many requests are for difficult, unnecessary, or pointless views such as radiographs of the sternum or coccyx or tomographic studies of the peripheral skeleton. Many examples of the correct approach to radiology are outlined in this book, and much unnecessary work will be avoided by taking note of them. For example, if a solitary osseous metastasis appears, a search for a primary site should begin with a chest x-ray. The search should progress to a number of contrast studies, starting with an intravenous pyelogram (IVP) and a barium enema study and continuing with an upper gastrointestinal (UGI) series and an oral cholecystogram (OCG) on the same day once the barium has been evacuated from the colon. If a mass in the abdomen has been delineated by an UGI series or an IVP, an ultrasonographic study will determine whether it is cystic, a computerized tomography (CT) scan will show its relationship to surrounding structures, and then, if still indicated, an angiogram may be performed.

Since diagnostic radiology advances so rapidly, clinicians would do well to consult the radiology department for up-to-date advice about clinical problems.

The X-Ray Report

The clinician's responsibility is to provide the x-ray department with the patient's name, age, and hospital identification number as well as an adequate clinical history. Often, a busy house officer will write "routine" or "pre-op" on the x-ray referral form for a patient who has some known major pathological condition that may appear on the radiograph. This practice should be discouraged; the patient is exposed to more radiation and pays a higher laboratory bill because the radiologist has not been given the relevant clinical information. The clinician should also specify exactly which part and which side of the body is to be x-rayed.

The *x-ray technologist's responsibility* is to make sure that the correct side of the designated part of the right patient is x-rayed and that adequate radiographs are taken in respect both to the angles obtained and to the quality of the picture. It is important for the technician to make sure that the radiograph is labelled correctly and that the contralateral side is x-rayed for comparison if indicated either clinically or radiographically. The technologist should consult the radiologist if there are any questions or problems.

The *radiologist's responsibility* is to check the films for technique as well as for the correct anatomical part and to make sure that they are of the right patient. Then the radiologist should read the films, comparing them to any relevant previous films if these are available and providing a lucid, readable, correct, and useful report regarding the presence or absence of a pathological condition. If possible, the report should not hedge but should be positive. If it proves impossible to be specific about a particular situation, possible differential diagnoses should be given, and further studies should be suggested. A good report should consist of a description of the findings, a comment on the differential diagnoses, a comment on other procedures indicated, a conclusion, and a brief "final impression" summarizing the main points of the report.

THE DANGERS OF RADIOLOGY

A brief discussion of the dangers of x-radiation and the current overuse of radiology is in order. It is known that large doses of radiation like those used in radiotherapy will cause tissue damage, but people forget that radiation damage appears to be largely cumulative. For a patient to have a chest x-ray every week is not only stupid but dangerous. A large number of the early radiologists had shortened life spans or died of leukemia, soft tissue sarcoma, or some other form of cancer. We do not know how small a dose of radiation can cause problems, although a number of recent studies have shown that the offspring of women who received a single plain film of the abdomen (KUB) while pregnant exhibit an increased incidence of leukemia many years later. Even more disturbing is the recent report of an increase in breast cancer in patients who received frequent chest fluoroscopy as part of the treatment for tuberculosis by repeated pneumothoraces in the 1930s.

Thus, there is evidence of direct damage (radiation burns, fibrosis, necrosis, and sarcomas) as well as "indirect" damage (leukemia, increased incidence of cancer, shortened life span, genetic damage, and chromosomal aberrations). The number of x-rays ordered for patients, particularly for younger ones, should be limited. Gonadal shielding should be used where feasible and appropriate. Physicians themselves should always wear lead aprons in fluoroscopy rooms and lead gloves if they help to position the patient under the main x-ray beam.

If a clinician gives careful thought to which x-rays to order for a particular patient, the number of unnecessary procedures will be curtailed. Most radiologists have a private list of what they consider to be useless or unnecessary x-rays. Here is a list of alternatives to radiological examination:

1. Do a rectal examination for hemorrhoids, not a barium enema.
2. Use a stethoscope on a patient with a cold, not a chest x-ray.
3. Take a clinical history for a patient with constipation; do not order a barium enema study without making sure the patient's colon is clear of feces.
4. Do not book too many patients into the outpatient clinic; physicians who do so seem to send more of their patients to the radiology department to "keep them happy."

One final comment: In Britain, patients receive half as many radiographs and undergo half as many surgical procedures per head of population as patients in the United States, yet the survival rate is the same. Use clinical acumen, not the x-ray beam.

CHAPTER 2

PLAIN FILMS

THE CHEST

Approximately 60 per cent of the workload of the average x-ray department is chest radiography. There are two routine views of the chest, but a number of other views of the lung fields and thorax are also of importance.

PA View

For a posteroanterior (PA) view of the chest, the patient is positioned with the x-ray tube about 6 feet behind and with the cassette in front. The patient is then requested to take and hold a deep breath, and the film is taken. Many different techniques and exposures are available, but it is the end result that counts. A good PA chest x-ray (Fig. 2–1A) should allow the vessels behind the heart to be seen as well as the vessels in the peripheral lung fields. In female patients, it should be possible to see the costophrenic angles and the lungs behind the breast shadows. The thoracic spine should be visible (particularly the pedicles and paraspinal lines). The trachea and carina should be seen, although often this is possible only when the film is held obliquely to the light–a useful trick for eliminating overlying soft tissue shadows.

This film is taken PA instead of "AP" (anteroposterior) because there is less magnification of the heart on the PA film. If a relatively accurate measurement of cardiac size is required, it is preferable to use the PA view. To measure the depth of inspiration, the ribs may be counted. Although many radiologists count the posterior ribs because they are easier to see, it is probably more accurate to count the anterior ones. A good PA film should show the diaphragms at the level of 5½ to 6½ ribs anteriorly or 10 to 11 ribs posteriorly.

Lateral View

The choice of a left or right lateral view is largely arbitrary and depends on the practice of the radiology department. The left lateral view is usually chosen because the heart lies closest to the film in this position. There are a number of ways to identify which side is which — for instance, the higher diaphragm is often the one farthest from the film (look for the gastric air bubble under the left hemidiaphragm), and the shape and contour of the ribs may also be helpful. Usually the arms of the patient are placed forward or above the head to remove the additional bone and soft tissue shadows that would otherwise obscure the lung fields on the lateral view (Fig. 2–1B).

Reading a Routine Chest Film

Although this is not meant to be a textbook of radiology, the chest x-ray is so important that a brief discussion of the normal x-ray is in order. It is also important to stress that since much of a physician's professional life is likely to be spent in looking at chest films, some sort of system is

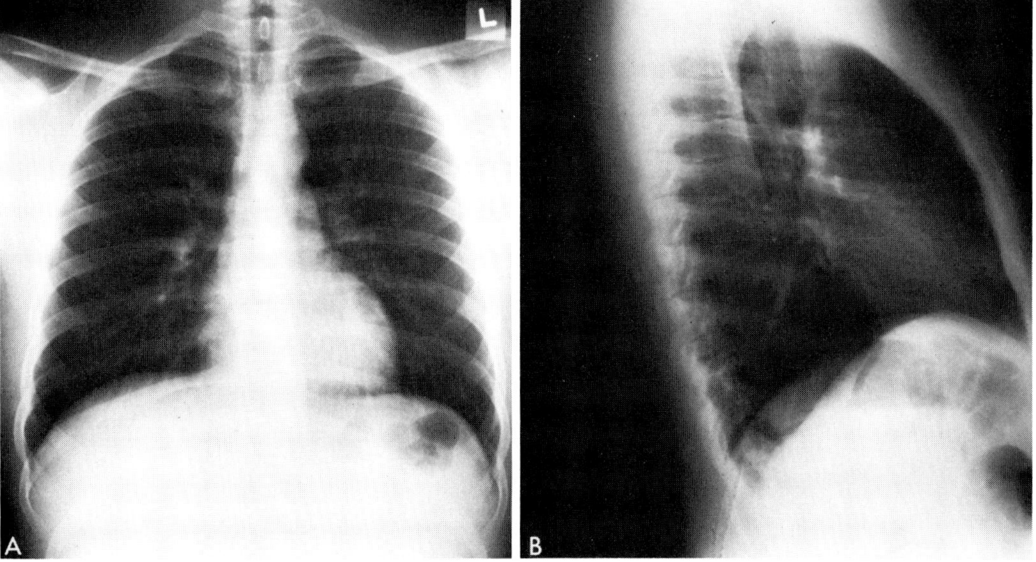

Figure 2–1. Normal chest. *A*, PA view. *B*, Lateral view. See text for explanation.

required to evaluate the findings. This is particularly true if there is an obvious lesion that strikes the eye immediately; a second lesion may be easily missed unless a systematic search is undertaken.

There are many different ways to review a chest radiograph, and every radiologist has his own method. The method recommended here is based on that of the late George Simon and has served the authors well for many years. The suggested order is: diaphragms (and below), heart, hila, superior mediastinum, lung fields, bones, and soft tissues. It really does not matter what system a radiologist adopts as long as he adheres to it.

On the PA view:

1. Diaphragms should be rounded, with the dome at least an inch above a line joining the costophrenic and cardiophrenic angles. The costophrenic angles should be sharp and clear-cut.

2. The heart should be less than half the width of the chest (the cardiothoracic ratio). Its maximum horizontal measurement should not be greater than 15.5 cm.

3. The center of the left hilum should be about an inch more cephalad (higher) than the right. Both the arteries (the lower part of each hilum) and the veins (the upper part) should be clearly seen.

4. The aortic knob should be visible without being prominent, the trachea should be seen to descend from the neck in a relatively straight line, and the carina should be sharply pointed.

5. The lung fields should be clear, with the vessels tapering to become almost invisible peripherally. The vessels in the lower zones should be somewhat larger than those in the upper zones. Look for the minor (horizontal) fissure, and remember the relative paucity of vessels in the normal right midzone.

6. The ribs and soft tissues should be symmetrical, and the pedicles of the thoracic spine should be visible.

On the lateral view:

1. The heart should be visualized with the inferior vena cava entering the right atrium and making an equilateral triangle with the diaphragm and the left ventricle.

2. The retrosternal air space should come two thirds of the way down the sternum.

3. The aortic arch should be smooth, without any areas of dilation.

4. The hila should be identified, and

the left mainstem bronchus should appear as a circular lucency. The left main pulmonary artery should run over and posterior to this, while the right mainstem artery should emerge from the mediastinum in front of it.

Additional Views of the Chest

Lordotic View

This view may be taken in a number of ways, but the end result is a radiograph that has thrown the clavicles off the apex of the lungs. The effect is achieved by positioning the patient or the x-ray beam at an oblique angle (Fig. 2–2). An apical lordotic view has two principal uses: visualization of the apex of the lung in suspected cases of tuberculosis or tumor and visualization of the mid-zones of the lung fields, in which a right middle lobe or lingular process such as pneumonia or scarring may be delineated.

Inspiration and Expiration Views

Views of the chest during inspiration and expiration are particularly useful if a small pneumothorax is suspected (Fig. 2–3). During expiration, the pressure in the lung goes down and the tension in the pneumothorax is relatively increased, so the pneumothorax will become more apparent.

Decubitus View

A decubitus view is useful if a patient has either an obvious pleural effusion or a suspected subpulmonic effusion. Placing the patient on one side (or both) causes the fluid to layer out unless it has become loculated (Fig. 2–4). A useful trick: If a peripheral or pleurally based lesion is to

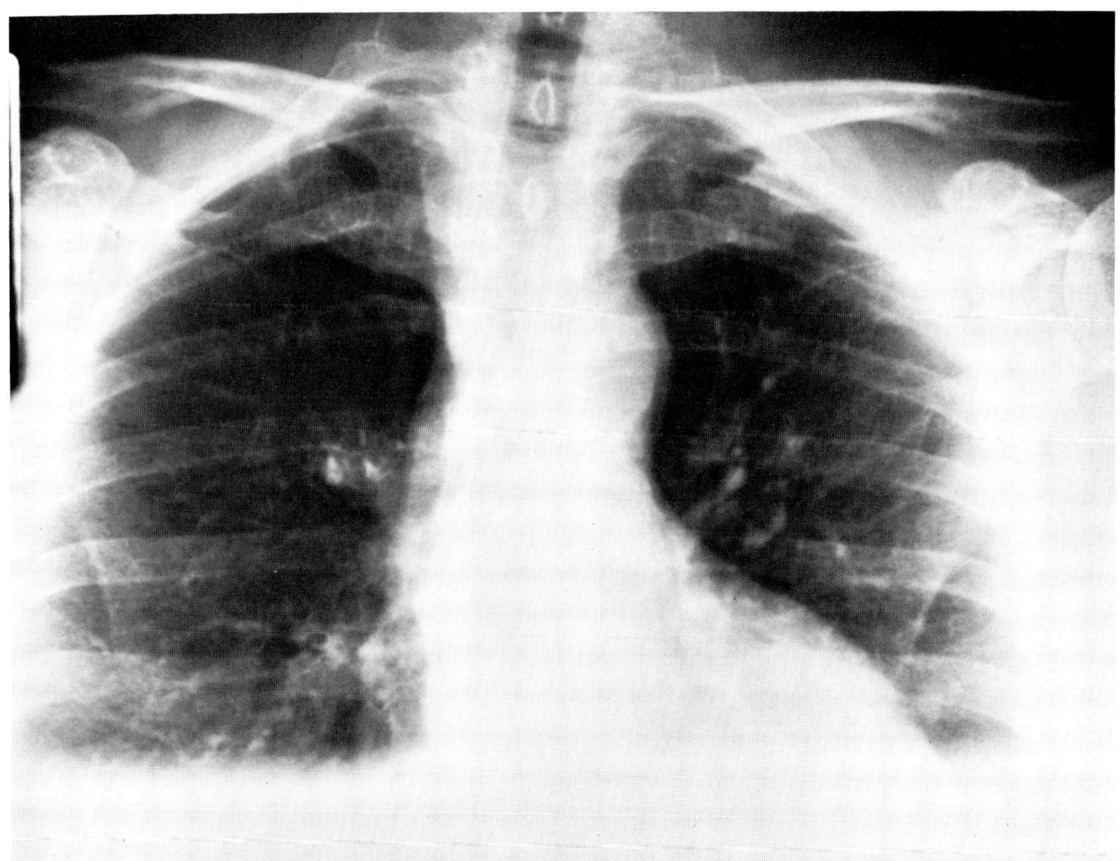

Figure 2–2. Normal apical lordotic view. This view was taken to exclude the possibility of tuberculosis in the apex of the lung in this 71-year-old man.

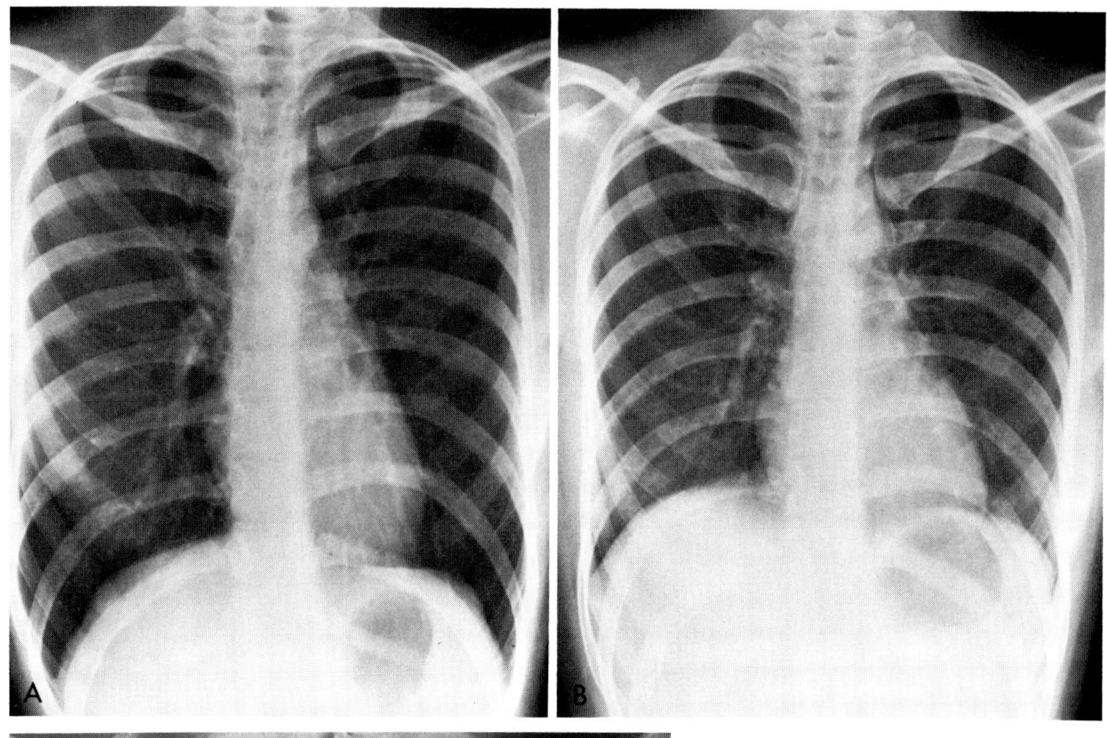

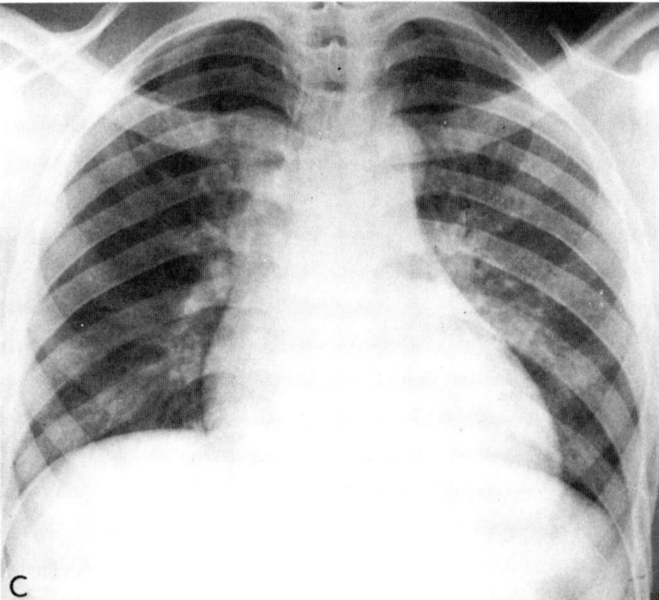

Figure 2–3. Normal inspiration (*A*) and expiration (*B*) views. See text for explanation. *C*. Fuller expiration view in a different (normal) patient.

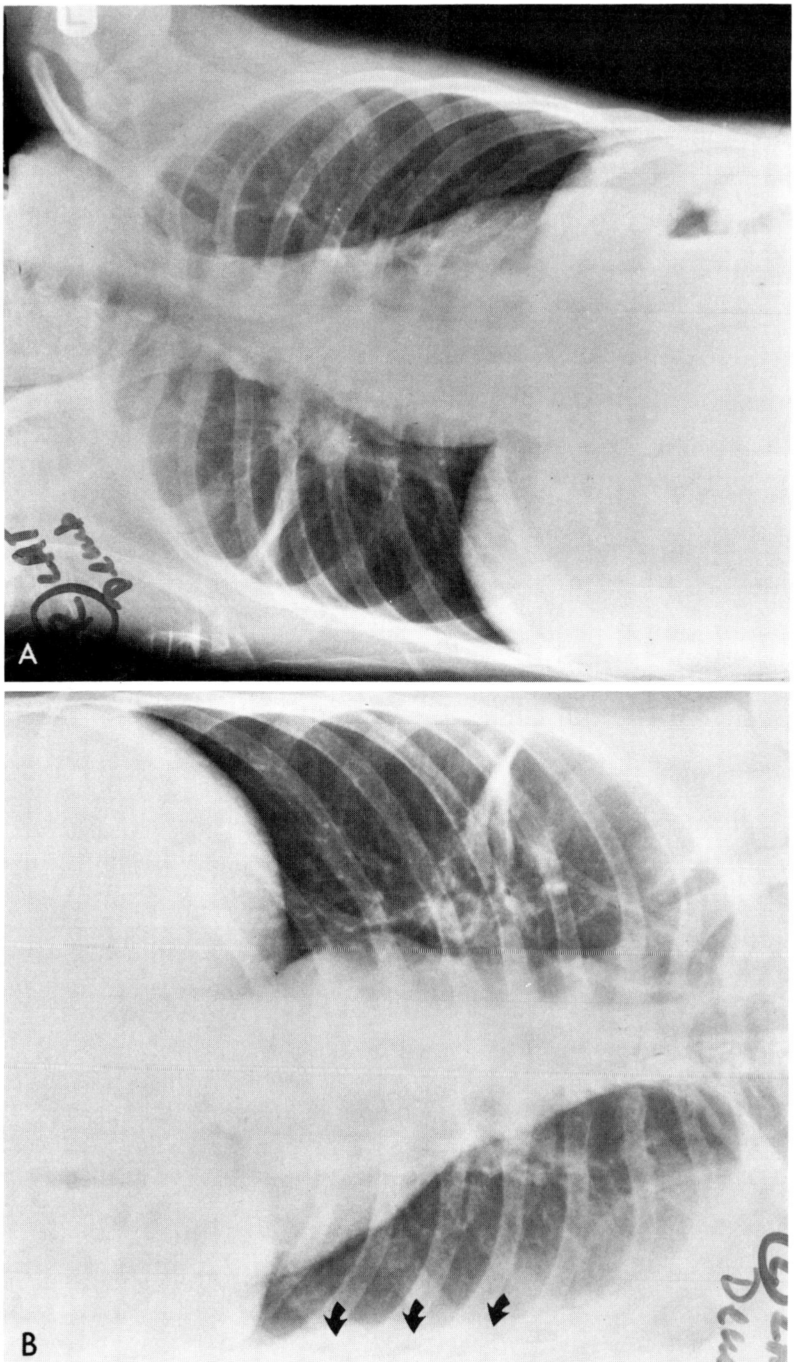

Figure 2–4. *A*, Right lateral decubitus view shows no free fluid on the right side in this young patient with suspected pulmonary emboli, although there is an area of atelectasis. *B*, Left lateral decubitus view shows layering out of fluid on the left side *(arrows)*.

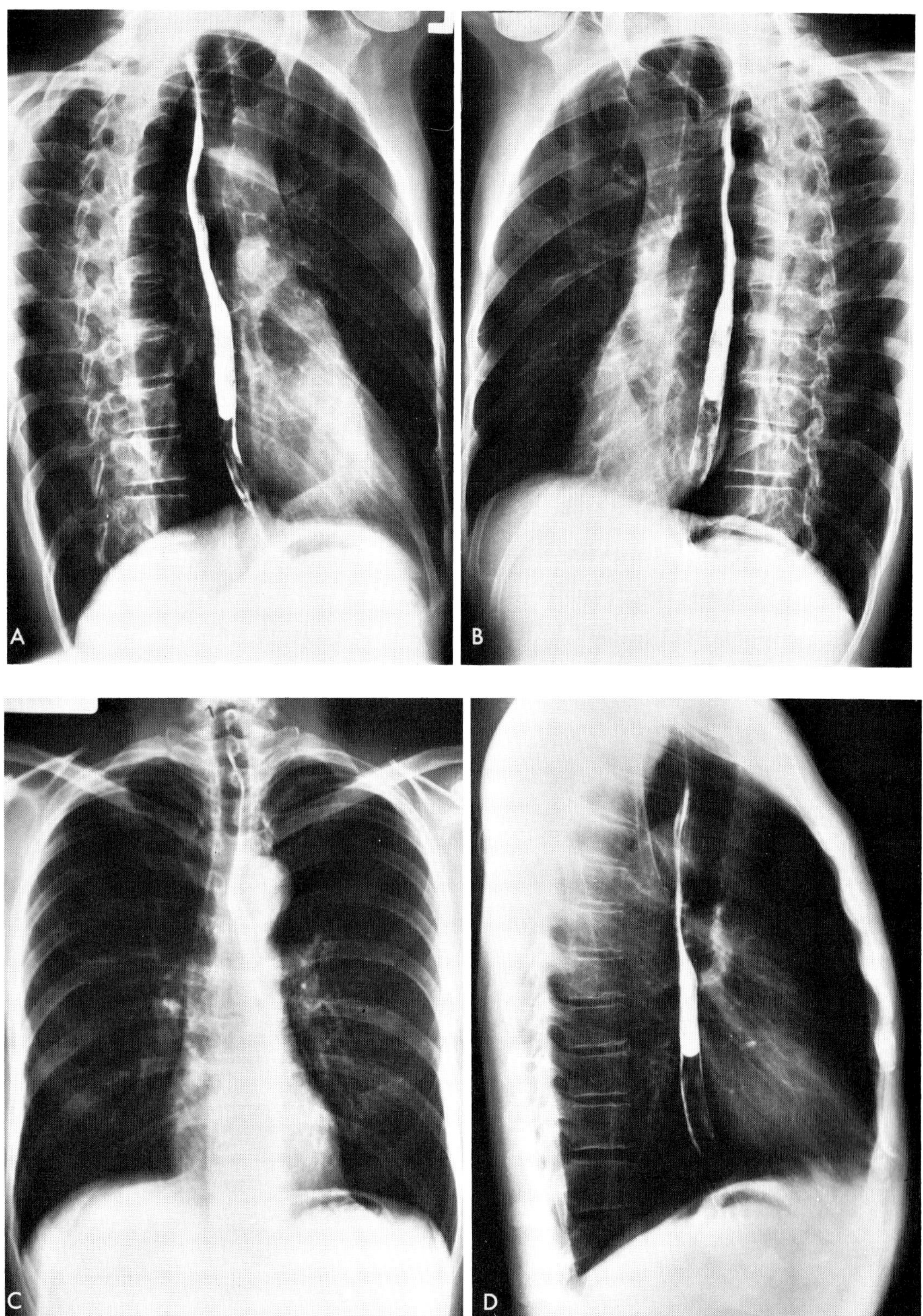

Figure 2–5. A normal "cardiac series." *A*, Right anterior oblique view shows the left atrium to advantage. *B*, On the left anterior oblique view, the aortic arch is unfolded and the left ventricle is well seen. *C*, Posteroanterior view. *D*, Lateral view.

some extent obscured by fluid, the patient should be tilted *away* from that side and the *opposite* decubitus view should be taken. This procedure clears the area of the lesion for better visualization.

Cardiac Series

To the routine PA and lateral views of the chest, a number of other views may be added to constitute a cardiac series. RAO (right anterior oblique) for the left atrium (Fig. 2–5A), LAO (left anterior oblique) for the right atrium (Fig. 2–5B), a lateral view with barium swallow for left atrial enlargement, and an overpenetrated PA view with barium are the most commonly used additional projections.

AP and Portable Films

For severely ill patients or those who cannot stand, it is often impossible to take a PA view, so an AP view with the cassette behind the patient may have to suffice (Fig. 2–6). This view does not allow the heart size to be accurately assessed, but it often provides enough basic information about the state of the lung fields and the presence or absence of pulmonary edema to be of use to the clinician. Supine portable films done at the patient's bed or in the intensive care unit are frequently difficult to interpret. It is always better to bring the patient to the radiology department where better quality films can be obtained.

Ribs

If specific views of the ribs are ordered, it is important that the patient, the clinician, the technologist, or the radiologist specify exactly which part of the rib cage is to be radiographed. Often, axial views and various oblique views are all that is necessary to show the area (Fig. 2–7). Only about 45 per cent of rib fractures are

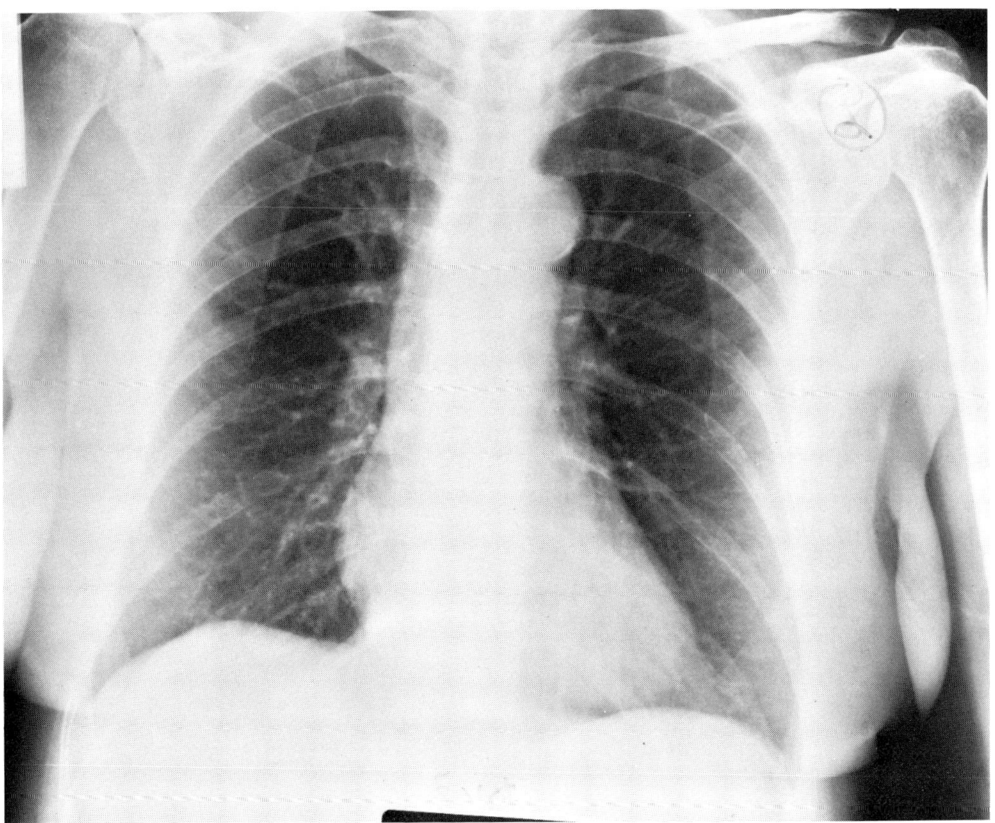

Figure 2–6. Normal AP view of the chest. Note that the heart is apparently enlarged because of the magnification but that the lung fields are well seen.

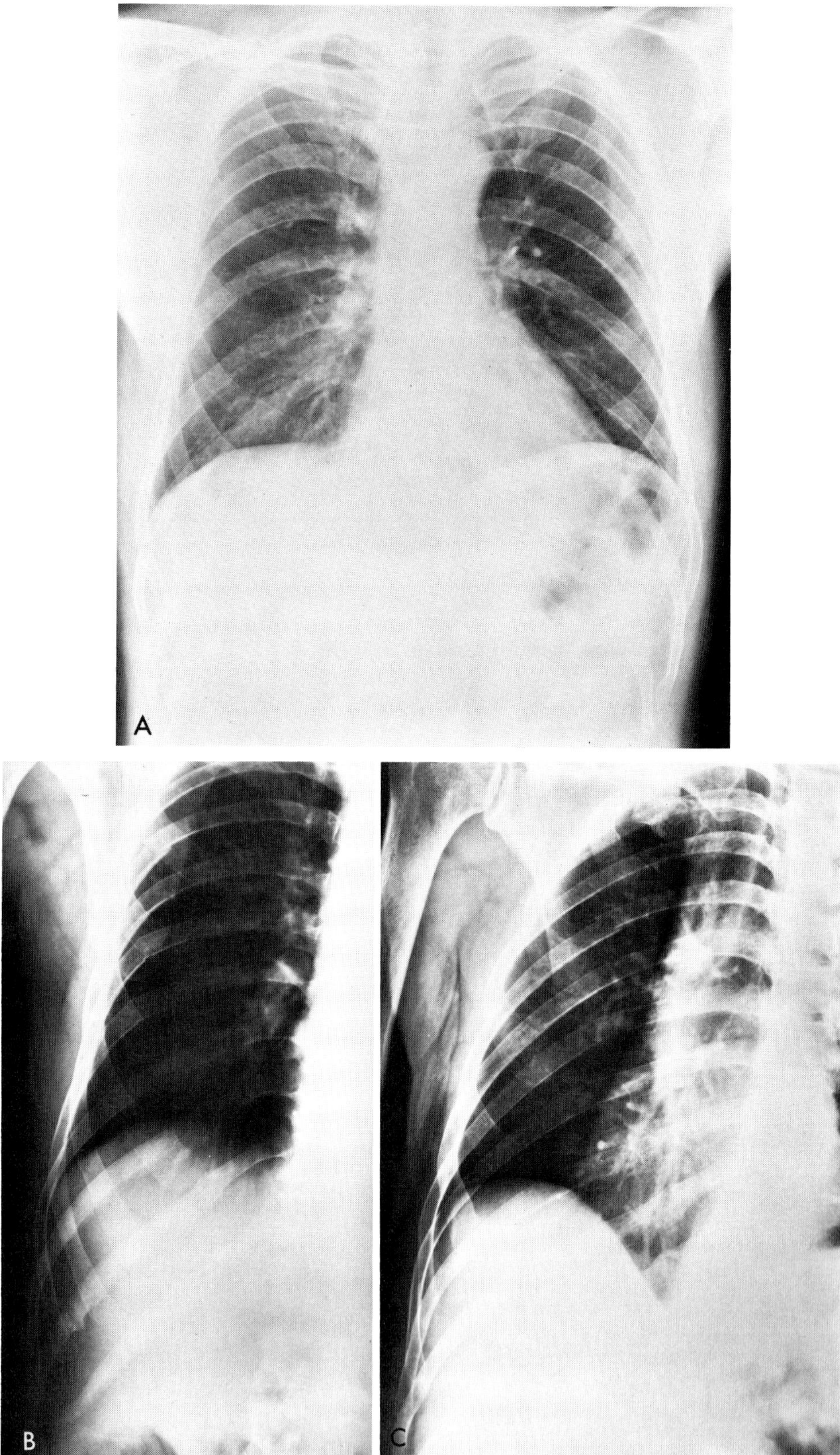

Figure 2–7. Oblique views of the ribs. An apparently normal chest x-ray (*A*) was taken of this 54-year-old man complaining of pain in his right side following a fall. Note that no pneumothorax is visible. Different oblique views (*B* and *C*) reveal at least four rib fractures – 5, 6, 7, and 8.

actually seen radiographically. The only important clinical feature is the presence or absence of pneumothorax. Demonstration of an actual rib fracture will not usually alter treatment; hence, some radiologists feel that a rib x-ray after minor trauma is a waste of time.

Sternum

The sternum and its articulations are particularly difficult to visualize. A lateral view is often useful, and oblique PA views (RPO) or tomograms may be necessary for an adequate view of the sternum. The sternoclavicular joints are often seen only by means of tomography.

Guidelines for the Clinician

1. Provide adequate clinical information for the radiologist, possibly by asking direct questions (for example: Is pulmonary edema present?).
2. Make sure the radiologist has access to previous films for comparison — even if they come from Timbuctoo.
3. It is sometimes necessary to repeat the x-ray using nipple markers if a small rounded density is seen in the lower lung fields on the first film.
4. Notice the difference between what can be seen on underexposed and overexposed films and what can be diagnosed on the basis of a well-exposed film.
5. Remember that the variation in normal is immense (just look at people's faces). Make allowance for this when reading chest x-rays.
6. Develop a systematic way of looking at all x-rays, particularly chest films.

THE ABDOMEN

There are two routine views of the abdomen and a number of variations. All of these will be discussed, but most departments take a plain abdominal radiograph before doing any contrast studies (IVP, UGI, BE, angiogram). The clinician can save the patient additional radiation dosage as well as additional expense by not ordering an extra film beforehand.

KUB, Supine and Erect

The origin of the abbreviation *KUB* is lost in the mists of time, but it appears to have been a common term in the 1930s. It was probably introduced about the time that intravenous pyelography became commonplace. The preliminary plain film of the abdomen covered the area of the Kidneys, Ureters, and Bladder; hence the abbreviation.

Supine and erect films of the abdomen are taken in most patients who have vague abdominal complaints, cramps, change of bowel habit, gastrointestinal bleeding, or similar abdominal disturbances. The supine film should include from about the level of the symphysis pubis to as high up the abdominal cavity as possible (Fig. 2–8A), whereas the erect view should include the domes of the diaphragms and should go down as far as possible (Fig. 2–8B). Thus, the whole peritoneal cavity will have been covered. If a perforated viscus is suspected, free air may be sought under the diaphragms.

Reading a KUB Film

Since the KUB is a frequently performed radiograph, a brief discussion of how it should be approached is included. Once again, it is important to develop a system of looking at abdominal radiographs and to adhere to it.

1. Check the overall appearance of the abdomen. Look particularly for calcifications, either gallstones or stones lying in the region of the kidneys, ureters, and bladder (Fig. 2–9). Are there calcifications in the regions of the liver, spleen, adrenals (Fig. 2–10), uterus (suggesting fibroids), or mesenteric lymph nodes (very common and usually without significance)? Is there vascular calcification or evidence of an aneurysm?
2. The bowel gas pattern should be looked at carefully. Is it normal, or is there too much gas, with distension in the loops of the small or the large intestine? Are there any air-fluid levels? If so, are they horizontal (ileus) or in different planes with a stepladder effect, suggesting obstruction (Fig. 2–11)? Check to see if the abdomen is featureless (with little or no

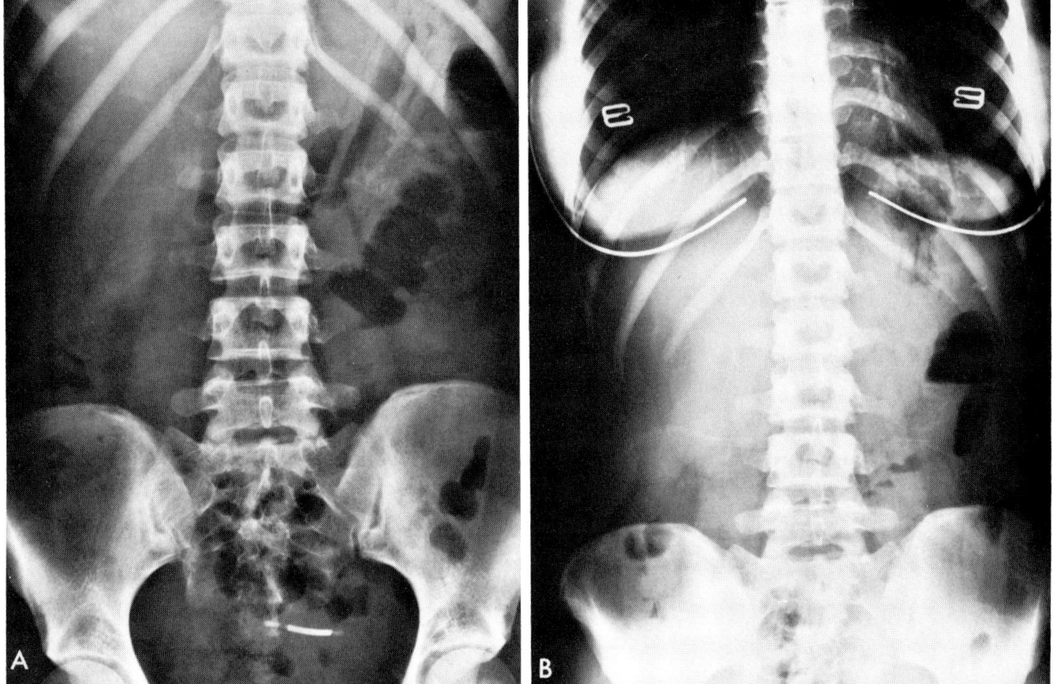

Figure 2–8. Normal KUB, supine view (*A*) and erect view (*B*). Note that an IUD can be seen on the supine view and that metallic parts of a supporting device are visible on the erect view. See text for explanation of how to approach a normal KUB.

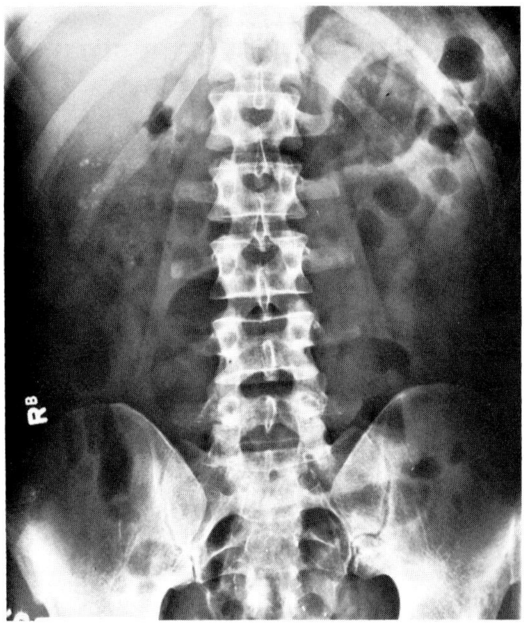

Figure 2–9. Renal calcification. This 35-year-old male had idiopathic hypercalciuria with nephrocalcinosis. Note the discrete calcifications overlying both kidneys, whose outlines can be clearly seen on this KUB.

gas), if there is too much fecal material, or if the gastric shadow is normal or distended. Also, check for any obvious displacement of a viscus.

3. The psoas muscle outlines should be visible and smooth.

4. The renal outlines are usually fairly easy to see. Are they smooth or irregular, enlarged or small, deviated or distorted (Figs. 2–9 and 2–10)?

5. The liver should be seen to fill most of the right upper quadrant and its lower margin should be clear-cut. Remember, however, that there are accessory lobes of the liver (Riedel's and the quadrate). It is difficult if not impossible to measure the hepatic size radiographically.

6. The spleen is usually fairly well seen, and its maximal longitudinal measurement, which is taken from the diaphragmatic dome to the tip, should not exceed 14 cm.

7. The soft tissues of the pelvis should be visible and the bladder and the rectal gas should be identified. Note the iliopectineal soft-tissue lines running parallel to the bony pelvis.

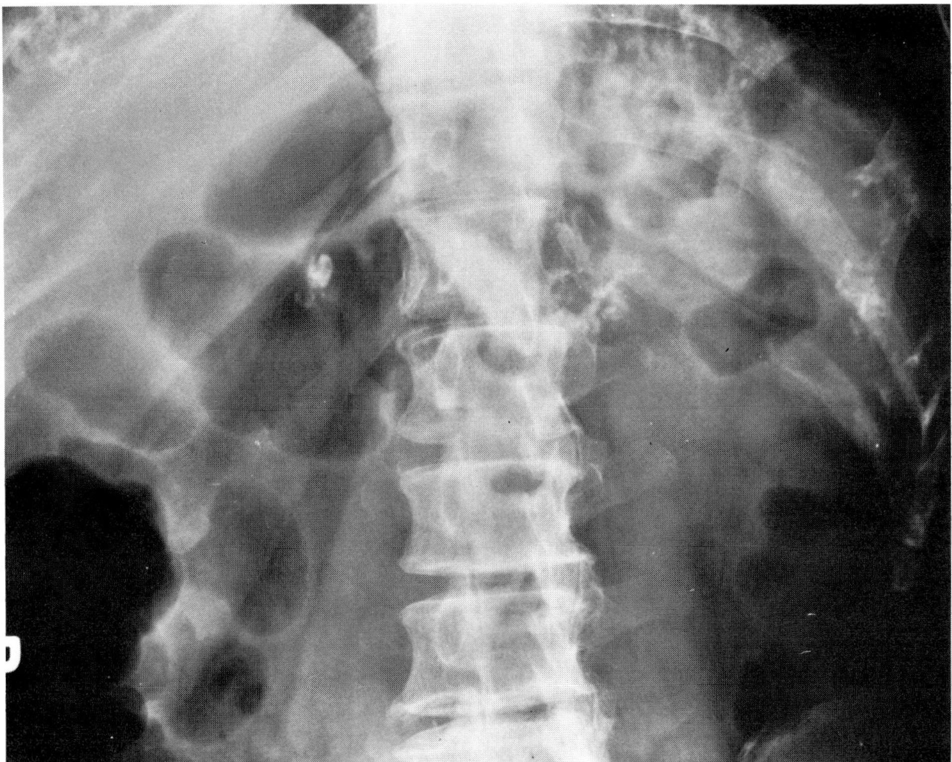

Figure 2–10. Adrenal calcification. Dense calcifications are visible above the upper poles of both kidneys, whose outlines can be clearly seen. The cause of the calcification in this 60-year-old man was thought to be tuberculosis.

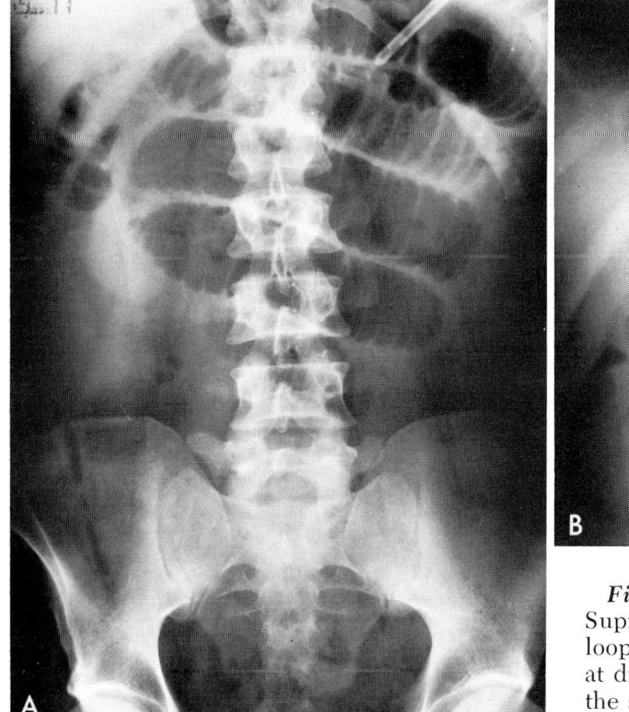

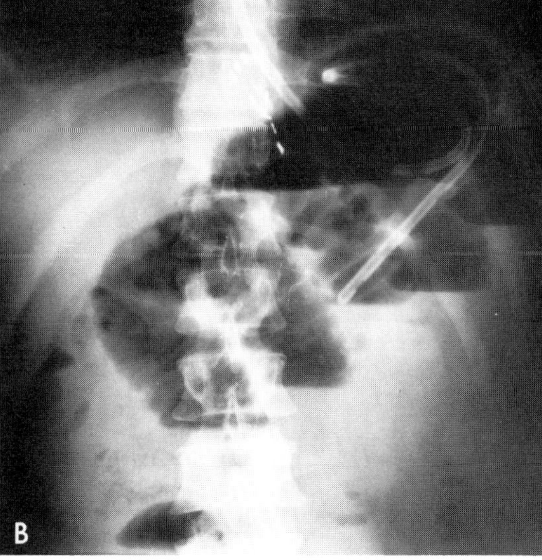

Figure 2–11. Intestinal obstruction. *A*, Supine view. *B*, Erect view. Note the multiple loops of distended bowel with air-fluid levels at different planes in the same loop. Note also the stepladder effect in *A*.

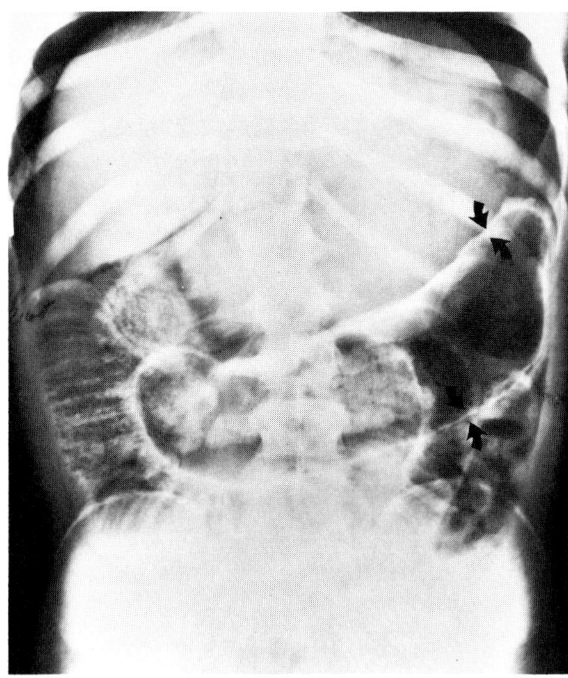

Figure 2–12. Free intraperitoneal air. In this extremely ill patient with intestinal perforation, the supine abdominal film shows distension of multiple loops of bowel and reveals *both* sides of the intestinal wall *(arrows)*, signifying free air in the abdomen.

8. Look for the flank stripes and for evidence of peritonitis or ascites.
9. Look for free air under the diaphragms or see if *both* walls of the intestine are visible; these signs have the same significance (Fig. 2–12).
10. The spine and pelvis should not be ignored. Look for the pedicles of the spine and the integrity of the pelvis. Look at the transverse processes in cases of trauma or splinting. Check the sacroiliac and hip joints, and assess the intervertebral disc spaces.

Additional Views of the Abdomen

It is often necessary to add extra radiographs to routine views of the abdomen, and in specific clinical situations, some of the following special views may prove useful.

Inspiration and Expiration Views

Views of the abdomen during inspiration and expiration are useful, for instance, if there is calcification overlying the region of the kidney. If the calcification and the kidney remain in the same relationship to each other when the patient breathes, the calcification is probably renal.

Decubitus Views

If a patient is too ill to stand for the erect film, decubitus films are frequently used to look for free air or air-fluid levels. Decubitus projections are useful in the assessment of flank stripes in cases of suspected peritonitis, although coned-down views of this area can be just as helpful.

Cross-table Lateral Films

There are two main indications for a cross-table lateral film, which is taken with a horizontal beam.

The view is used to look for free air and to determine the presence of an aneurysm of the abdominal aorta. (Obviously, the wall must be calcified in order for an aneurysm to be identified with certainty, and a lateral tomogram may have to be used to confirm the diagnosis.)

Prone Films

Although there are a number of indications for a prone KUB, the most important ones are looking for rectal air (primarily in children) and looking for evidence of regional enteritis during a barium study (the abdomen is compressed in a prone view, thus separating the loops of the small bowel).

Oblique Views of the Abdomen

Occasionally, it is necessary to identify renal outlines or to localize calcifications within the kidneys, and oblique views may be helpful. They are also used in searching for evidence of a retroperitoneal tumor, because the psoas muscle outlines can be more easily seen on these projections.

Coned-down Views of RUQ

Evidence of gallstones or of calcification in the gallbladder wall is more easily seen on coned-down views of the right upper quadrant (Fig. 2–13).

Inverted View

This special view is not recommended for adults weighing over 600 lbs! The inverted view is used for neonates with imperforate anus (Fig. 2–14). By holding the baby up by the legs and placing a penny or thimble in the anal dimple, the distance between the exterior and the distal air-filled bowel lumen can be determined. This will help the surgeon to plan the operation, because the air in the bowel will rise as high as it can go.

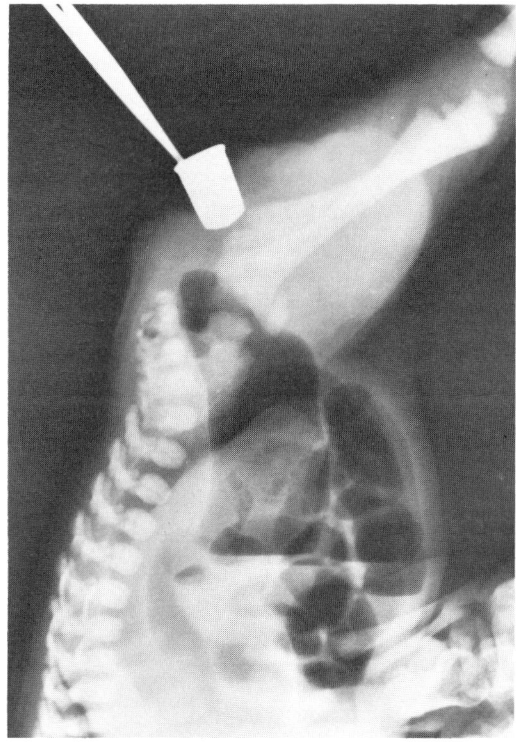

Figure 2–14. Inverted view of a neonate with rectal atresia. A thimble is placed in the anal dimple and the child is held by the legs until the bowel gas reaches as distally as it can go. The distance between the two shadows represents the length of the atresia.

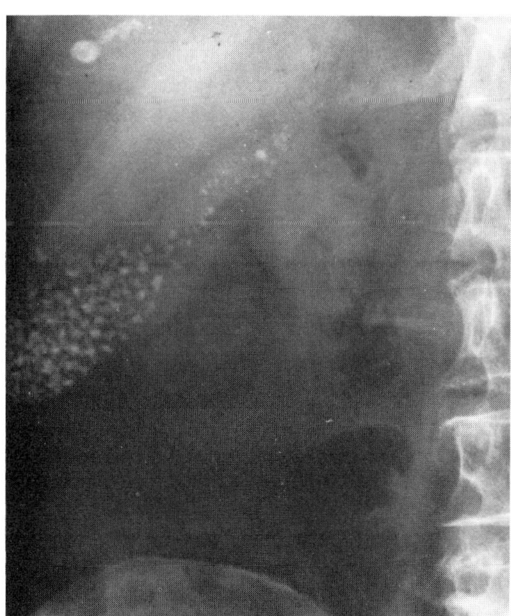

Figure 2–13. Coned-down view of the right upper quadrant reveals multiple calcified gallstones.

THE UPPER EXTREMITY

For clarity, discussions of the arm and of the leg will begin with the distal part of the extremity and move proximally; thus, in the arm we begin with the fingers and end with the shoulder girdle.

Fingers

Usually, an AP and a lateral or oblique view are taken to look for a fracture or a foreign body in the fingers. A magnification view may sometimes be helpful. If there is any suspicion of fracture, particularly before the epiphyses fuse, an x-ray of the corresponding finger on the opposite hand may be useful.

The Hand and Wrist

There are 29 bones visible on a radiograph of the wrist and hand (Fig. 2–15). For most common situations, however, only one or two views are required to evaluate any pathological condition.

Both AP and PA views may be useful for evaluation of the hand and wrist. The PA view is often more comfortable for the patient. Both these views should be taken with the other hand for comparison, preferably on the same film. This is particularly important in cases of metabolic bone disease, arthritis, and various forms of dysplasia. The lateral film is often taken, but in our experience this view is rarely of any help for evaluating disease of the metacarpals and fingers; lateral films can be very useful, however, for patients with dislocations involving the wrist.

Oblique views are sometimes useful in the early evaluation of arthritis (particularly rheumatoid arthritis) or in location of a foreign body in the soft tissues. On the whole, these projections of the hand serve to evaluate the metacarpals and wrist as well as the phalanges, but special views of the carpus are available. Oblique views are helpful in the evaluation of the first carpometacarpal joint, which is frequently the first joint in the hand to be involved by osteoarthritis. Coned-down PA and oblique views of the wrist for patients with ulnar or radial deviation of the hand allow evaluation of most of the bones in the carpus (Fig. 2–16). There is also a series of oblique and lateral views of the carpal scaphoid (os naviculare) that is useful in assessing a scaphoid fracture. If no definite fracture can

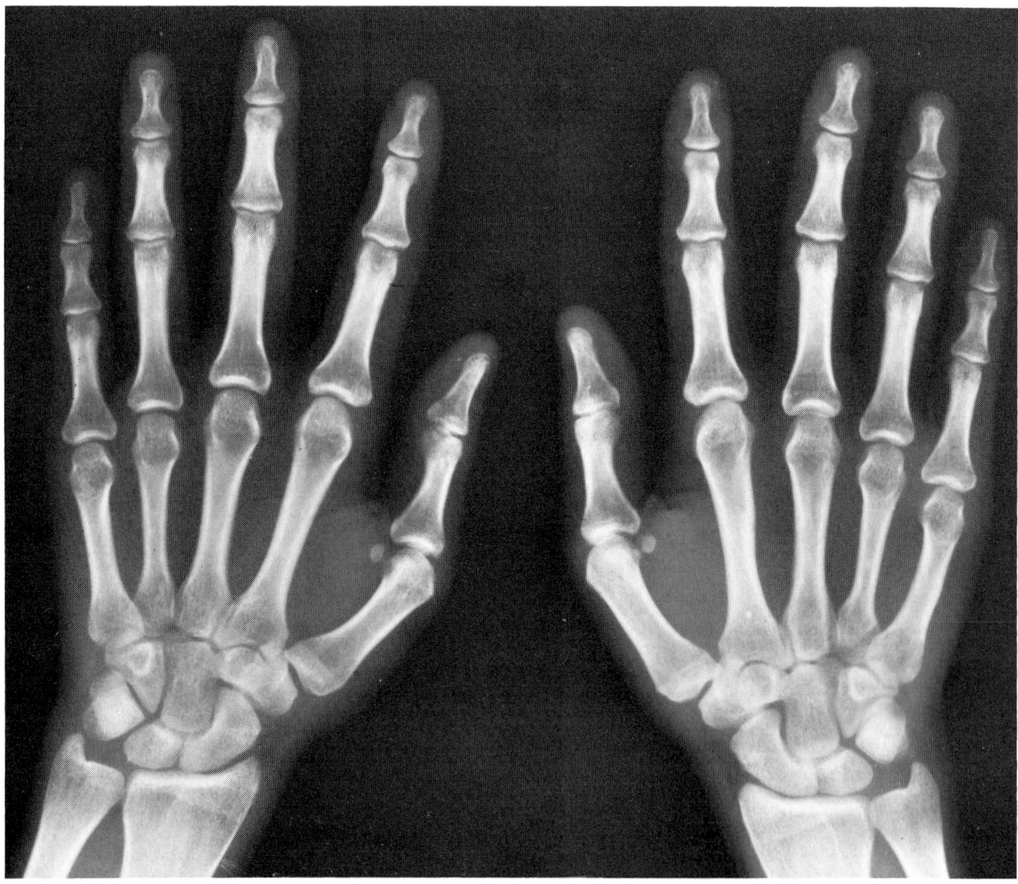

Figure 2–15. Normal hands, PA view. See text for explanation.

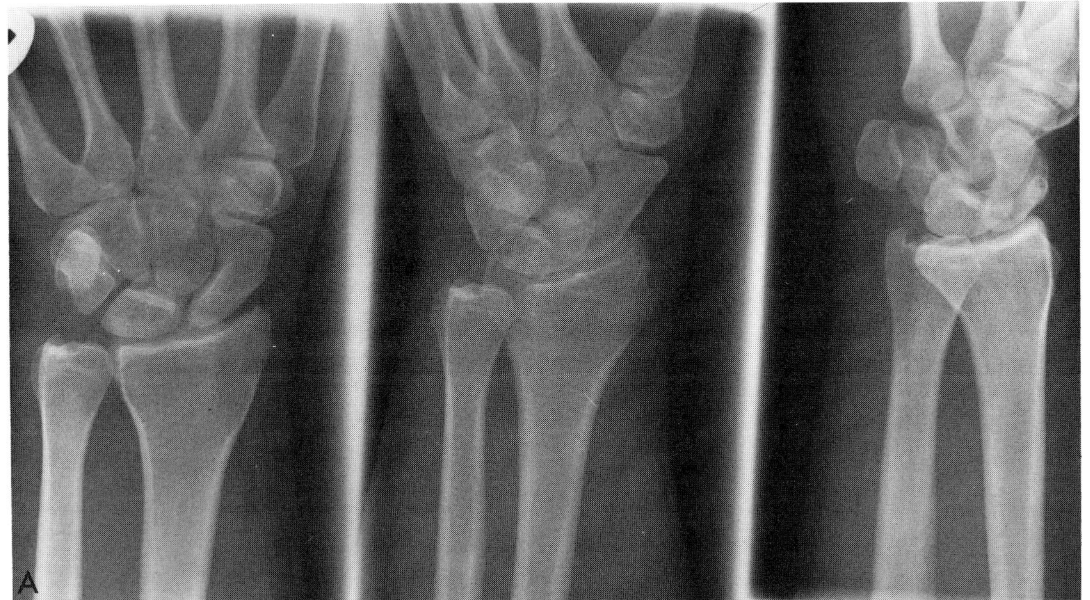

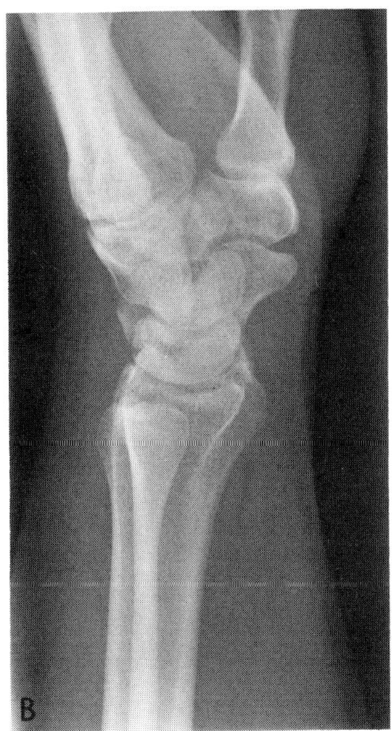

Figure 2–16. Normal coned-down oblique views of the wrist to show the carpal bones. Note particularly the appearance of the navicular bone.

be identified on the initial film, it is often wise to repeat the radiographs in seven to ten days. Finally, a carpal tunnel view may be taken to evaluate the soft tissues that lie in the carpal tunnel between the navicular and greater multangular bones and the pisiform bone and the hook of the hamate. There are at least three methods of taking this x-ray; in the authors' opinion, however, the carpal tunnel view rarely provides any useful information.

Forearm

X-rays of the forearm should cover both the elbow joint and the wrist, because the concept of a "ring of bone" should be considered. Thus, if there is a fracture of the midshaft of the ulna, a fracture or dislocation of the radius should be sought. Often it is a dislocation of the radial head at the elbow, known as a *Monteggia fracture-dislocation.* An AP view with the elbow in

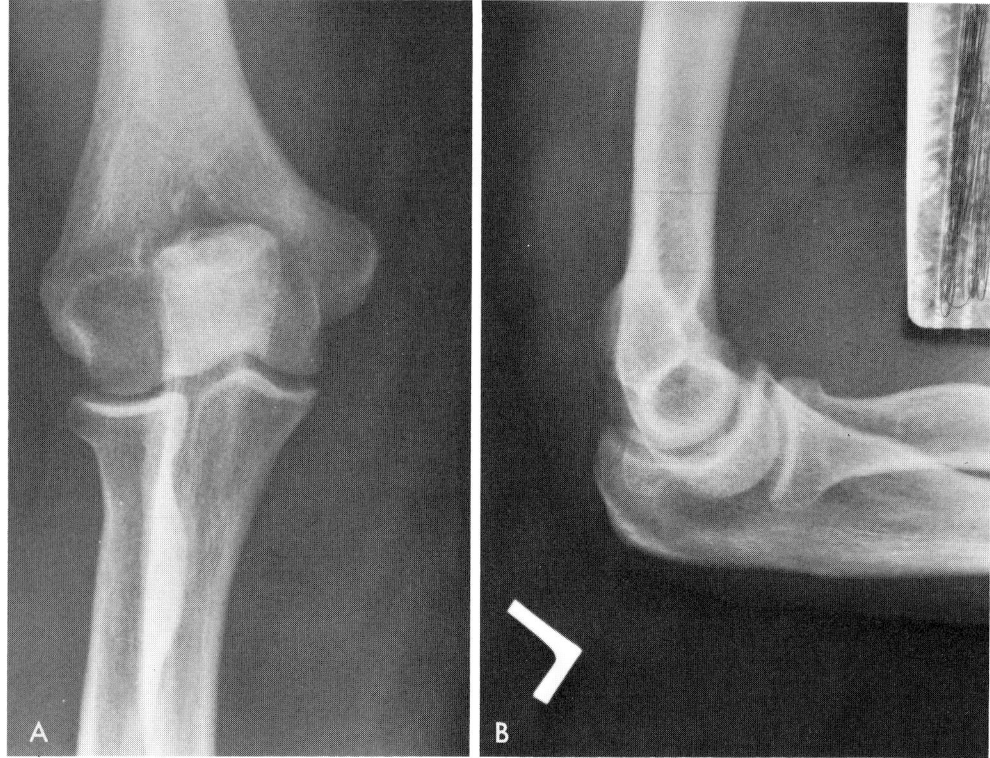

Figure 2-17. Normal elbow, AP view (*A*) and lateral view (*B*). Look particularly for the presence of fat pads and for discrete fractures of the radial head.

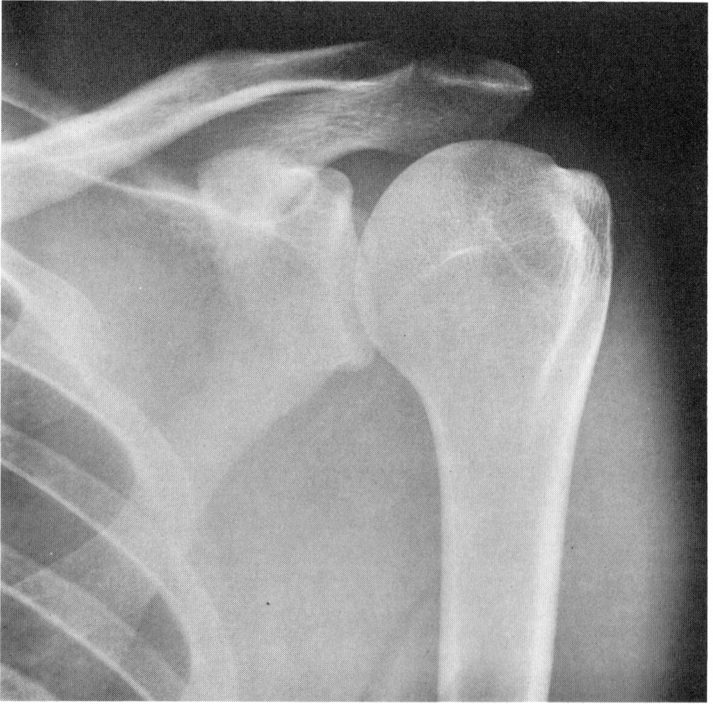

Figure 2-18. Normal shoulder. Note the relationship of the clavicle, scapula, and humeral head.

correct anatomical alignment and a lateral view are generally required.

Elbow

A number of views of the elbow are useful in assessing alignment or looking for fractures or evidence of arthritis. An AP position with the elbow joint extended is most frequently used (Fig. 2–17A). For assessment of the radial head in suspected fractures, however, an AP view with the elbow extended to about 120° is preferable; for better assessment of the lower humerus (in supracondylar fractures, for example), the same 120° view may be taken with the film parallel to the humerus instead of the radius. In the lateral position (Fig. 2–17B), the fat pads should be sought. Although the anterior fat pad may occasionally be visible normally, the posterior one is never seen unless there is a joint effusion, in which case a fracture of the radial head must be suspected (Fig. 1–3). Oblique views of the elbow are useful in looking for discrete fractures, particularly of the radial head.

Humerus

X-rays of the humerus should include the shoulder and the elbow joints. AP and lateral projections are usually the only views necessary.

Shoulder Joint

The shoulder joint represents a complex radiographic situation, and the choice of views depends on the pathologic condition that is suspected. If calcific tendinitis or bursitis is suspected, it is best seen on AP views in both internal and external rotation; the exposure should be such that the soft tissues are clearly visible (Fig. 2–18). A lateral view is useful in searching for fractures or dislocations; it may be performed either as a transthoracic view, which is often difficult to interpret, or as an oblique view with the film cassette against the shoulder laterally and the beam passing through the middle of the medial scapular edge (Fig. 2–19). The humeral head can be seen to lie at the midpoint of the y-shaped scapula. In anterior dislocation, the humeral head lies under the glenoid margin and coracoid process. If there is a posterior dislocation, the humeral head lies behind the spine of the scapula.

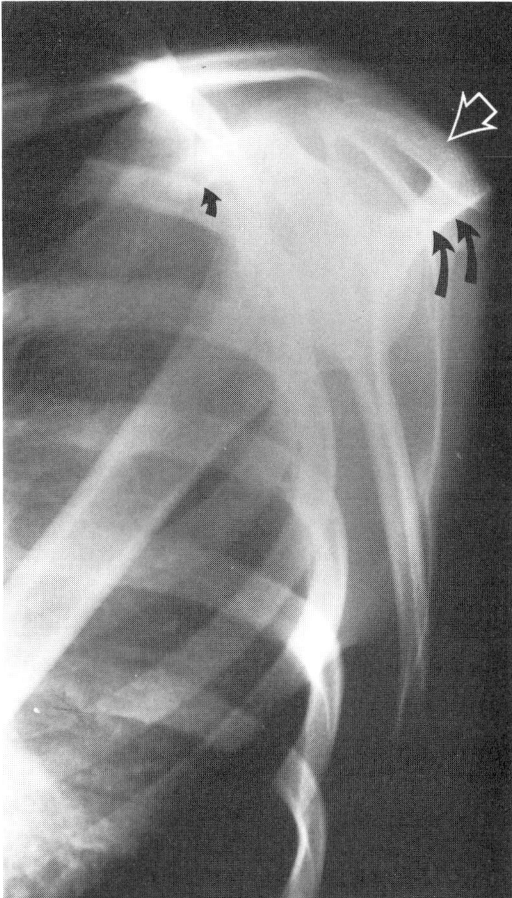

Figure 2–19. Oblique view of the shoulder joint. This radiograph is actually an axial view of the scapula, but it is a very good demonstration of the relationship of the humeral head to the glenoid. Note the position of the coracoid process *(single arrow)*, scapula spine *(double arrows)*, and acromion *(hollow arrow)*.

Axial views can also achieve visualization of a dislocation, but the patient may be experiencing too much pain to abduct the arm sufficiently for the radiograph to be taken. On the AP views, an anterior dislocation of the shoulder is usually obvious, with the humeral head lying below and medial to the glenoid fossa; however, in posterior dislocations, the humeral head often dislocates directly posteriorly, thus appearing to be in place on the AP view. For patients in whom shoulder dislocations are suspected, it is imperative to perform a lateral, oblique, or axial view of the shoulder as well as an AP view.

Acromioclavicular Joint

The acromioclavicular joint is usually radiographed in an AP position only. If subluxation or dislocation is suspected, however, films of *both* acromioclavicular joints should be taken with the patient holding a 10-pound weight in each hand.

Scapula

The scapula is often difficult to radiograph, but a reasonable AP view can be achieved by having the patient put the hand on the head with the elbow in a ventrolateral position. A lateral view like that taken for shoulder dislocation is possible and may also be taken by having the patient put the forearm on the head and shooting obliquely through the scapula.

Clavicle

Two angled PA or AP views with the beam angled 20° above or below the horizontal and going through the center of the clavicle are all that is usually required for this joint. Special views of the acromioclavicular joint have already been discussed; the sternoclavicular joint is often seen satisfactorily only with tomography.

THE LOWER EXTREMITY

Toes

AP and lateral views of the toes may be taken using small dental films for patients with suspected fractures. More often than not, however, the whole foot is x-rayed.

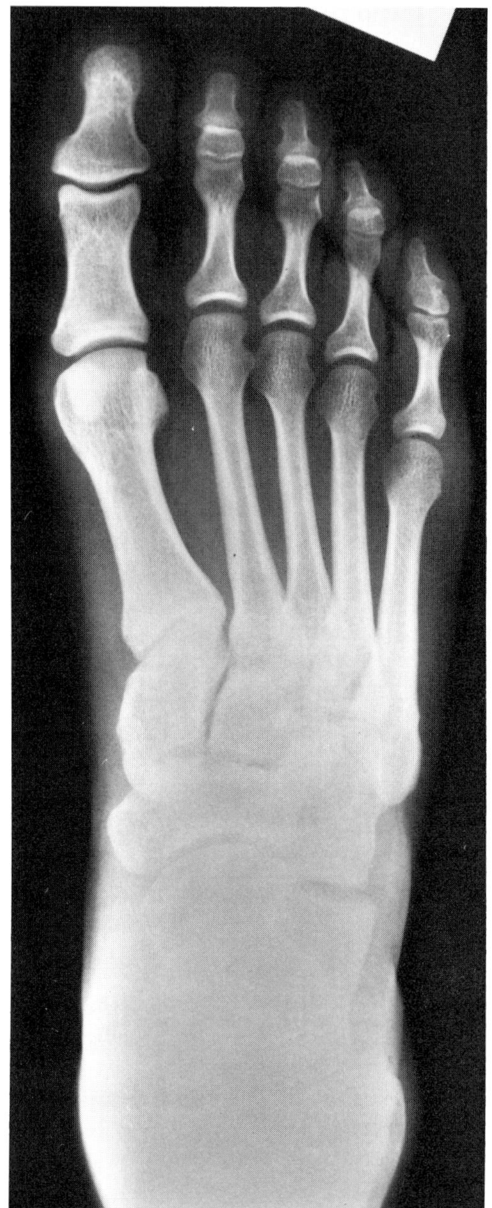

Figure 2–20. Normal AP view of the foot. See text for explanation.

Foot

An AP or supero-inferior view and a lateral view are taken for patients with suspected fractures, arthritis, metabolic bone disease, and osteomyelitis and also for diabetic patients who develop diabetic osteopathy (Fig. 2–20). These radiographs allow evaluation of the two arches of the foot. The "weight-bearing arch" runs through the talus, os calcis, cuboid, fifth metatarsal, and first through fifth metatarsal heads. The other arch, for "springing," runs through the talus, os calcis, talus, navicular bone, cuneiform bones, and first metatarsal and into the metatarsal heads and the toes. Sometimes oblique views of the foot are also useful in the search for discrete fractures of the metatarsals as well as for evidence of erosive changes in the tarsus that may occur in early rheumatoid arthritis.

Heel

Many special views of the os calcis or the calcaneum are possible, but a true lateral view will demonstrate the insertion of the Achilles tendon and the origin of the plantar aponeurosis, either of which may be the site for spurs in degenerative arthritis or erosions in ankylosing spondylitis and rheumatoid arthritis. Oblique views may be useful in the assessment of fractures of the calcaneum. The subtalar joints may be shown by means of special oblique views taken with the lower leg rotated medially 45° and the main beam entering at an angle of 10°, 20°, or 40° through the talocalcaneal joints. The Harris view, taken with the heel against the film and the beam entering through the sole of the foot at a 60° angle to the horizontal, is a useful projection for looking at the body of the calcaneum in cases of trauma.

Ankle

Three views of the ankle should be sufficient: an AP view, a lateral view (Fig. 2–21A), and an oblique AP view with medial rotation of the lateral malleolus away from the fibulotalar joint to demonstrate the ankle mortise and the tibiotalar joint satisfactorily (Fig. 2–21B). Other oblique views

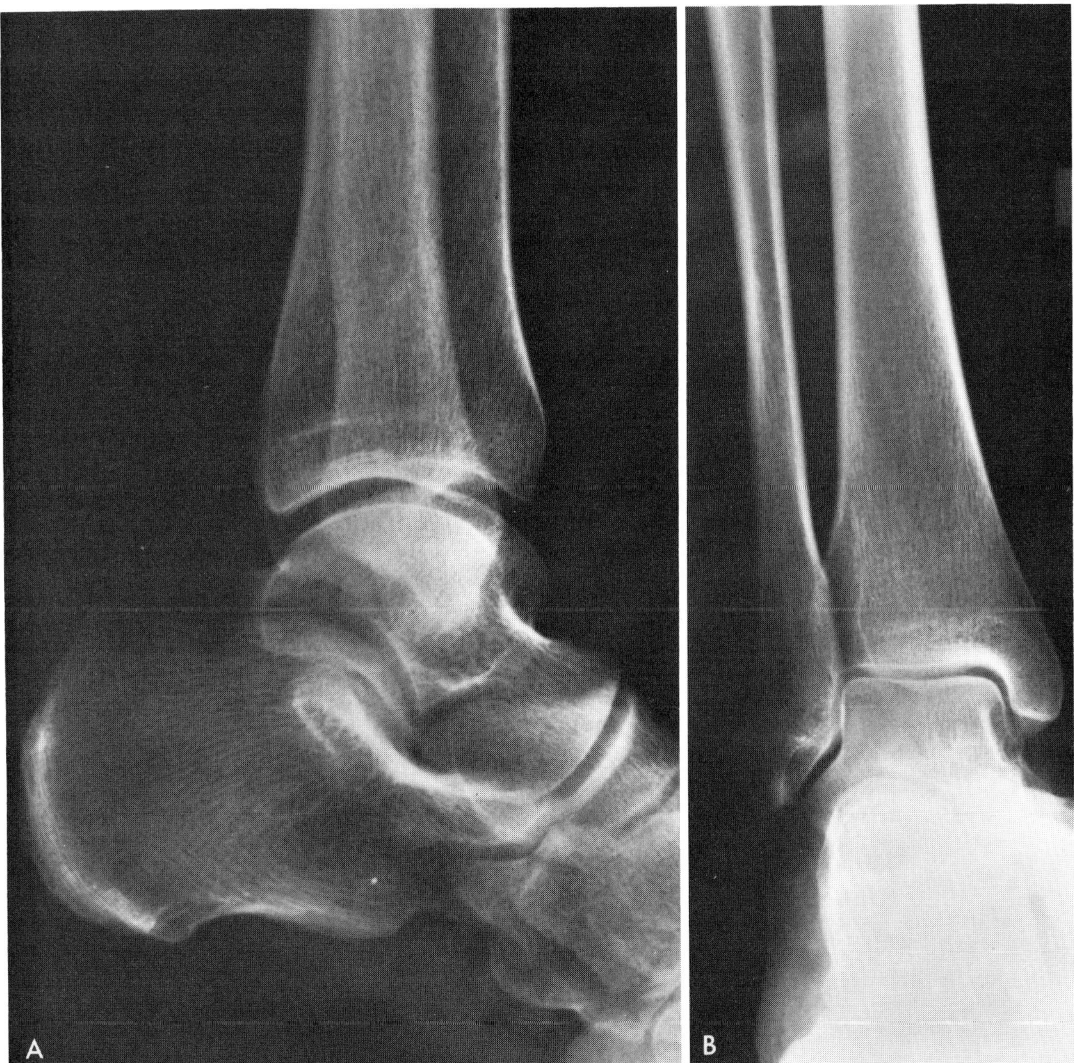

Figure 2–21. Normal ankle. *A*, Lateral view. *B*, Normal mortise view, which is achieved by angling the normal AP view obliquely so that the lateral malleolus is rotated off the fibulotalar joint.

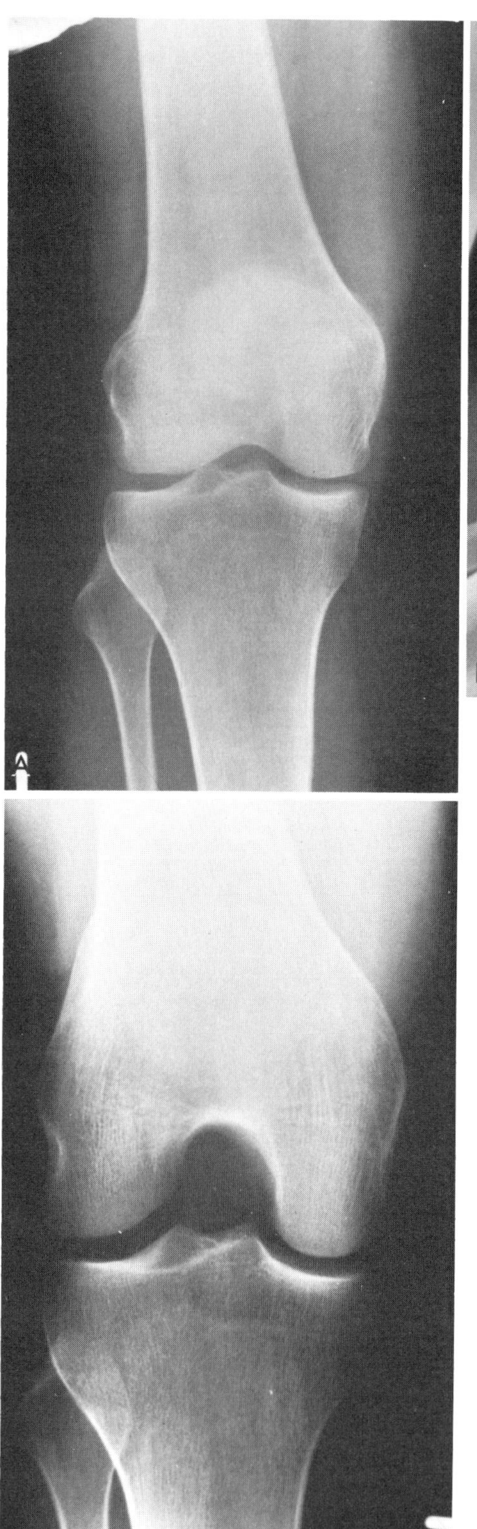

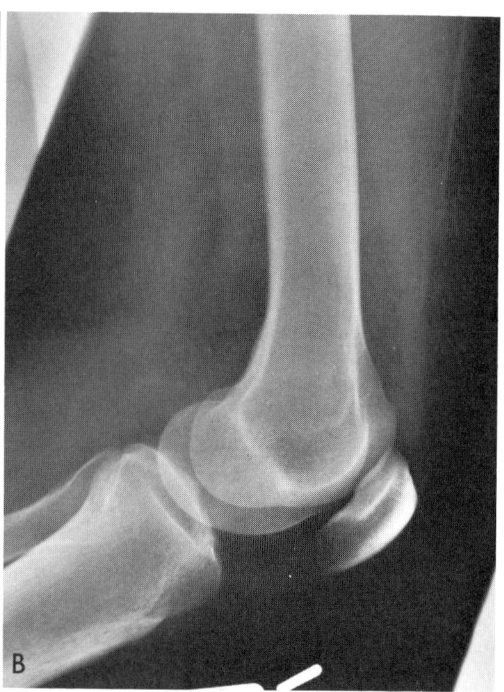

Figure 2–22. Normal knee. *A*, AP view. *B*, Lateral view. *C*, "Tunnel" view. Note the contours of the normal intercondylar notch.

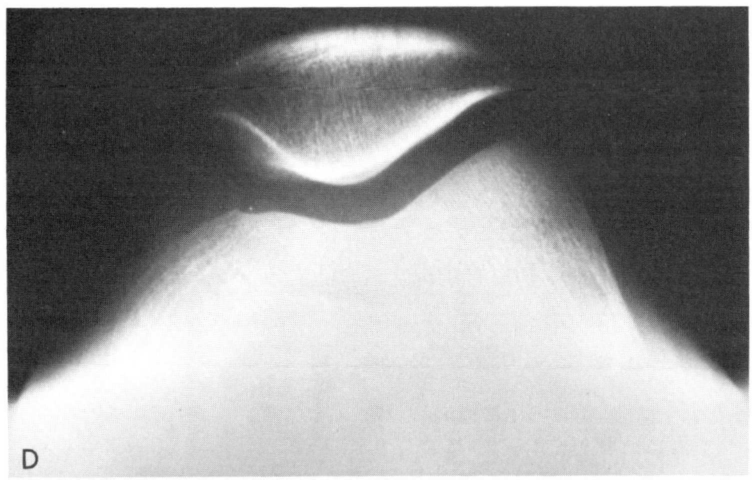

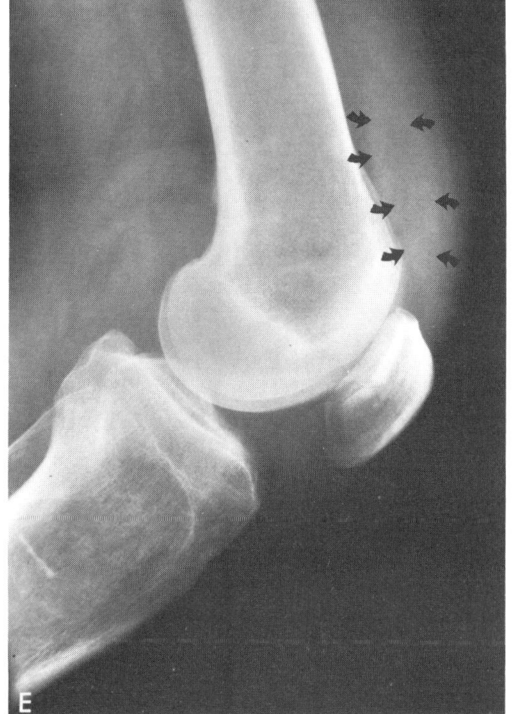

Figure 2–22. *Continued.* *D*, "Skyline" view. Note the shape of the patello-femoral articulation; the lateral part of the patella has a longer and more horizontal surface than the medial surface. *E*, This lateral view of a different patient (a 52-year-old woman) shows an effusion *(arrows)*.

may be necessary if a subtle fracture is suspected.

Lower Leg

Radiographs of the lower leg should include the full length of both the tibia and the fibula as well as the knee and ankle joints (another "ring of bone"). For example, if an isolated fracture of the lower tibia is seen on views of the ankle, it is imperative to x-ray the full length of the fibula. AP and lateral views of the lower leg should suffice, although the lateral view may be taken two ways: with either the knee or the ankle positioned truly laterally.

Knee

An AP view with the knee fully extended (Fig. 2–22A) and a lateral view with the knee flexed to about 30° (Fig. 2–22B) are the usual views taken of the knee in cases of minor trauma. In patients with larger effusions or major trauma, a cross-table lateral view is useful for looking for fat-fluid levels within the effusion, which indicate a significant fracture. In order to assess the knee joint properly, however, a so-called "tunnel view," an AP view with the knee flexed at 90° (Fig. 2–22C), helps to visualize the intercondylar notch, which may become widened and eroded in hemophilia, rheumatoid arthritis, tuberculosis, and villonodular synovitis. "Skyline views" of the patella may be taken, with the knee flexed, usually to about 40° (Fig. 2–22D) but sometimes at a different angle. In this view, the beam passes axially through the patella, facilitating assessment of the patellofemoral joint in cases of chondromalacia patellae, recurrent dislocation, and arthritis. Oblique views of the knee and patella are occasionally useful, but in any patient with arthritis, a radiographic evaluation of the knee joint is not complete until "weight-bearing" views of both knees are taken with the patient standing. No assessment of the integrity of the articular cartilage of the knee is complete without this view.

Femur

Radiological evaluation of the femur is complete only when the hip and knee joints are included. An AP view is often the only one required, but occasionally a lateral view may be of help. The male genitalia should be shielded where possible and relevant.

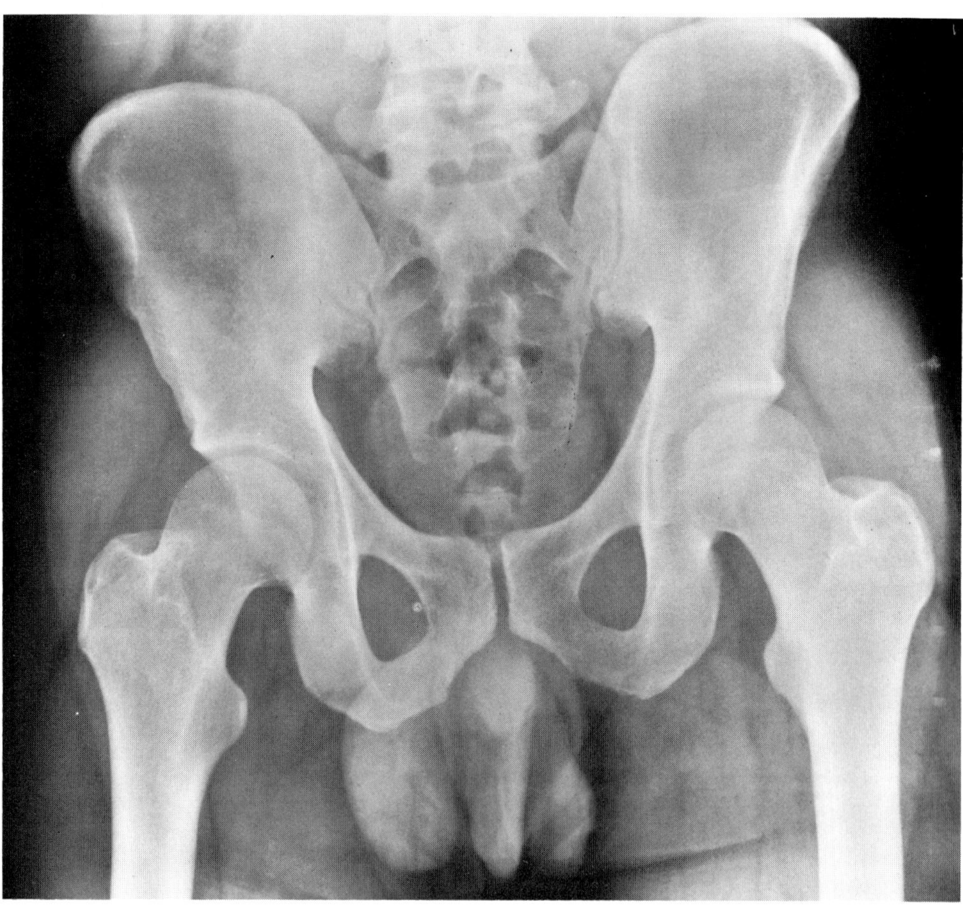

Figure 2–23. Normal pelvis. See text for explanation.

Pelvis and Hip Joints

An AP view is the usual single view taken of the pelvis (Fig. 2–23). This should include the lower lumbar spine, the sacrum and coccyx, the sacroiliac joints, the symphysis pubis, both hip joints, and the femoral necks as well as the bones of the pelvis. Close-up views of the symphysis are occasionally useful for postpartum females in whom infection is suspected and for males with chronic prostatitis. For the hip joint proper, a straight AP view and a "frog-leg" lateral view are useful to assess the femoral articular cartilage and the integrity of the femoral head, in cases of suspected avascular necrosis, for example. The "frog-leg" view is so called because the patient is instructed to keep his heels together and to abduct his hips so that his knees are apart, a position similar to that of a frog, and designed to bring the weight-bearing surface of the femoral head into the plane of the x-ray beam (Fig. 2–24). A "true lateral" view of the femoral neck is useful in patients with suspected fractures, in cases of internal fixation of old fractures, and in patients with total hip replacements. This is performed by having the patient flex the knee 90° and abduct the femur and placing the film behind the hip. Other special views of the hip joint are requested by the orthopedic surgeon for specific disorders such as congenital dislocation of the hip (CDH), subluxation, and slipped capital femoral epiphysis, but these lie outside the scope of this book.

It is desirable to shield both the male and female genitalia, particularly with younger patients or patients for whom repeated studies of the pelvis are indicated. Shielding of the ovaries, however, will often conceal the sacroiliac joints, and poorly placed shielding of the testicles may obscure the symphysis pubis or even a hip joint. Thus, a compromise often has to be reached by both the clinician and the radiologist with respect to proper shielding and the attainment of the best possible radiographs.

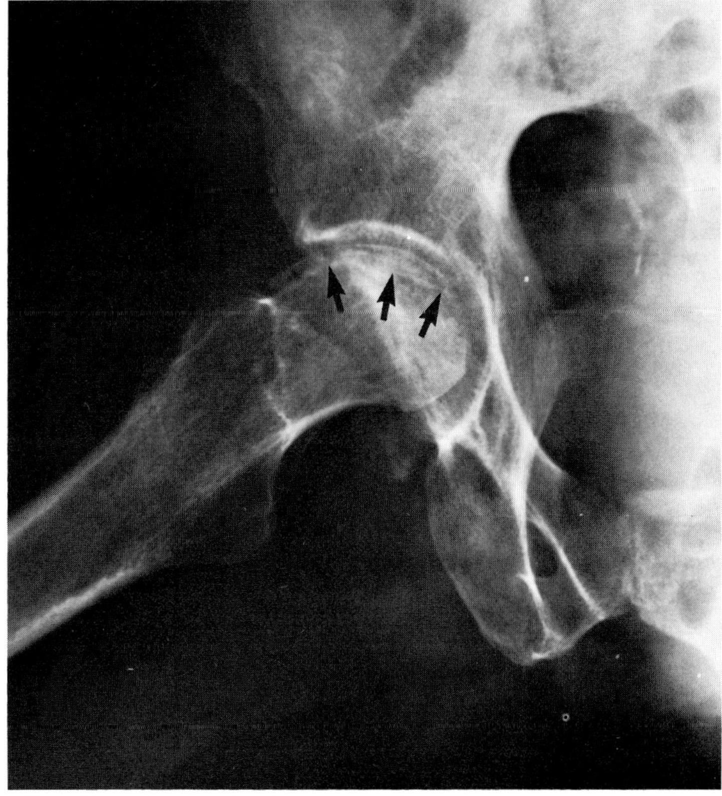

Figure 2–24. Frog-leg view of the hip. In this 40-year-old man receiving long-term steroid therapy, the normal AP view failed to show any abnormality of the femoral heads. This frog-leg view shows the subchondral fractures typical of avascular necrosis *(arrows)*.

THE SPINE

Cervical Spine

Routine views of the cervical spine include an AP projection in neutral position, a lateral view, and two oblique views to show the intervertebral foramina (Fig. 2–25). These are performed by rotating the whole body 45° or by angling the beam 45° from the lateral position. When the patient faces left, the *right* foramina become visible, and when the patient faces right, the *left* foramina become visible.

Other views of the cervical spine that may be taken include an AP open-mouth

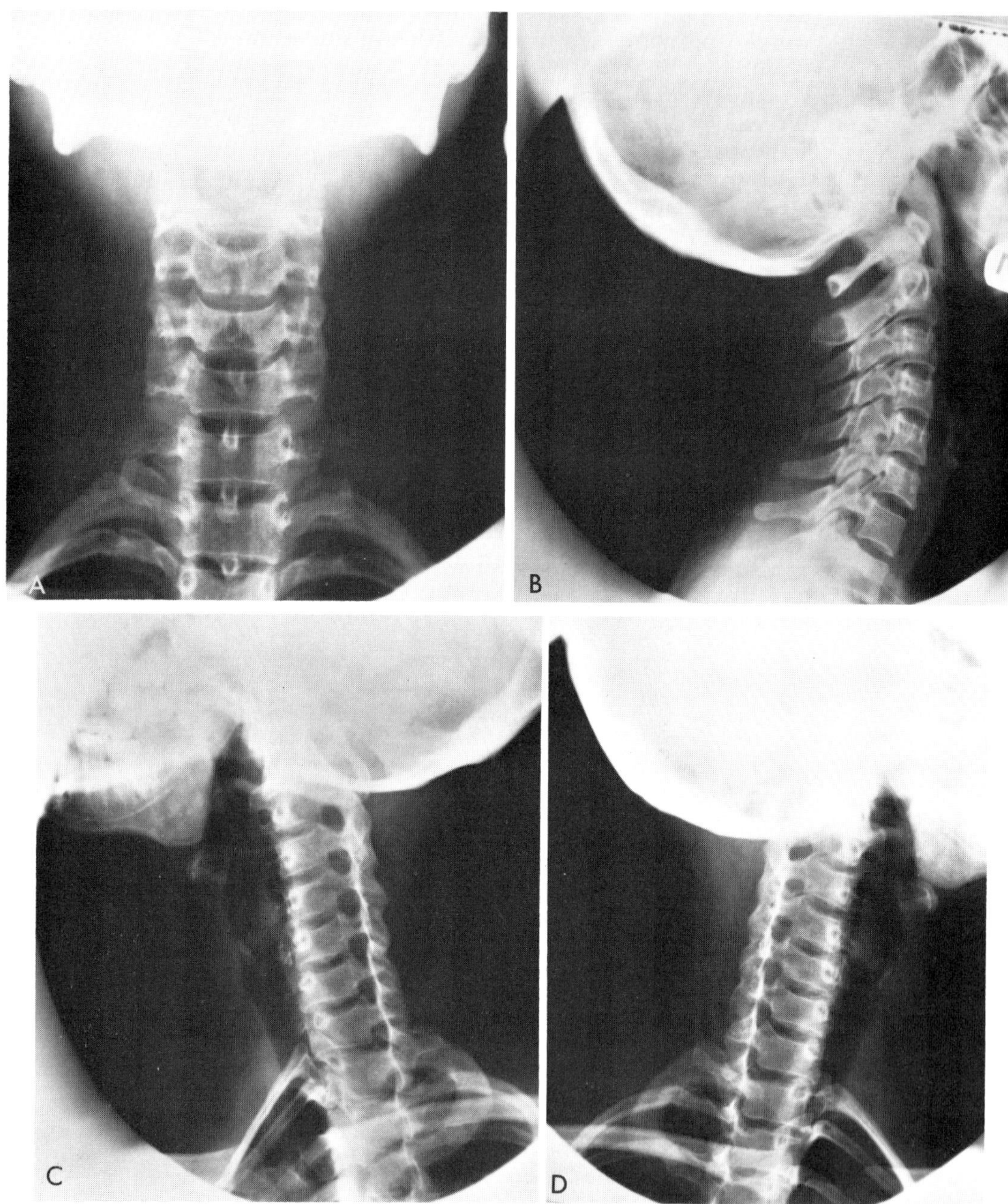

Figure 2–25. Normal cervical spine. *A*, AP view. *B*, Lateral view. *C*, Right oblique view. *D*, Left oblique view. See text for explanation.

view of the odontoid peg, which is useful in cases of suspected fracture or subluxation of the atlanto-axial articulation. Flexion and extension lateral views are used for patients with rheumatoid arthritis in whom subluxation of the atlanto-axial joint is suspected. The normal space between the posterior aspect of the anterior arch of the atlas and the anterior margin of the odontoid is 2 mm. These projections should be taken with great care in cases of suspected subluxation because of the danger of paralyzing or pithing the patient. Pillar views of the lateral masses are useful in patients with suspected fractures of the neck. These are performed by placing the head at a 45° angle and angling the x-ray beam at a 30° angle towards the head, with the patient in

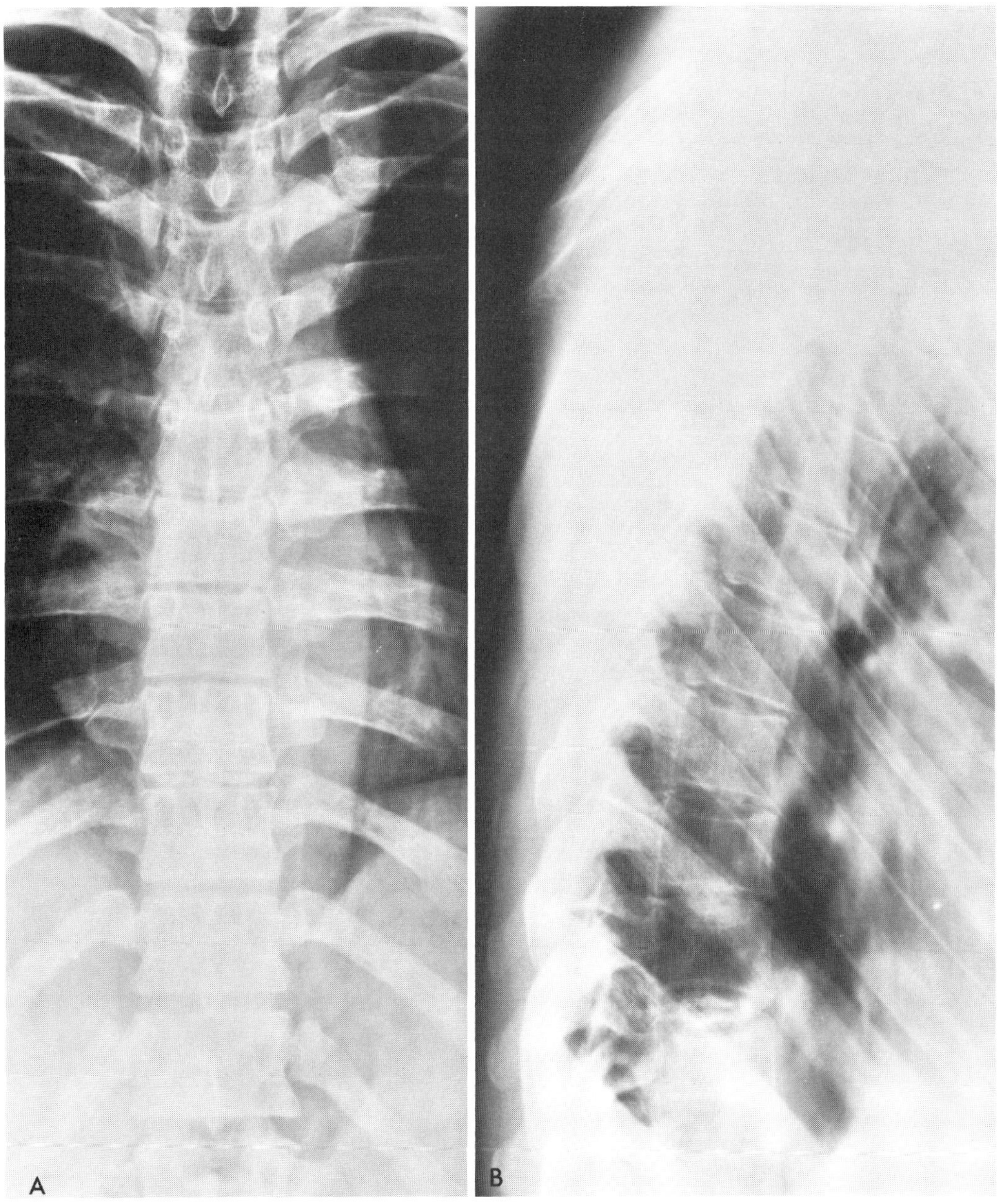

Figure 2–26. Normal thoracic spine *A*, AP view. *B*, Lateral view. See text for explanation. Note the disc calcification at the T9–T10 level.

the PA position. A lateral "swimmer's" view of the lower cervical and upper thoracic spine is achieved by having the patient place one arm slightly anterior and upward and the other posterior and downward (like a swimmer doing the crawl); this placement removes most of the overlying bone and soft tissues from the picture.

Thoracic Spine

AP and lateral views of the thoracic spine are usually taken (Fig. 2–26). The "swimmer's" view is a useful projection for the upper part of the thoracic spine. This may be combined with an inclined AP view of the lower cervical and upper thoracic spine to facilitate evaluation of this region. Oblique views are sometimes ordered for evaluation of the foramina, but these projections rarely provide any useful information.

Lumbar Spine

A routine survey of the lumbosacral spine for metastatic disease should probably consist only of AP and lateral views (Figs. 2–27A and 2–27B). If trauma or a congenital anomaly is suspected, however, left and right oblique views should also be taken, this time with the patient rotated to the side of the foramen (Fig. 2–27C). If spondylolisthesis (anterior or, occasionally, posterior slippage of one vertebra upon the next) is visible on the lateral projection, the possibility of spondylolysis (a break in the pars interarticularis) must be excluded. Spondylolysis is relatively easy to see; all one must look for is a "collar on the Scottie dog" (Fig. 2–27D). A coned-down lateral view of L5/S1 is often taken in addition to AP and lateral views, because disc disease is common at this level and because on the overall films of the whole lumbar spine this area is often obscured.

Sacrum and Coccyx

The routine AP view of the sacrum is taken with the x-ray beam entering at an angle of 20° cephalad, but a 10° caudad AP view may also be taken. This is best done after the patient has emptied the bladder.

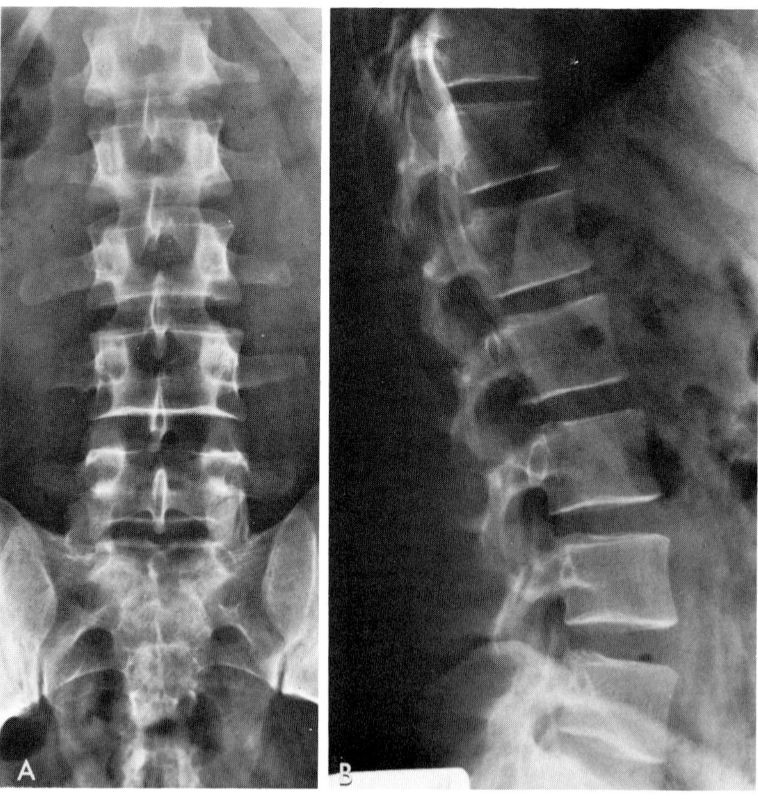

Figure 2–27. Normal lumbar spine: *A*, AP view. *B*, Lateral view.

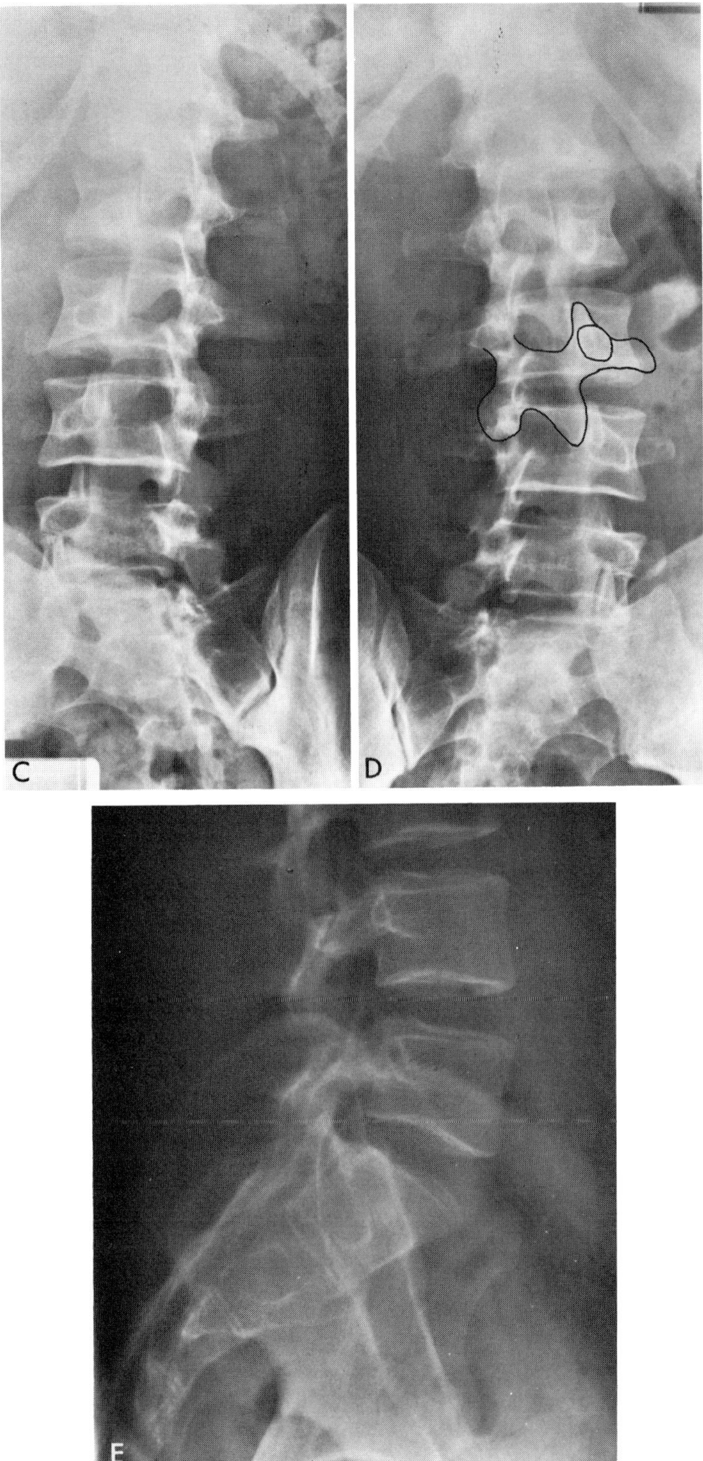

Figure 2–27. Continued. *C* and *D*, Oblique views with drawing of "Scottie dog." *E*, Coned-down lateral view of L5 S1. Can you work out the anatomy of the Scottie dog?

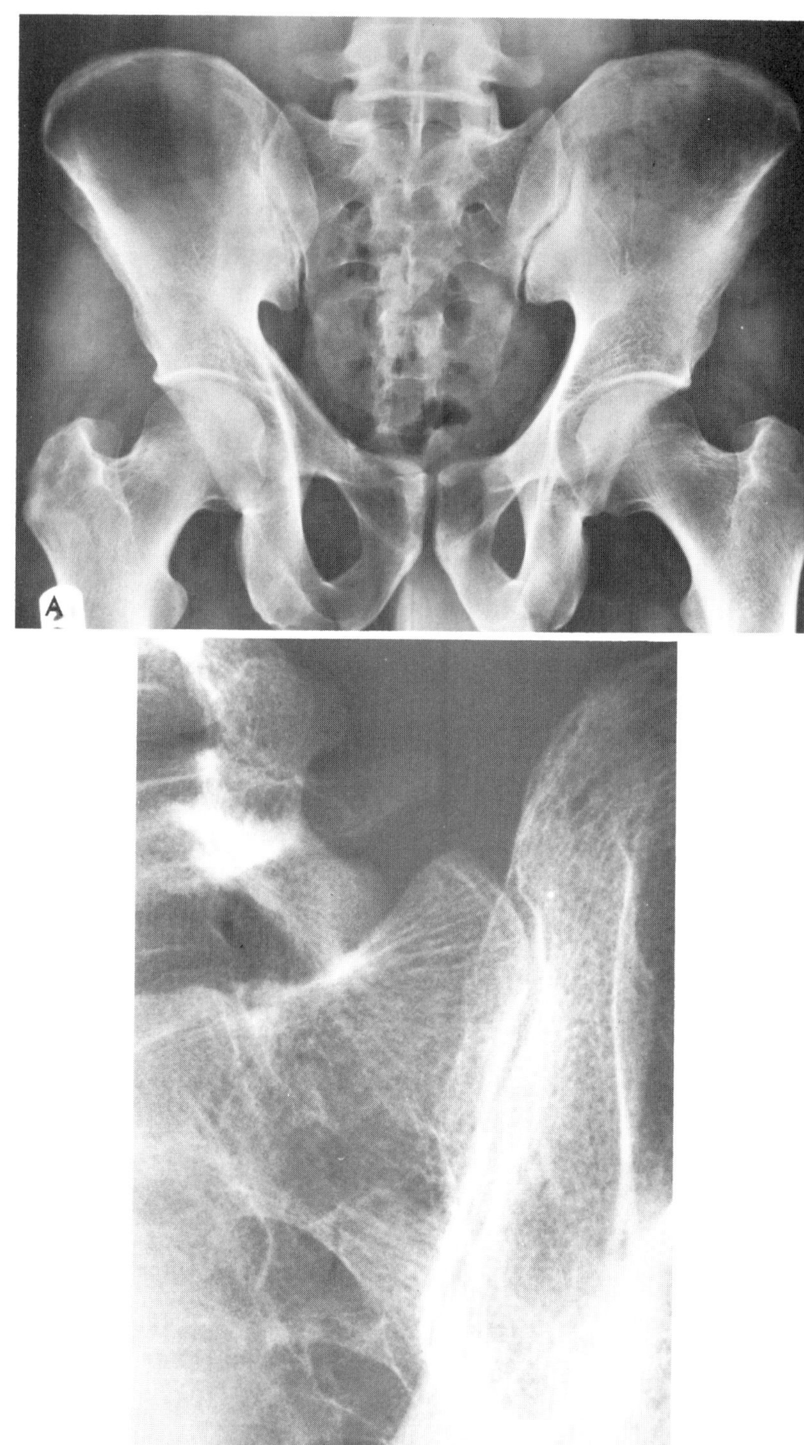

Figure 2–28. Sacroiliac joints. *A*, Normal pelvis view. *B*, Normal oblique view.

A lateral view is useful in looking for fractures of the sacrum, but tomography is usually required to confirm a sacral lesion such as a tumor or metastasis. Coned-down views of the coccyx are a waste of time, because the diagnosis of a coccygeal fracture or dislocation can be made clinically with great ease — and the use of a finger cot.

Sacroiliac Joints

On most pelvic radiographs, the sacroiliac joints are visualized, but since the joints are inclined at a 35° angle away from the midline, oblique AP views are extremely useful and should always be performed for both sides (Fig. 2–28). An AP view with the beam inclined 10° caudad is often helpful. For example, if early ankylosing spondylitis is suspected, an AP view of the pelvis with oblique views of the sacroiliac joints would be an appropriate radiological work-up.

THE SKULL AND HEAD

There are many clinical indications for performing x-rays of the skull, including trauma, infections, tumors, and intracranial bleeding. The most common indication is undoubtedly suspected injury, which is often minor; for medico-legal reasons, it has become fashionable to take five or more views of the skull. It has been shown conclusively that this series is really unnecessary because a single lateral view will suffice. If there is evidence of major trauma, however, all the routine views are essential, and any other special views or studies that are clinically indicated should also be taken. It is important to realize that the choice between a single view and a routine skull series is made by the clinician.

Routine Views of the Skull

There are five basic views of the skull.

The PA view is taken at a 25° angle to the baseline between the orbit and the external auditory meatus with the patient's face against the film (Fig. 2–29A). It is important that all loose objects or metal paraphernalia be removed (this includes hairpins, glasses, and dentures, although the patient with a glass eye may be allowed to leave it in). The PA view is a useful view in which to look for the overall symmetry of the skull as well as for fractures or midline shift. It also provides a good picture of the maxillary antra, nose, mastoids, and floor of the sella.

The AP view is taken with the back of the patient's head against the film, and the beam enters at an angle of 25° to the orbitomeatal line (Fig. 2–29B). The AP film can be used to show the features visible on a PA view, but it also shows us the frontal sinuses and is especially useful in looking for midline shift.

The lateral view is taken with the affected side toward the film (Fig. 2–29C), but some radiology departments take both left and right lateral views routinely. This is an excellent view for looking for fractures, evidence of raised intracranial pressure, and calcification in the pineal gland as well as abnormalities in the sinuses, mandible, and upper cervical spine.

The Townes view is an inclined half-axial projection taken at a 35° angle to the orbitomeatal line. It should project the dorsum sellae into the foramen magnum (Fig. 2–29D). This view is useful in looking for symmetry, midline shift, fractures of the calvarium, and abnormalities of the mastoids.

The base or axial view is taken at a 90° angle to the orbitomeatal baseline, with the x-ray beam entering through the neck just under the chin and the film under the patient's head (Fig. 2–29E). This is the best routine view for looking at the base of the skull, since the atlantoaxial articulation, the mastoid air cells, the sinuses, the foramina, and the mandible are all well visualized.

Although the clinical uses of all these views will be illustrated later, one comment seems appropriate here. A midline shift may be measured by finding the pineal gland on a routine view (if it is calcified) and measuring from it to the inner table of the calvarium on either side; a 2 mm difference is allowed for normal skulls (Fig. 2–30). An alternative method is to draw a line from the top of the odontoid peg to the vertex (sagittal suture). This line

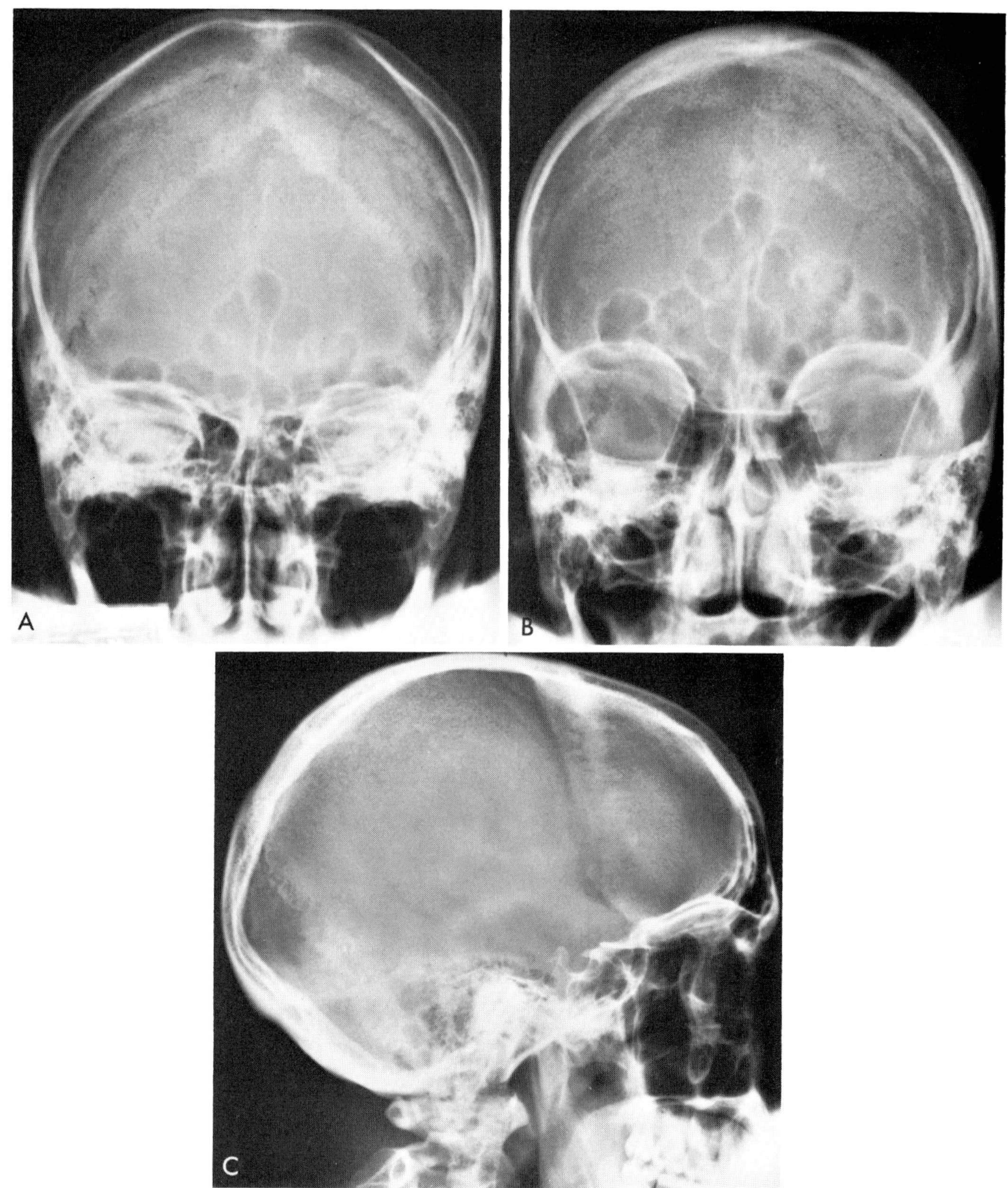

Figure 2–29. Normal skull. *A*, PA view. *B*, AP view. *C*, Lateral view.

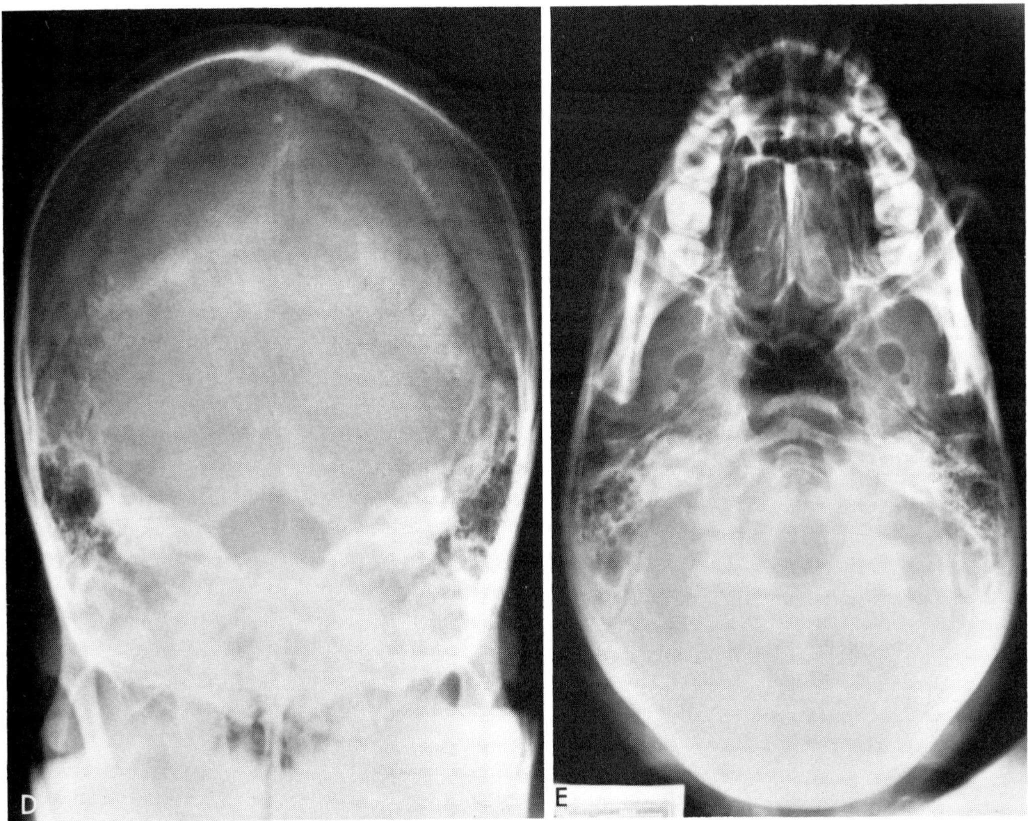

Figure 2–29. Continued. *D*, Townes view. *E*, Base view. See text for explanation.

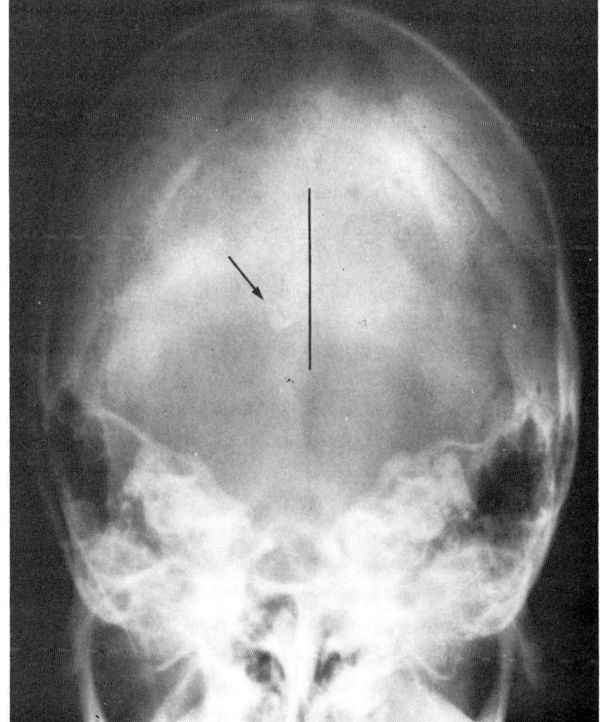

Figure 2–30. Townes view of skull to show midline shift of calcified pineal gland *(arrow).*

should transect the normal pineal with a difference no greater than 2 mm.

Special Views of the Skull

Of the many non-routine views of the skull, one in particular may be of use in specific circumstances. The lateral view taken with a horizontal x-ray beam will show air-fluid levels in the sinuses (particularly the sphenoid) or in the skull itself, and the atlanto-axial joint is usually also clearly visualized.

Many other special views of the facial bones and specific areas of the skull are available, but most of these are so specialized that they lie outside the scope of this book. Those most frequently used are views of the sella turcica and of the optic canals.

Views of the Sella Turcica

A coned-down lateral view and a coned-down PA view will provide information on the integrity of the floor of the sella and the dorsum sellae or show evidence of enlargement of the sella. Although many measurements of the sella may be made, the most useful parameters are its length (8–10 mm with a mean of 10 mm), width (12–20 mm with a mean of 16 mm), and height (6–10 mm with a mean of 8 mm), giving an average area of 600 cu mm. However, tomography is often necessary for the final evaluation of pathologic conditions of the sella.

Views of the Optic Canals

At least five techniques for visualizing the optic canals have been developed for looking for tumors or other abnormalities of the optic nerve. Basically, they are all oblique views taken in two different planes of obliquity: 20° or so from the orbitomeatal line and 20 to 30° from the midline. Both optic canals should be x-rayed when a tumor is sought, because the radiograph of the unaffected side can serve as normal comparison.

Routine Views of the Head

Paranasal Sinuses

Three or four views are usually taken of the sinuses. For the PA view, although similar to the PA view of the skull, the film is inclined at a 30° angle toward the forehead, allowing all the sinuses to be seen (Fig. 2–31A). The lateral view, similar to the lateral view of the skull, is coned down to the region of the sinuses (Fig. 2–31B). The axial or base view is similar to the axial view of the skull but is also coned down (Fig. 2–31C). The Waters view is an inclined PA projection with the mouth open and the film inclined 15° forward (Fig. 2–31D). This provides a good view of the orbits as well as the frontal and maxillary sinuses. It is useful in looking for air-fluid levels, and the sphenoid sinus can be seen through the open mouth.

Sinusitis may be demonstrated by blurring of the normally clear-cut bony margins of the sinuses, thickening of the mucosa, the presence of air-fluid levels (Fig. 2–32), or opacification of the entire sinus. Retention cysts and polyps have smooth rounded margins and do not affect the underlying osseous margins, whereas mucoceles and most tumors can destroy the bone.

Nose

Often, lateral views and an axial view will suffice to look for nasal fractures. On the whole, fractures of the nose will run at right angles to the anterior margin of the nasal bones, whereas suture lines are inclined to run parallel with it.

Zygomatic Arches

The zygomatic arches are often best shown in the axial view of the skull, but special tangential views are available if a fracture is suspected.

Mandible

The temporomandibular joints are radiographed in an inclined lateral position, but many alternative projections are possible. Both sides of the mandible should always

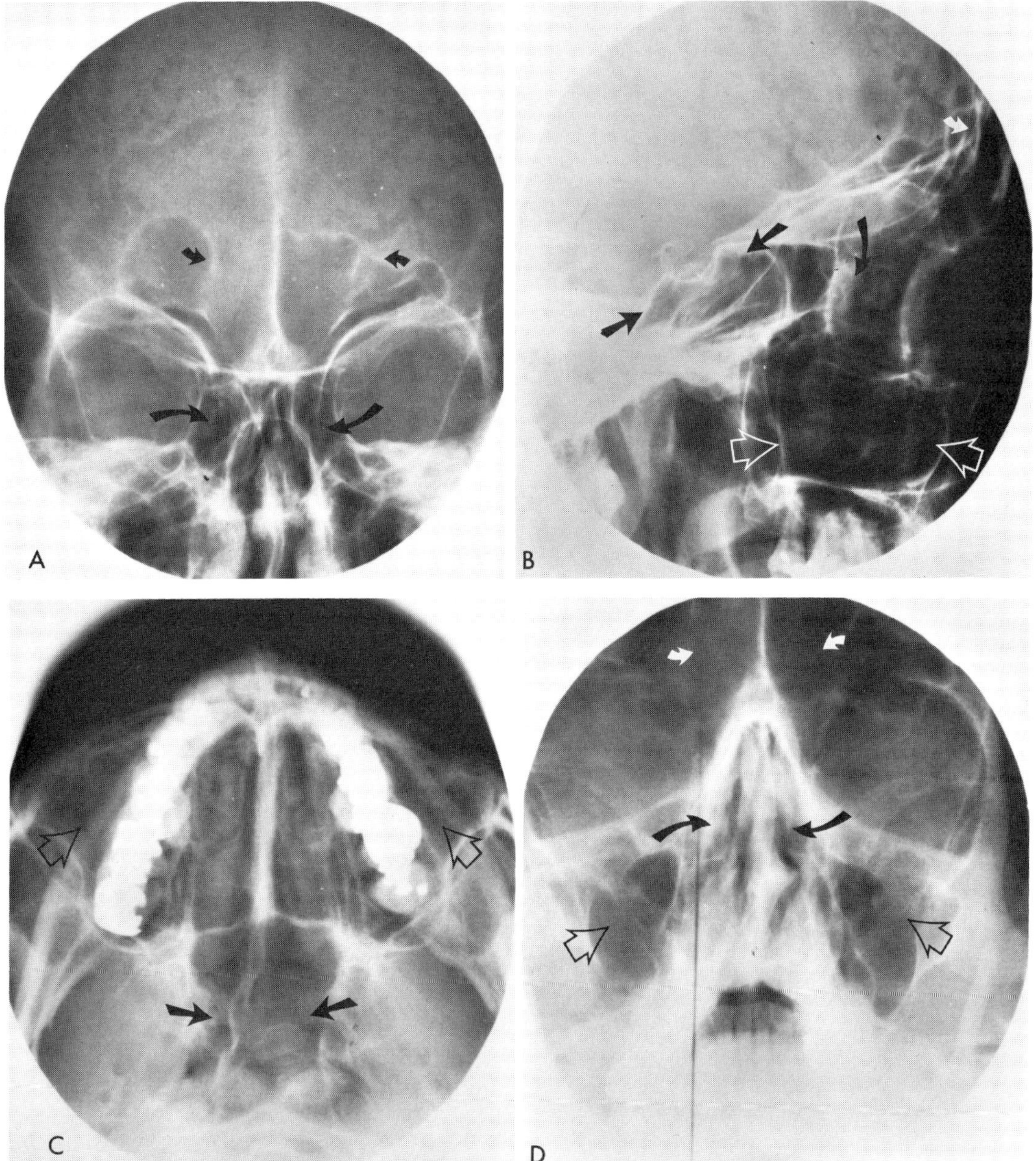

Figure 2–31. Normal sinuses. *A*, PA view. *B*, Lateral view. *C*, Base view. *D*, Waters view. These views demonstrate the frontal *(small arrows)*, ethmoid *(curved arrows)*, maxillary antra *(hollow arrows)*, and sphenoid *(straight black arrows)* sinuses.

be taken, and open-mouth and closed-mouth views are usually considered essential. The PA view of the mandible is similar to the PA view of the skull, although the Panorex has now made this view unnecessary. The Panorex is a special rotating x-ray film and tube that circles the patient's head and produces a panoramic radiograph of the whole mandible, including the dentition; this radiograph is frequently used by dentists. Oblique AP views of the mandibular rami and the condyles are sometimes indicated in cases of suspected fracture. Lateral views are useful in assessing the extent of osteomyelitis or of tumors in the floor of the mouth.

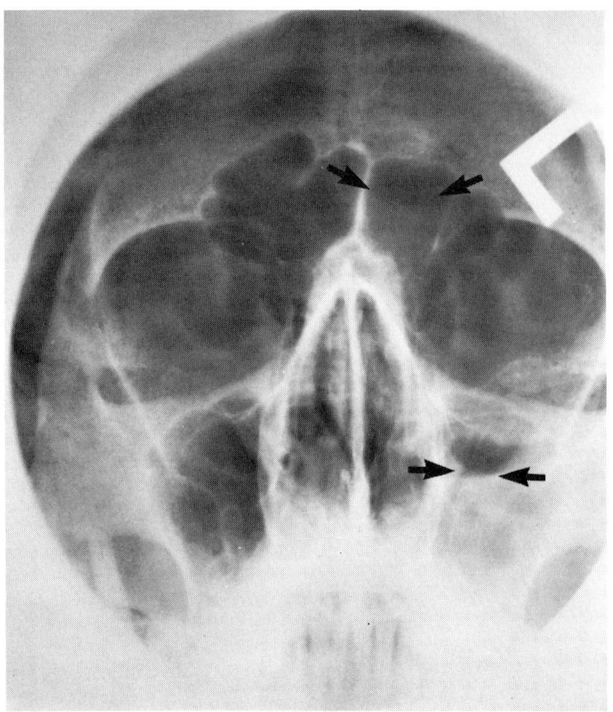

Figure 2–32. Erect Waters view of a patient with sinusitis. Note the air-fluid levels in the frontal sinus and left maxillary antrum *(opposing arrows).*

Orbits

Fractures of the orbit or a tripod fracture of the floor of the orbit, zygoma, and maxillary antrum is common. Both fractures involve a "ring of bone," so if one fracture can be identified with certainty, additional fractures must be sought. Tomography is often necessary, but many plain film views are available. A PA view similar to that taken of the skull will show the orbit. A Waters view similar to that of the paranasal sinuses will outline the floor of the orbit very clearly. Oblique views are useful for looking for foreign bodies as well as for identifying fractures of the zygomatic arch. The special views of the optic canals previously described are also essential when looking for tumors.

Mastoid Air Cells and Inner Ear

Many views are possible for looking at this region, but the projections more commonly taken are a base view, a Townes view, and an inclined AP view that projects the internal auditory canal through the orbits (Fig. 2–33A) and is particularly useful in looking for evidence of an acoustic neuroma. A Stenvers view, an oblique lateral projection showing the mastoid air cells as well as the internal ear, is particularly useful (Fig. 2–33B). A large number of other variants of this oblique position such as the Mayer and Chaussé views are also helpful.

SPECIAL RADIOGRAPHIC SURVEY FILMS

Metastatic Bone Survey

Most osseous metastases involve the axial rather than the peripheral skeleton. Sometimes, a routine metastatic survey is requested because the clinician thinks there are no bony metastases but wishes to make sure. An isotope bone scan is a much more accurate way of achieving this aim. Any "hot spots" may be subsequently radiographed to exclude the possibility of other lesions such as those seen in arthritis or Paget's disease, which will also produce a positive scan. If bony metastases are shown to be present and radiographs have been requested as a baseline, as a follow-up, or as a measure of the efficacy of therapy, the following views are sug-

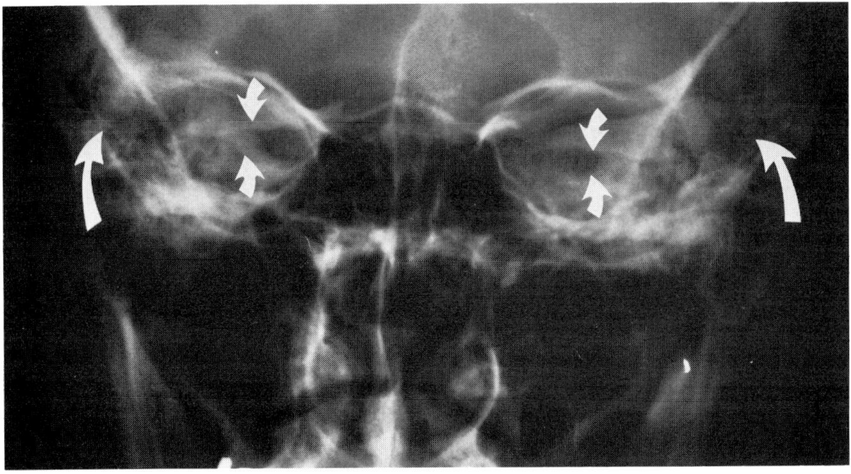

A

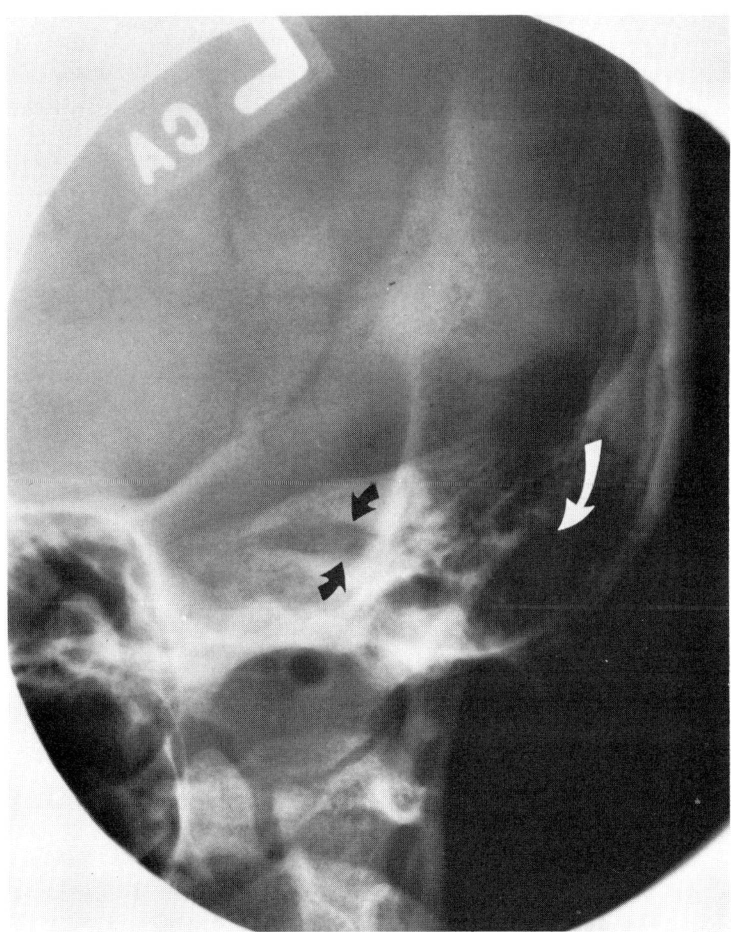

B

Figure 2–33. Normal internal auditory canals. *A*, Inclined AP view through the orbits. *B*, Stenvers view showing the normal internal auditory canals *(small arrows)* and the mastoid air cells *(large arrows)*.

gested, although these may vary from department to department:

1. Lateral skull.
2. AP and lateral thoracic spine.
3. AP and lateral lumbar spine.
4. AP pelvis.
5. PA chest — if no recent film available.
6. Radiographs of other parts of the skeleton if there is any clinical indication such as pain or swelling.

Hyperparathyroid Bone Survey

In both primary and secondary hyperparathyroidism, there are certain specific skeletal manifestations. In cases of hypercalcemia or other forms of metabolic bone disease, the following radiographic views are suggested:

1. PA view of hands and wrist — magnification view if possible.
2. Lateral lumbar spine.
3. AP pelvis.
4. AP acromioclavicular joints.
5. PA chest — if no recent film available.

Joint Survey

Views used in a joint survey depend on the type of arthritis suspected, but a useful survey should include the following:

1. PA of hands and wrists.
2. Lateral elbows.
3. AP shoulders.
4. AP pelvis.
5. AP and lateral knees.
6. AP ankles.
7. AP and lateral feet.

Scoliosis Series

For patients who have a severe kyphoscoliosis, it is often necessary to take full-length films of the entire spine, either separately or with a long (36-in) cassette. The choice of views will vary depending on the orthopedist, but a spine series should include:

1. AP at rest and with traction.
2. AP with left and right lateral tilt (bend).
3. Lateral views at rest and with traction.
4. Lateral views in full flexion and full extension.

Leg-length Films

Leg-length films are required in a number of situations, including the follow-up of a leg fracture for a child in whom the growth may have been accelerated or retarded, in cases of scoliosis, or in cases of congenital anomalies. The pelvis has to be straight, with the anterior-superior iliac spines parallel to each other and the film. Either a long (36-in) cassette may be used, with or without a metal ruler or grid for measurement, or two separate films may be taken, with a metal ruler between the legs for measurement. Thus, the leg lengths can easily be compared by measuring, for example, from the symphysis pubis to the medial femoral condyles to the medial malleolus, and any joint abnormalities can be discovered at the same time.

Stress Films of Joints

For any joint that shows clinical evidence of ligamentous laxity, subluxation, or dislocation, stress films should be taken. If it is a paired joint, the process must be repeated on the normal side to provide a "control" for comparison. Stress films of the ankles and knees are taken to look for collateral ligament tears. The cervical spine can be radiographed in flexion and extension, and in cases of suspected subluxation, the acromioclavicular joint may be placed under stress by having the patient carry a weight.

Pelvic Measurement

Measurements of the pelvic inlet and outlet during the latter stages of pregnancy are now only rarely performed. They have been superseded by ultrasonographic examination, in which there is no danger of radiation damage.

CHAPTER 3

DIAGNOSTIC RADIOLOGY: CONTRAST STUDIES

Many metallic substances appear on radiographs: plates in the skull, pacemakers and their wires, joint prostheses, hairpins, money, keys, and hearing aids. Even old injection sites in the buttocks are often visible, relics from the period when arsenicals and bismuth were used in the treatment of syphilis.

Although technically all heavy metals are denser than soft tissue, only one, barium, is in common use in diagnostic radiology. Barium is employed for gastrointestinal studies. The dense contrast agents containing iodine are used for most other radiographic procedures. The purpose of opacifying hollow viscera is to be able to diagnose disease processes. Without the use of contrast agents, fluid-filled intestine, ureters, and bladder are not visible because they are surrounded by soft tissues of similar radiodensity.

BARIUM

Barium was first used as a contrast agent in 1910. Initially used for many special procedures, including cystograms and retrograde pyelograms, barium is now employed mainly for studies of the gastrointestinal tract. Barium occurs naturally in the ground as barite and is mined in Canada, South Africa, and the Soviet Union. It is purified and refined and often flavored to make it more palatable.

Barium is innocuous and inert and can be used safely in nearly all circumstances. If it should be aspirated, the patient will usually cough most of it up, and the remainder will be taken care of by the macrophages. If barium enters the peritoneal cavity through a perforation, for instance, it does no direct harm, although there are two side effects: it is more difficult at operation for the surgeon to "mop up" than gastric juices, and it can cause local granulomas and adhesions that make reoperation more difficult. For patients with suspected intestinal perforation, an iodinated water-soluble contrast agent (for example, Gastrografin) should be used.

Barium is routinely used for the evaluation of the gastrointestinal tract. It is now common to use only a small amount of thick barium to coat the mucosa and then to distend the viscus with air. For the upper gastrointestinal tract, a gas-producing substance such as bicarbonate powder or crystals (in the old days a soda pop was used) is given to the patient to drink. For the lower tract, a small hand pump attached to the enema catheter inflates the colon. These procedures are known as *double-contrast studies*. The mucosa is well-coated with barium, and gas distends the lumen of the bowel. This is an excellent way of demonstrating discrete mucosal lesions such as small colonic polyps or early gastric carcinomas.

Many radiologists routinely use various forms of relaxants to decrease peristalsis, and either Buscopan or glucagon may be given intravenously just before the study begins. This will often allow better visualization of the mucosa of the stomach, duodenum, and small bowel because of the lack of peristalsis and the concomitant dilatation of the lumen of the bowel. (The patient is also instructed to eat or drink nothing after midnight of the previous day so that the stomach and small intestine are empty for the study.)

Barium Swallow (Esophagogram)

At least two views should be taken of the mouth and pharynx during the process of swallowing barium while the patient is in the upright position. PA and lateral views under fluoroscopic control are the usual projections. The column of barium should be observed as it travels the whole length of the esophagus until it goes through the gastroesophageal junction (Fig. 3–1). Note should be made of any holdups, strictures, constricting lesions, or diverticula. Then the patient should be placed flat; a number of alternative positions are available (for instance, prone oblique on the right side). As the patient swallows more barium, particular attention should be paid to the gastroesophageal junction for signs of reflux from the stomach into the esophagus or of a hiatus hernia. The esophageal motility should be observed; in the patient with one of the scleroderma-like syndromes, there is usually loss of normal esophageal peristalsis, and the barium is inclined to remain in the midesophagus when the patient is supine and there is no pull of gravity to help it down. Normally, there are two forms of peristalsis in the esophagus: *primary peristalsis*, the major forward force of contraction, and *secondary peristalsis*, the smaller waves. Tertiary contractions are abnormal, although they frequently occur in old age, in free gastroesophageal reflux, and in disorders of esophageal motility.

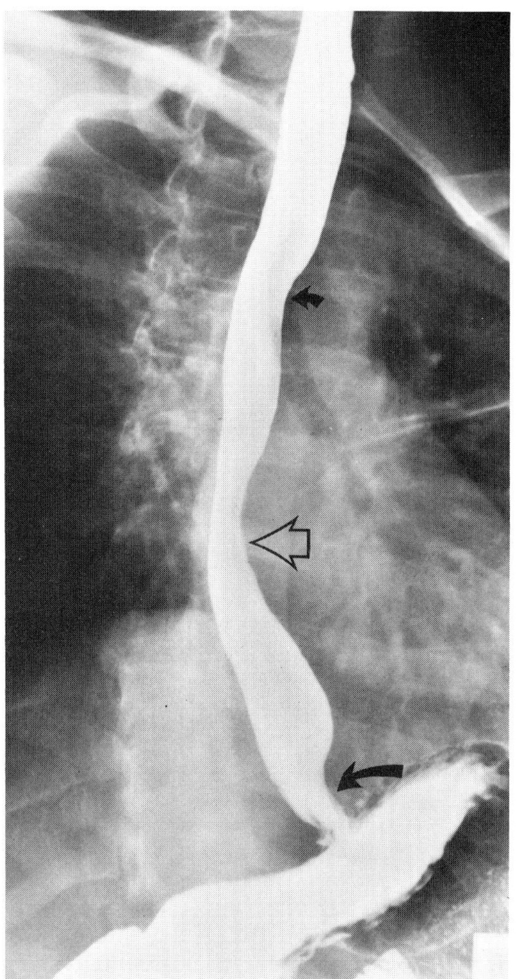

Figure 3–1. Normal esophagus, prone oblique RAO view. After the patient drinks barium while in the prone oblique position, the whole length of the esophagus can be seen. Note that there are three normal indentations on the barium-filled esophagus—the cricopharyngeus, the aortic arch *(small arrow)*, and the diaphragmatic hiatus *(large arrow)*. This 46-year-old man also has indentation caused by an enlarged left atrium *(hollow arrow)*.

Upper Gastrointestinal Series (UGI)

Although patients with digestive problems should have an esophagogram, greater attention should be paid to the stomach, duodenum, and proximal small intestine. The stomach should be adequately distended, either with barium alone (using 9 to 15 ounces of barium) or with a double-contrast technique. Radiographs of the stomach must reveal all its surfaces (Fig. 3–2). Usually, oblique supine views and erect views are taken, as well as radio-

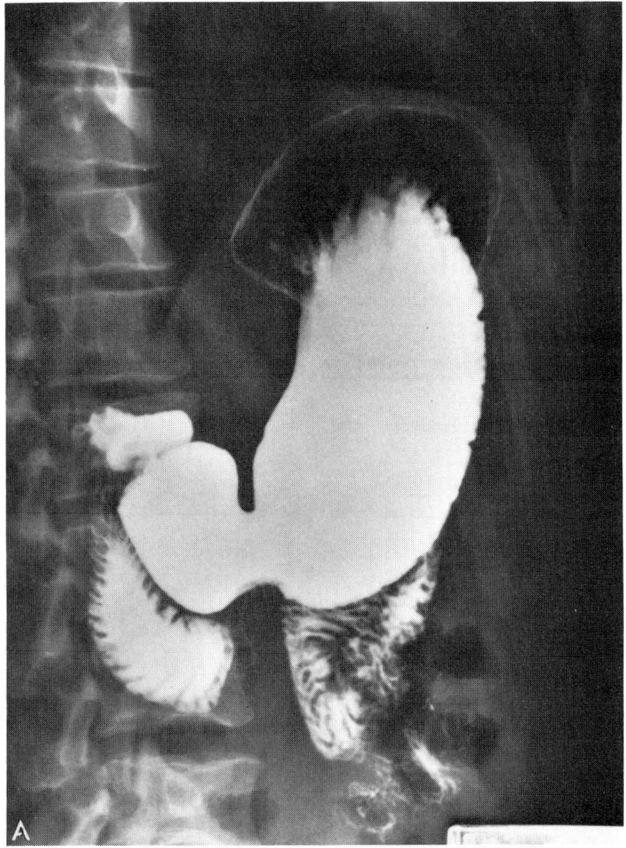

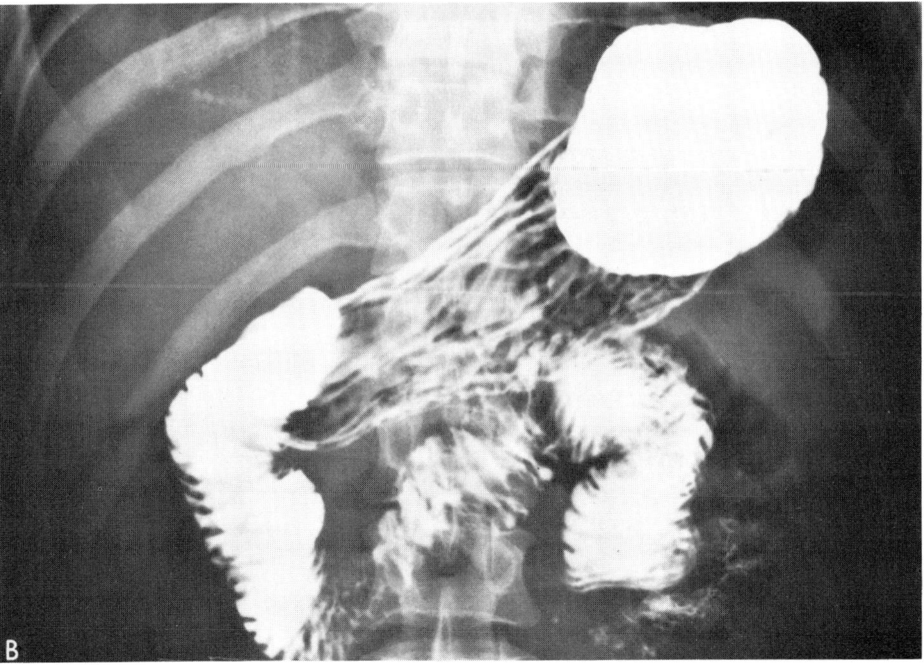

Figure 3–2. Normal stomach, an oblique view (*A*) and a supine view (*B*). Note the fundus distended with both gas and barium, the body of the stomach with the mucosal pattern (*B*), and the pylorus, duodenal cap, and duodenal sweep.

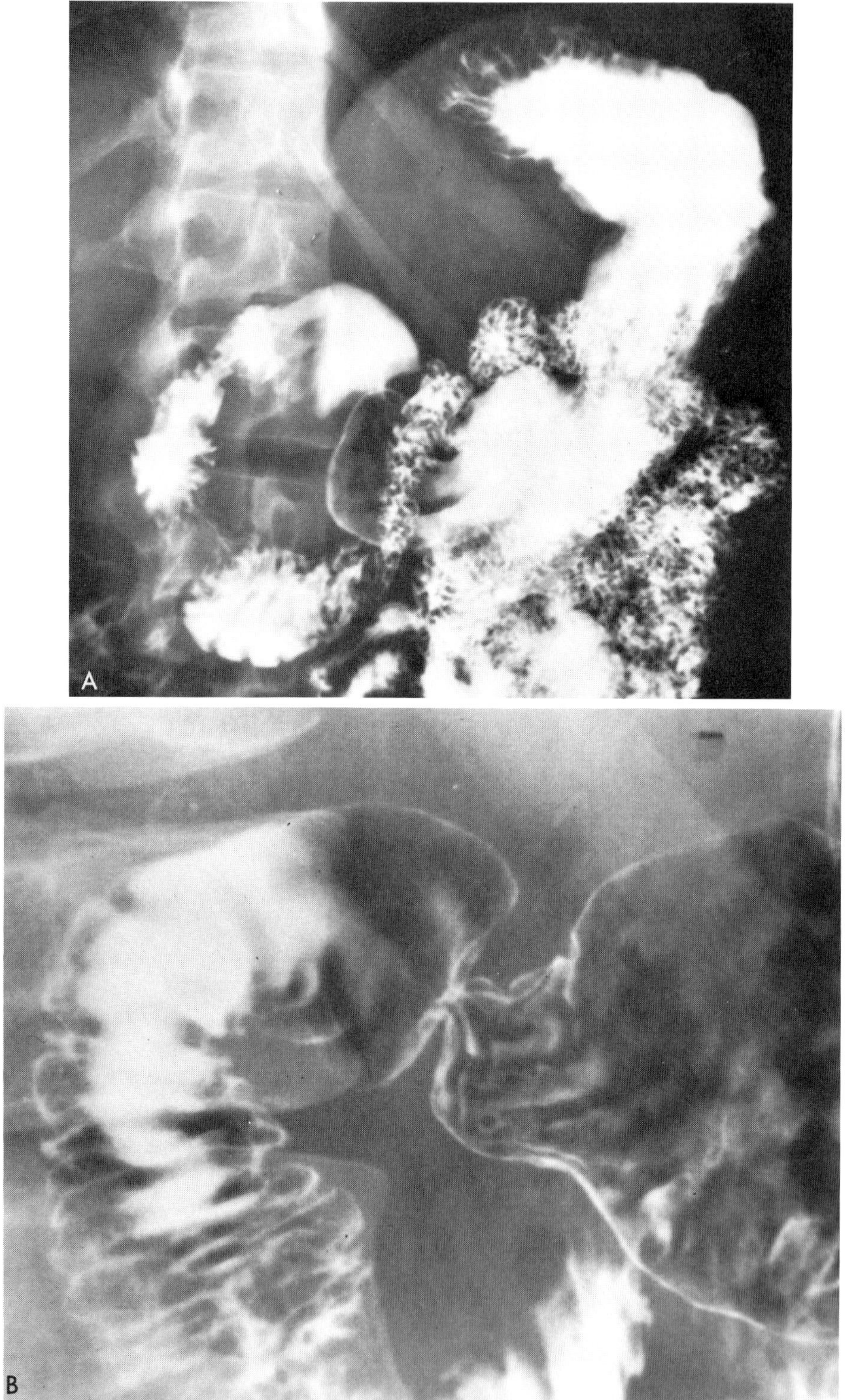

Figure 3–3. Normal duodenum. *A*, Barium-filled duodenum. *B*, Air-filled duodenal bulb.

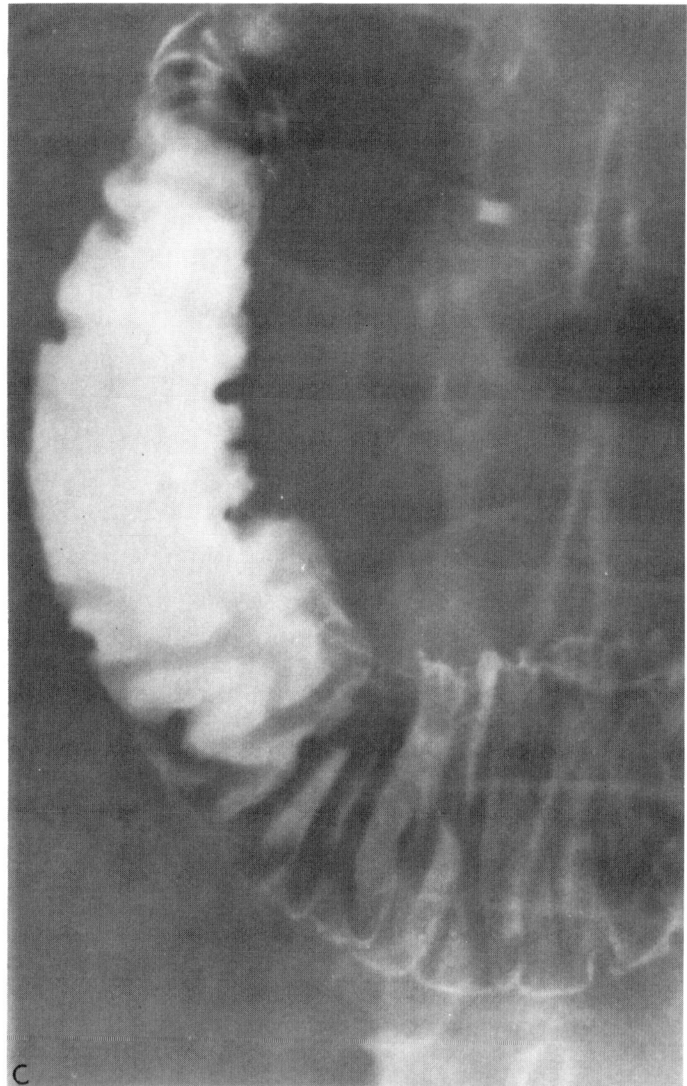

Figure 3–3. *Continued.* *C*, Hypotonic duodenogram. The conical shape of the duodenal bulb is well shown both barium-filled and with air relief. The duodenal sweep is best seen with hypotonic duodenography. Note the peristalsis and the normal filling of the small intestine on the barium-filled view.

graphs of the patient in the Trendelenburg position (head down), which causes the fundus of the stomach to be distended. If, however, a lesion behind the stomach is suspected, such as a carcinoma in the tail of the pancreas, a true lateral view of the stomach may also be useful. The duodenum is best shown barium-filled with the patient in the LPO position or air-filled with the patient in the supine RAO position (Fig. 3–3).

Small Bowel Follow-Through (SBFT)

A delayed film is often taken at the end of the upper gastrointestinal series to show the proximal loops of the jejunum. A formal small bowel follow-through is indicated in patients with unexplained diarrhea, abdominal cramps, malabsorption syndromes, or unexplained gastrointestinal bleeding. A routine upper gastrointestinal series is performed, and the patient is then

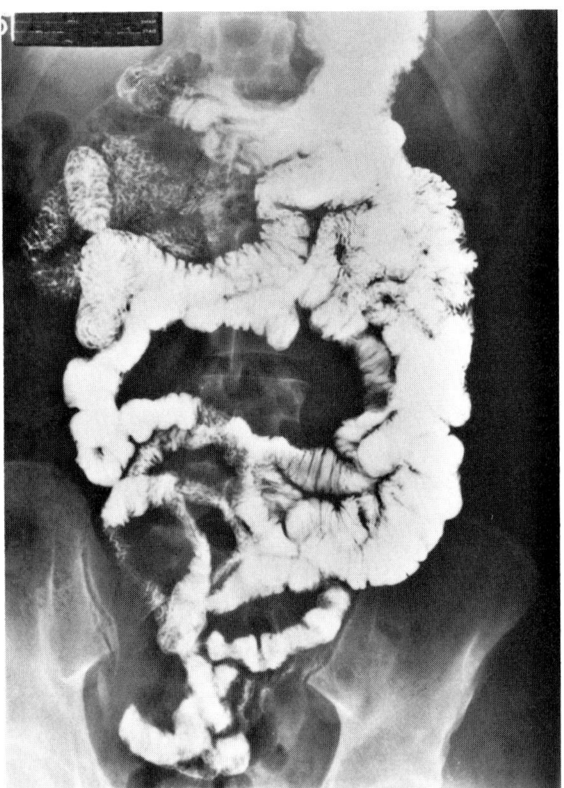

Figure 3–4. Normal small bowel follow through. Note the barium is filling both jejunum (which has a feathery mucosal pattern in the upper part of the picture) and the ileum (which has a more organized appearance and has obvious peristaltic waves). Some barium remains in the stomach.

given more barium (10 to 16 ounces), sometimes with Gastrografin added to speed up the transit time. (An iodine-containing contrast agent, Gastrografin is hypertonic and stimulates peristalsis.) Films of the whole abdomen, often with the patient prone so that the loops of bowel are spread apart, are taken at half-hour intervals or more frequently if clinically indicated (Fig. 3–4). If a mass or other abnormality becomes apparent or when the ileocecal region is identified, spot films with compression are indicated. The normal transit time from the mouth to the cecum varies from 45 minutes to 6 or 8 hours. If a specific malabsorption syndrome is suspected, the offending substance, such as lactose or gluten, may be added to the barium. A characteristic abnormal mucosal pattern can be visualized, and the transit time will be much shorter (in celiac disease, for example, there is often a slow transit time when barium is used alone).

Barium Enema

It is rarely possible to delineate the colon with a barium swallow study. Thus, it is necessary to perform a barium enema when one is looking for abnormalities of the large intestine. The double-contrast technique is preferred for the colon. The patient is instructed to have a light lunch the day preceding the examination and then to drink lots of fluids for the remainder of that day. Caster oil, mineral oil, or a laxative is given 15 to 18 hours before the examination, and the patient does not eat until after the barium enema has been completed.

The conscientious radiologist inserts the tube himself (preferably after having performed a rectal examination to exclude the possibility of local mass lesions), and the

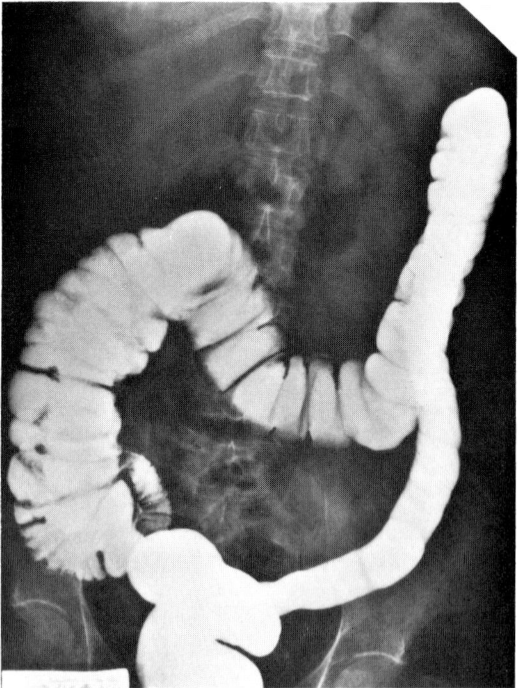

Figure 3–5. Normal barium enema. A single-contrast barium enema shows reflux of barium into the terminal ileum, as well as the cecum, entire colon, and rectum.

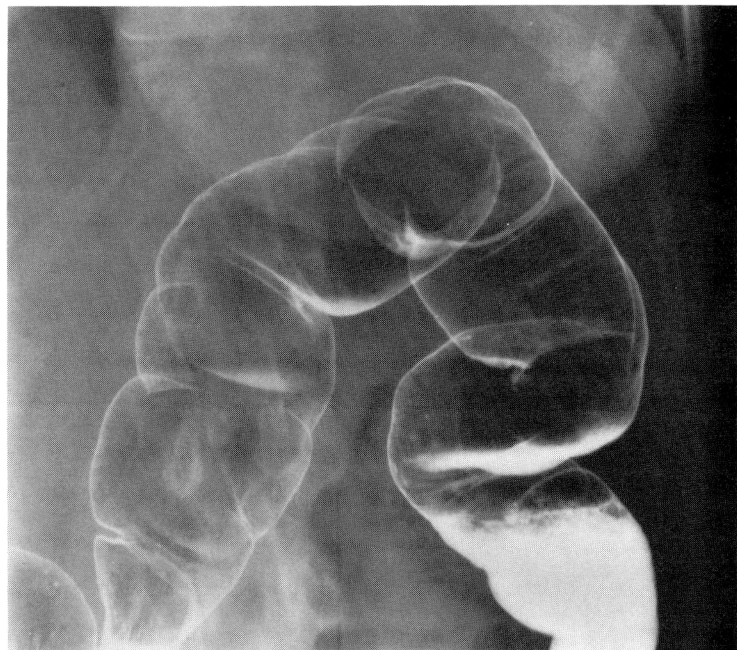

Figure 3–6. Normal splenic flexure. In this double-contrast, barium enema, note the excellent visualization of the mucosa.

barium slowly fills the colon from the rectum to the cecum. The radiologist should then make sure the cecum is adequately filled. Ideally the appendix should fill out or there should be slight reflux into the terminal ileum (Fig. 3–5). If a double-contrast technique is used, barium should be run up only to the splenic flexure, and air should be introduced, allowing gravity to pull the column of barium into the cecum as the air distends the lumen behind the barium. Many radiologists use relaxants (Buscopan or glucagon) to decrease colonic peristalsis and thus reduce the discomfort the patient may experience.

Radiographs of the following structures are usually sufficient:

1. Rectum (lateral and prone angled views).
2. Sigmoid (usually supine RAO).
3. Descending colon and splenic flexure (erect LAO, as in Figure 3–6, or prone RPO).
4. Transverse colon (straight KUB).
5. Ascending colon and hepatic flexure (erect RAO or prone LPO).
6. Ileocecal valve (compression views).

The patient is then allowed to evacuate the colon and a final film is taken to demonstrate the mucosal pattern clearly.

Hypotonic Duodenography

When single-contrast barium studies without relaxants were in common use, it was frequently impossible to visualize the duodenal sweep adequately. Hypotonic duodenography has been developed, in which the duodenum is paralyzed, so that peristalsis ceases in patients in whom lesions of the head of the pancreas (tumors or pancreatitis) are suspected. Paralysis is achieved locally by introducing a tube into the duodenum via the mouth and injecting local anesthetic directly into the duodenum before instilling barium or air to distend the duodenal sweep (see Figure 3–3C). An alternative method is to give an intravenous injection of Probanthine or Buscopan and then have the patient swallow the contrast agent. Hypotonic duodenography has largely fallen into disuse as a separate procedure because of the current widespread use of intravenous relaxants and of double-contrast upper-gastrointestinal techniques.

IODINATED CONTRAST AGENTS

The first attempts to introduce positive contrast agents other than barium were

TABLE 3–1. Frequently Used Contrast Agents

TRADE NAME	GENERIC NAME
Diatrizoate Group	
Renografin (Squibb, U.S.A.)	Diatrizoate meglumine and diatrizoate sodium
60	60% solution
76	76% solution
Reno-M (Squibb, U.S.A.)	Diatrizoate meglumine
30	30% solution
60	60% solution
Renovist (Squibb, U.S.A.)	Diatrizoate sodium and diatrizoate meglumine injection
Hypaque Sodium 50% (Winthrop, U.S.A./G.B.)	Diatrizoate sodium, 50% solution
Hypaque Meglumine 60% (Winthrop, U.S.A./G.B.)	Diatrizoate methylglucamine, 60% solution
Hypaque-M (Winthrop, U.S.A./G.B.)	Diatrizoate methylglucamine and diatrizoate sodium
75	75% solution
90	90% solution
Urografin (Schering, G.B.)	Diatrizoate meglumine and diatrizoate sodium, available in 30%, 60%, and 76% solutions
Iothalamate Group	
Conray (Mallinckrodt, U.S.A./May & Baker, G.B.)	Iothalamate meglumine, 60% solution
Conray-30 (Mallinckrodt, U.S.A./May & Baker, G.B.)	Iothalamate meglumine, 30% solution
Conray 400 (Mallinckrodt, U.S.A./May & Baker, G.B.)	Iothalamate sodium, 66.8% solution
Angio-Conray (Mallinckrodt, U.S.A.)	Iothalamate sodium, 80% solution

made in 1905 using colloidal suspensions of heavy metals, but it was not until 1930 that the first relatively safe water-soluble iodinated contrast agent was introduced. When it was discovered that this substance was excreted by the kidneys, intravenous pyelography was born. Initially, small volumes of contrast agent were used (10 to 20 ml) but dosages have increased so that at present, 1 ml per kg is used. Most contrast agents contain either the sodium salt or the meglumine salt of the iodinated compound (Table 3–1). Water-soluble iodinated contrast agents are, of course, used for clinical procedures other than urography, such as general and neuroradiological angiography.

TABLE 3–2. Adverse Reactions to Intravenous Contrast Agents

Minor Reactions	
Flushing and a feeling of warmth	Arm pain
Nausea	Facial edema
Vomiting	Headache
Lightheadedness	Sweating
Itching	Dizziness
Swelling of salivary glands	Urticaria
	Chills
Moderate Reactions	
Hypotension	Bronchospasm
Refractory skin rash, urticaria, or edema	
Major Reactions	
Severe hypotension	Cardiac arrest
Loss of consciousness	Shock
Pulmonary edema	Convulsions
Laryngeal edema	Oliguria or anuria
Cardiac arrhythmias	Bronchospasm

There is one danger in using contrast agents containing iodine: some patients are allergic to iodine. Although minor side-effects are quite common following intravenous injections of iodinated contrast agents, major side-effects are fortunately rare (Table 3–2).

Intravenous Pyelography (IVP)

In the standard intravenous pyelogram, an iodinated contrast agent is injected intravenously and is followed radiographically through the urinary tract until it leaves the body. The actual sequence of films will vary according to the radiologist's preference and the radiology department's practice as well as the patient's clinical situation. The indications for intravenous pyelography include: hematuria, flank pain or mass, alterations in the pattern of urination (particularly in older patients with possible benign prostatic hypertrophy or cystoceles), passing of stones or gravel, and hypertension. An IVP may also be performed as part of the search for the primary site of a malignancy.

The patient is instructed not to eat after 6 P.M. the evening preceding the procedure, although fluids are not restricted. A mild laxative is usually given the night before to cleanse the bowel as much as possible. Initially, "scout" films are taken, which may be a single KUB (Fig. 3–7), inspiration and expiration views of the renal areas, or a KUB with oblique views of the kidneys. The contrast is injected either as a bolus or as an intravenous infusion; the choice of method appears to make little difference to visualization of the urinary tract.

Films of the renal areas are taken at intervals, initially in a predetermined sequence which is routinely performed, for example, one, three, and five minutes; one, two, three, four, and five minutes; or one and five minutes. The one-minute film, which may be combined with tomographic examination, provides a view of the intense filling of the renal parenchyma and is known as the *nephrogram phase* (Fig. 3–8). The three-minute (Fig. 3–9) and five-minute films should show filling of the calyces, and the five-minute film may be followed by oblique views (Fig. 3–10).

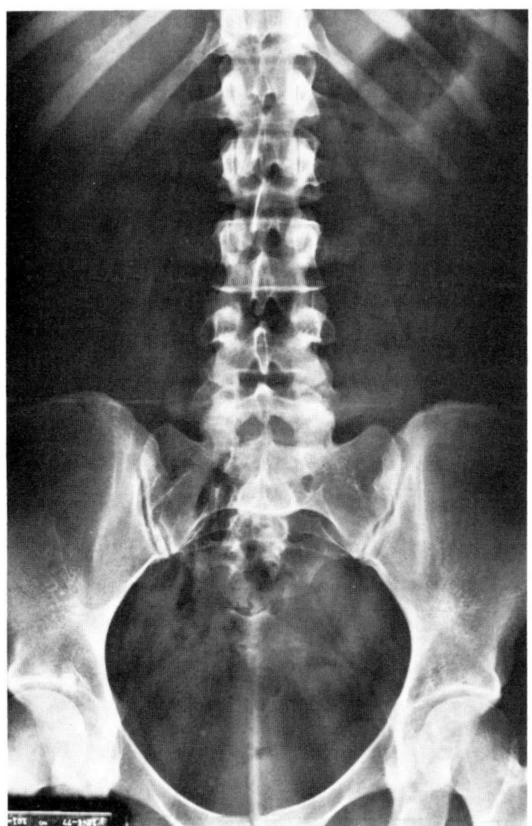

Figure 3–7. Normal scout film (KUB) for an IVP.

Frequently, a KUB with or without oblique views of the renal areas is then taken, and some form of compression of the ureters is used to demonstrate the whole upper urinary tract. The compression may be natural, by having the patient lie prone, or, more usually, induced, by applying a compression band consisting of a tight belt with two rubber balloons which compress the ureters at the pelvic brim. After three to six minutes of compression, the band is removed and a radiograph is taken immediately which should demonstrate the whole urinary tract from the calyces to the bladder (Fig. 3–11). If everything has been visualized, the patient is requested to empty his bladder, and a postvoid film of the bladder is taken to evaluate residual urine and inspect the bladder mucosa.

This progression of films may be altered, increased, or curtailed, depending on the clinical circumstances. For example, in a patient with a stone obstructing a ureter, delayed films are necessary to demonstrate the exact level of obstruction. If the patient has benign prostatic hypertrophy or bladder problems, the bladder is allowed to fill more so that its base can be visualized. For young female patients with acute pyelonephritis, only a few films of the renal areas are needed. Few early films are required for patients with severe renal failure, but films as late as 12 to 24 hours after injection are frequently needed.

Should the renal outlines, renal parenchyma, or calyceal pattern be poorly seen, tomographic examination is mandatory; in fact, many departments use tomography routinely as part of the intravenous pyelographic procedure (Fig. 3–12). If tomography is going to be used, however, an initial scout tomogram is useful, as much to locate the level of the kidneys as for any diagnostic purpose. Tomograms are then per-

Text continued on page 55

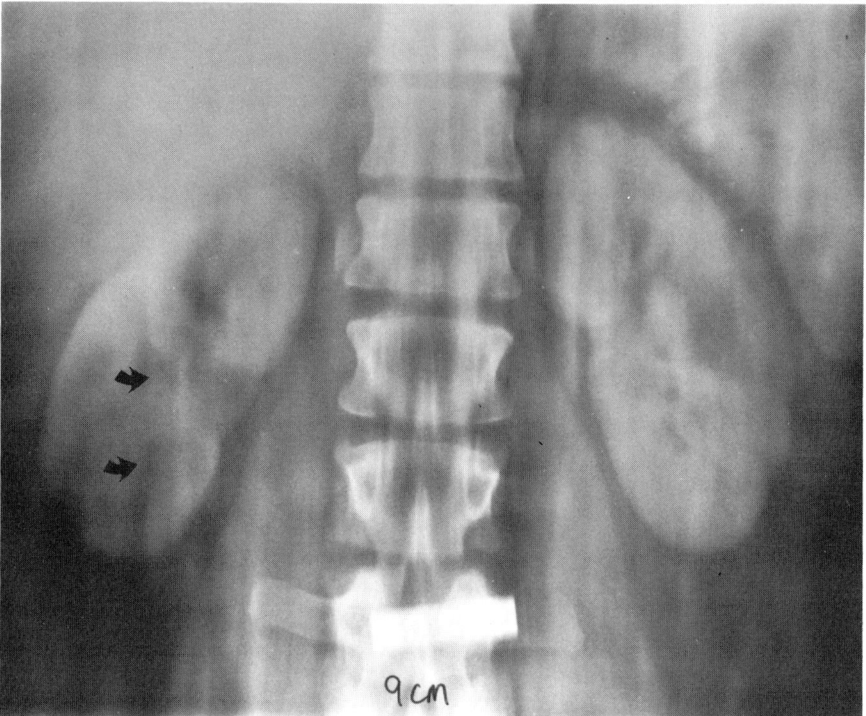

Figure 3–8. Nephrogram phase, one-minute tomogram. Note the opacification of the renal parenchyma and early filling of the centrally lying calyces with the perirenal fat in between (*arrows*).

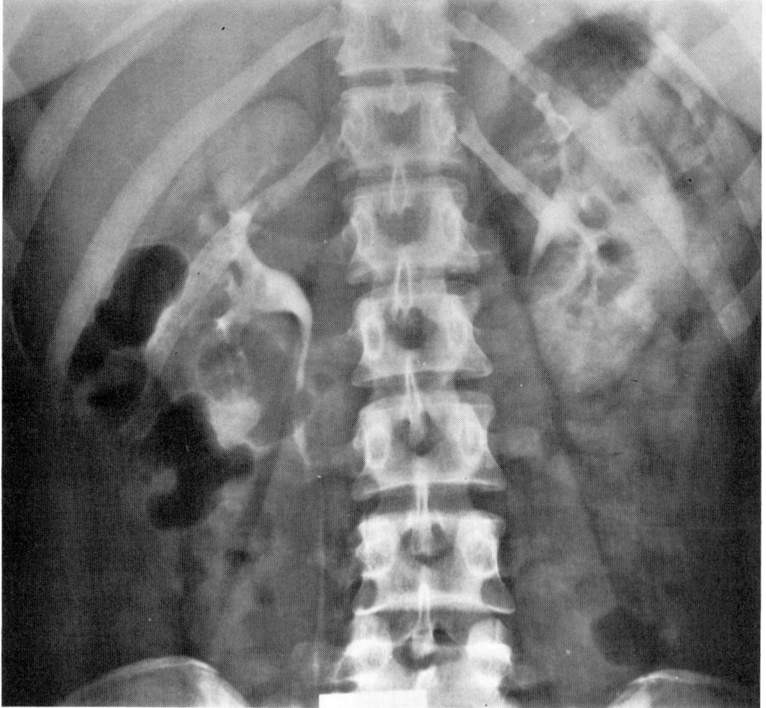

Figure 3–9. Normal three-minute IVP film. The calyces and renal pelvis are filled, and the right ureter is opacified.

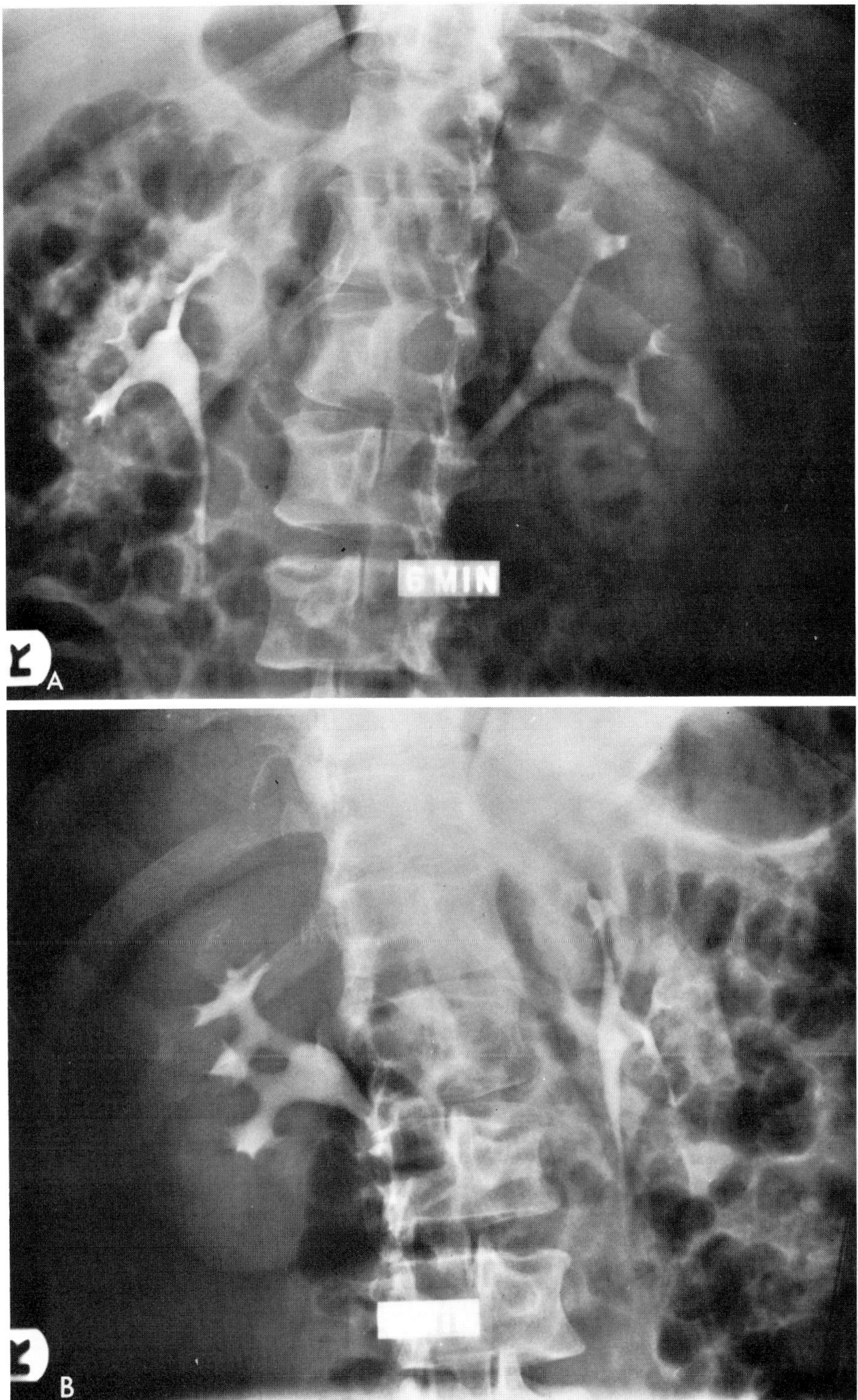

Figure 3–10. Normal six-minute IVP films, left anterior oblique view (*A*) and right anterior oblique view (*B*). These views are used to better delineate the calyces and renal pelvis because the bowel gas is shifted from in front of the kidneys.

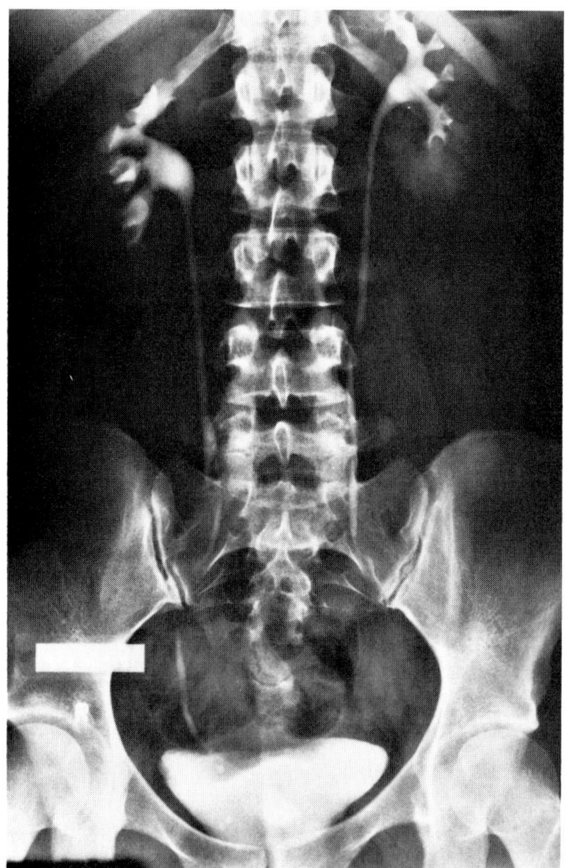

Figure 3–11. Normal postcompression 15-minute IVP film. This shows the whole of the renal tract, including the full length of both ureters.

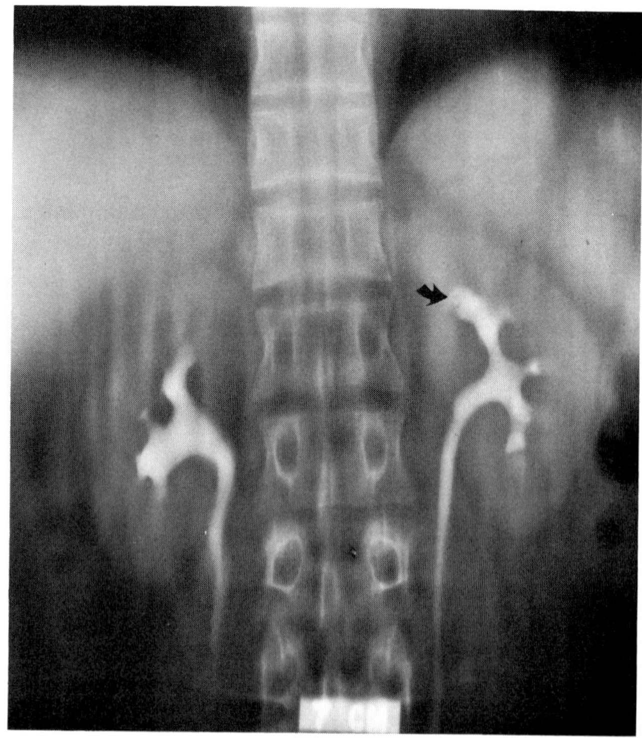

Figure 3–12. Tomography of the kidneys. This 38-year-old man presented with sterile pyuria. An IVP showed an irregularity of the left upper pole papilla, which was confirmed on tomography (*arrow*); the cause proved to be tuberculosis.

formed wherever clinically required, usually at one minute and ten minutes, to visualize the renal parenchyma, renal outline, and calyces on one film.

Basically, the IVP should be tailored for each patient, with the judicious use of oblique and prone films, compression bands, and tomography as required.

Certain other special techniques are available and can be performed in addition to a standard IVP.

1. If the bolus of contrast is injected rapidly, visualization of all the abdominal organs, including the liver, spleen, and abdominal aorta, may be achieved (a "bodygram"), particularly in infants and thin adults.

2. Oblique films of the vesicoureteric junction should be done, particularly in patients with suspected calculi.

3. Fluoroscopic examination of the ureters provides an opportunity to observe peristalsis.

4. Lateral films of the abdomen will demonstrate anterior displacement of the ureters (or even kidneys) in retroperitoneal tumors and lymphoma, for example (Fig. 3–13).

5. Special views (often oblique views and tomograms) are needed to show a transplanted kidney sitting in the pelvis.

6. Delayed films may be performed to show the exact site of ureteric obstruction from a stone or pelvic tumor. This is best achieved by having the patient stand, because the contrast agent is heavier than urine.

7. Fluoroscopy or radiographs taken while the patient is voiding may serve as a "poor man's" vesicourethrogram; usually, however, the concentration of contrast is so poor that the urethra is not adequately visualized.

It is of interest that the iodinated contrast agents are excreted by the liver and the intestinal wall in total or partial

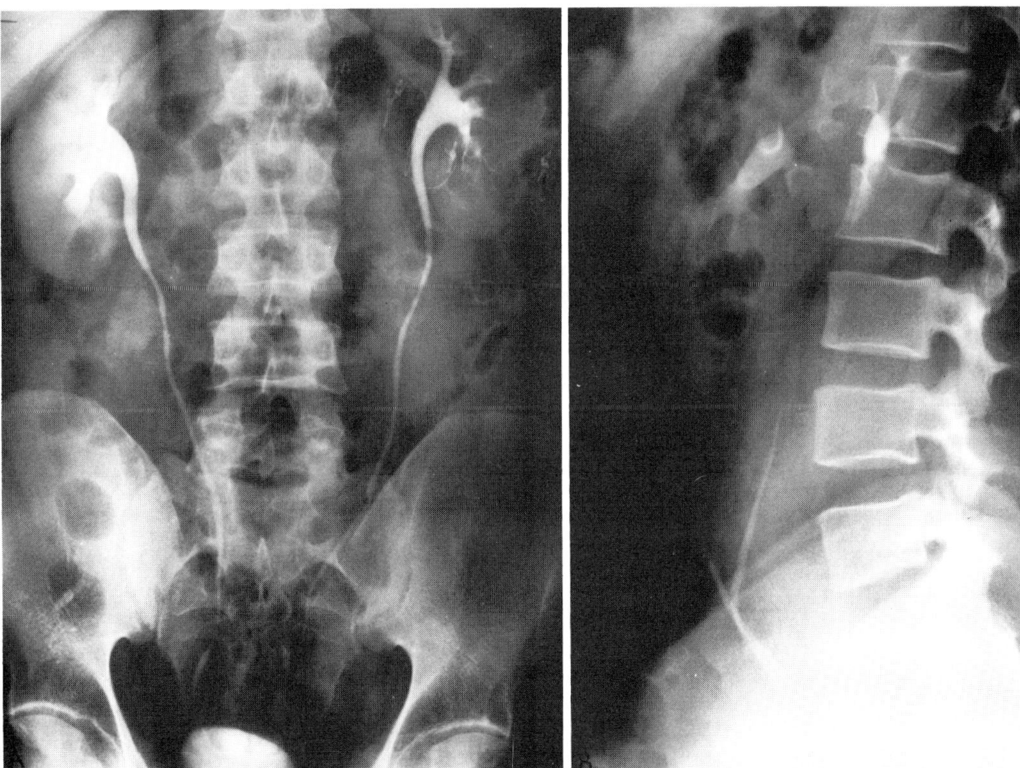

Figure 3–13. Retroperitoneal lymphoma, AP (*A*) and lateral (*B*) IVP films. These views show lateral displacement and irregular course of both ureters as well as distortion of the bladder in this 28-year-old man with lymphoma. The lateral view shows marked anterior displacement of both ureters away from their normal course, which is adjacent to the anterior aspect of the lumbar vertebral bodies.

renal failure. This is a very slow process, however, and should not be chosen as a method of removing the contrast agent in a severely debilitated patient with renal failure.

Special Urological Procedures Using Iodinated Contrast Agents

Retrograde Pyelography

It is often necessary to achieve better visualization of the ureters and the renal collecting system than intravenous pyelography can provide. Positioning a catheter in a ureter (or one in each ureter) allows a retrograde pyelogram to be performed (Fig. 3–14). Although the original retrogrades were performed prior to 1920 using barium, iodinated contrast agents are now used, and 6 to 8 ml are injected into each side. A word of warning: During retrograde pyelography, about 5 per cent of the contrast agent is absorbed parenterally; thus, this is *not* a suitable alternative to IVP for a patient with a known severe allergy to contrast media.

The indications for retrograde pyelography are many, although the high doses of contrast agent now used during routine intravenous pyelography have made adequate visualization of the lower urinary tract possible in the vast majority of patients. Retrograde pyelography is still useful in investigating and documenting a mass in the renal pelvis, in evaluating the extent of damage caused by papillary necrosis, and in observing the distortion and deviation of the ureters and looking for areas of narrowing or direct involvement in patients with retroperitoneal fibrosis or retroperitoneal tumors. For patients with renal failure, it is necessary to catheterize only one side to determine whether the underlying cause is obstruction, chronic pyelonephritis, chronic glomerulonephritis, or polycystic kidneys.

One other indication for retrograde pyelography is non-visualization on an IVP of one kidney and its ureter. The urologist often performs cystoscopy and cannulation of the "missing" ureter and injects contrast agent under fluoroscopic guidance. This may reveal renal ectopia (frequently, the kidney overlies the sacrum and is there-

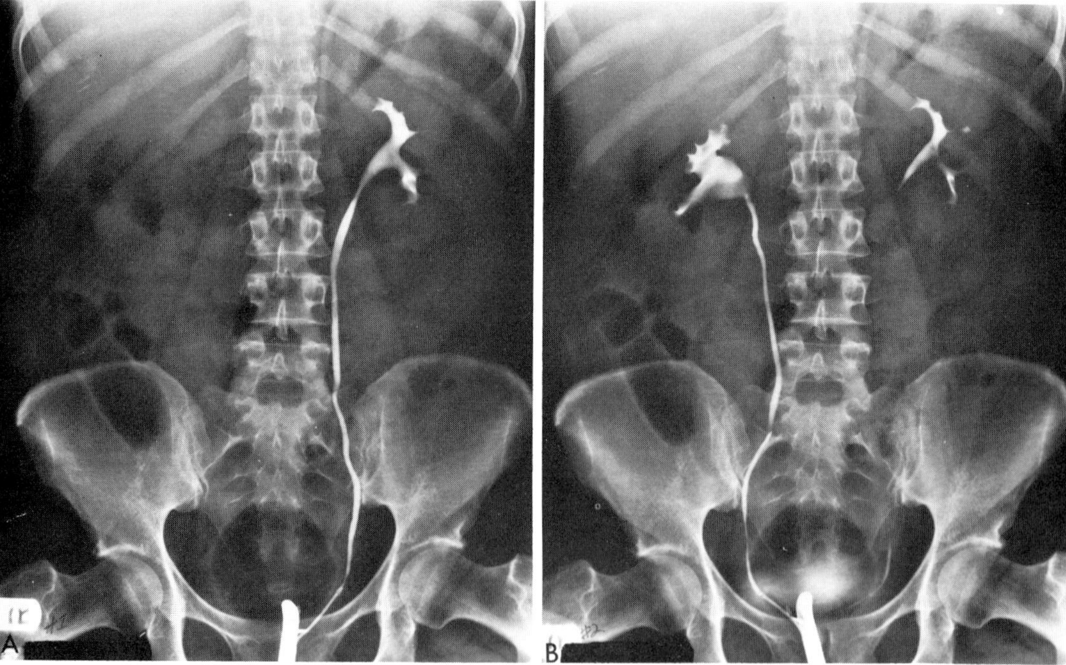

Figure 3–14. Retrograde pyelography, left ureter (*A*) and right ureter (*B*). After hysterectomy, this 44-year-old woman was having intermittent hematuria. An IVP was normal, as was a retrograde pyelogram. The "hematuria" was actually a bloody vaginal discharge.

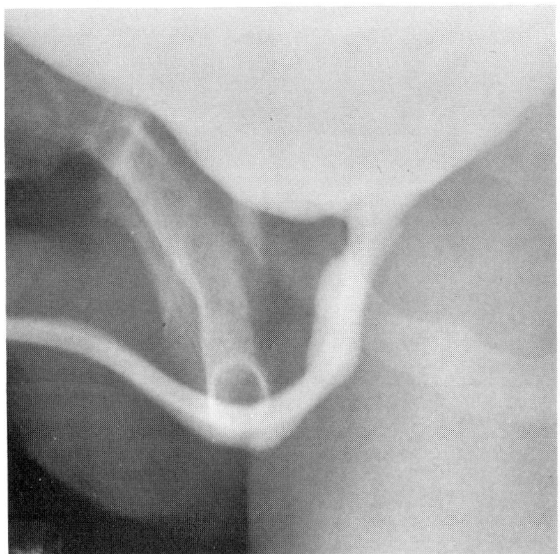

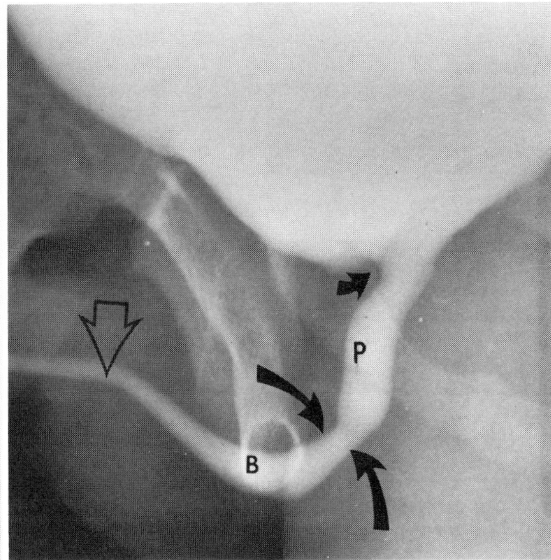

Figure 3–15. Normal VCUG. The base of the bladder and the urethra are well seen. The urethra is divided into the internal sphincter (*small arrow*), the prostatic urethra (*P*), the external sphincter or membranous urethra (*large arrows*), the bulbous urethra (*B*), and the penile urethra (*hollow arrow*).

fore difficult to see on the IVP) or renal atrophy.

Cystography, Urethrography, and Voiding Cystourethrography (VCUG)

Three procedures may be used to demonstrate the lower urinary tract: cystography, urethrography, and voiding cystourethrography. The cystogram is performed by catheterizing the patient and filling the bladder with iodinated contrast material warmed to body temperature. The resulting film allows the radiologist to examine the bladder wall (for thickness, trabeculae, diverticula, or masses), to evaluate prostate size and the prostatic bed following a subtotal prostatectomy, and to check for the presence and extent of vesicoureteric reflux.

In a VCUG, the patient is asked to void and spot films are then taken (Fig. 3–15). Should the patient manage to void successfully under fluoroscopic observation, radiographs are best taken with male patients standing in a 45° LAO position and with female patients lying or sitting on the fluoroscopy table. A VCUG will demonstrate the urethra and any defects, strictures, or other abnormalities. In men, the area of the prostate and the degree of narrowing of the prostatic urethra may be assessed. Residual urine may be measured; this should be negligible in women and under 20 ml in men.

An alternative method for a male patient employs an instrument that clamps onto the end of the penis, blocking the external urethral orifice but allowing direct filling via a catheter. This technique gives excellent visualization of the urethra and is useful for patients who are impossible to catheterize because of posttraumatic or postinfective strictures or who have severe benign prostatic hypertrophy.

Other Special Genitourinary Procedures Using Iodinated Contrast Agents

Loopogram. If the bladder has been removed and an ileal loop has been constructed in its place, a retrograde study of this loop (a *loopogram*) will allow visualization of reflux into the ureters and evaluation of any obstruction or other abnormality.

Nephrostogram. Direct studies of the renal pelvis may be performed if the patient has a nephrostomy tube in place. The nephrostomy is usually used to decompress the renal pelvis in cases of severe lower ureteric obstruction from a pelvic tumor or calculi. Most of these patients have severe hydronephrosis. In a *nephrostogram*, contrast is instilled through the tube; the resulting film can demonstrate the degree of ureteral obstruction.

SINOGRAM AND FISTULOGRAM. In patients who have draining wounds, contrast agent can be injected under fluoroscopic guidance into the sinus tract to determine the extent of the underlying abscess cavity and to demonstrate communication between the tract and bowel loops. A fistulogram is performed by catheterizing the viscus with the highest intrinsic pressure. For example, the bladder would be catheterized in patients with suspected fistulae between the bladder and the vagina or uterus (often caused by cancer).

SEMINAL VESICULOGRAM. There are two methods of performing a seminal vesiculogram: direct injection into the vas deferens in the scrotum and cannulation of the prostatic utricle. With the injection of the contrast agent, the seminal vesicles and vasa may be seen (originally oily media was used, but water-soluble agents are used now). The seminal vesiculogram, which is rarely performed today, is indicated in patients with tumors, congenital anomalies, or chronic infections (particularly tuberculosis and venereal disease).

HYSTEROSALPINGOGRAM. It is frequently important to investigate the female genital tract; injection of a contrast agent into the cervix to opacify the uterus and fallopian tubes for fluoroscopic examination is known as *hysterosalpingography* (Fig. 3–16). Oily contrast agents cause less peritoneal irritation and produce better radiographs but are not absorbed, whereas the water-soluble agents are absorbed but cause slightly more pain. The primary indication for this procedure is assessing the patency of the fallopian tubes of an apparently infertile patient. Retrograde injection of the contrast agent into the uterus fills the normal fallopian tubes. Contrast should spill from the fimbria into the peritoneal cavity. Blockage of one or both of the tubes (often caused by infection) is evidenced by the lack of free spillage, and the level of obstruction is usually well seen. A second indication for hysterosalpingography is suspicion of a tumor, either in the uterus or cervix (benign fibroids or malignant carcinomas) or in the soft tis-

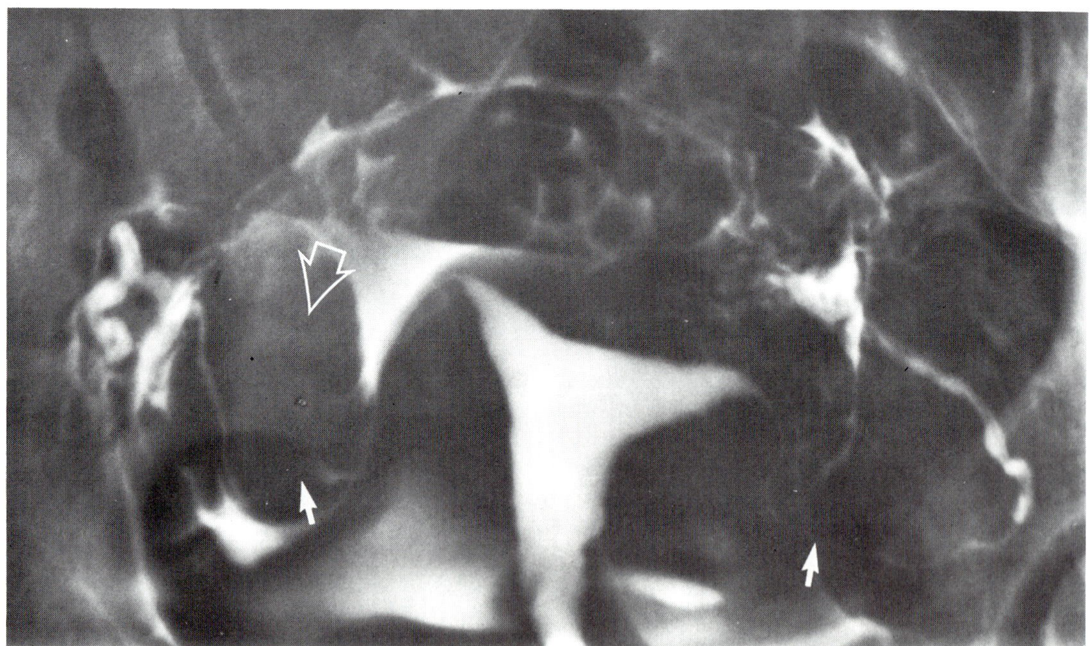

Figure 3–16. Normal hysterosalpingogram. The tip of the catheter is in the cervix, and there is good filling of the normal triangular uterus. Both fallopian tubes are filled (*small arrows*), and there is free bilateral spillage of contrast into the peritoneal cavity, which on the right appears to outline an enlarged ovary (*hollow arrow*).

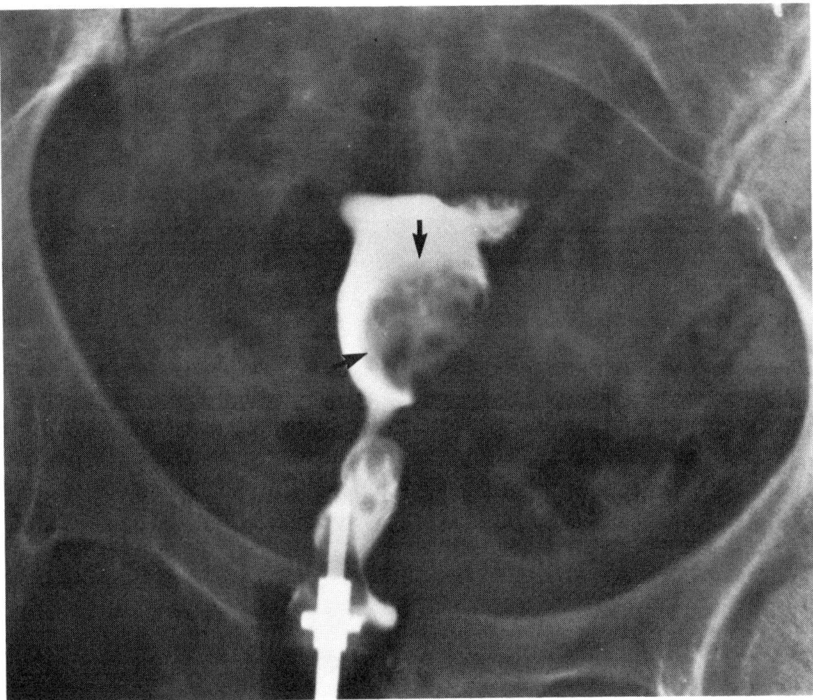

Figure 3–17. Abnormal hysterosalpingogram with mass. A large polypoid mass is seen in the lower portion of the uterus (*arrows*), and there is no filling of the tubes. At biopsy the mass was found to be endometrial carcinoma.

sues of the pelvis. Most female patients who present with unexplained bleeding or a pelvic mass will undergo hysterosalpingography (Fig. 3–17).

Other Procedures Using Iodinated Contrast

The study of the gallbladder and biliary tree was facilitated by the discovery that labelling bile salts or bile acids with iodine makes observation of the excretion by the liver of these substances possible. The first cholecystograms were performed in the 1930s; since then, both the oral and the intravenous methods of opacification of the biliary tract have become more sophisticated (Table 3–3).

The indications for a contrast study of the biliary tract include right upper quadrant pain, clinically suspected gallstones, pyrexia of unknown origin (PUO), and jaundice. The jaundice, however, must not be too severe, or a total failure of opacification will occur. Usually, a bilirubin level of more than 1.5 mg per 100 ml precludes oral cholecystography, and a level of more than 4 mg per 100 ml precludes intravenous cholangiography, even with the use of tomography and delayed films (normal bilirubin level is 0.3 to 1.1 mg per 100

TABLE 3–3. Commonly Used Oral Cholecystographic Contrast Agents

AGENT	TRADE NAME	PERCENTAGE OF ORGANICALLY BOUND IODINE	PREPARATION AND FORM
Iopanoic acid	Telepaque (Winthrop)	66.7	0.5 g tablet
Ipodate calcium	Oragrafin Calcium (Squibb)	61.7	3.0 g granules
Ipodate sodium	Oragrafin Sodium (Squibb)	61.4	0.5 g capsule
Sodium tyropanoate	Bilopaque Sodium (Winthrop)	57.4	0.75 g tablet
Iocetamic acid	Cholebrine (Mallinckrodt)	62.0	3.0 g tablets

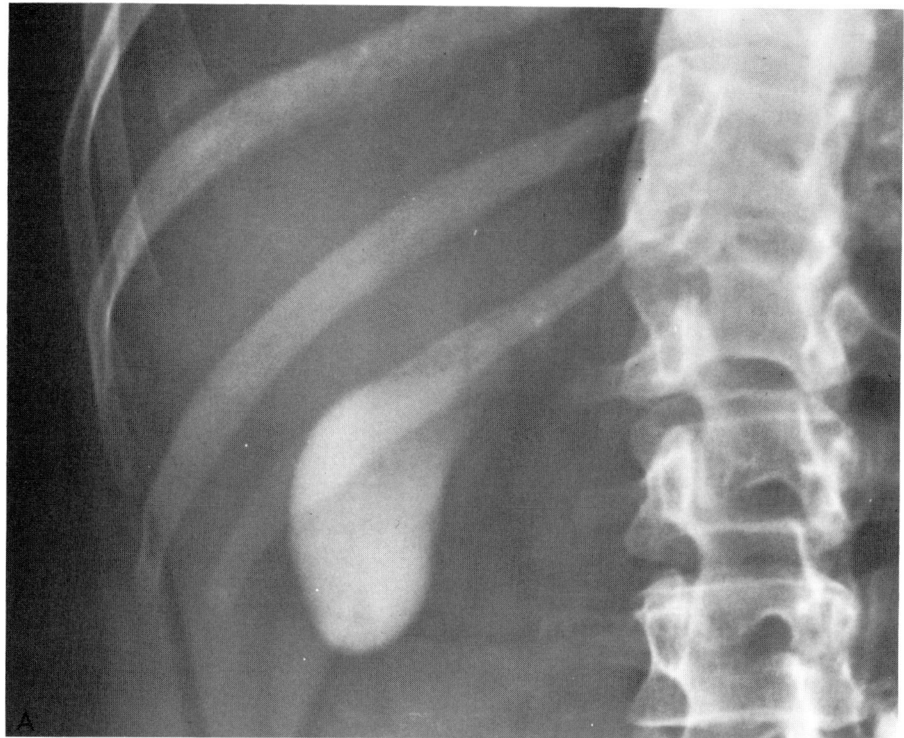

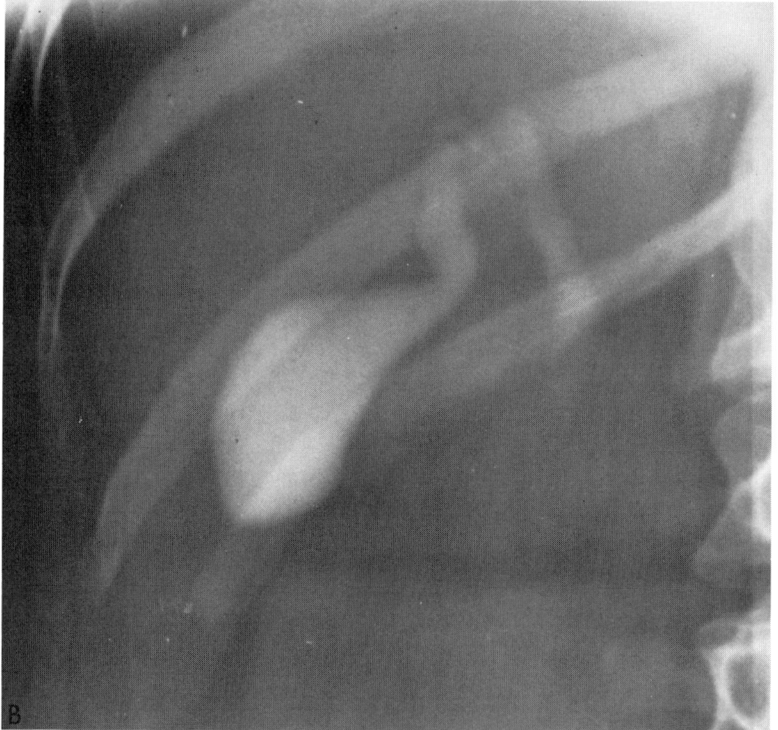

Figure 3–18. Normal oral cholecystogram. *A*, Right upper quadrant coned-down view. *B*, An early film following a fatty meal demonstrates contraction of the gallbladder and visualization of the cystic duct and common bile duct.

ml). As in all studies involving iodinated contrast agents, there is a risk of side-effects; in fact, the majority of patients undergoing intravenous cholangiography will experience nausea, and vomiting is quite common. Particular care must be taken for people with known allergies.

Oral Cholecystogram (OCG)

It is important that a plain film of the abdomen be taken before any contrast study, including oral cholecystography. Most patients, however, will have had a KUB or other preliminary film prior to an IVP or UGI; if not, a KUB, often in conjunction with a coned-down view of the right upper quadrant, should be taken. The oral cholecystogram is frequently combined with other procedures, particularly an upper gastrointestinal series, since the two contrast studies do not usually interfere with each other.

The patient is given iodinated contrast agent in tablet form to be taken the night before the OCG and is instructed to remain on a fat-free diet. This procedure should cause a normal gallbladder to become opaque the following day. A KUB and a coned-down right upper quadrant radiograph are usually taken initially (Fig. 3–18). If necessary, a number of spot films of the gallbladder region are also taken, with fluoroscopic treatment to separate the biliary tract from overlying bowel gas shadows and the rib cage. If a fluoroscope is not available, a right lateral decubitus view will usually achieve the same result.

The oral cholecystogram will demonstrate gallstones (Fig. 3–19), although sometimes it is necessary to stand the patient up to allow very small gallstones to "layer out" by finding their own level of buoyancy (Fig. 3–20). Congenital abnormalities such as duplication of the gallbladder or a phrygian cap may be demonstrated. Chronic inflammation of the gallbladder (cholecystitis) is associated with smallness and scarring, often with stones and with gallbladder nonvisualization. Tumors of the gallbladder can also be demonstrated, particularly benign adenomyosis, which is probably related to chronic inflammation. Carcinoma of the gallbladder usually leads to nonfunction of the organ and hence cannot be demonstrated on oral cholecystography.

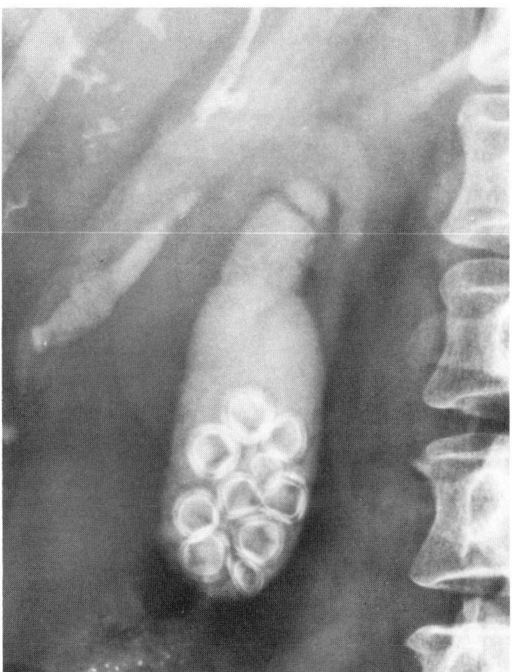

Figure 3–19. Oral cholecystogram. Multiple facetted opaque gallstones are present in a well-opacified gallbladder.

Non-visualization of the gallbladder on the first oral cholecystogram may occur for any number of reasons, and the patient should be given a second dose of tablets and the radiographic procedure should be repeated on the following day. (This is known as a *second-day* or *double-dose procedure*.) Third and subsequent doses are of no additional value; if the gallbladder cannot be visualized on the second-day radiograph, an intravenous cholangiogram is indicated for the vast majority of patients. If the patient is considered an unlikely candidate for gallbladder disease (in which case the study should probably not have been done in the first place), a second oral cholecystogram can be performed two to four weeks later. If the patient has indeed taken the tablets and if the tablets have been absorbed properly (i.e., no contrast agent remains in the stomach or colon), non-visualization implies gallbladder disease. Non-visualization of the gallbladder following two doses

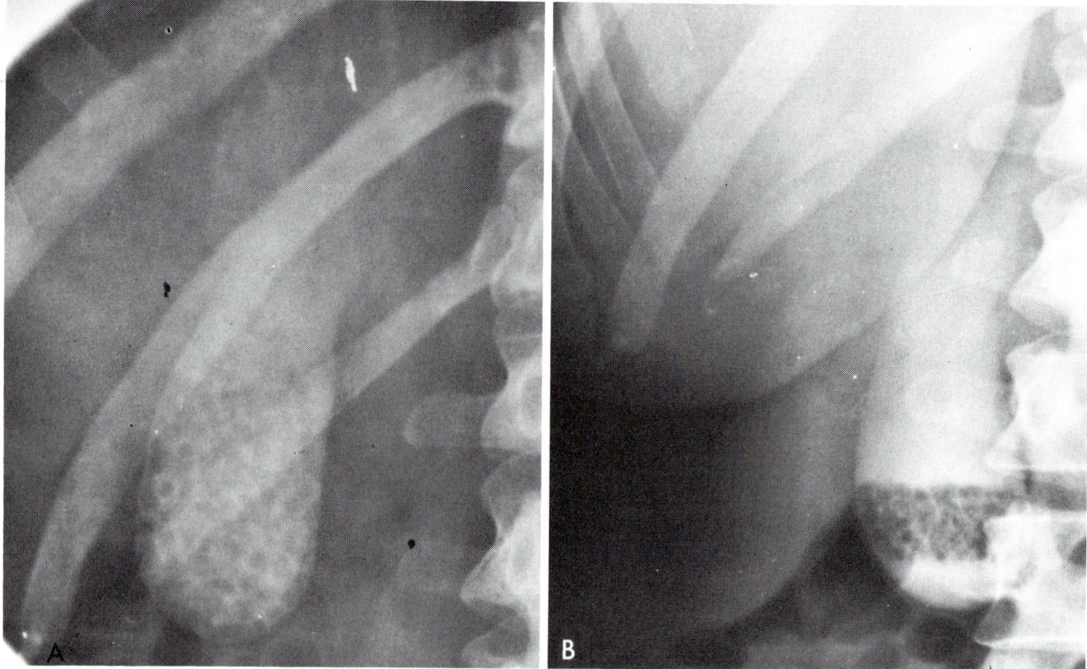

Figure 3–20. Oral cholecystogram, supine view (*A*) and erect view (*B*). Multiple tiny radiolucent stones have layered out in the opacified gallbladder.

of tablets is an absolute indication for an intravenous study in patients in whom biliary tract disease is suspected.

One final comment concerns the use of fatty meals. In some radiology departments, the oral study includes giving the patient a fatty meal. A film is taken 20 to 30 minutes later, and a normal gallbladder should contract considerably. Failure to contract implies failure of gallbladder function and infiltration of the wall by either fibrosis or tumor. Ingestion of a fatty meal should also cause the bile to become concentrated, making small stones easier to see and accentuating any signs of adenomyosis. The main indication for the use of a fatty meal, however, is that after contraction of the gallbladder, it is often possible to visualize the common bile duct (Fig. 3–18B).

Intravenous Cholangiogram (IVC)

Intravenous study of the biliary tract is usually indicated for the patient whose gallbladder was not visualized on oral cholecystography, the patient with increasing jaundice, the patient who has had a cholecystectomy, and the patient whose common bile duct is of clinical interest rather than the gallbladder itself (for instance, if carcinoma of the head of the pancreas is suspected). A scout film is essential; a KUB or a coned-down view of the right upper quadrant *plus* a scout tomogram should always precede the injection of a contrast agent for an IVC. Slow injection of 20 to 40 ml of Cholegrafin should enable the common bile duct and biliary tree to be visualized in most normal people within 20 to 30 minutes (Fig. 3–21). Tomography is mandatory.

A plain film of the right upper quadrant is taken after 20 minutes. If the biliary tract is visualized (and sometimes even if it is not), a set of tomograms is taken to cover the whole length of the common bile duct and its branches as well as the gallbladder region. Plain films are also taken at 40 minutes and 60 minutes, if necessary, and tomographic examination is performed. If there is still inadequate visualization or non-visualization at 1 hour, plain films are taken at

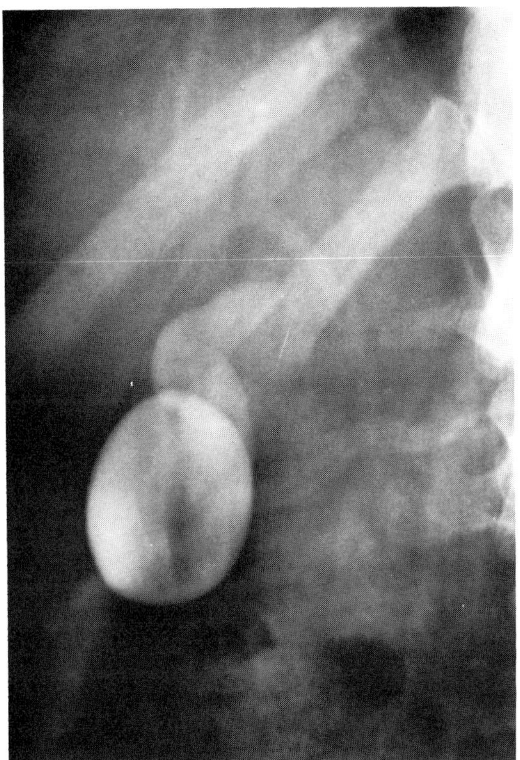

Figure 3–21. Normal intravenous cholangiogram. Note the appearance of the hepatic biliary radicles and common bile duct. There is a typical "mixing artifact" in the opacification of the gallbladder, caused by the difference in density of bile and the contrast agent.

2 hours, 4 hours, and even occasionally at 12 hours and 24 hours.

Visualization of the common bile duct virtually always occurs at some stage of the procedure (at which time tomograms are essential), unless the bilirubin is over 4 mg per 100 ml, in which case the procedure should not have been attempted in the first place. The common bile duct, cystic duct, and hepatic biliary tree can often be seen well with good tomographic films, and often a delayed film (at 12 or 24 hours) will show some opacification of the gallbladder itself. Failure of the gallbladder to become opacified on an intravenous cholangiogram does not imply gallbladder disease. A stone or obstruction at the lower end of the common bile duct is well shown on an intravenous cholangiogram, the stone having an upward facing meniscus and a carcinoma a downward facing one. Involvement of the bile ducts by primary or metastatic tumors, the effects of chronic infections or cholangitis, and the presence of parasites may also be shown on an intravenous cholangiogram (Fig. 3–22).

Special Procedures for the Biliary Tract

INTRAOPERATIVE CHOLANGIOGRAPHY. When the surgeon has removed the gallbladder for stones, intraoperative cholangiography is performed. Placing a catheter into the common bile duct while the patient is on the operating table and injecting water-soluble contrast allows any residual stones in the hepatic ducts or in the common bile duct to be seen; the surgeon then removes them (Fig. 3–23).

T–TUBE CHOLANGIOGRAPHY. An extension of intraoperative cholangiography, T-tube cholangiography may also be performed. After the gallbladder has been removed, the surgeon places a T tube in the midportion of the common bile duct. Ten

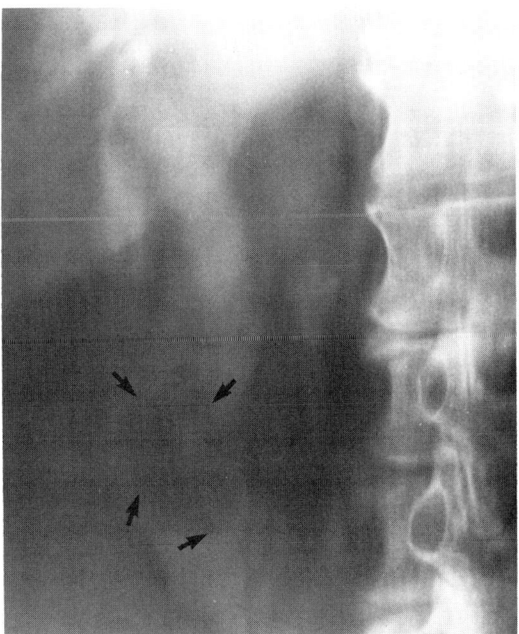

Figure 3–22. Intravenous cholangiogram showing a villous adenocarcinoma of the ampulla of Vater. A mass defect (*arrows*) can be seen within the contrast-filled duodenum. Note that the common bile duct is somewhat distended.

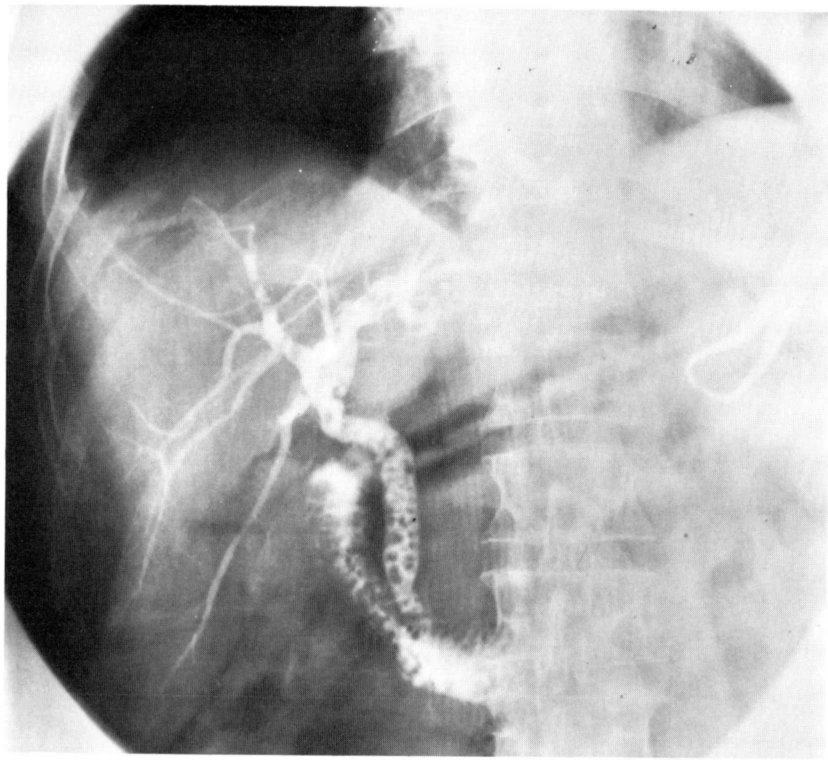

Figure 3–23. Intra-operative cholangiography. Multiple small stones are seen in the common bile duct and hepatic biliary tree while the patient is still in the operating room, thus allowing immediate surgical removal of the stones if clinically indicated.

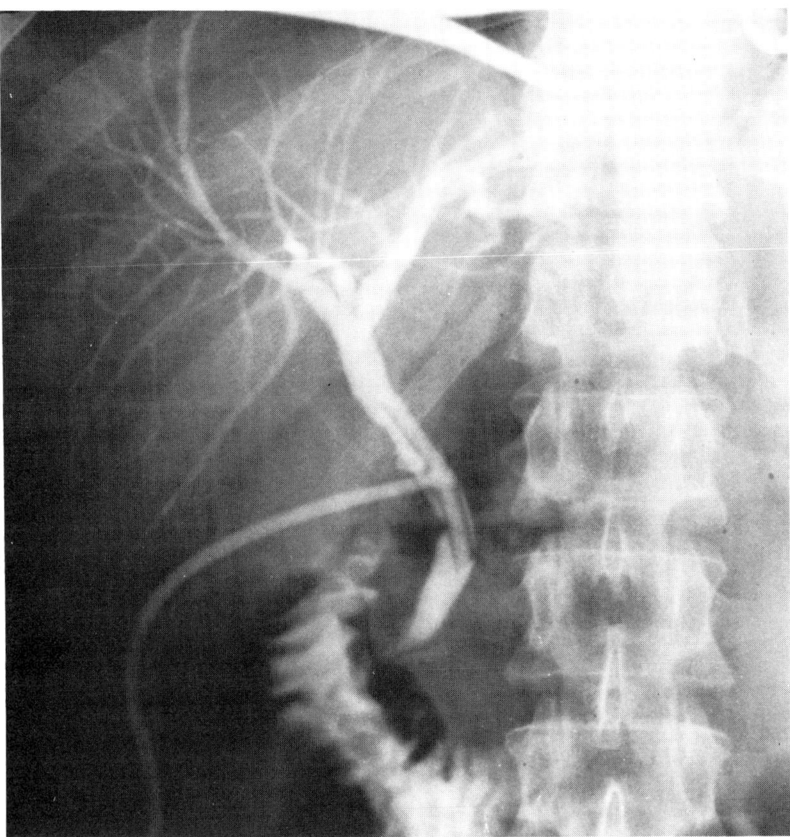

Figure 3–24. Normal T-tube cholangiogram. Note the normal common bile duct and hepatic biliary tree as well as the free flow of contrast into the duodenum.

days after operation, retrograde injection of a water-soluble contrast agent is made into the tube, after all air bubbles have been removed from the system. The contrast agent outlines the common bile duct and biliary tree, and any residual stones or fistulae may be seen (Fig. 3–24). An ideal T-tube study demonstrates the whole of the biliary tree as well as free flow into the duodenum.

ENDOSCOPIC RETROGRADE CHOLANGIOPANCREATOGRAPHY. In retrograde pancreatic cannulation, a fibro-optic endoscope is positioned at the ampulla of Vater so that opacification of the pancreatic ducts, the common bile duct, or both can be achieved. Although this procedure is usually used for pancreatitis or pancreatic carcinoma, a retrograde injection into the biliary tree provides much useful information.

DIRECT PERCUTANEOUS TRANSHEPATIC CHOLANGIOGRAPHY. In direct percutaneous transhepatic cholangiography, a needle is placed in the liver to puncture a biliary duct, and contrast agent is injected into the biliary tract. This procedure produces beautiful radiographs. Because of the danger of bile leak on the withdrawal of the older large needle, direct percutaneous transhepatic cholangiography was usually done only with patients in whom an exploratory laparotomy had already been scheduled. With the current use of a skinny needle, however, no such precautions are necessary. Direct percutaneous transhepatic cholangiography is indicated if the bilirubin level is too high for an intravenous cholangiography or if the IVC yields inadequate information for documentation of obstruction.

CHAPTER 4

SPECIAL PROCEDURES

TOMOGRAPHY

Ever since the first radiograph was taken, radiologists have tried to "focus" the x-rays at a particular point or in a particular plane, thus blurring out unwanted shadows like those of gas overlying the kidneys or a rib overlying a density in the chest. It was eventually discovered that this effect could be achieved by moving the x-ray tube and the film simultaneously in opposite directions. This method of radiography has acquired many names — *planigraphy, laminography,* and *body section radiography* — but *tomography* is the term most often used today and it is the one used in this book. There are many indications for tomographic study. As a basic rule, however, if plain radiographs fail to show *any* abnormality, tomographic examination will be a waste of time.

Tomography can be performed using a variety of different motions of the tube and film, and each radiology department has its own technique. *Autotomography* is a technique that requires the patient to move in a predetermined way so that only one plane of his body remains stationary with respect to the radiographic film during exposure. It is useful in two clinical situations: During an air encephalogram, if the patient rotates his head axially, the midline structures (third and fourth ventricles) remain focused in relation to the film. Much more frequently, autotomography is used for the dorsal spine. As the patient breathes during exposure, the ribs and soft tissues of the thorax move and blue on the image, but the spine remains stationary and in focus.

Chest

Lung Fields

Tomography can be used to better define the margins of a mass, to look for a cavitation in an area, segment, or mass, to check for calcification in a mass or the pleura, and to search for small intrapulmonary metastases from the skeleton, skin, soft tissues, and the female genital tract (Fig. 4–1). Many radiologists are of the opinion that searching for unsuspected metastases using chest tomography is an exercise in futility, unless there is some suspicion of a lesion on PA and lateral chest x-rays. Tomographic study of the chest can cover the whole chest from front to back or can be coned down to a particular area, for example, the apical regions when tuberculosis is suspected.

Hilum and Mediastinum

Tomography is particularly useful in searching for lymphadenopathy or a mass in the hila or the central mediastinum (Fig. 4–2). Tomography can also be used to look at the lower trachea and carina as well as the main pulmonary bronchi and

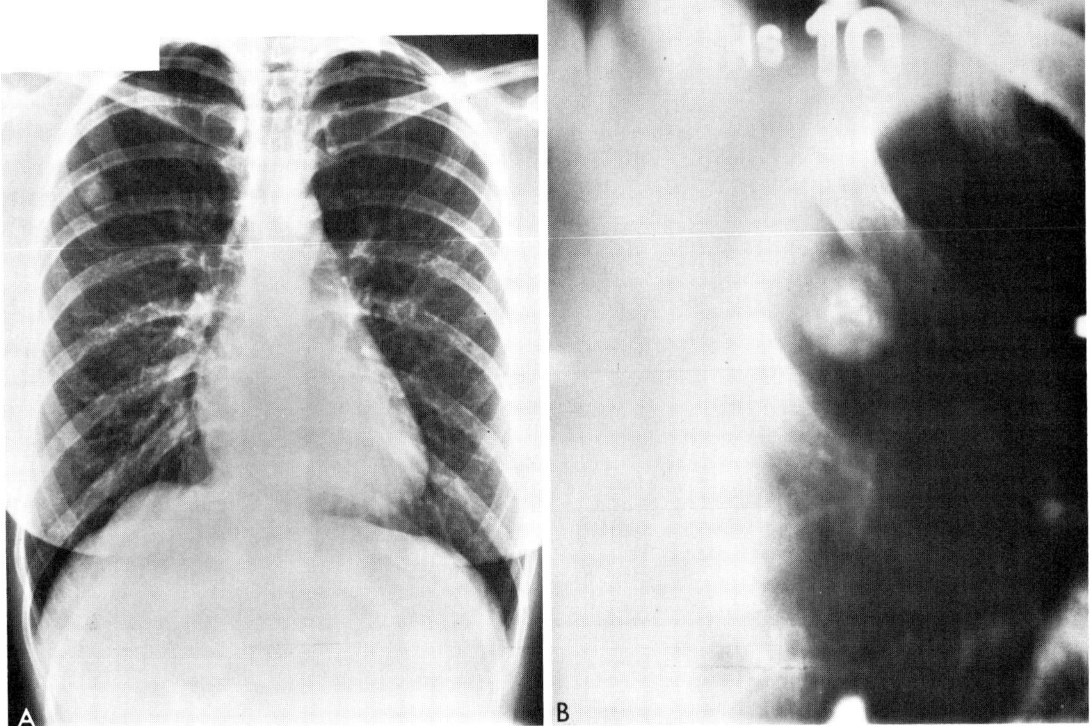

Figure 4–1. A mass in the chest, routine PA x-ray (*A*) and tomogram (*B*). This 23-year-old patient was asymptomatic, but a routine chest x-ray revealed a 2-cm solitary nodule in the right upper lobe. Tomography demonstrated central calcification. A thoracotomy confirmed that this was a benign granuloma.

their branches for widening of the otherwise acute angle of the carina or for evidence of tumor, constriction, stenosis, encasement, and erosion, which are often associated with a mass. Since tomographs are usually obtained with the patient supine, the azygos vein is distended in this position and lies within the curve of the right upper lobe bronchus so that it resembles a mass. For certain bronchi (for example, the right middle lobe and left lingula), oblique tomography in the plane of the bronchus is used.

Bony Thorax

Often, oblique views of the ribs fail to show enough detail, and tomography is requested. It is not particularly useful except for visualizing the lower posterior ribs, but these can also be well seen on standard views of the abdomen. With respect to the sternum and sternoclavicular joints, tomography may be useful because this area is difficult to visualize satisfactorily on plain films.

Abdomen

Intravenous Pyelography

Tomography is frequently used during routine intravenous pyelography. Tomograms are performed at the early stages of the procedure (*nephrotomography*) and then at later stages to better delineate the renal calyces. Tomography is used prior to the injection of contrast agent to ascertain if calcification lies within the kidneys (Fig. 4–3A). In patients who have a high serum creatinine and are in renal failure, tomography may be the only way to estimate renal size and shape as well as provide a clue to the primary cause of the renal failure (Fig. 4–3B). Tomography is used to outline the geography of polycystic kidneys to determine whether a renal pelvic irregularity is a mass, stone or blood clot, and to determine the nature of mass lesions in the kidney, such as benign cysts or hypernephromas. (See the discussion on ultrasonic evaluation of the kidney, Chapter 6.)

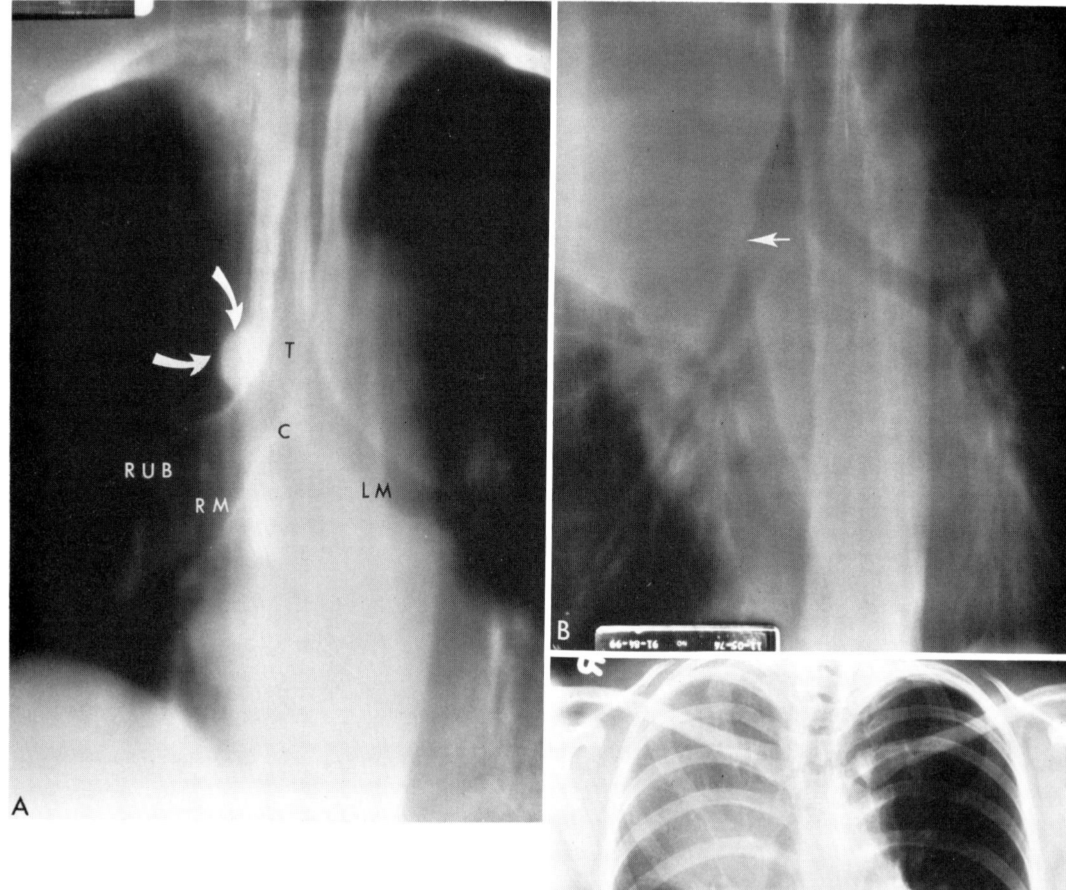

Figure 4–2. The hilum. *A*, Tomogram of a normal patient. Note the trachea (T) with the sharply pointed carina (C) at the division into the left (LM) and right (RM) main stem bronchi. The right upper lobe bronchus (RUB) branches off immediately. Note also the enlargement of the azygos vein (*long arrows*) caused by the fact that the patient is lying supine for tomography. *B* and *C*, Tomogram and PA chest x-ray of a 21-year-old female with a right upper lobe mass. Note that the right upper lobe bronchus is missing (*arrow*). This patient had Hodgkin's disease.

Intravenous Cholangiography

Tomography is an essential part of intravenous cholangiography and is used to delineate the common bile duct, the biliary radicals, and even the gallbladder when opacification is poor on plain films.

Examination of the Adrenal Glands

Tomography is used to evaluate masses in the suprarenal area with or without the use of intravenous contrast as part of an intravenous pyelogram. Tomographic examination can document the site of abdominal

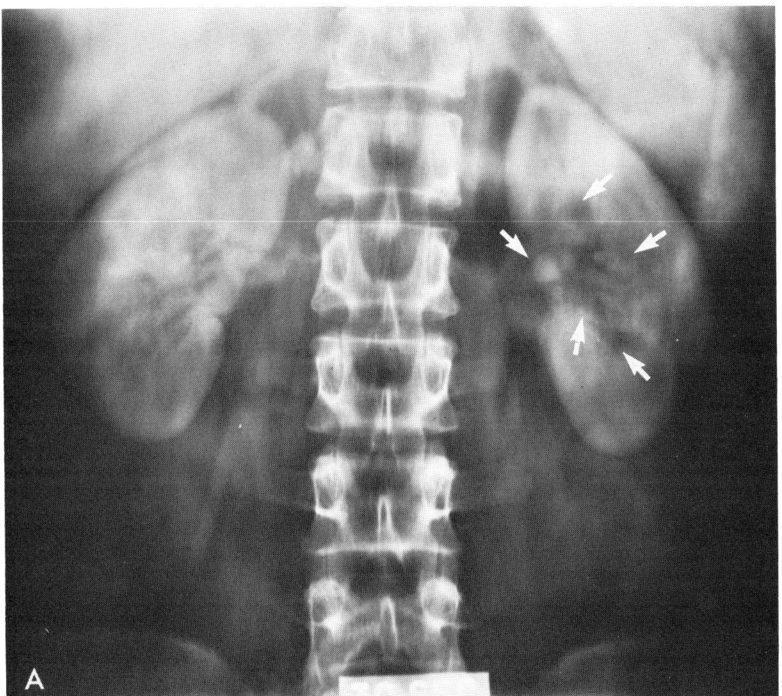

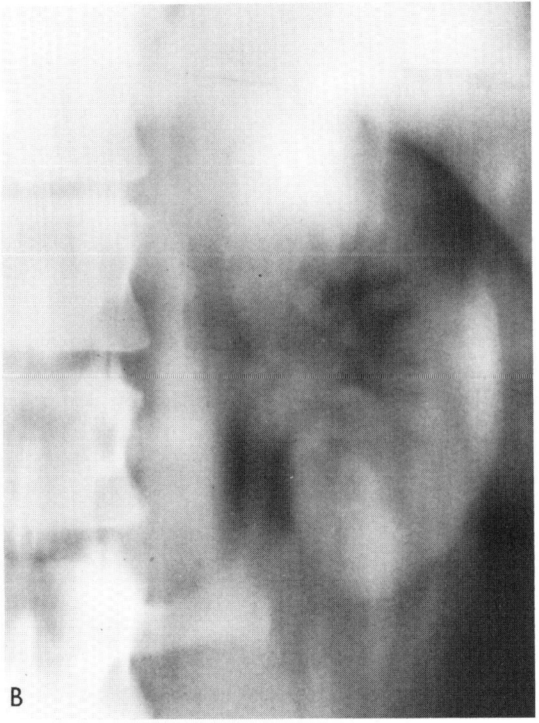

Figure 4–3. Tomography of the kidney. *A*, A normal nephrotomogram reveals the smooth outline of the kidneys with increased density around the edge of the renal cortex as well as early filling of the calyces and renal pelvis, which can be visualized because they are in a bed of lucent peripelvic fat (*arrows*). *B*, Abnormal nephrotomogram. This rather small kidney with an irregular cortex and apparently small calyces was found in a 47-year-old man with renal failure due to chronic glomerulonephritis.

calcification in a patient with Addison's disease or a history of tuberculosis.

Tomography is also part of *retroperitoneal air insufflation,* in which air or carbon dioxide is injected into the soft tissue plane between the rectum and the coccyx, clearly outlining the kidneys and the adrenal glands. Recently, however, angiography has replaced retroperitoneal air insufflation as the procedure of choice.

Tomography of the Abdomen

Lateral tomographs of the abdomen have been used in the investigation of suspected abdominal aortic aneurysms in order to find calcification within the wall and to delineate aneurysm size.

Spine and Long Bones

Tomography can be used to better delineate any pathological lesion in the skeleton. But it has been used particularly in osteomyelitis involving the spine or tumors involving the long bones. Other indications for tomography include assessing microfractures and compression fractures in elderly people, checking the position and stability of various prosthetic devices, and evaluating the healing of fractures in which exuberant callus hides the fracture line. Tomography is usually not indicated for the peripheral skeleton because good plain film radiography with or without magnification studies supplies adequate information.

Skull and Face

Tomography can be used to better show the extent and significance of fractures of the orbits and facial bones (Fig. 4–4). The procedure is also used to delineate the sella, particularly when looking for evidence of a pituitary tumor, such as erosions, double floor, or enlargement. Tomography is used to investigate the internal auditory canals and inner ear for evidence of acoustic neuroma, otosclerosis, infection, or congenital anomalies. Finally, tomography can be used to evaluate the extent of damage in a basal skull fracture.

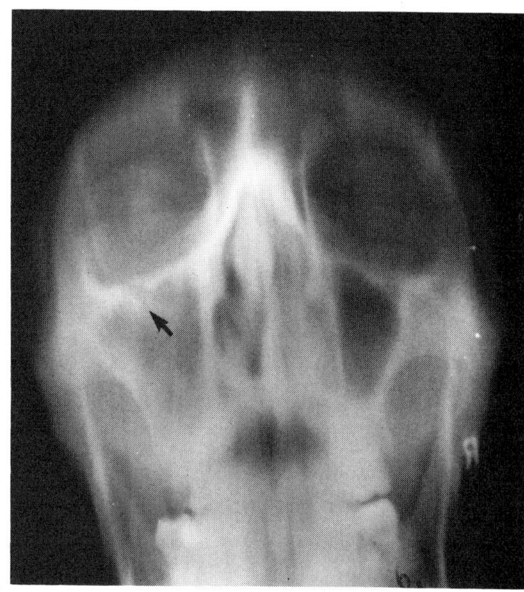

Figure 4–4. Tomography of the face. A fracture through the orbital floor (*arrow*) as well as opacification in the left maxillary antrum can be seen in this young man following an automobile accident.

FLUOROSCOPY

There are many situations in which being able to observe the patient rather than a still radiograph is extremely helpful. It is usually desirable to record the radiographic findings in a permanent way, and there are a number of different methods of managing this. The easiest and most common method is to take spot films as the fluoroscopic procedure progresses; these can be taken at different depths of respiration or at differing angles of obliquity. Most radiology departments are equipped with cineradiography or videotape, either of which can be used to record findings. With cineradiography, which is now mainly used for various cardiac applications, there is often some delay in processing the films. Videotapes are excellent for instant playback and so have become popular for studying the lower urinary tract, looking at barium studies, and observing joint function. Since many of the fluoroscopic procedures discussed here are the subjects of complete monographs, these brief notes are only meant to be an introduction to the subject.

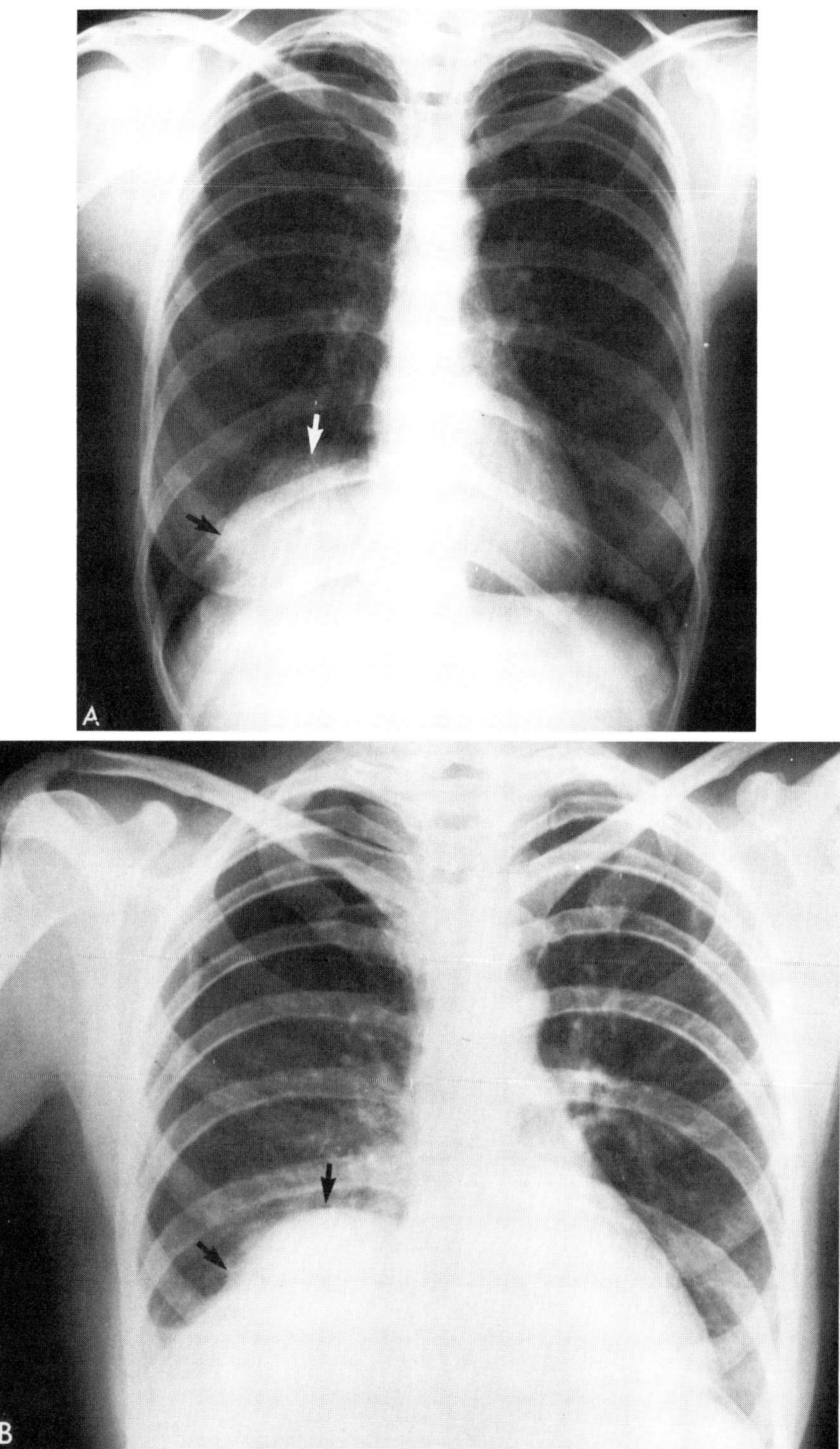

Figure 4–5. Fluoroscopy of a pericardial cyst, inspiration view (*A*) and expiration view (*B*). There is a large "mass" in the right cardiophrenic angle (*arrows*) that changes shape with respiration, getting larger on inspiration. This finding is typical of a pericardial springwater cyst.

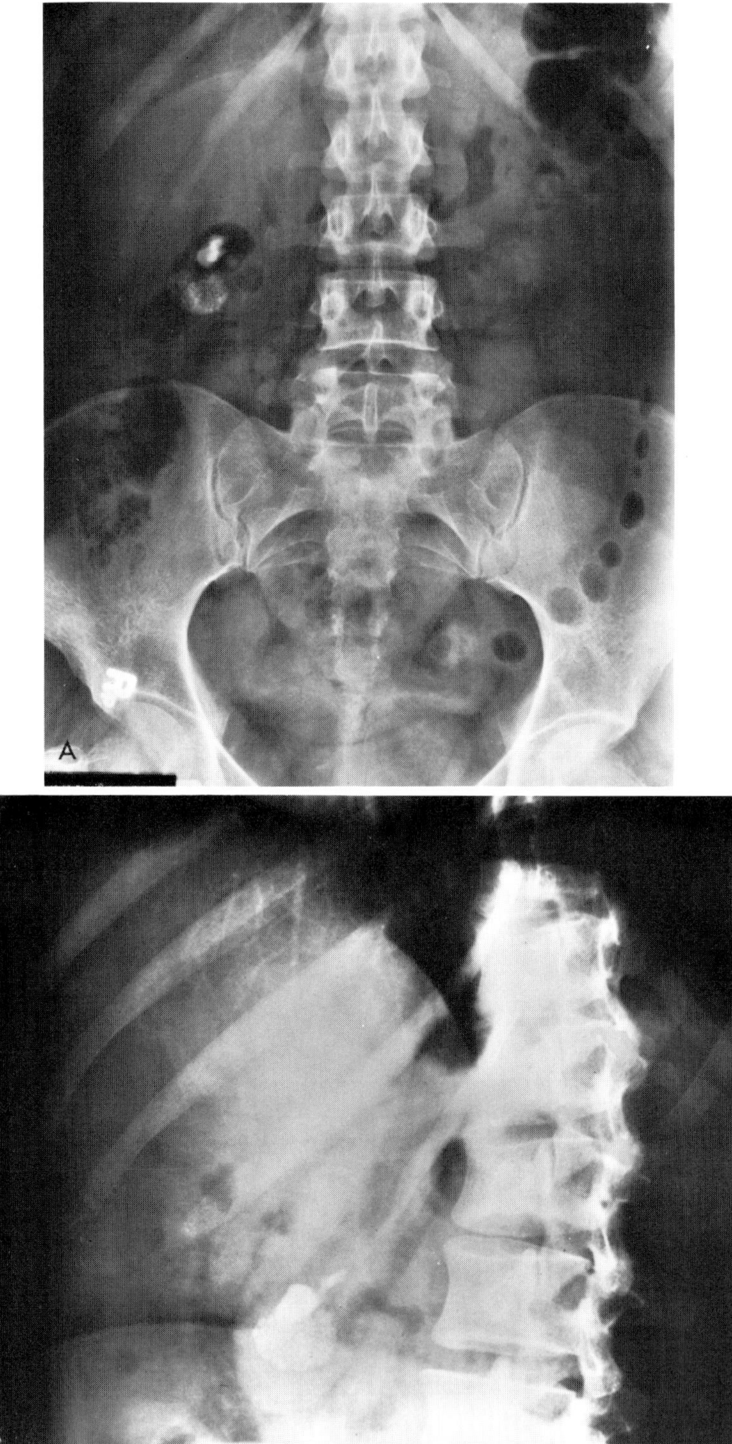

Figure 4–6. Fluoroscopy of renal calcification, expiration view (*A*), and inspiration view (*B*). Note that calcification lies in the right upper quadrant in this 34-year-old woman and looks like gallstones. On inspiration, however, the calcification is seen to lie within the kidney.

Chest

Fluoroscopy is used to observe the motion of the diaphragms to see if they move equally and freely. Similarly, fluoroscopy is used to observe a suspected pericardial cyst (springwater cyst), which becomes larger on inspiration and smaller on expiration (Fig. 4–5). Fluoroscopy is also used to observe the hila during respiration and to exclude the possibility of discrete tumors or lymph node masses as well as to differentiate between large vessels and nodes.

Fluoroscopy can be used to identify small pulmonary nodules and to see if they contain calcification. The procedure is also used to locate the position of a density or nodule seen on plain films, to determine, for instance, if it lies within the intrapulmonary tissues, pleura, soft tissues, or skin. Fluoroscopic investigation also enables one to verify pleural calcification, to observe both pleural and pericardial effusions, and to differentiate between pleural fibrosis and effusions as well as between a loculated effusion and a solid mass.

Looking for evidence of air trapping, in a young child with asthma or chronic bronchitis, for instance, is facilitated by fluoroscopy. This is particularly helpful in the evaluation of a patient with a suspected foreign body in a bronchus which may act as a ball valve and lead to air trapping.

Fluoroscopic investigation of the heart is also possible, to see if there is calcification, particularly around the mitral and aortic valves and coronary arteries or within a left ventricular thrombus. It can be used to observe evidence of dyskinetic segments of the ventricular wall or of left ventricular aneurysm (a suggestive sign of left ventricular aneurysm is squaring off of the ventricle on the PA chest radiograph). Fluoroscopy can be used to observe cardiac function, to assess chamber size, and to see if the ventricles are contracting adequately.

Abdomen

Fluoroscopy is used to identify the position of intra-abdominal calcifications, not only in the region of the gallbladder but also near the kidneys and adrenal glands (Fig. 4–6). During an intravenous pyelogram, fluoroscopy can be used to observe the kidneys and ureters and to watch ureteric peristalsis. It is also helpful in documenting intraureteral location of suspected calculi.

Fluoroscopy is also an integral part of *voiding cystourethrography* (VCUG). This procedure is performed by inserting a catheter into the bladder of a patient, filling the bladder with contrast material, and having the patient void. Fluoroscopy is used to observe the filling and emptying of the bladder, to check for vesicoureteric reflux, to measure the thickness of the bladder wall, to assess the size of the prostate, and to watch the urethra while the patient is voiding and to measure the residual urine.

Fluoroscopy is used to observe contrast being injected into an abdominal sinus or fistula; the depth to which the contrast goes and whether it communicates with a viscus help to determine the extent and significance of the lesion. This procedure is known as *sinography* (Fig. 4–7).

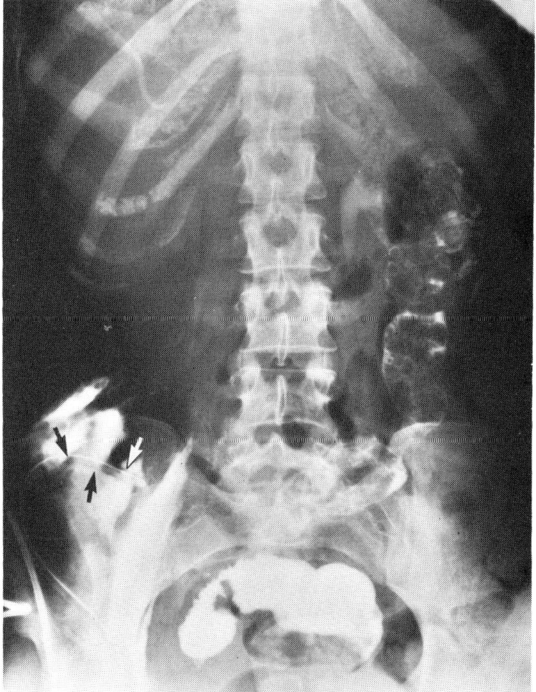

Figure 4–7. Sinogram, KUB. This 24-year-old woman developed a mass in the right lower quadrant of the abdomen that spontaneously discharged. For a sinogram, the catheter was positioned in the sinus (*arrows*) and contrast material was injected. A large abscess cavity is outlined that is displacing normal bowel loops. There is also filling of both large and small bowel from this abscess cavity. At operation, this patient was found to have regional enteritis.

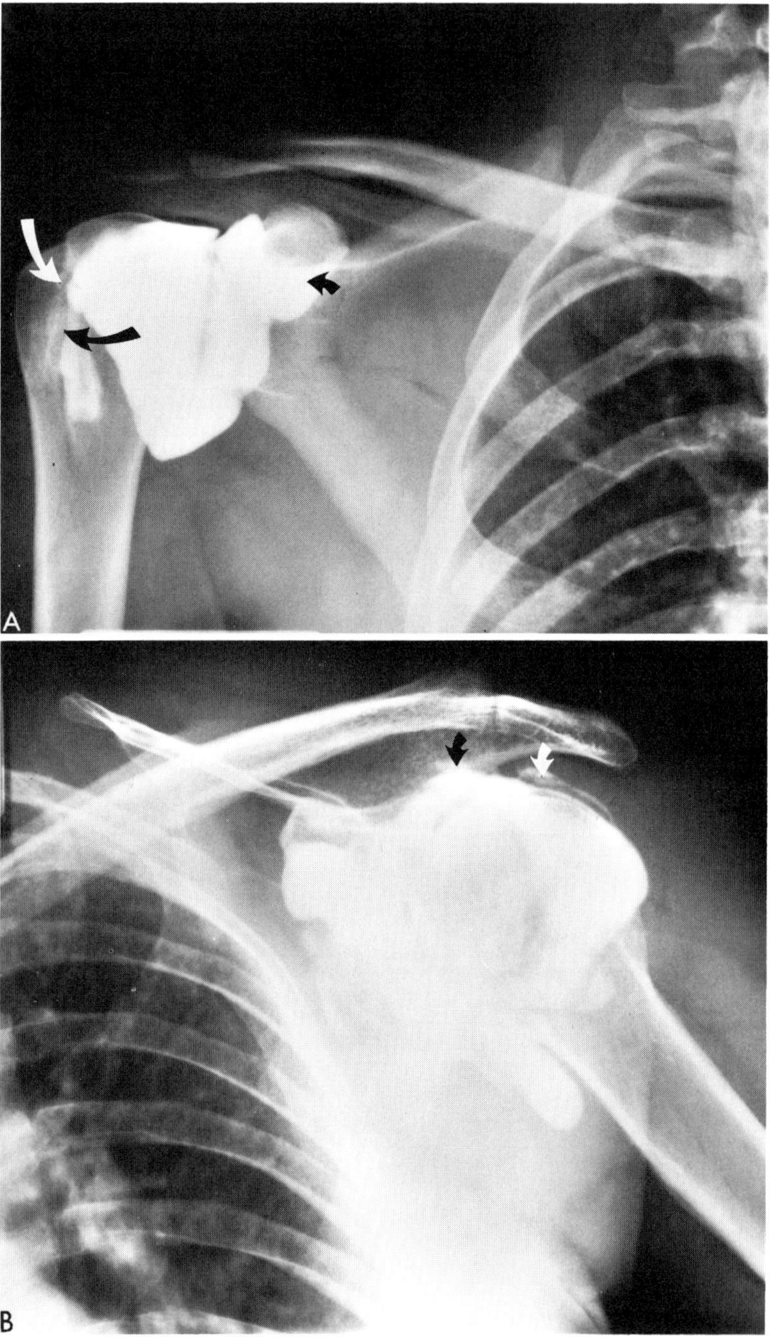

Figure 4–8. Arthrography. *A*, The normal shoulder joint is demonstrated with the subcoracoid recess (*small arrow*). Some contrast material has run down the biceps tendon sheath, and the tendon itself shows up as a lucency (*long arrows*). *B*, In this shoulder, contrast material has run superiorly out of the joint capsule in two places (*arrows*); this represents a partial tear of the rotator cuff.

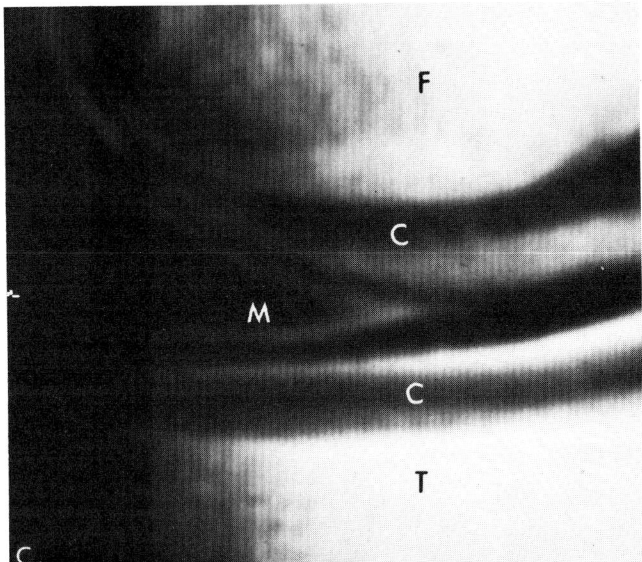

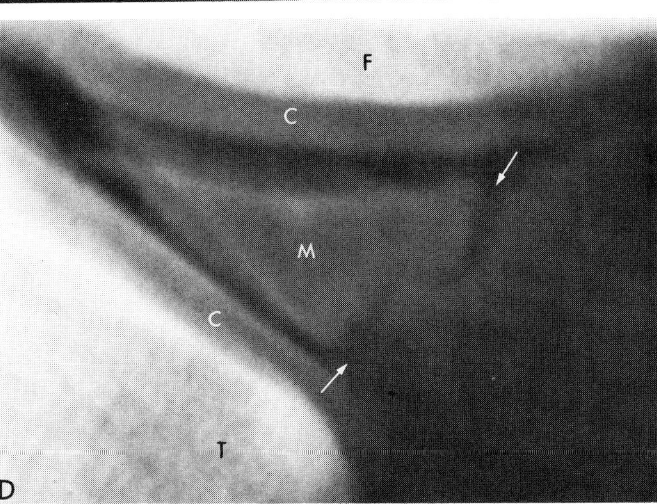

Figure 4–8. Continued. *C*, In the normal knee, the meniscus (M) and the articular cartilage (C) are well shown at arthrography; the normal meniscus appears as a smooth triangle. The femur (F) and tibia (T) are also visible. *D*, When the meniscus (M) becomes torn, as in this knee, it appears truncated or an actual tear may be seen (*arrows*).

Fluoroscopy is an essential part of a *T-tube cholangiogram.* It is used to observe the flow of contrast down the common bile duct into the duodenum after a gallbladder operation in which a cholecystectomy has been performed and the surgeon has left a T-tube in the common bile duct. Fluoroscopic observation is used to see if any stones have been left behind and to determine whether the hepatic biliary tree is normal.

Skeleton

Fluoroscopy is also an essential part of an *arthrogram.* After injection of contrast material alone or, more usually, air and contrast material (*double-contrast arthrography*), fluoroscopic observation is made and spot films are used to look at the integrity of the articular cartilage, to see if there are any loose bodies present, and to check for capsular or synovial tears (for instance, in looking for rotator cuff tears in the shoulder). Suspicion of meniscal tears in the knee is by far the most common indication for arthrography (Fig. 4–8). Arthrography can be performed on any joint in the body, including the wrist, fingers, acromioclavicular joints, and temporomandibular joints as well as the joints more commonly examined, such as the knees, hips, shoulders, and ankles.

Fluoroscopy is used to study the function of joints, particularly in patients with arthritis or with injury involving a joint, to see if one bone is impinging on another. Fluoroscopy can be used to observe the effect of stress on unstable joints. It also can be used to observe motion (or the lack of it) following internal fixation and joint replacement.

There are many indications for fluoroscopic observation of the motion of the spine. This procedure is often performed for patients with severe rheumatoid arthritis and suspected atlantoaxial subluxation. After surgical fusion, usually in the lumbar region, fluoroscopy can be used to look for evidence of solid fusion. Assessment of the relative rotatory and straight motions of the spine during tilting is made with fluoroscopic observation in patients with scoliosis.

Fluoroscopy is used when sinograms are performed on patients with chronic osteomyelitis who have a chronic draining sinus to see if there is any direct communication between the skin and the underlying bone.

Skull

In examinations of the skull, fluoroscopy can be used to localize a foreign body, particularly in the orbit, to identify an unusual line or density seen on the plain films and to evaluate suspected fractures. The procedure is also an integral part of transsphenoidal hypophysectomies.

Other Uses of Fluoroscopy

Fluoroscopic observation can be used to assist with the placement of tubes anywhere in the body, such as central venous pressure lines, endotracheal tubes, Swan-Ganz catheters, and Sengstaken-Blakemore tubes. Fluoroscopy is used during endoscopic procedures, particularly in the placement of a tube into the pancreatic duct, and helps with the injection of contrast material to outline the pancreatic and common bile ducts. This procedure is known as *endoscopic retrograde cholangiopancreatography (ERCP).*

SPECIAL PLAIN FILM RADIOGRAPHIC TECHNIQUES

Stereoscopic Radiography

There are a number of ways to enhance an image and thus improve on the information contained on a radiograph. One method is to take two plain radiographs of the same object with the x-ray tube in slightly different positions. (A similar technique was used for early three-dimensional movies, in which the observer wearing red and green glasses could see a "three-dimensional" image because a red image and a green image were superimposed on each other.) By taking a radiograph of the pelvis, for example, and taking a second film with the x-ray tube moved 6 to 10 inches either laterally or cephalad, two similar images are obtained that can be viewed together on a special light box with crossed prisms to produce a three-dimensional image. A light box is not necessary, however; if the radiologist crosses his eyes as he looks at the two radiographs hung side by side, he will be able to see a three-dimensional image. Stereoscopic radiography has largely fallen into disuse, but there are still some orthopedic applications, such as locating bone fragments in a comminuted fracture of the shoulder or of the pelvis and hip joint.

Magnification

The thought of being able to magnify the image and see more detail has intrigued radiologists for at least 60 years. Unfortunately, the focal spot size in the ordinary x-ray tube is so large that it is impossible to magnify an image more than 1½ to 2 times without loss of detail. If magnification greater than this is attempted, blurring will occur. There are two solutions to this problem. One is to use secondary optical magnification (a magnifying glass). This is possible only if the film provides a high-resolution image. High-resolution images are achieved by using special intensifying screens and films or by using mammographic or industrial films. It is possible to achieve a 5× optical magnification by this means. The second and more recent solution is to use an x-ray tube with a small focal spot (*microfocus spot tube*). Primary magnification is achieved by moving the film away from the patient or, better, by placing the patient closer to the x-ray tube. This system of imaging is still in its infancy, but it is anticipated that magnification radiography will be used for angiography (particularly neuroradiological and renal), skeletal work (particularly for metabolic bone diseases and orthopedic problems), pediatric applications (including respiratory distress syndrome, suspected fractures, and congenital anomalies of the base of the skull), and mammography.

Subtraction

If a normal radiograph, on which air is black and bone is white, is processed in a special way, it can be reversed, so that bone is black and air is white. In fact, the radiographs in many European textbooks of radiology have black bones and white air. If one performs an angiogram and then reverses the image, the blood vessels will appear black. If the original film taken without contrast material is superimposed on the reversed image taken with contrast material and a copy of the two is made photographically, the white and black bones will be superimposed on each other and will apparently disappear, the black and white air will apparently disappear, and one is left with black blood vessels on a light grey background. This procedure is called *subtraction* and is particularly useful in cerebral arteriography and also for detecting leaks of contrast material around a metal joint prosthesis.

Angiography

The basic concept behind angiography is to deliver a large enough bolus of contrast material into the correct place at a fast enough rate for the contrast to be observed opacifying blood vessels or chambers of the heart. The actual technique by which this is achieved need not concern us here in any detail, although the Seldinger method of positioning a catheter is so neat that it is worth going to watch an angiogram being performed. A needle is inserted into the vessel (normally the femoral artery or vein), and a flexible guidewire is inserted through the needle into the vessel. The needle is removed and a catheter is slid up around the guidewire and into the vessel. The catheter and guidewire are then correctly positioned, the wire is removed, and contrast agent is injected rapidly through the hollow catheter.

There are really two phases of an angiographic investigation. A preliminary series of films is taken of the general area following injection of contrast material into a major vessel. Then, selective catheterization of one or more specific vessels is usually undertaken. For example, in assessment of a pancreatic tumor, a preliminary aortogram with the catheter inserted at about the level of T10 gives an outline of the basic vascular anatomy and shows any obvious abnormalities. The initial films are followed by selective catheterization of the celiac axis and its branches to allow selective visualization of the pancreas itself. The contrast material is followed through to the venous drainage of the tissue or organ involved, and some assessment can be also made of this. Records of the study may be made in a number of different ways: on multiple rapid-sequence single films using a film changer, on cineradiographic film (particularly for coronary and cardiac studies), or on videotape. Remember, too, that the use of water-soluble contrast agents provides a "free" pyelogram, as the contrast is excreted by the kidneys.

Visceral angiography and peripheral angiography are discussed in this section; neurological angiography is dealt with in the following section. Let us begin with a few basic facts: Atheroma manifests itself as irregular plaques on the intima and is associated with narrowing of the lumen of the vessel to the point of actual stenosis. Tumors, both primary and metastatic, produce new blood vessels (*neovasculature*). They may also encase and distort normal vessels, and they often have a large capillary bed, thus causing them to "light up" on angiography. Aneurysms are usually obvious, although some of them may be filled with thrombi. Infections are also associated with increased vascularity. Final-

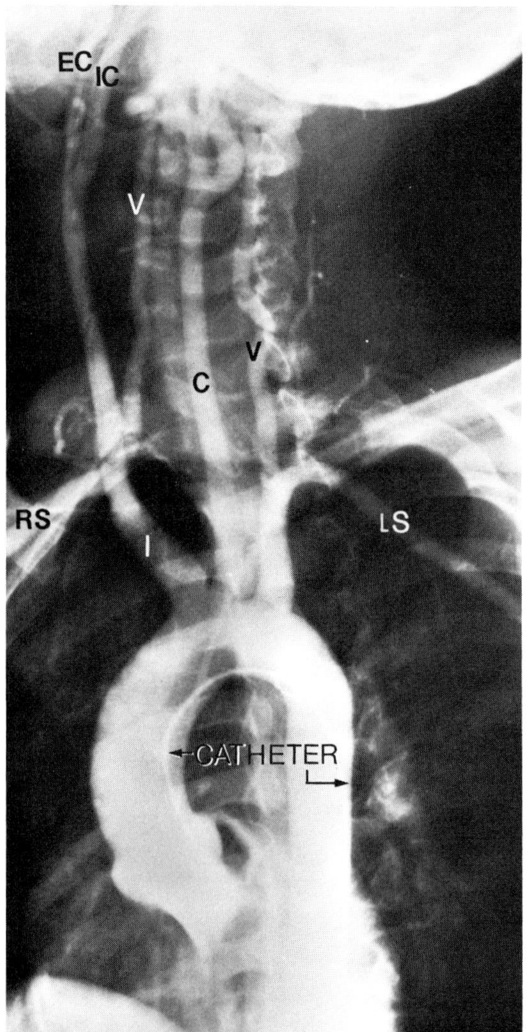

Figure 4–9. Normal arch aortogram. The catheter, which has been inserted in the aorta from below, shows as an opaque thread within the lumen of the vessel. The cusps above the aortic valve can be seen. The arteries are also visible: on the left, the left carotid (C), the left subclavian (LS), and the left vertebral (*black* V) arteries; on the right, the innominate artery (I) and its branches—the right subclavian (RS), the internal carotid (IC), the external carotid (EC), and the right vertebral (*white* V) arteries.

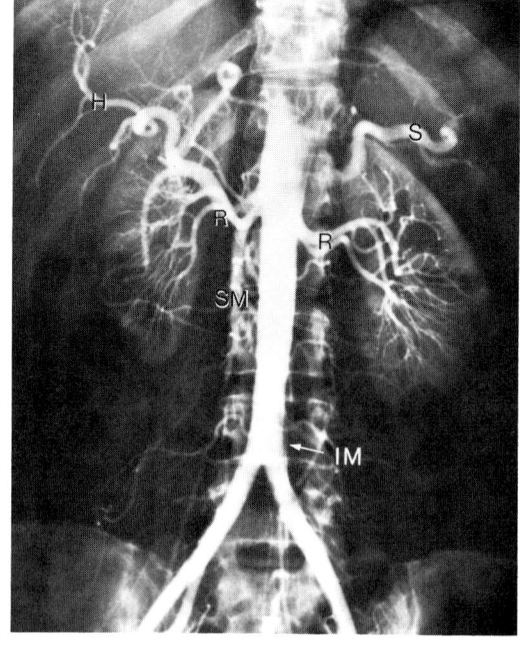

Figure 4–10. Normal abdominal aortogram. The catheter has been inserted from below, and the angiogram demonstrates the celiac axis with the splenic artery (S) and hepatic artery (H), as well as both renal vessels (R), the superior mesenteric artery (SM), and the inferior mesenteric artery (IM). The aortic bifurcation and the iliac arteries are also well seen.

ly, bleeding points can be identified by the puddles of contrast outside the normal confines of the vessel (in the lumen of the bowel, for example), and efforts can be made to halt the hemorrhage by injecting blood clot or Gelfoam directly through the catheter to the site of bleeding.

Thoracic Aortography

In thoracic aortography, the catheter is positioned in the aortic root, usually from below (Fig. 4–9). This procedure is useful in assessing the degree of atheroma, determining the size and position of aneurysms (and, with a dissecting aneurysm, locating the point at which the blood reenters the lumen, especially in relationship to the origin of the renal arteries), and looking for stenoses in the major vessels to the head and neck. Thoracic aortography may also be performed as a preliminary study for selective catheterization of the small vessels in the neck, such as the arteries supplying the parathyroid and thyroid glands, or in the chest, such as the bronchial arteries. The procedure can also be used to assess congenital anomalies of the aortic arch itself, including coarctation.

Abdominal Aortography

The abdominal aorta can be reached either from below or via a translumbar direct-puncture technique. Opacification of the aorta below the diaphragm allows visualization of the celiac axis (which is the origin of the splenic, left gastric, and hepatic arteries), the superior and inferior mesenteric arteries, the renal arteries, the lumbar and phrenic arteries, and the run-off into the iliac vessels (Fig. 4–10). Abdominal aortography is useful in assessing aneurysms, atheromata, and stenoses and in searching for evidence of primary or secondary tumors involving the liver, pancreas, kidneys, adrenals, and retroperitoneal structures. In a patient with suspected ischemic bowel disease, the blood supply to the colon can be assessed. In a patient who is bleeding, either from a perforated ulcer or following significant trauma (e.g., a fractured pelvis), the bleeding site can be identified and attempts can be made to cause thrombosis in the vessel, a process that often entails leaving the catheter in place and taking another angiogram as much as 48 hours later.

Renal Arteriography

Renal arteriography is useful in looking at the renal vessels for atheroma, stenosis, or fibromuscular hyperplasia (Fig. 4–11). In patients with hypertension, the size and contour of the main renal arteries can be observed, as can the ramification of the intrarenal vessels. With magnification, even the small intralobular arteries become visible. Renal arteriography is useful in assessing the function of a renal transplant as well as in looking at arterial and venous anastomoses. Arteriography can be employed in differentiating between renal cysts and tumors, in looking for infarcts, arteriovenous malformations, and aneurysms (either single or multiple, as in periarteritis nodosa, for example), and also in investigating renal anomalies and ectopic kidneys. If the contrast is observed as it passes through to the venous side, the possibility of renal vein thrombosis may be confirmed or excluded.

Peripheral Arteriography

The major clinical indication for a study of the peripheral vessels is suspected atheroma and arteriosclerosis in the legs (Fig. 4–12). This procedure is usually performed using a lower aortic injection to demonstrate the aortic bifurcation and the iliac and femoral vessels as well as the run-off into the popliteal arteries and the vessels of the feet. In patients with severe premature peripheral vascular disease, Buerger's disease should be suspected; signs of this condition are multiple occlusions associated with corrugations of the main vessels and "corkscrew" collaterals. Patients with Raynaud's phenomenon in the arms from whatever cause are usually investigated with arteriography. In both upper and lower limbs, emboli are sought in patients with acute ischemic changes of a limb. Arteriovenous malformations are arteriographed prior to surgery, and soft-tissue tumors are often investigated angiographically to observe the origins and ramification of their blood supply. Finally, peripheral arteriography is used to check dialysis

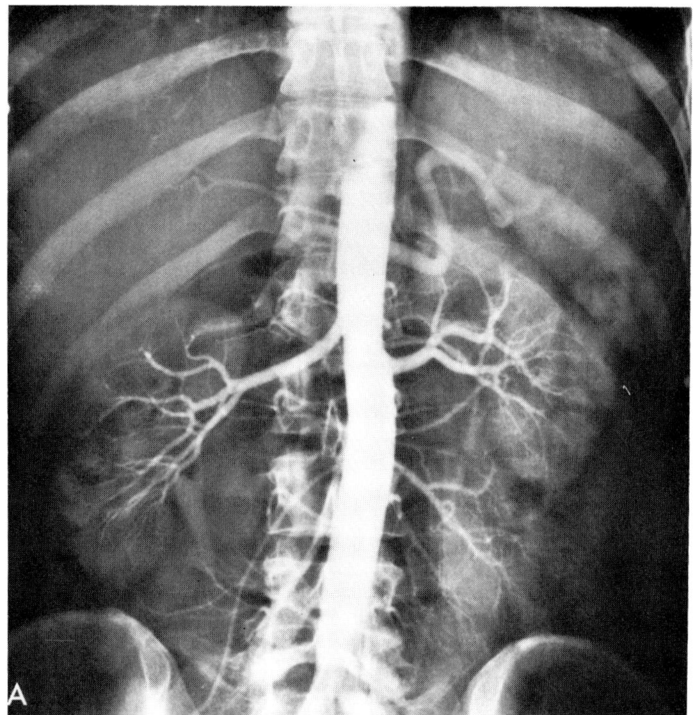

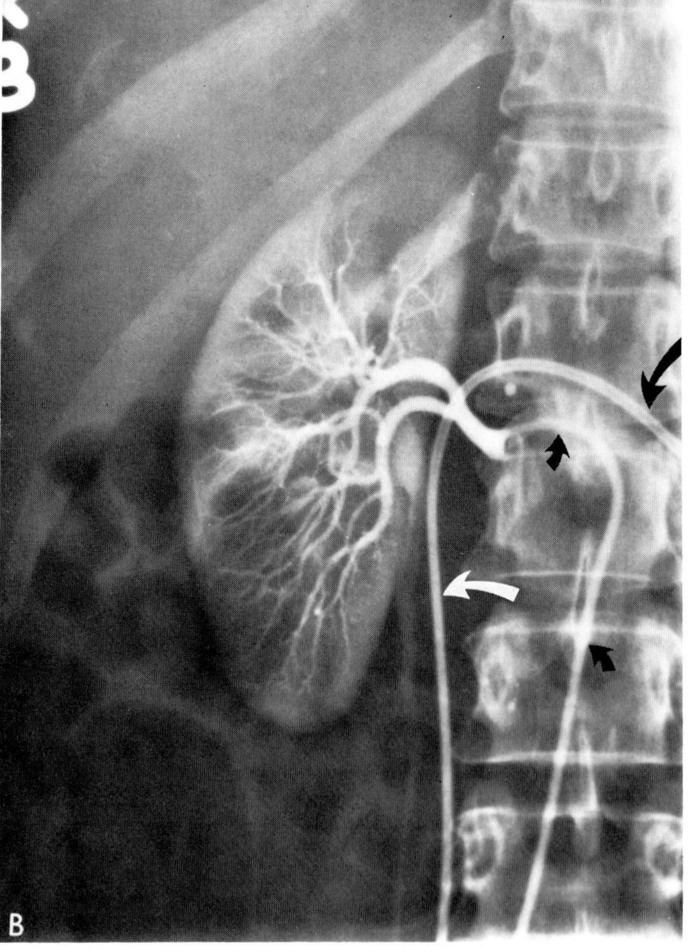

Figure 4–11. Renal arteriography. *A*, The aortogram is normal. Note the single renal artery on the right and the double renal artery on the left. *B*, Selective right renal arteriogram. The catheter is placed directly into the right renal artery (*small arrows*), and better visualization of the intrarenal vessels is obtained. The other catheter is in the inferior vena cava and left renal vein (*large arrows*). Note the excretion of contrast by the kidney (a "poor man's pyelogram").

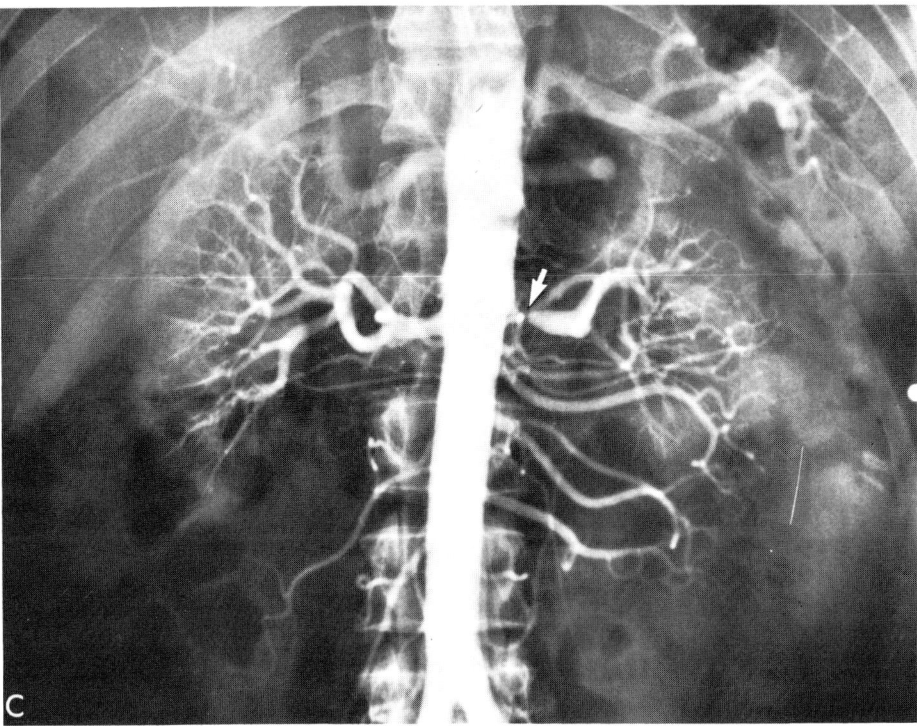

Figure 4–11. Continued. *C*, Aortogram of renal artery stenosis. The stenosis of the left renal artery is clearly seen (*arrow*). There is some poststenotic dilatation, which is due to a physiological phenomenon associated with significant stenosis. Note that the left kidney is smaller in this 45-year-old male with a long history of hypertension.

shunts to see whether they are still patent or have become thrombosed.

Pulmonary Angiography

Studies of the pulmonary vasculature are primarily done for patients with suspected thromboembolic disease. The catheter is usually introduced into the inferior vena cava or through the heart into the pulmonary arteries. Selective catheterization of specific pulmonary arteries can be obtained. With pulmonary angiography, the pulmonary arteries and pulmonary veins can be clearly seen as can the chambers of the heart (Fig. 4–13). Pulmonary angiography can also be used to diagnose pulmonary arteriovenous malformations, total or partial anomalous venous return, and arteriovenous fistulae.

Cardiac Angiography

Angiography of the heart is done mainly for two reasons: to investigate congenital heart disease, such as tetralogy of Fallot transposition of great vessels, tricuspid atresia, truncus arteriosis, and coarctation, and to investigate left to right shunts, such as atrial septal defects, ventricular septal defects, and patent ductus. It is also used for the examination of congenital and acquired valvular diseases — aortic stenosis (both supra- and sub-valvular), aortic regurgitation, pulmonary stenosis, mitral stenosis or regurgitation, and tricuspid valve disease (Fig. 4–14). Cardiac angiography is also useful for investigation of left atrial myxoma and confirmation of ruptured chordae tendineae.

Coronary Arteriography

After the initial aortic root study, selective arteriography of the coronary arteries is used for the investigation of angina, in looking for changes of arteriosclerosis or occlusion as well as in identifying coronary artery fistulae or aneurysms (Fig. 4–15).

Venography

The study of veins in the leg is important in the differential diagnosis of pain in

Text continued on page 86

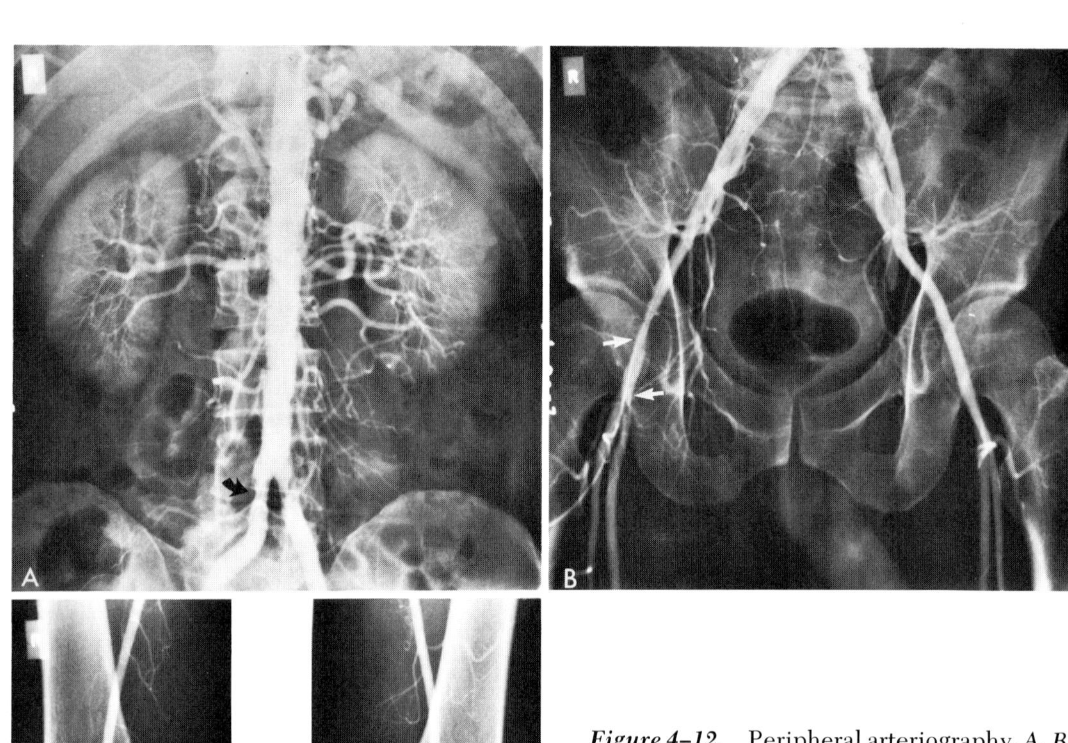

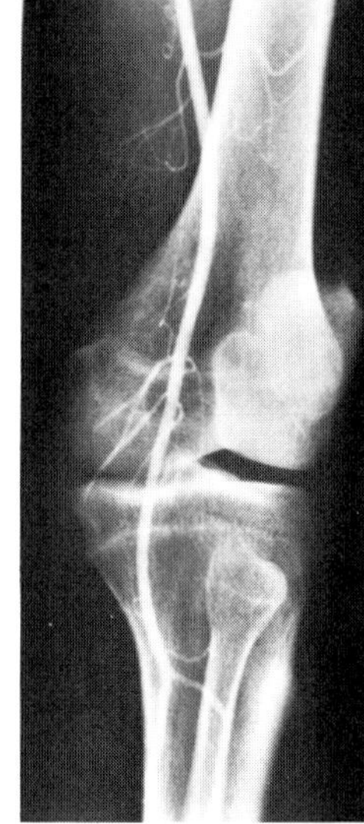

Figure 4–12. Peripheral arteriography. *A*, *B*, and *C*, Normal aorto-femoral arteriogram. These films show excellent filling from the aorta down to the knees in this 48-year-old male, although there are some arteriosclerotic plaques in the lower aorta (*arrow*) and at the origins of the common iliac arteries. The femoral artery and its branches are normal; the catheter can be seen entering the right femoral artery (*small arrows*).

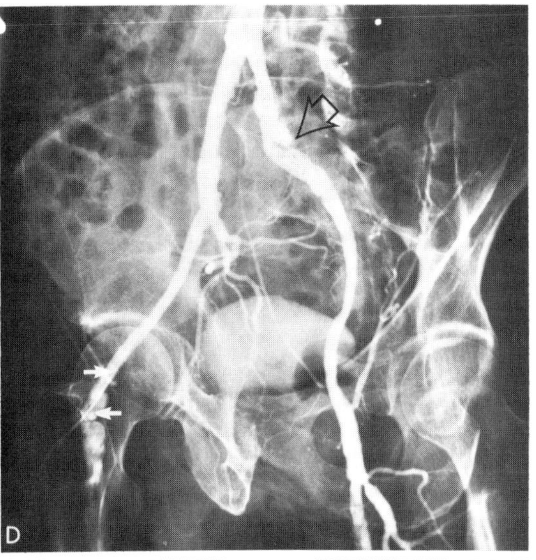

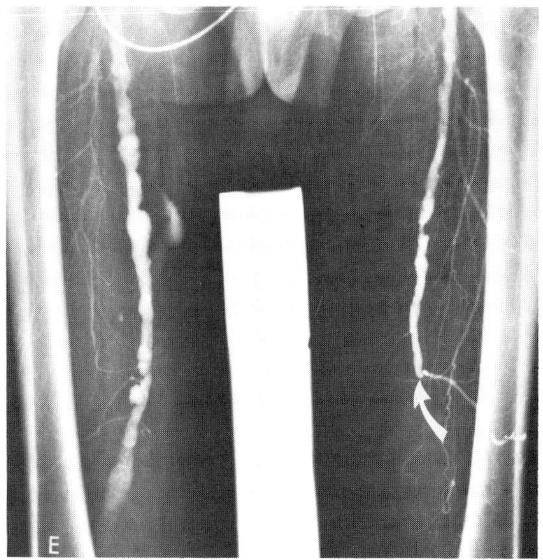

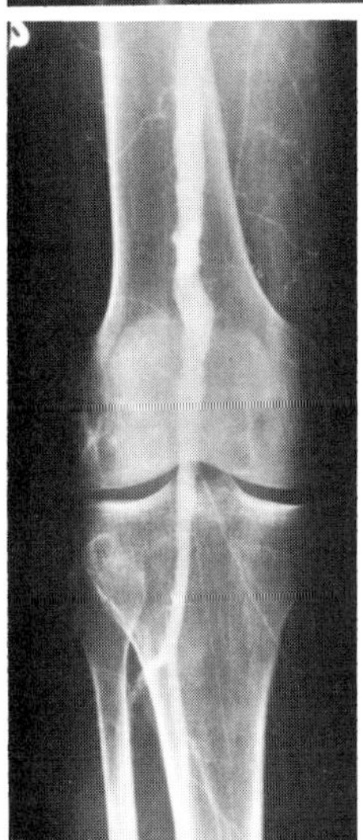

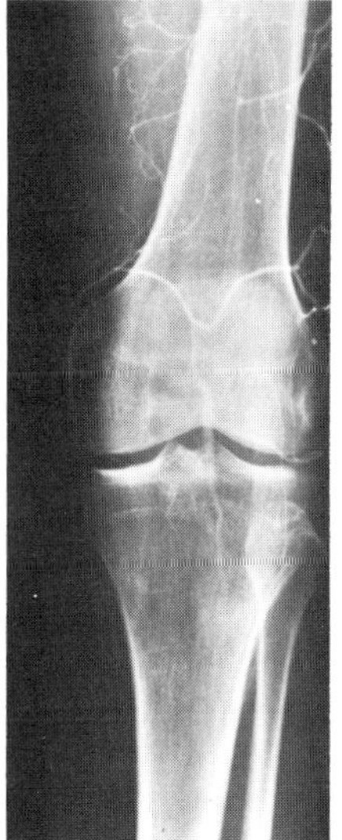

Figure 4–12. *Continued.* *D*, *E*, and *F*, Aortofemoral arteriogram of a patient with severe arteriosclerotic disease. There is complete occlusion of the left internal iliac artery at its origin (*hollow arrow*) and of the left superficial femoral artery (*large arrow*), with reconstitution of the left popliteal artery via collateral vessels. The beading of both femoral arteries is pronounced, although the vessels on the right are patent. The catheter can be seen entering the right femoral artery (*small arrows*).

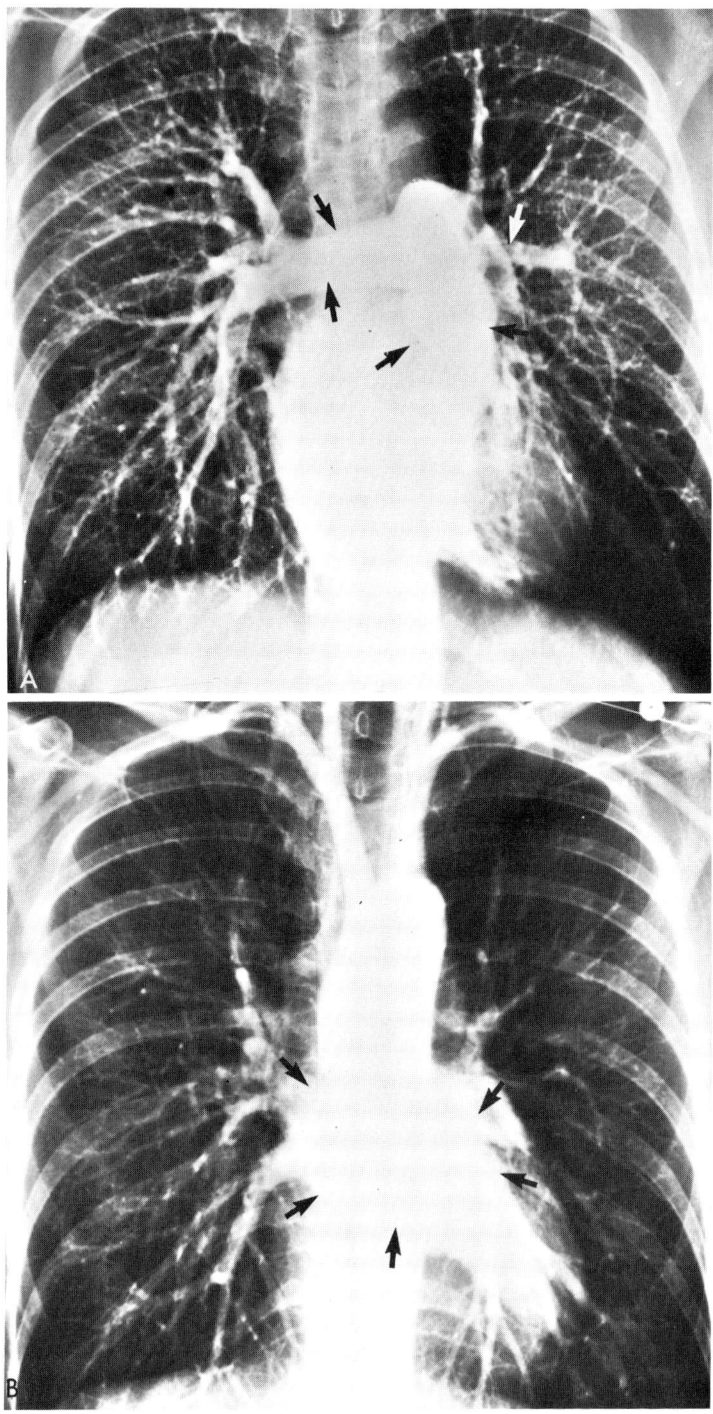

Figure 4–13. Normal pulmonary angiogram, arterial phase (*A*) and venous phase (*B*). The injection is made into the right side of the heart and the main pulmonary artery, and the division into the left and right pulmonary arteries (*arrows*) and the ramifications of the arteries out into the lungs are well seen. In the venous phase (*B*), the venous return to the left atrium (*arrows*) is at a lower level than the main arterial bifurcation. Note the relatively equal distribution of both arteries and veins in the lung fields.

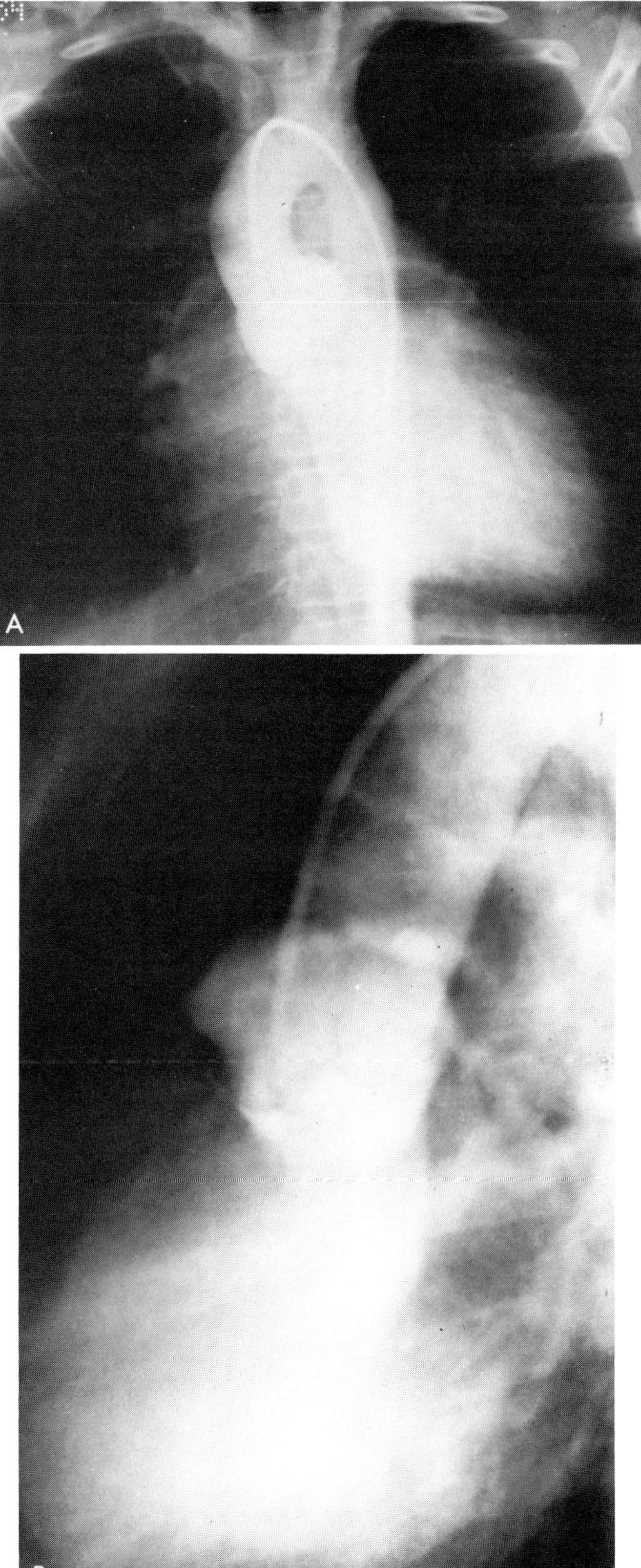

Figure 4–14. Angiogram demonstrating aortic insufficiency, AP view (*A*) and lateral view (*B*). This 10-year-old boy with ventricular septal defect and aortic regurgitation had been followed for many years. The catheter is placed in the aortic root. Marked aortic regurgitation into a dilated left ventricle is apparent. Little shunting into the right heart can be seen.

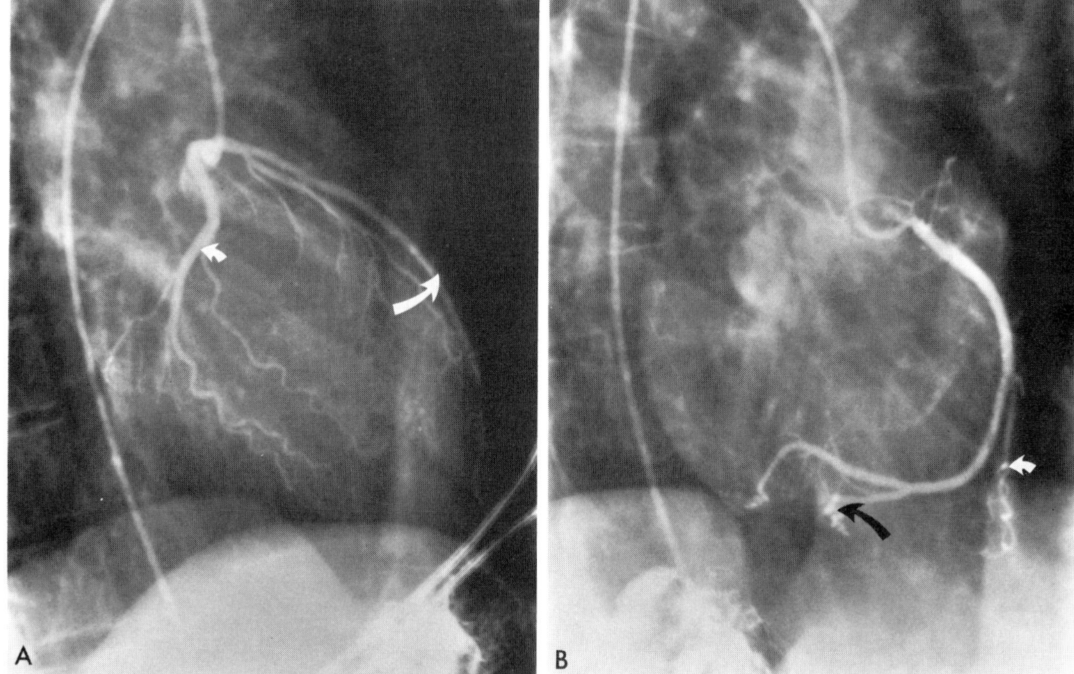

Figure 4–15. Normal coronary arteriogram. *A*, Left coronary artery in RAO projection. The catheter is in the left main coronary artery, and the two branches can be clearly seen: the circumflex (*small arrow*) and the left anterior descending arteries (*large arrow*). *B*, Right coronary artery in a steep RAO projection. There has been selective catheterization of the origin of the artery, and the posterior lateral branch to the left ventricle can be seen (*small arrow*) as well as the posterior descending branches (*large arrow*).

the calf and in the search for the origin of emboli. Occlusions due to thrombophlebitis can be easily demonstrated with this procedure. Venography is also used for the investigation of varicose veins and the preoperative evaluation of perforating veins. In the arm, venography is useful in looking for axillary vein thrombosis or in assessing the superior vena caval syndrome, which is caused by obstruction secondary to tumors, mediastinitis, or superior mediastinal masses. Inferior vena caval obstruction can be identified using lower limb venography, and renal vein thrombosis may be visualized by means of a selective catheterization technique in the inferior vena cava itself (Fig. 4–16). This method may also be utilized to evaluate renal vein renin levels or to selectively sample the adrenal venous blood in searching for elevated catecholamine levels in patients with suspected pheochromocytomas. Finally, the investigation of the portal venous system can be achieved in a number of ways, including direct splenic puncture and transhepatic portal venography. This is important in the identification of esophageal and gastric varices in patients with portal hypertension and cirrhosis.

Neuroradiology

For many years, neuroradiology was the only separate subspecialty within the discipline of diagnostic radiology. Although it is somewhat confusing to separate cerebral arteriography from general angiography and myelography from the other procedures using iodinated contrast material that were outlined in the previous chapter, the degree of sophistication required by neuroradiologists suggests that it is easier to consider neuroradiological procedures as a separate entity. Moreover, although the advent of computerized tomographic (CT) scanning has revolutionized the whole field of radiology, it is as a *noninvasive* neuroradiological technique that CT scanning has found its principal use. (For a

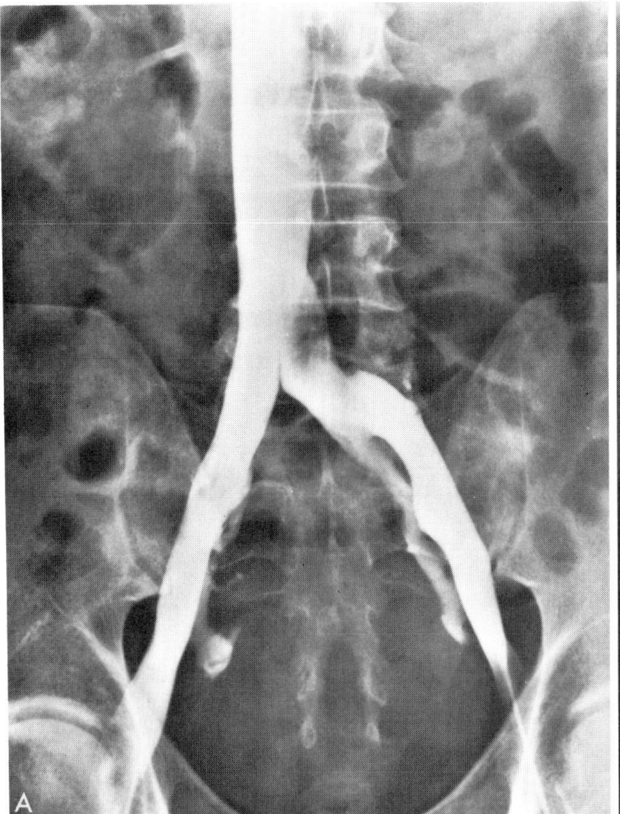

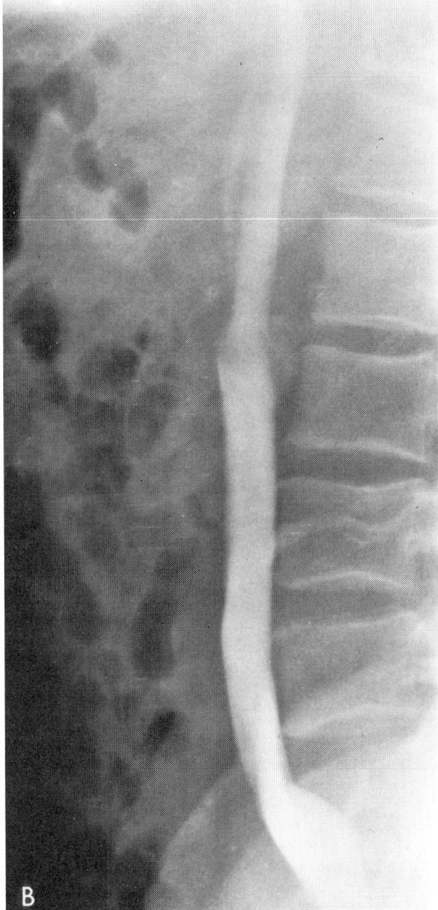

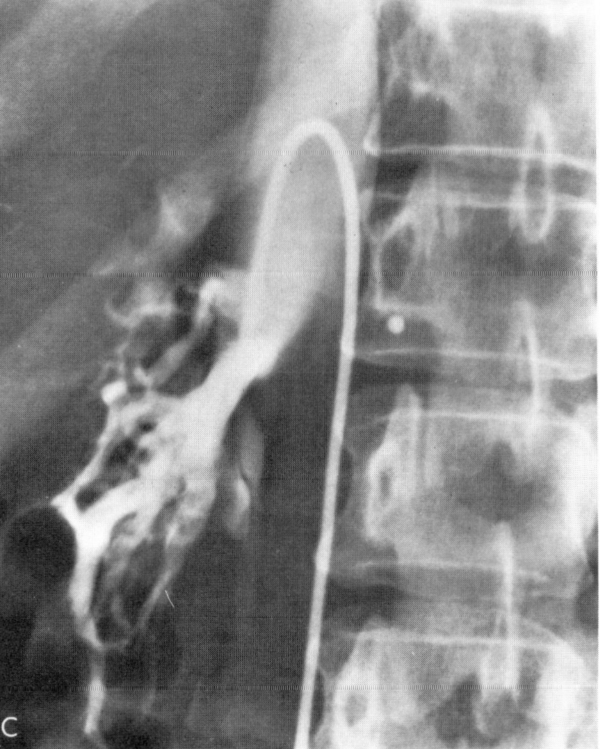

Figure 4–16. Venography. *A*, Normal AP view. Injection of contrast material into the iliac veins will demonstrate the normal inferior vena cava. *B*, The lateral view is the other most useful projection for visualization of the vena cava. *C*, The renal veins, however, require selective catheterization. The filling defects are caused by nonopacified blood from other veins entering the system.

discussion of computerized tomography, see Chapter 7 and page 93.)

Myelography

An intrathecal injection of a contrast agent into the spinal subarachnoid space results in a myelogram (Fig. 4–17A). In the majority of myelograms, positive contrast material is used, in the form of an iodinated oil or a water-soluble opaque material (a more recent development that obviates the need to remove the contrast at the end of the procedure). Air can also be used as a contrast agent, and air myelography can be extremely useful in investigating spinal lesions that involve the cervical cord or in evaluating pediatric spinal injuries. Air myelography is usually performed in association with tomography. One primary indication for myelography is suspected disc disease (Fig. 4–17B), but it can also be used for localizing primary and secondary tumors of the spinal cord and for demonstrating a total or partial block of the subarachnoid canal. With this procedure, it is

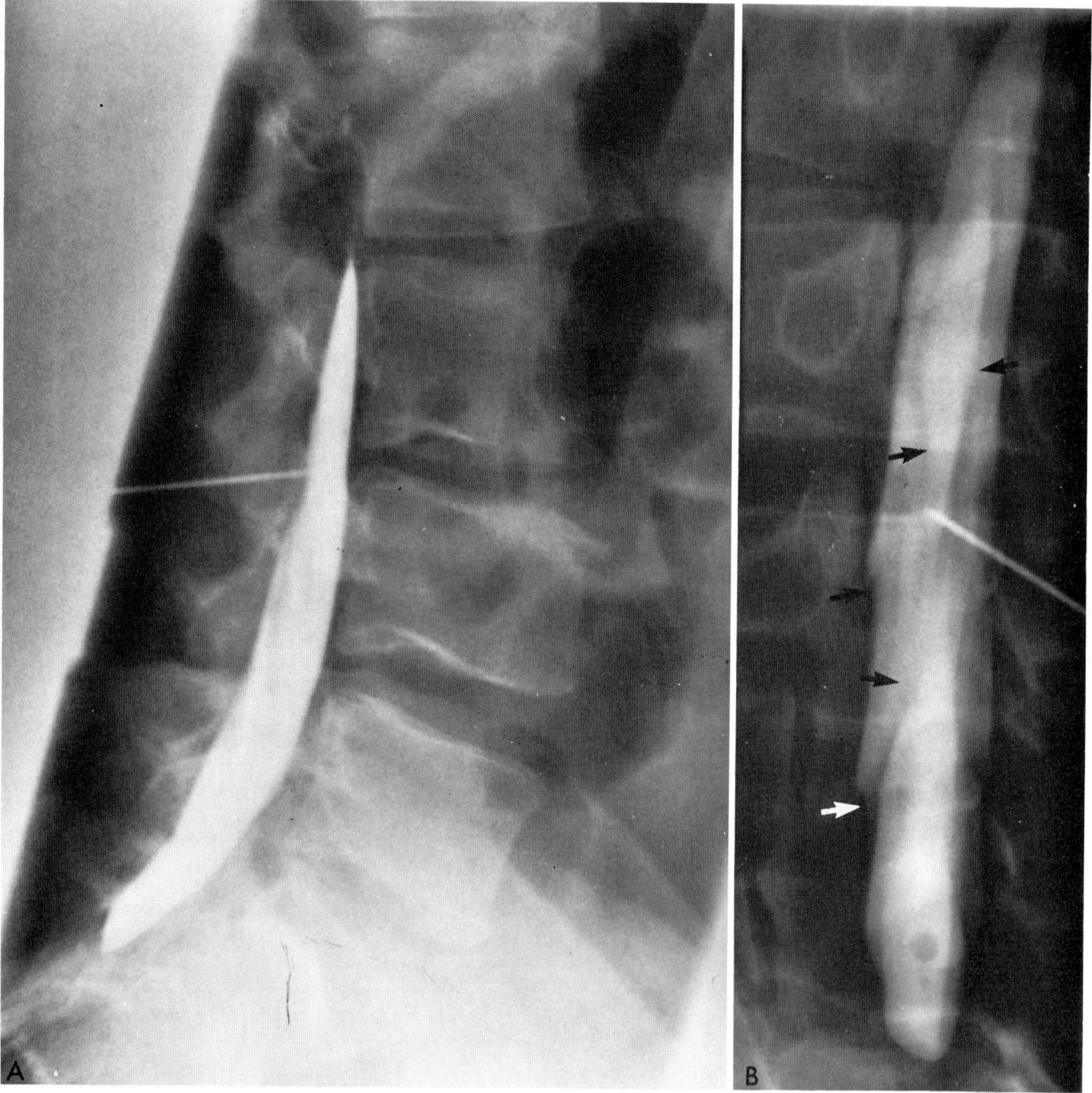

Figure 4–17. Normal myelogram, lateral view (*A*) and RAO view (*B*). The lumbar puncture needle has been inserted in the space between L3 and L4 and contrast has been injected. At this level, the spinal canal "proper" has ended, and all that can be seen are the nerve roots (*arrows*).

possible to distinguish intradural from extradural lesions and intramedullary from extramedullary masses. Contrast is most often injected into the lumbar region, and if iodinated oil is used, the needle either is left in place or is reintroduced to remove as much of the oil as possible. (The oil is removed for fear of its causing arachnoiditis, although this fear is more prevalent on the American subcontinent than in the rest of the world.) The cervical approach for myelography using a lateral C1–2 injection or a cisternal puncture is utilized for delineating the upper margins of lesions of the spinal cord in patients with complete block that makes a lower route for contrast injection impossible. Myelography can be supplemented by other procedures such as iliolumbar (spinal) venography and discography.

Cerebral Arteriography

Preliminary studies such as precede angiographic studies of other parts of the body are rarely performed before cerebral arteriography. A high thoracic aortic injection (a "four-vessel" study) may, however, precede selective catheterization of intracranial vessels. With this examination, it is possible to assess the main branches of the aortic arch supplying the head. Selective catheterization and opacification of the carotid arteries demonstrates the anterior and middle cerebral arteries. Selective opacification of the vertebral arteries as they arise from the subclavian arteries demonstrates the basilar and posterior cerebral arteries. Usually, simultaneous AP and lateral rapid-sequence films are taken following the injection of contrast material, allowing one to see the cerebral circulation in two planes (Fig. 4–18). Frequently, cerebral angiography is performed using subtraction techniques with or without magnification.

Cerebral arteriography is used for the delineation of arteriovenous malformations, aneurysms, bleeding points, infarcts, and tumors. This procedure will define the degree and extent of arteriosclerotic involvement not only of the arteries supplying the brain but also of those located in the cerebrum itself. Although CT scanning is now widely used in the evaluation of intracerebral lesions, angiography is still done because it gives information (detailed vascular anatomy, for example) not supplied by the CT scanner. CT scanning has largely replaced angiography in the investigation of subdural hematomas and cerebrovascular accidents (produced by infarcts or hemorrhages), except when the process is acute and there is a possibility of surgical intervention.

External carotid arteriography is performed to look for evidence of temporal arteritis. In addition, this procedure is useful for the investigation of the blood supply to facial tumors, for looking for vascular and facial anomalies prior to plastic surgery on the face, for searching for meningeal blood supply to intracranial tumors, and for embolization in the treatment of intractable epistaxis.

Cerebral venous opacification is usually achieved by following on sequential films the contrast agent that was injected intra-arterially as it passes to the venous side. There are some exceptions. In cavernous sinus venography, for example, which is part of the investigation of sellar and suprasellar tumors, opacification of the cavernous sinuses is achieved by injection of the contrast agent into the supraorbital veins, by direct puncture of the sagittal sinus with secondary opacification of the associated cerebral sinuses, or by retrograde injection of the jugular vein.

Pneumoencephalography

Before the advent of CT scanning, the best way to outline the cerebral ventricles and intracranial cisterns was to delineate them using air as the contrast agent. Pneumoencephalography was useful for localizing neoplasms, evaluating congenital anomalies, and investigating hydrocephalus (Fig. 4–19). Although the procedure is now performed less frequently, pneumoencephalography is still indicated for the delineation of sellar and parasellar abnormalities. Running air into the basal cisterns of the brain allows the area of the suprasellar cistern and related structures to be clearly visualized.

During the procedure, the patient sits erect. Air is introduced into the spinal canal via a lumbar puncture needle and is allowed to rise into the cranium. Moving the patient's head in different positions makes it

Text continued on page 93

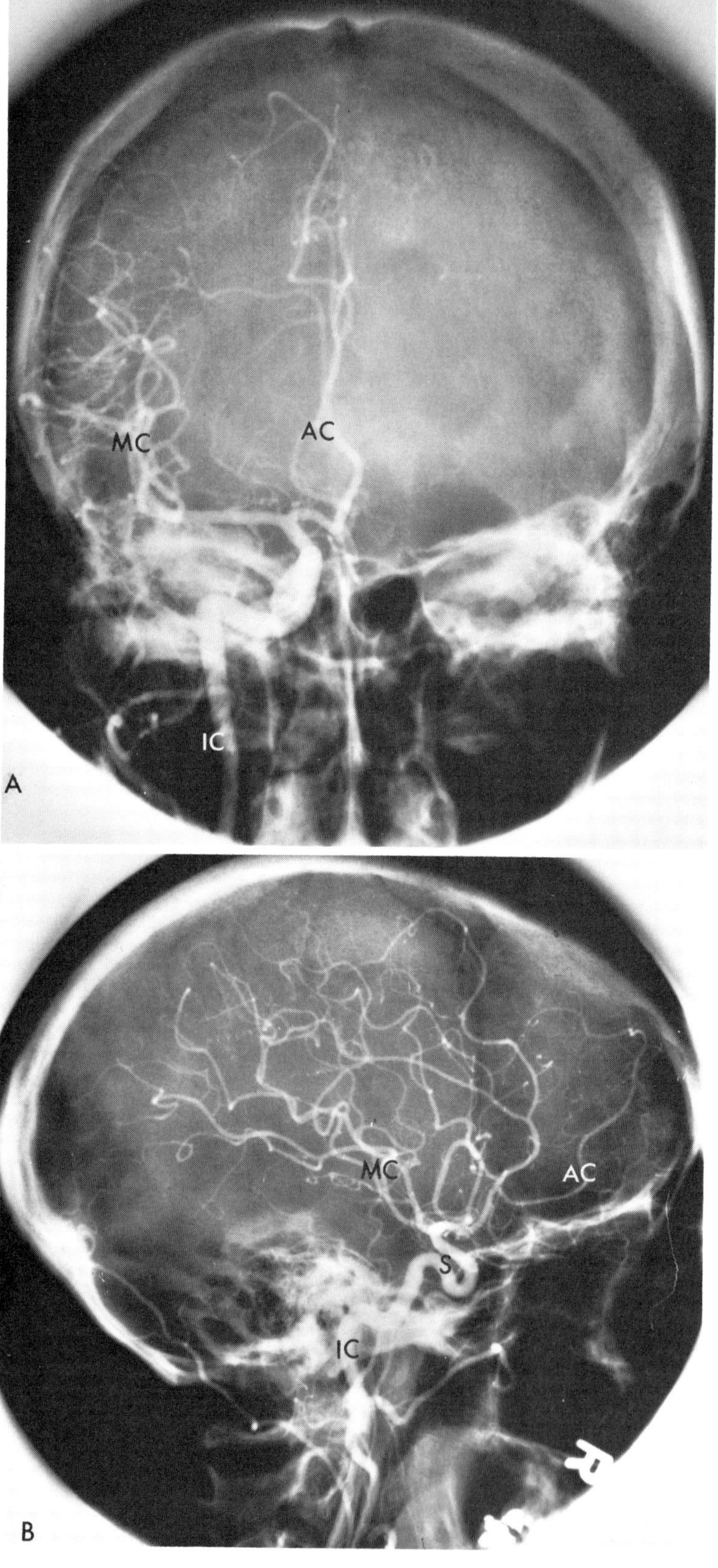

Figure 4–18. Normal carotid arteriogram, frontal view (*A*) and lateral view (*B*). The contrast is injected into the common carotid artery. On the frontal (AP) view, the opacified internal carotid artery (IC) is seen to extend into the skull and to bifurcate into the anterior cerebral (AC) and the middle cerebral (MC) arteries. The lateral view shows the tortuosity of the carotid artery around the sella (carotid siphon, S) before the artery divides into the two vessels. Note the fan-shaped appearance of the middle cerebral group of vessels.

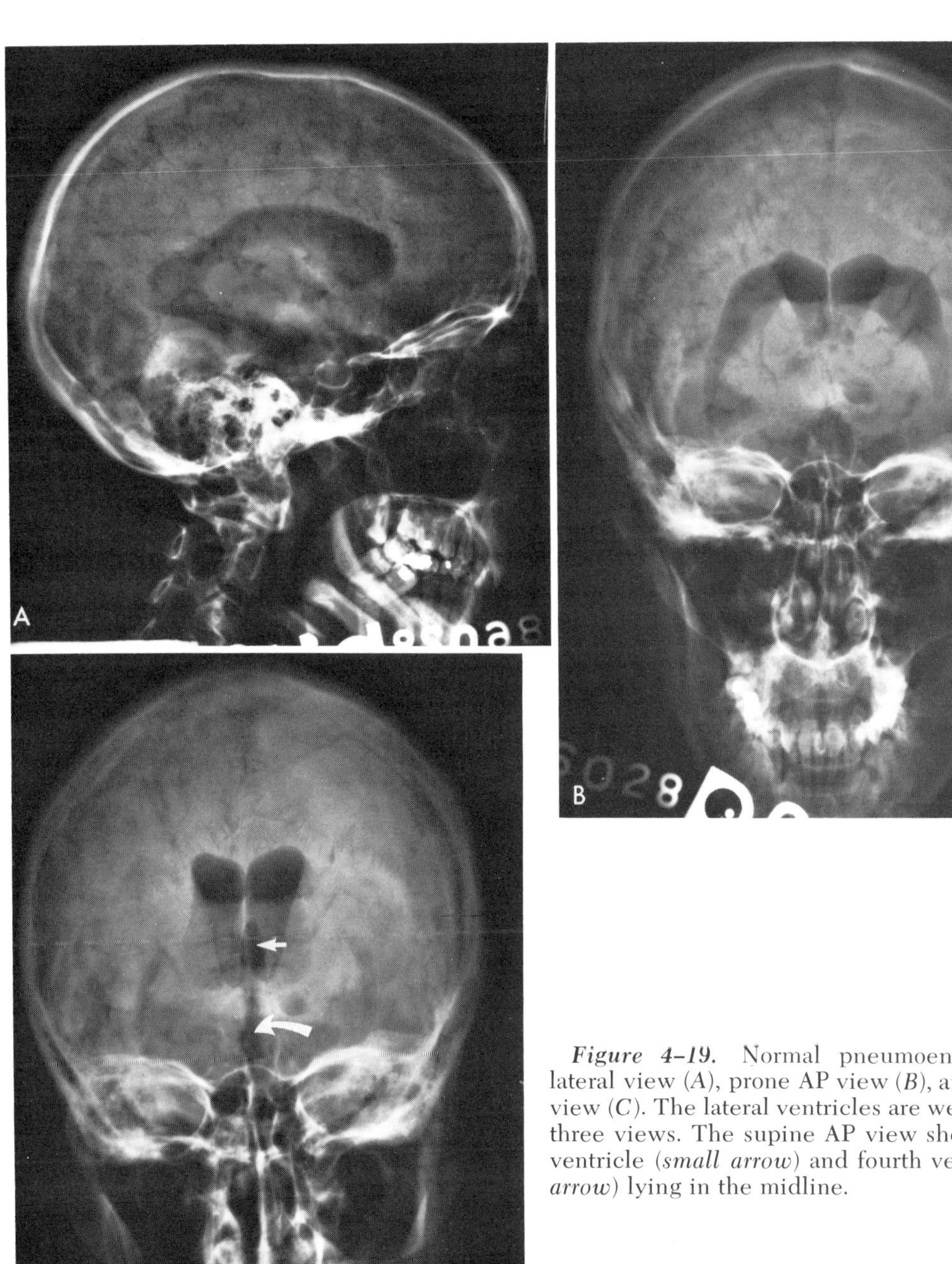

Figure 4–19. Normal pneumoencephalogram, lateral view (*A*), prone AP view (*B*), and supine AP view (*C*). The lateral ventricles are well seen on all three views. The supine AP view shows the third ventricle (*small arrow*) and fourth ventricle (*large arrow*) lying in the midline.

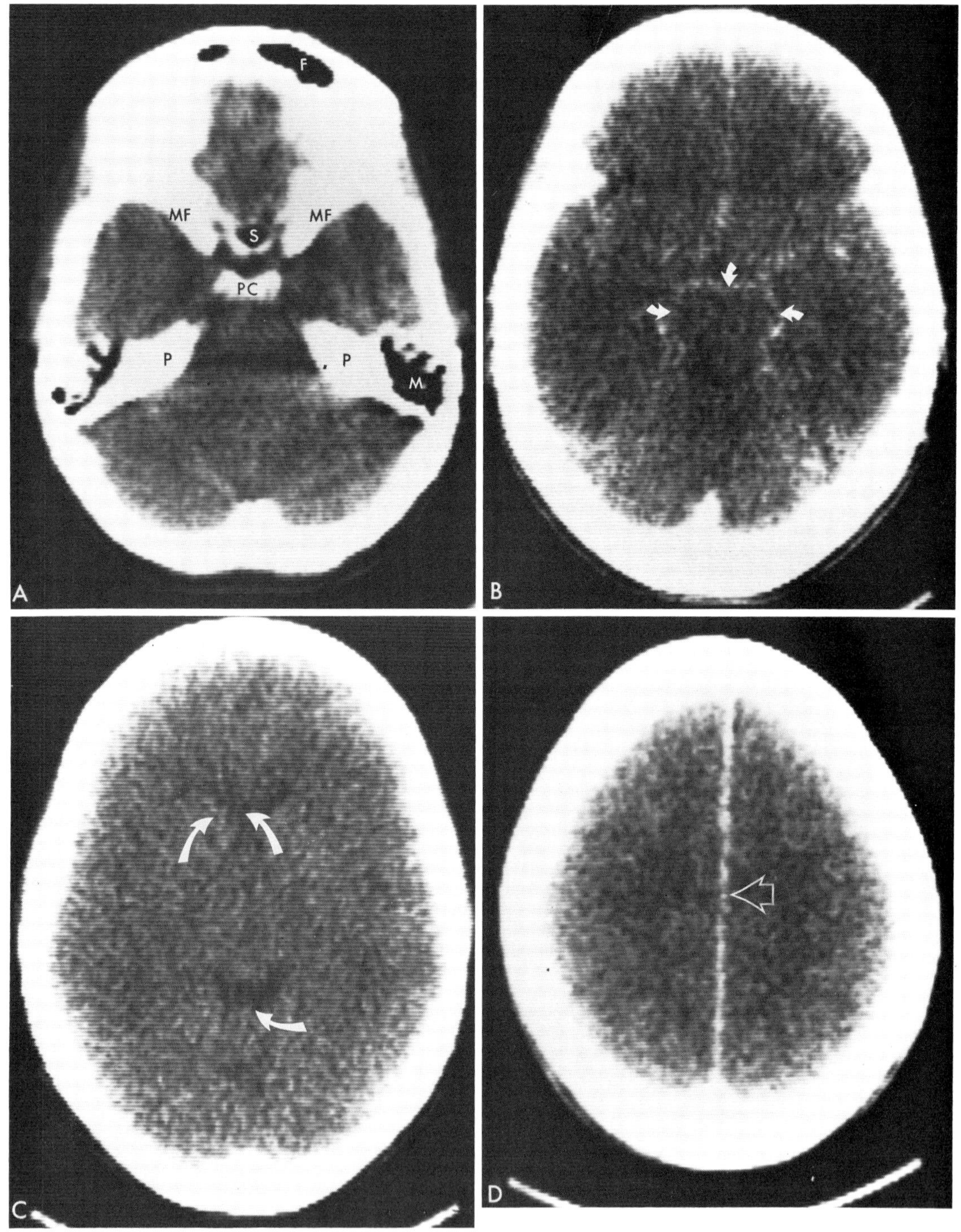

Figure 4–20. Normal CT scan of brain. Four scans from the base of the skull cephalad. *A*, The mastoid air cells (M), petrous pyramids (P), posterior clinoids (PC) and sella, air in sphenoid sinus (S), anterior margins of middle fossa (MF), and air in the frontal sinus (F) are all seen. *B*, Contrast material enhanced a scan at a higher level, showing opacification of the circle of Willis (*arrows*). *C*, At a still higher level, the ventricles can be seen as areas of diminished absorption coefficient (*arrows*). *D*, At the uppermost level, opacification of the superior sagittal sinus is seen. (*hollow arrow*).

possible to move the air selectively from one ventricle to another to provide visualization of the desired cistern or of the convexity of the brain.

An alternative to pneumoencephalography, *ventriculography,* is occasionally still indicated for investigation of suspected internal obstructive hydrocephalus. In this procedure, air is injected directly into the lateral ventricle. The reason for performing a ventriculogram rather than an air encephalogram is the danger of precipitating herniation of the cerebellar tonsils through the foramen magnum, which may occur if a lumbar puncture with fluid withdrawal is performed in a patient whose intracranial pressure has increased. Positive contrast ventriculography can also be performed, but it is rarely used today.

Computerized Tomography

Computerized tomography (CT scanning) has changed the face of radiology, especially neuroradiology. CT scanning produces what amounts to anatomical slices of the brain that can be studied without the patient's having to undergo any more painful procedure than an intravenous injection of an iodinated contrast agent (Fig. 4–20). The scientific principle of CT scanning is discussed in Chapter 7; basically, the technique allows us to differentiate tissues of only slightly differing density such as cerebrospinal fluid, grey and white matter, and neoplasms. Differentiation between blood-containing areas and avascular areas can be enhanced greatly by the intravenous injection of iodinated contrast material. Indications for CT scanning of the brain are the same as for neuroradiology. CT scanning is especially useful as a screening procedure for subsequent neuroradiological investigation of the patient. Indications for the use of CT scanning therefore include: suspected tumors (to determine size, location, and often, type), hemorrhage and infarction (old or recent), cortical atrophy, hydrocephalus, intracranial malformations and calcifications, cranial abscesses (for which serial studies will show the effects of treatment), and virtually any suspicious central neurological signs and symptoms.

Although CT scanning has largely supplanted cerebral arteriography and pneumoencephalography, a number of indications for these studies still remain. Arteriography is used in the diagnosis of vascular disorders, atherosclerosis, arteriovenous malformations, aneurysms, and emboli. Air studies are still indicated in the investigation of sellar lesions and internal hydrocephalus.

OTHER SPECIAL PROCEDURES

Bronchography

Instilling an opaque material into the trachea and bronchial tree allows visualization of the outline of the major and minor bronchi. This can be achieved using barium, iodinated oily media, or powdered tantalum, and the contrast can be instilled through tracheal catheterization or percutaneous transcricoid injection. Bronchography is useful for demonstrating evidence of bronchiectasis, bronchial obstruction, and other deformities as well as for investigating patients with chronic bronchitis to ascertain the degree of damage, distortion, bronchial dilatation, and mucous plugging (Fig. 4–21). Bronchography is performed in patients whose chest x-rays suggest bronchiectasis or chronic middle lobe syndrome and patients with unexplained densities and fibrosis, particularly in the lower zones. This technique seems to have become less popular, probably because of the development of fibro-optic bronchoscopy and brush or needle biopsies as well as the decline in incidence of the postinfective sequelae of infections and tuberculosis of the lungs.

Laryngography

Indications for laryngography include alteration of phonation, change of voice, chronic hoarseness, spitting up blood, dyspnea, pain and swelling in the throat, and difficulty in swallowing. A laryngogram is performed by anesthetizing the patient's oropharynx and larynx and coating the laryngeal area with an opaque oily material (Dionosil). The contrast agent is usually dropped into the larynx through a curved cannula, which is inserted with flu-

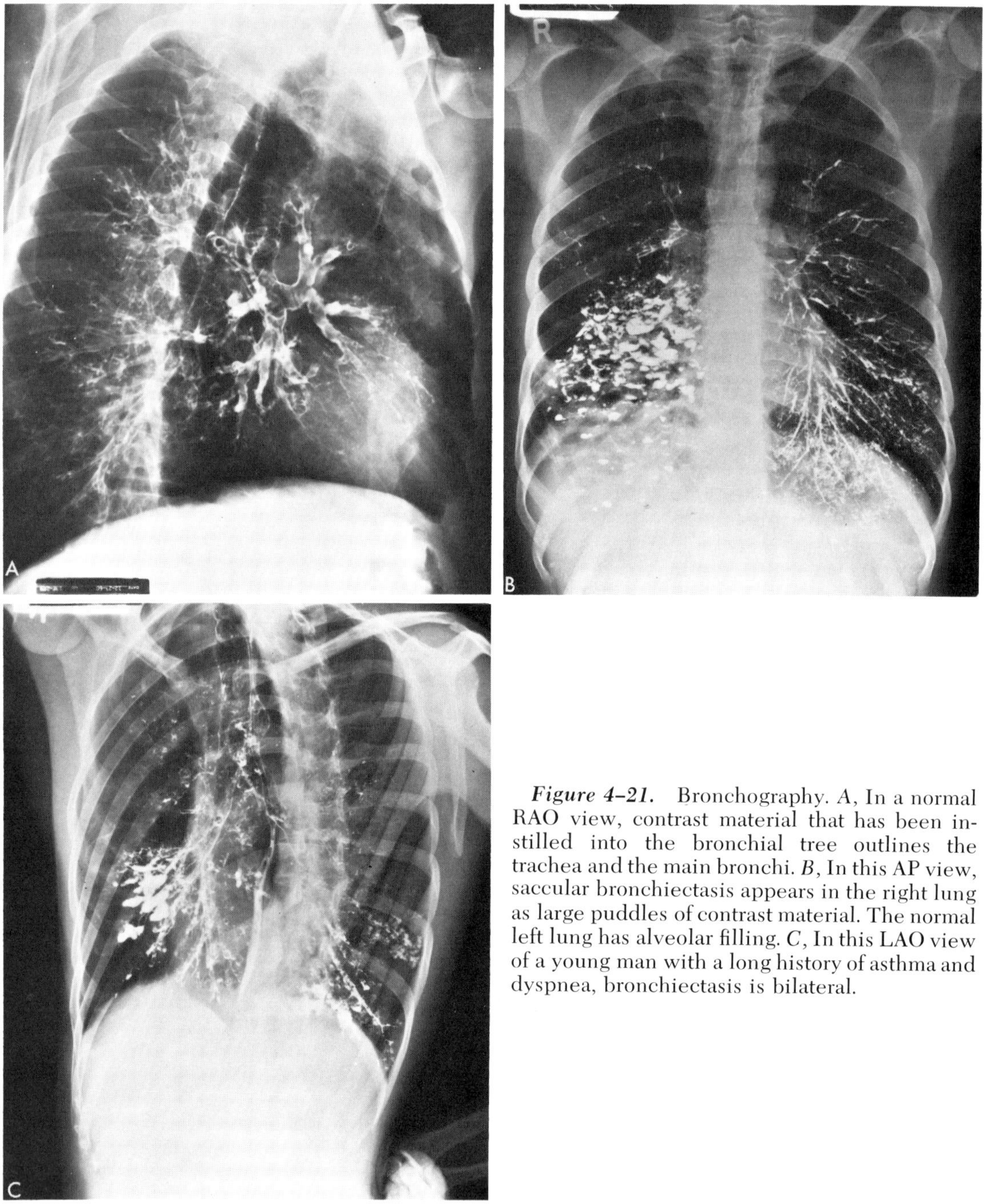

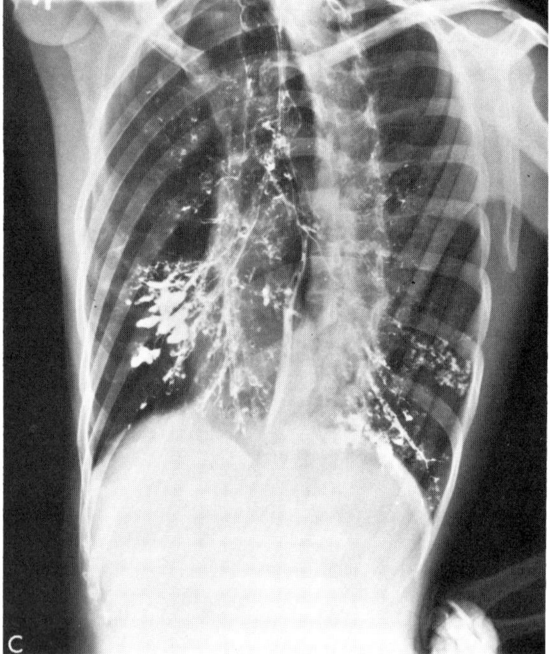

Figure 4–21. Bronchography. *A*, In a normal RAO view, contrast material that has been instilled into the bronchial tree outlines the trachea and the main bronchi. *B*, In this AP view, saccular bronchiectasis appears in the right lung as large puddles of contrast material. The normal left lung has alveolar filling. *C*, In this LAO view of a young man with a long history of asthma and dyspnea, bronchiectasis is bilateral.

oroscopic guidance. A laryngogram provides visualization of the whole larynx, including the pyriform sinuses, valleculae, true and false cords, as well as laryngeal tumors or other abnormalities, particularly those involving the cords or adjacent tissues (Fig. 4–22).

Sialography

The clinical indications for sialography (radiographic examination of the salivary glands) include alteration in the pattern of salivation, intermittent or sustained salivary gland swelling, presence of a mass

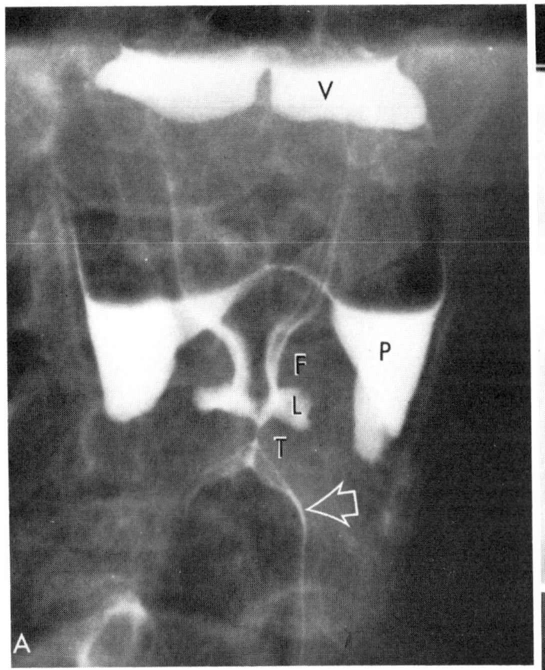

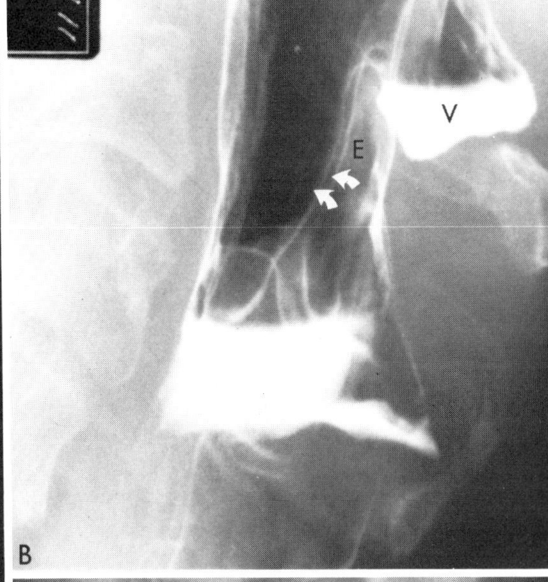

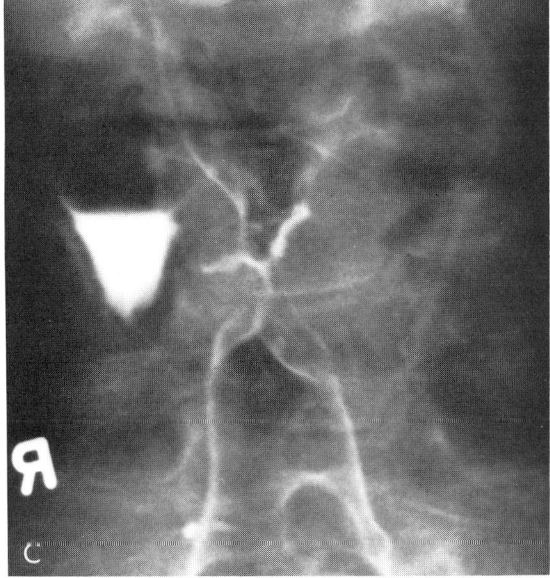

Figure 4–22. Laryngography. *A* and *B*, Normal AP and lateral views. Contrast material is seen pooling in the vallecula (V) at the base of the tongue. On the lateral view (*B*), the epiglottis is visible (E). Good distension of the pyriform sinuses (P) and delineation of the ariepiglottic folds (*arrows*) may be seen. Contrast material delineates both the true (T) and false (F) vocal cords, with the laryngeal ventricles (L) lying between them. Contrast material has also outlined the upper trachea (*hollow arrow*). *C*, This AP view shows distortion of the normal anatomy caused by a squamous cell carcinoma of the left vocal cord.

within a salivary gland, and calcifications related to the salivary glands. Calculi, both small and large, may be shown in the glands or ducts where they can obstruct. There may be alterations in the parenchyma of the glands, such as occurs in Sjögren's syndrome. A mass (benign or malignant) may be demonstrated by distortion of the normal arborization within the gland itself. Sialectasis may also be present. This is equivalent to bronchiectasis and has similar causes such as abnormal secretions or congenital abnormalities. Injecting an oily contrast agent into either Stensen's or Wharton's duct makes it possible to opacify the parotid or submaxillary salivary glands (Fig. 4–23). Sialography is rarely performed on the sublingual glands because they often have multiple ducts.

Lymphography

There are two main indications for lymphography, or lymphangiography: checking the integrity of the lymphatic system

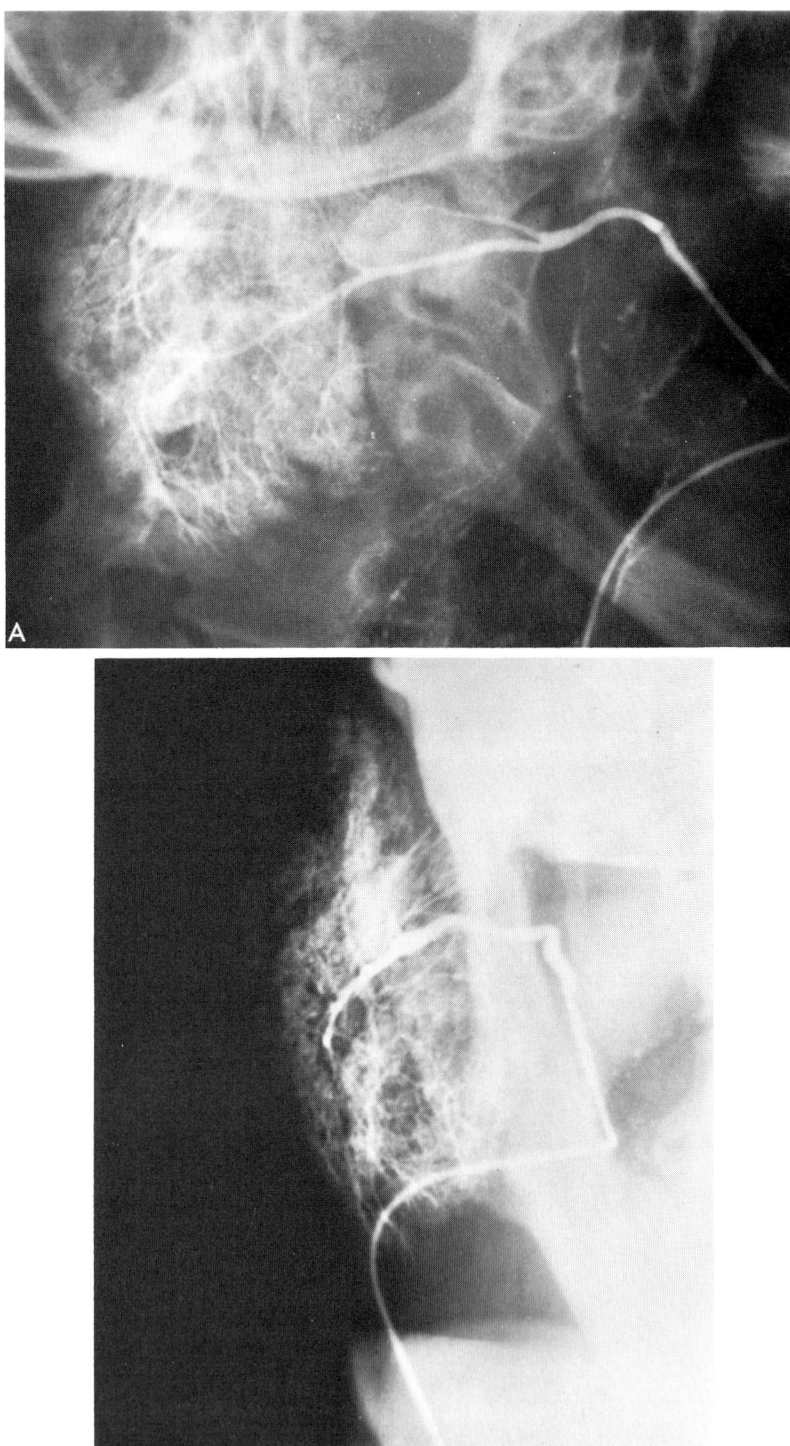

Figure 4–23. Sialography of the parotid gland, lateral view (*A*) and AP view (*B*). The normal duct and gland are shown. Note the extensive arborization within the gland.

itself, as in parasitic disease (elephantiasis), and much more commonly, investigating tumors (either lymphoma or metastatic spread of cancer). The procedure is also used in looking for evidence of retroperitoneal tumors and of distortion or displacement of the lymph nodes by secondary pressure effects or by direct involvement. Lymphography is usually performed for visualization of the abdominal lymph nodes. Iodinated oil is slowly injected into a lymph vessel on the dorsum of each foot, opacifying the lymphatics of the leg, the inguinal regions, the lymphatics of the iliac area, and the retroperitoneum up to the thoracic duct (Fig. 4–24A). The contrast agent slowly accumulates and a 24-hour plain abdominal radiograph should show almost total opacification of the pelvic and para-aortic lymph nodes. Lymphoma classically produces enlarged "foamy" nodes, whereas metastases produce filling defects (Fig. 4–24B). Pressure effects of retroperitoneal tumors may also be observed. It is unwise to interpret the appearance of lymph nodes below the inguinal ligament, because those nodes in the groin often become enlarged or inflamed in association with infections of the leg or toes or around the buttocks.

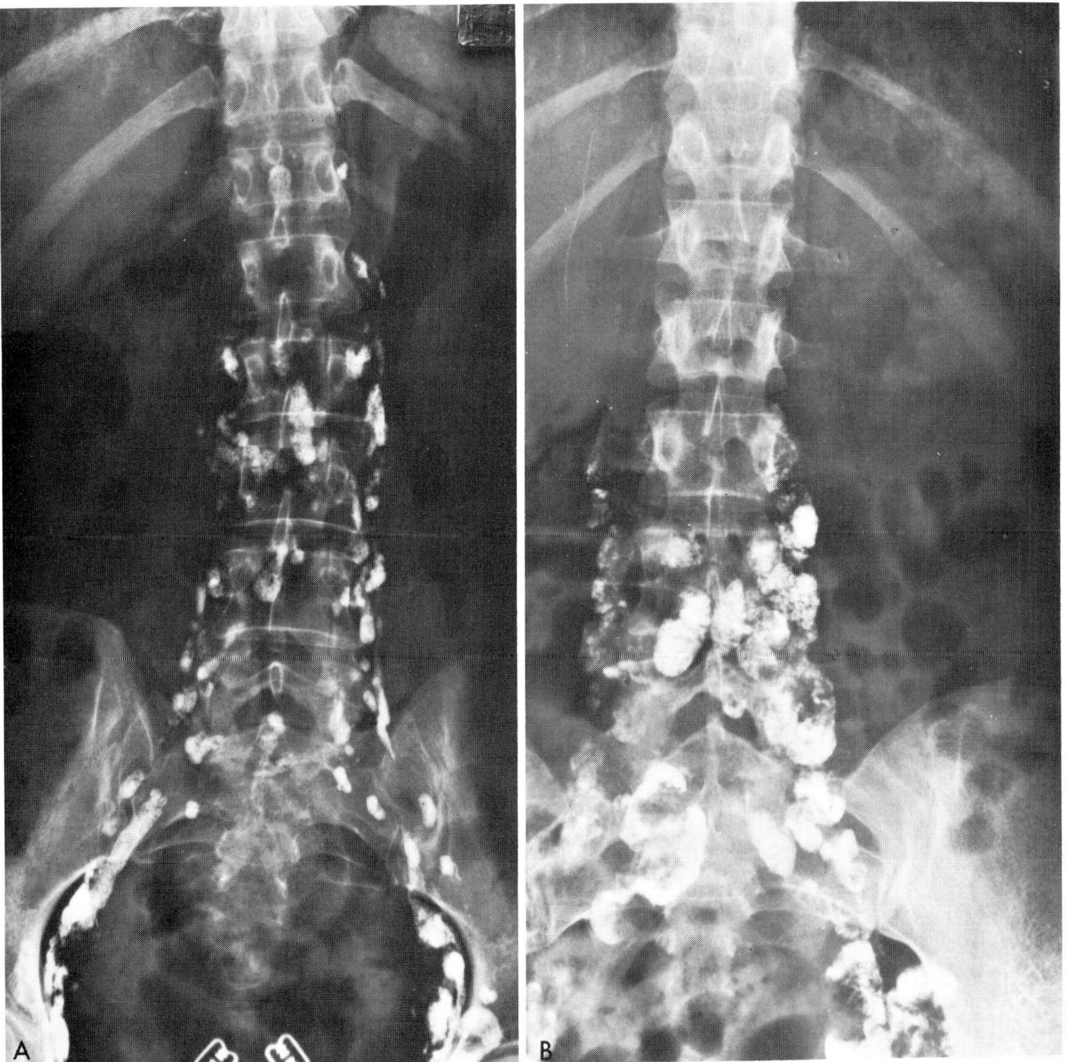

Figure 4–24. Lymphography. *A*, A normal 24-hour film from a lymphogram demonstrates small, well-circumscribed lymph nodes with a homogeneous appearance. *B*, In lymphoma, the lymph nodes enlarge and become "foamy," as occurred in this female patient with Hodgkin's disease.

Discography

Although most of the radiological information concerning a slipped disc can be obtained from the plain films, myelography, or spinal venography, it is occasionally necessary to confirm the pathological changes by an injection of water-soluble contrast agent directly into the disc space (Fig. 4–25). This is achieved by using a long lumbar needle and approaching from a position just lateral to the midline. Usually, three or more disc spaces are injected. In a normal patient, the contrast agent appears as a puddle at the end of the needle, demonstrating the integrity of the annulus fibrosus. In a ruptured disc, however, the contrast seeps out either anteriorly or posteriorly, and the diagnosis is easy to make. Discography is now rarely performed, possibly owing to the risks of infection or of causing further damage or to the difficulty of interpreting the results.

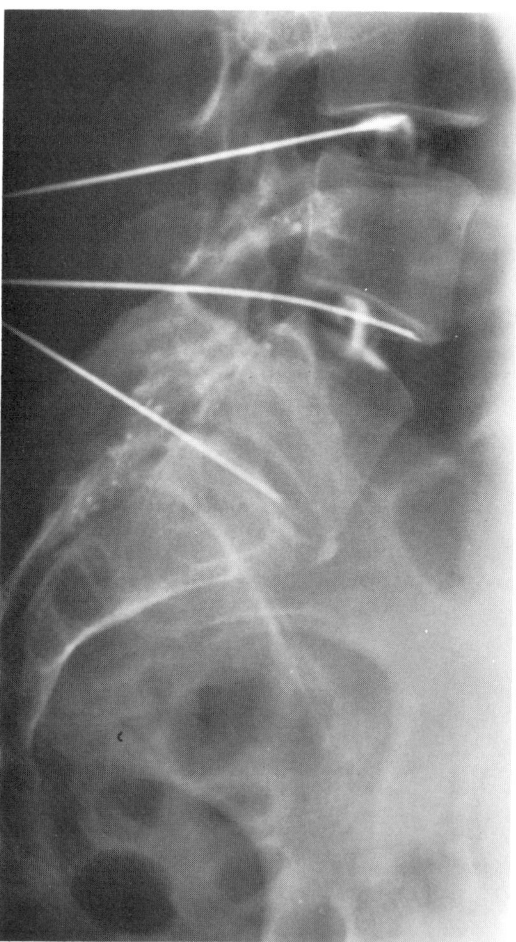

Figure 4–25. Normal discography. Needles have been inserted into the disc spaces at the L3–4, L4–5, and L5–1 levels. Contrast material is seen as a puddle in the central part of each disc space.

Mammography

Although mammography is performed using only plain films, it is generally considered to be a special procedure. The indications for mammography include a mass in the breast, painful nodularity, change in shape of the breast, and nipple discharge. Mammography should be performed in two planes: with an axial (top to bottom) view and a lateral view (Fig. 4–26A and 4–26B). Special x-ray tubes, special films, and even special processing techniques are used. The aim is to produce high-resolution radiographs of the breast with the smallest radiation dose possible. Unfortunately, radiographic mammography is still associated with a high-radiation dose and so should not be performed indiscriminately. Screening populations of women who are susceptible to breast cancer every 6 months is reasonable, but mammography should probably not be used as a routine screening technique on women under 50. Radiographically, one looks for distortion of the parenchyma, a single large mass, which is probably malignant, or multiple masses and cysts, which usually represent chronic mastitis, fibrocystic disease, or fibronodular disease, all of which are benign (Fig. 4–26C). Supportive radiographic evidence for breast cancer includes large blood vessels, skin thickening (which can be seen clinically as "peau d'orange"), microcalcifications, and loss of definition of the margins of the mass. Unfortunately, marked physiological changes occur in breast tissue; whereas the young female breast is fairly solid and homogeneous, age causes fatty involution to occur throughout the breast parenchyma, ultimately leaving only the stroma and ductal systems visible within a large mass of fatty tissue. Thus, a breast cancer is often hidden in this changing background, and mammograms require as much expertise to interpret as most special films.

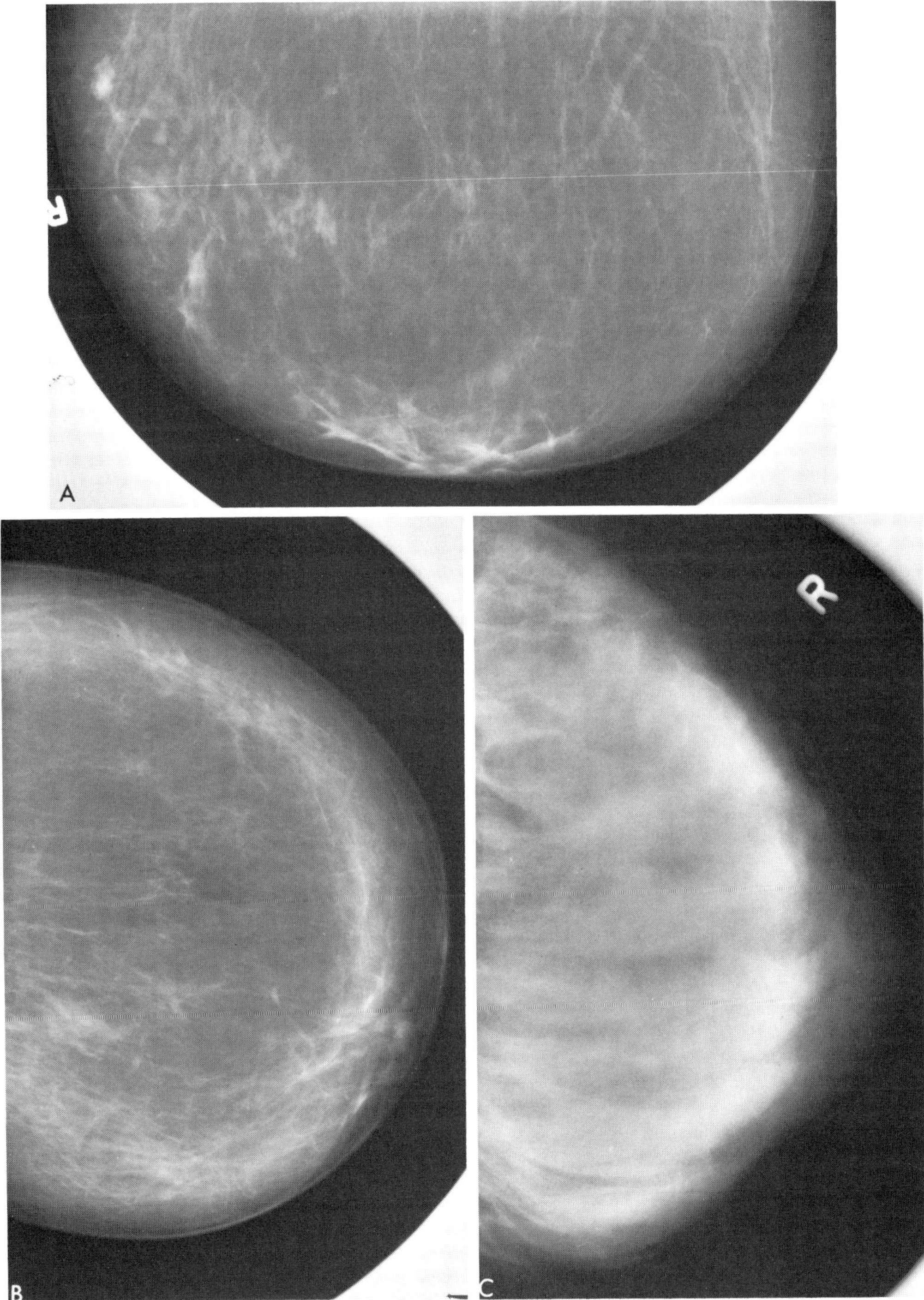

Figure 4–26. Normal mammography. *A* and *B*, Superoinferior and lateral views of a postmenopausal patient. Fat has largely replaced the denser tissue seen in the breasts of younger patients. The solid calcification seen on the lateral aspect in the superoinferior view was found to be benign. *C*, Normal breast of a patient of childbearing age.

Interventional Radiography

Traditionally, radiologists have been diagnosticians, but more and more investigative procedures are now being performed with radiological guidance. Biopsies of many of the organs in the abdomen are easier to perform if the organ is visible fluoroscopically. The first such biopsies were done on the kidneys (particularly renal cyst puncture after an intravenous pyelogram to ascertain if the lesion was indeed a benign cyst). Liver punctures were performed to enable percutaneous transhepatic cholangiography to be done, and more recently, needle biopsies of the pancreas under ultrasonographic guidance have become common. The reason is not hard to find: these are relatively noninvasive procedures and in a large percentage of cases are diagnostic, thus saving the patient from having to undergo a laparotomy. Lung biopsies used to be done "blind," on the basis of the findings on the plain chest x-ray, but now lung biopsies are mainly done under fluoroscopy. Whether a needle or brush is used depends on the lesion to be biopsied. Fibrooptic bronchoscopy may also be performed using fluoroscopy so that the tip of the bronchoscope can be directed into the specific area of interest. Finally, bone biopsies under fluoroscopic guidance are also becoming more common, to investigate peripheral lesions such solitary lytic metastases from an unknown primary site and to examine the spine, often for possible infection.

Additional Radiological Procedures

Many other special radiological procedures have been performed. Some procedures are in vogue for just a short time, whereas others are used routinely for years. For the sake of completeness, a few will be mentioned here:

1. Diagnostic pneumothorax is used to demonstrate adhesions or pleural masses.
2. Diagnostic pneumoperitoneum demonstrates masses in either the upper or lower abdomen, with the patient in the Trendelenburg position. This is a particularly useful technique for visualizing the uterus and ovaries in laparoscopy and colposcopy.
3. Studies of the lacrimal ducts by direct cannulation reveal calculi, stenoses and tumors.
4. Direct contrast studies of the paranasal sinuses demonstrate polyps, mucoceles and tumors; this procedure is virtually never performed now.
5. Radiological assistance is often used to localize foreign bodies.
6. Localization of the intrauterine fetal abdomen is useful for exchange transfusions.

CHAPTER 5

NUCLEAR MEDICINE

by William D. Kaplan, M.D.

Radionuclide imaging involves the use of unstable atoms, which disintegrate to release energy in the form of gamma rays. Selected organ systems can be imaged when these energetic atoms are coupled to substances that undergo normal physiological processing in a patient. For example, the spleen sequentially removes damaged red cells from the bloodstream. Therefore, if some of a patient's red cells are damaged, are tagged with a radioactive substance and then are reintroduced into the circulation, an image of the spleen can be produced on a screen or film.

Although it is possible to evaluate almost any organ in the body using radionuclide techniques, the liver, spleen, bones, urinary tract, lungs, heart, thyroid, and brain are the organs most frequently investigated in a modern nuclear medicine department.

Production of the radionuclide image ("scan") begins with the emission of gamma rays from an organ and their interaction with a sodium iodide crystal. If the crystal is small (1 inch in width), it must be moved back and forth over an organ such as the thyroid gland in order to image the entire gland; hence the term *scan*.

More recently, a larger crystal (15 inches in width) has been incorporated into an instrument known as a *gamma camera*. This instrument's advantage over the scanner is that large organs can be imaged in a single view (Figure 5–1). The larger surface area can also be used to gather information of a dynamic nature. Function studies facilitate quantitation of a number of physiological processes, such as cardiac blood flow, pulmonary ventilation and perfusion, and renal function.

LIVER–SPLEEN IMAGING

Liver-spleen examinations account for between 30 and 50 per cent of the radionuclide imaging studies performed in clinical nuclear medicine departments. The major diagnostic purposes for which liver-spleen scanning can be used include estimating organ size, investigating diffuse parenchymal diseases (such as seen in alcoholism, hepatitis, and infiltrative tumors), looking for possible space-occupying lesions (such as abscesses, cysts, and neoplasms), as well as following the changes in size of metastases in response to chemotherapy (Figure 5–2).

As opposed to static images, scanning makes it possible to take rapid sequence pictures after intravenous or intra-arterial radionuclide injection to assess the degree

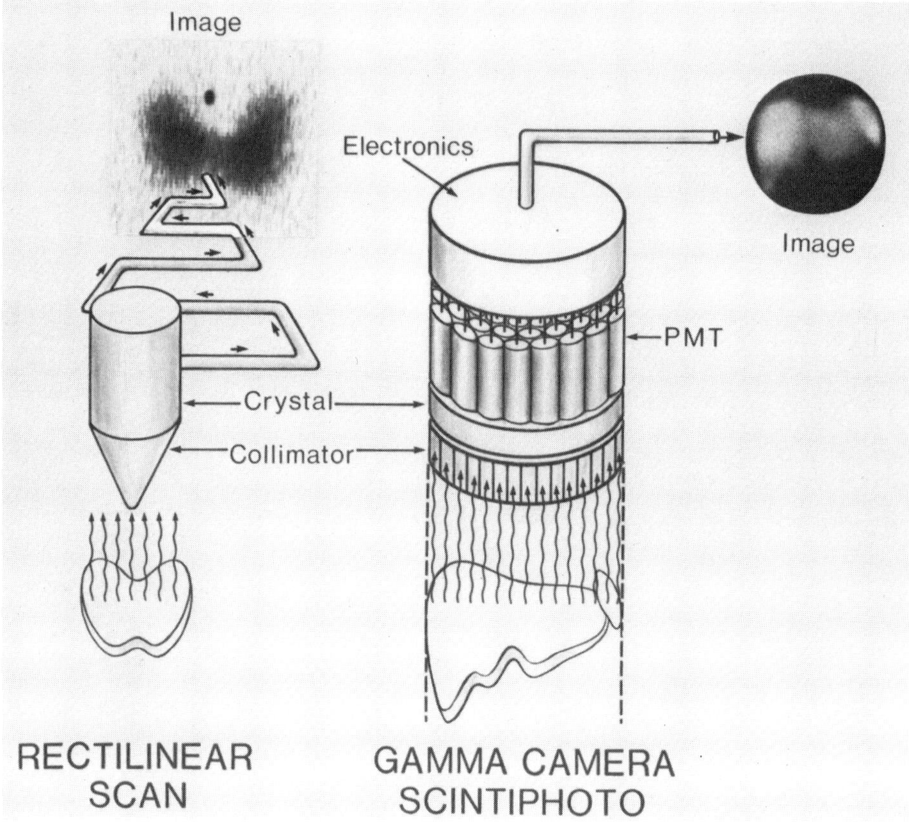

Figure 5–1. Diagrammatic representation of a scanner and a gamma camera. On the left is a conceptual image of a rectilinear scanner. Gamma rays emanating from the thyroid gland enter the "pinhole" collimator to interact with a sodium iodide crystal. Light is produced within the crystal and is converted to electrons in the photomultiplier tube. The crystal moves back and forth over the patient's neck to create the "scan" of the thyroid gland seen at the top. The larger surface area of the crystal in the gamma camera (on the right) allows a large organ such as the liver to be imaged without "scanning"; a representative resultant image is seen at the far right.

of vascularity of intrahepatic lesions. The infusion of radioaggregates in patients receiving intra-arterial infusions of chemotherapeutic agents via hepatic artery catheters has been shown to be of value in assessing the distribution of these agents. This technique allows catheters to be placed for optimal therapeutic effect (Figure 5–3).

The radionuclide evaluation of the hepatobiliary tree can be achieved either as a complementary study or as a supplement to other diagnostic radiological liver studies. The major indications for this procedure are in the differential diagnosis of complete versus incomplete biliary obstruction, and in the further evaluation of focal hepatic defects seen on standard Technetium-99m–sulfur colloid liver scans (Figure 5–4). The agents used are either Iodine-131 (^{131}I) Rose Bengal, which closely resembles Bromsulphalein (BSP) in structure, or Technetium labeled iminodiacetic acid compounds (^{99m}TcHIDA). The advantage of the technetium labeled agents is that they allow visualization of the biliary tree when the serum bilirubin is above 1.5 mg per 100 ml, the point at which oral cholecystography is not helpful. In children, these agents can help in identifying choledochal cysts and are useful in evaluating biliary atresia.

Since the sensitivity, or true positivity rate, of a liver scan in the detection of hepatic abnormalities is greater than 85 per cent, this study should be one of the first procedures used in evaluating patients with po-

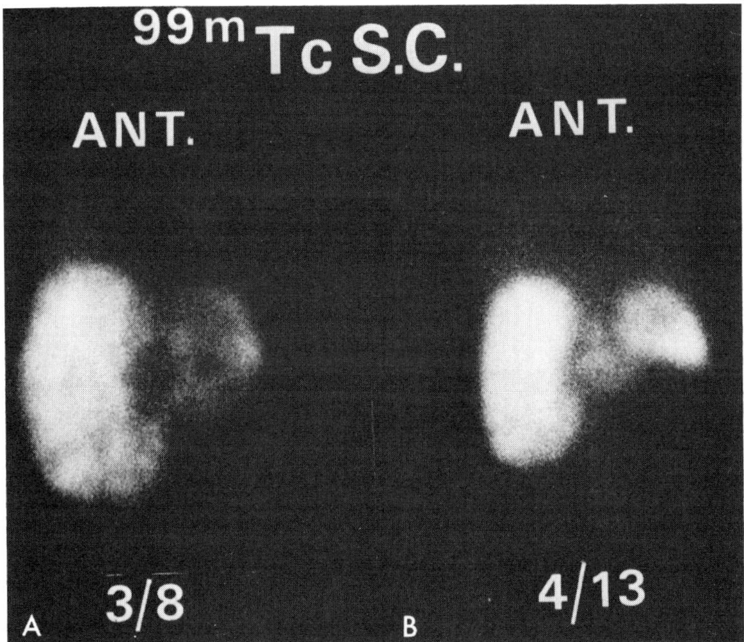

Figure 5–2. Response of metastases to chemotherapy. Two anterior views of the liver and spleen taken after ^{99m}Tc-sulfur colloid administration are seen. *A*, There is an enlarged liver with a large focal defect interposed between the right and left lobes as well as a smaller defect in the left lobe. *B*, After five weeks of chemotherapy, there is marked decrease in the overall size of the liver as well as significant resolution of the two intrahepatic defects.

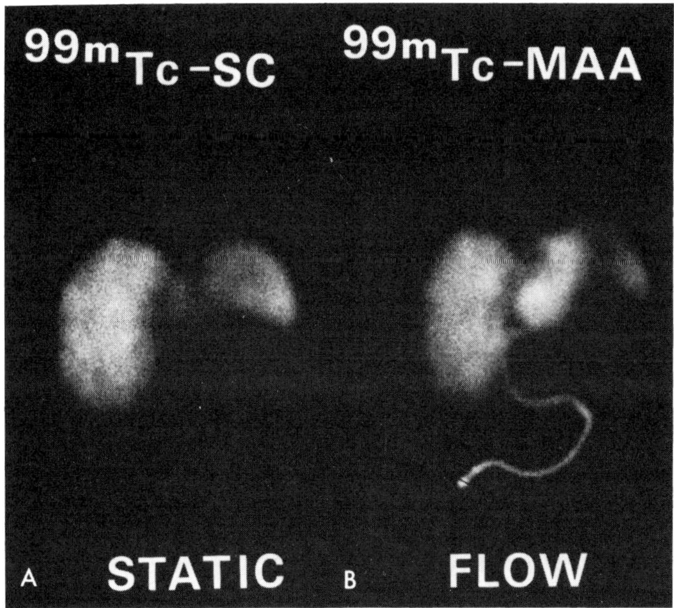

Figure 5–3. Static and dynamic imaging of a liver tumor. *A*, A large focal defect interposed between the right hepatic lobe and the spleen is seen to occupy most of the left lobe. *B*, After a slow infusion of ^{99m}Tc-macroaggregated albumin through a hepatic artery catheter, the bulk of the tracer can be seen to flow through the area of tumor. As one might expect, this patient responded well to intra-arterial chemotherapy.

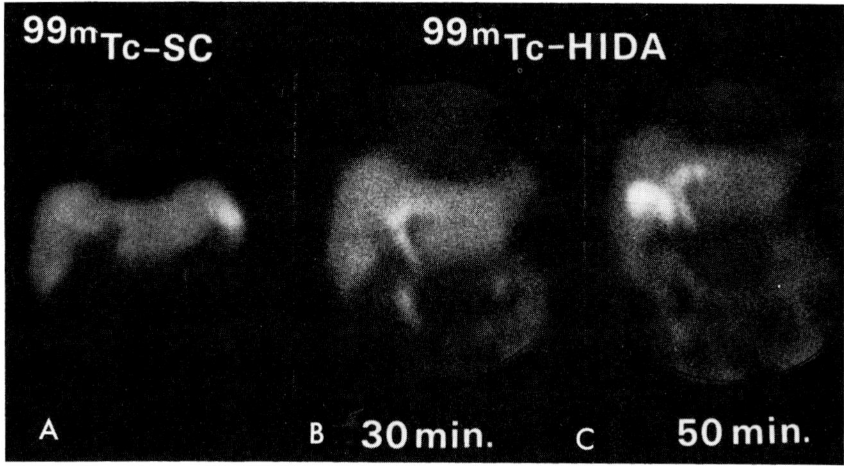

Figure 5–4. Demonstration of the patency of the common bile duct. *A*, An image taken with ^{99m}Tc-sulfur colloid shows a large focal defect in the region of the porta hepatis. *B*, A 30-minute ^{99m}Tc-HIDA image shows a portion of the defect, which can be attributed to the hepatic duct. *C*, On a 50-minute ^{99m}Tc-HIDA image, the gallbladder can be seen to fill the remainder of the defect. In addition, extensive activity inferior to the liver and throughout the gastrointestinal tract signals patency of the common bile duct.

tential hepatic disorders. If the scan shows a single defect, an ultrasound study should then be performed to determine whether the finding is related to normal anatomy; if the finding is a true abnormality, the ultrasound study will show whether the defect is cystic or solid before percutaneous biopsy is performed. On the other hand, a radionuclide liver scan that shows multiple focal defects or demonstrates diffuse parenchymal disease does not require confirmation.

BONE SCANNING

By means of bone scanning, minimal alterations in skeletal blood flow and bone turnover can be detected weeks or months before changes in bone can be seen on a radiograph. For identifying abnormal skeletal lesions, the gamma camera is the instrument of choice (Figure 5–5).

In approximately 80 per cent of cases, the radiographs and bone scan demonstrate identical findings: Both are normal or both are abnormal. In 15 per cent of cases, the bone scan shows abnormalities not visible on the x-rays, such as discrete metastases, early osteomyelitis, or changes related to a stress fracture. In 5 per cent of patients, the radiographs show an abnormality, and the scan is normal. For example, in "burnt out" metastatic lesions such as the osteoblastic metastases seen in prostatic carcinoma, the x-rays demonstrate what has happened *previously* (the metastases are apparent), but the bone scan indicates that there is no active bone turnover (Figure 5–6). Radiographs may show evidence of slow-growing lesions in which bone repair keeps up with bone resorption or of predominantly lytic lesions such as those seen in multiple myeloma.

Thus, the sensitivity of the bone scan suggests that when a skeletal pathological condition is suspected, a radionuclide study should be performed initially and radiographs should then be taken of areas that are positive on the scan as well as those that are negative on scan but clinically symptomatic.

There are a number of indications for bone scanning apart from the search for metastases. The evaluation of *delayed union of fractures* may be achieved by performing a bone scan, since absence of radionuclide uptake in the region of the fracture implies nonunion. In over half of patients with *stress fractures*, the initial radiograph may be normal but the bone scan usually shows evidence of abnormality within 48 hours; the bone scan can therefore serve as an excellent guide to treatment. A normal scan and radiograph imply that no fracture has occurred.

In *osteomyelitis* a positive bone scan can

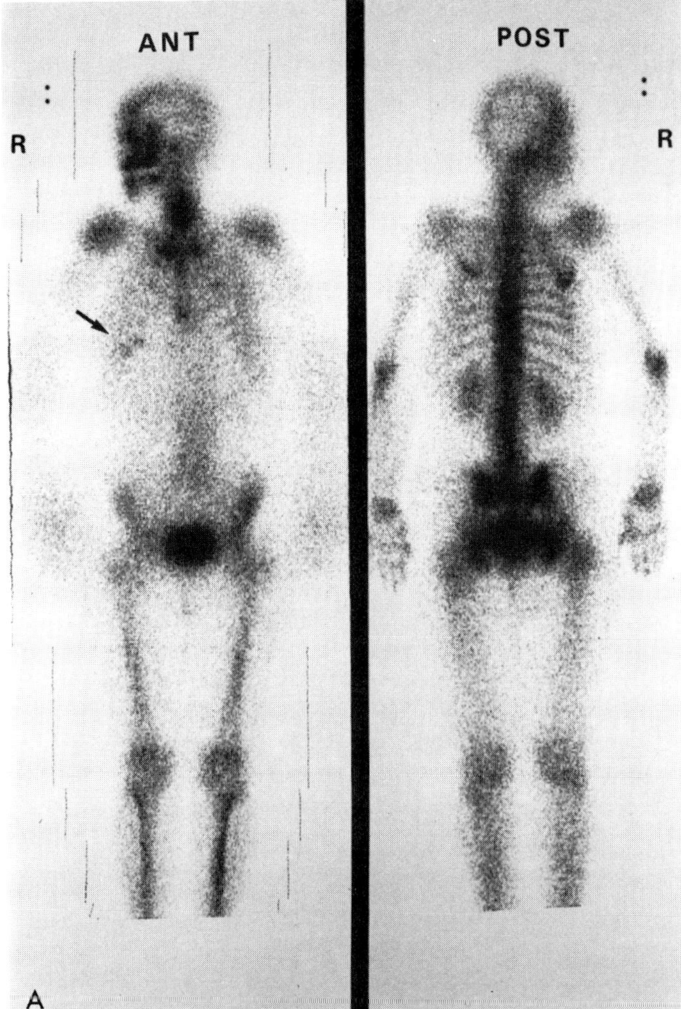

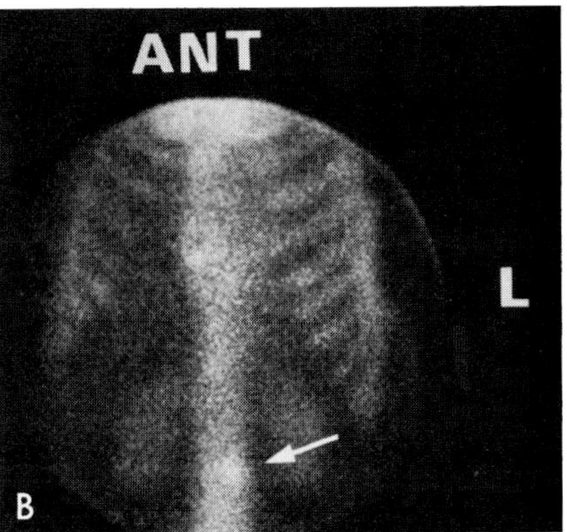

Figure 5–5. Skeletal metastases. *A*, A total-body rectilinear bone scan in both anterior and posterior views shows a suspicious area in the region of the right anterior thorax (*arrow*). *B*, On an anterior view of the thorax taken with the gamma camera, increased uptake is again noted in the anterior lower ribs on the right. An additional abnormality in the midlumbar spine (*arrow*) was compatible with the signs of metastasis seen on x-ray. Note that this focus was not appreciated on the total-body scan views.

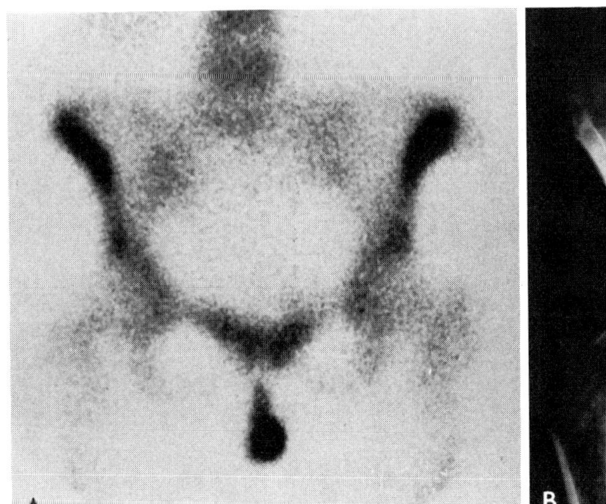

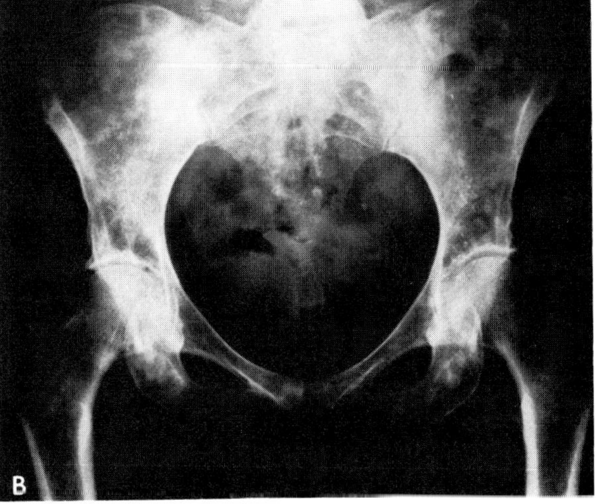

Figure 5–6. "Burnt out" metastases. *A*, On an anterior gamma camera image of the pelvis of this patient, who is known to have prostatic carcinoma, increased activity can be seen bilaterally on the anterior iliac crest. Otherwise, this scan seems normal. *B*, A pelvic x-ray obtained on the same day shows numerous "burnt out" metastatic lesions throughout the pelvis and the proximal femora.

pre-date radiographic changes by days to weeks; in fact, with immediate antibiotic therapy, there may never be radiographic evidence of infection. Two to three weeks after adequate therapy has begun, a bone scan may be normal.

In a child complaining of hip pain for whom routine radiographs are normal, bone scanning may give the only indication of femoral head avascularity; a bone scan should therefore be an integral part of the clinical evaluation of patients presenting with symptoms of possible Legg-Perthes disease. Similarly, in an adult patient with *avascular necrosis* of the femoral head, a bone scan may demonstrate a wedge-shaped defect in the epiphysis significantly sooner than abnormalities may be found on a radiograph (Figure 5–7).

Now that prosthetic surgery is commonly performed, *evaluation of a hip prosthesis* is of major concern. An abnormal bone scan may be the earliest postoperative indicator of potential clinical problems in patients who have received total hip replacement. Persistent activity around the acetabular and femoral components six months after surgery is abnormal and can be associated with infection or prosthetic loosening (Figure 5–8).

The sensitivity of radionuclide bone imaging for detecting skeletal abnormalities has made the procedure an integral part of the evaluation of patients with skeletal disease. It must be remembered, however, that although the bone scan is extremely sensitive, it is not specific and does not provide any morphological information. Thus, the correct work-up for a patient with symptoms or signs of skeletal abnormality requires correlation of the bone scan with radiographs.

RENAL IMAGING

Radionuclide studies of the kidneys provide much useful information. Tracer evaluation is well suited to assessment of three critical areas: renal blood flow, renal function, and vesicoureteral reflux.

Perfusion studies to assess blood flow are easily performed following intravenous administration of ^{99m}Tc-labeled renal agents. Rapid sequence imaging taken anteriorly when assessing a transplant or posteriorly when assessing both kidneys (Figure 5–9), delineates patency of the renal artery and vein and defines areas of ischemia or infarction.

Renal function studies are generally performed using ^{131}I-Hippuran. Normal patients show peak renal activity approximately five minutes after radiotracer

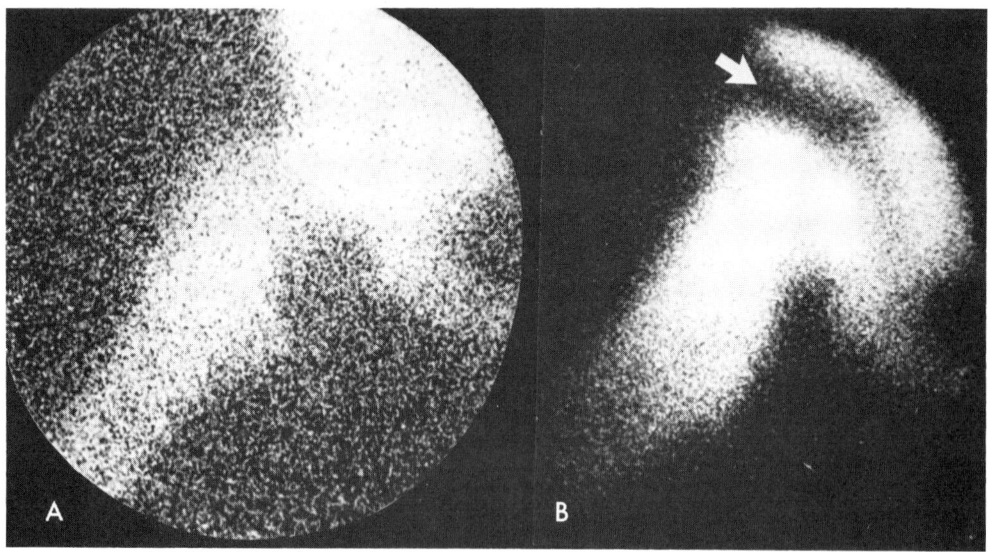

Figure 5–7. Avascular necrosis. *A*, A "pinhole" view of an externally rotated proximal femur is normal. *B*, A similar view of another patient shows avascular necrosis of the femoral head. Note the wedge-shaped defect in the epiphysis (*arrow*).

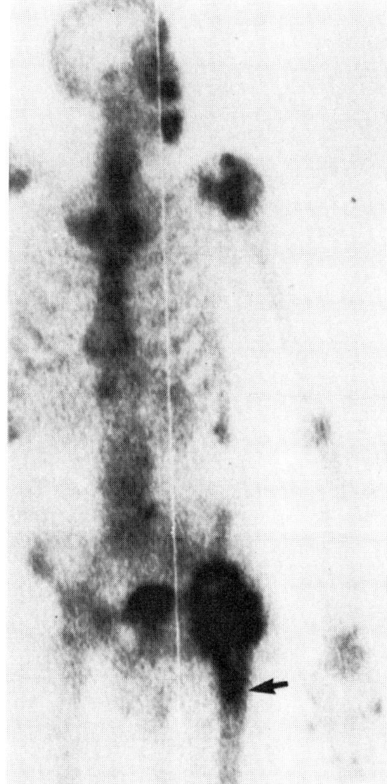

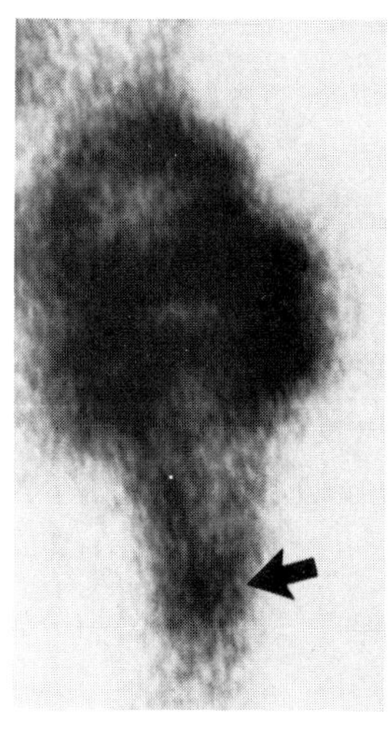

Figure 5–8. Loosening of a total hip prosthesis. This view was taken approximately one year after the patient had total left hip replacement. There is marked radionuclide uptake in both the acetabular and femoral compartments. Uptake near the femoral compartment (*arrows*) has most often been associated with loosening of the prosthesis.

administration; activity usually falls to one half of peak value about ten to fifteen minutes later. Studies of this type allow a functional comparison between the left and right kidneys (Figure 5–10).

Function studies can also be used to assess the viability of a renal transplant. Transplant rejection is associated with decreased uptake and secretion of radionuclide as well as irregular uptake within the

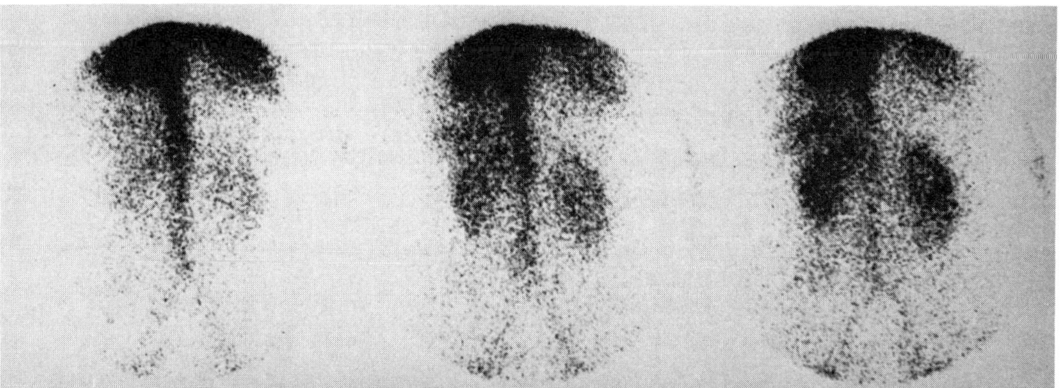

Figure 5–9. Normal renal perfusion studies. Posterior images of the abdomen were obtained sequentially at 1-second intervals after administration of a ^{99m}Tc renal agent. The abdominal aorta can be seen bifurcating into the iliac arteries, and increasing uptake of radiotracer is apparent within both kidneys. Uptake superior to the patient's left kidney, which is on the left of this image, represents radionuclide in the spleen and the left ventricle of the heart.

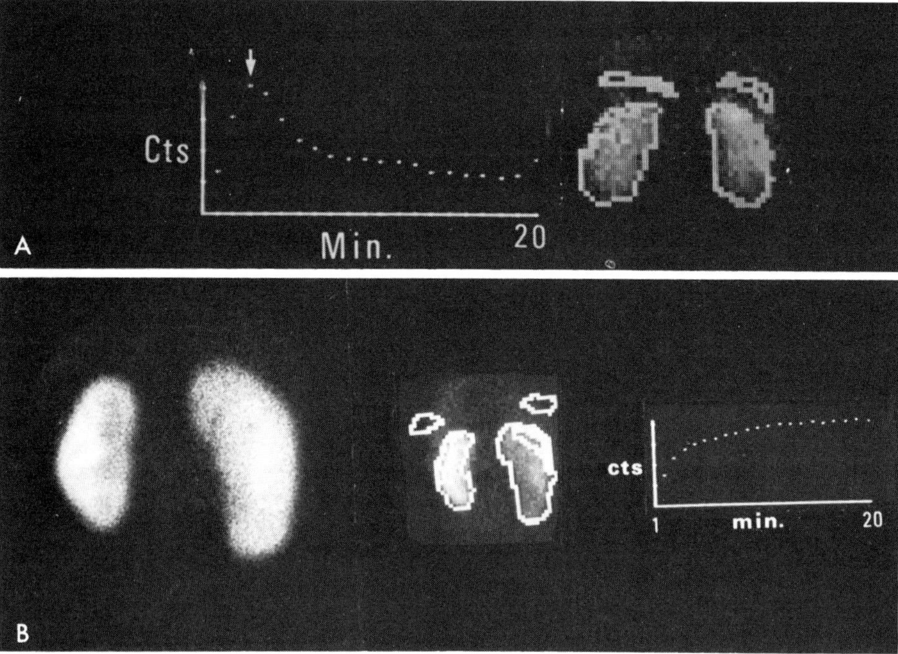

Figure 5–10. Renal function studies. *A*, The graph on the left shows the relationship of time and activity count within a computer-defined area overlying the kidney. The arrow indicates the peak activity time, which is 3 minutes for this patient; the amount of agent present in the area is reduced to one-half peak value at about 8 minutes. On the right is a computerized representation of the area being studied. *B*, On the left is a high-resolution posterior view of the kidneys. Right-sided hydronephrosis accounts for the discrepancy in renal size. The center picture is a computerized representation of the same area showing the overlying regions of interest. The graph on the right shows the relationship of time and activity count; this information was obtained from the abnormal right kidney. There is continuous uptake of radionuclide with time and no evidence of an excretory phase. (Courtesy of S. Ted Treves, M. D., of Children's Hospital Medical Center.)

renal parenchyma. Occurrence of these findings shortly after transplantation suggests rejection, but their occurrence later is compatible with tubular necrosis.

Vesicoureteral reflux is present in many children who are evaluated for recurrent urinary tract infection. Although intravenous pyelography, cystoscopy, and voiding cystourethrography are the diagnostic procedures commonly used in evaluating this condition, both indirect and direct radionuclide cystography have been shown to be valuable adjunctive studies. The indirect approach is performed by administering the radioisotope intravenously and imaging the kidneys and urinary bladder as during a perfusion study. In the direct approach, radionuclide voiding cystourethrography is performed by introducing ^{99m}Tc as pertechnetate in saline solution into the urinary bladder via a catheter. Unlike x-ray studies, the radionuclide VCUG allows continuous monitoring of both the filling and voiding phases so that rapid and transient reflux can be detected (Figure 5–11).

It has been calculated that 100 direct radionuclide cystography studies can be performed for the same radiation dose incurred in a single roentgenographic examination. Thus, the radionuclide technique is an excellent way of periodically re-evaluating the lower urinary tract.

LUNG SCANNING

Pulmonary imaging is achieved by the intravenous injection of aggregated radiolabelled human serum albumin. The aggregates, slightly larger than red cells, are trapped in the pulmonary capillaries. Patients are injected while supine to eliminate the normal apex-to-base gradient of blood flow and to encourage more homogeneous distribution of the aggregates for optimal anterior and posterior imaging. The most

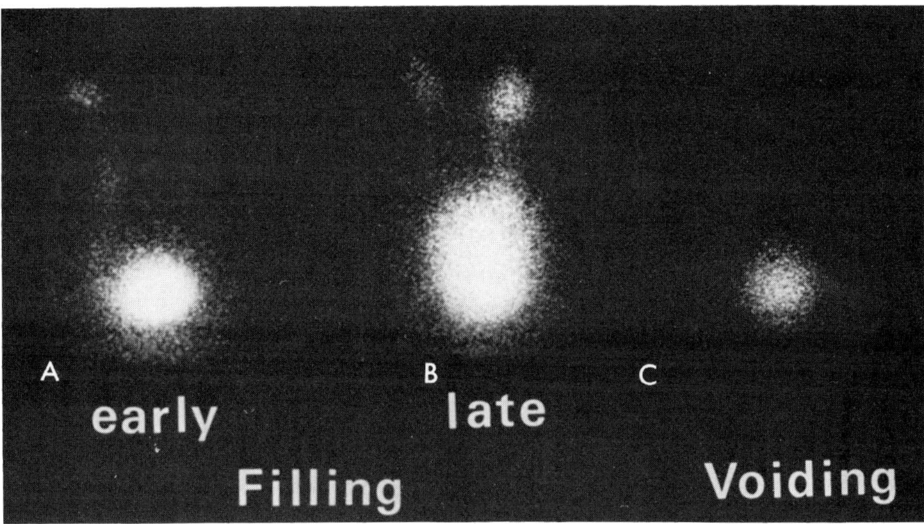

Figure 5–11. Direct radionuclide voiding cystourethrography. *A*, The anterior image of the pelvis taken during the early phases of bladder filling shows reflux to the level of the patient's right renal pelvis. *B*, During the later phases of bladder filling, bilateral renal reflux is seen. *C*, The image taken during the voiding phase shows no evidence of vesicoureteral reflux. (Courtesy of S. Ted Treves, M. D., of Children's Hospital Medical Center.)

common indication for perfusion lung scanning is suspicion of pulmonary emboli.

The characteristic perfusion defects in pulmonary emboli are large, approaching segmental or lobar dimensions (Figure 5–12). Multiple small subsegmental defects and defects that have ill-defined margins and cross anatomical boundaries are more frequently associated with entities such as congestive heart failure and chronic obstructive lung disease.

The use of a radioactive gas such as xenon-133 has improved diagnostic accuracy in detecting pulmonary emboli. Ventilation studies are performed by continually imaging the patient as a single breath of radioxenon gas is inhaled. Large or segmental perfusion defects that are shown to ventilate on a single breath of radioxenon are probably due to pulmonary emboli (Figure 5–13). A normal perfusion and ventilation lung scan excludes the possibility of a significant pulmonary embolus.

It is important to take a chest radiograph in conjunction with the radionuclide scan, particularly if the results of the tracer study are positive. If the chest x-ray is normal and a defect is seen on the lung scan, there is a high probability of pulmonary embolism. An abnormal scan is also seen in patients

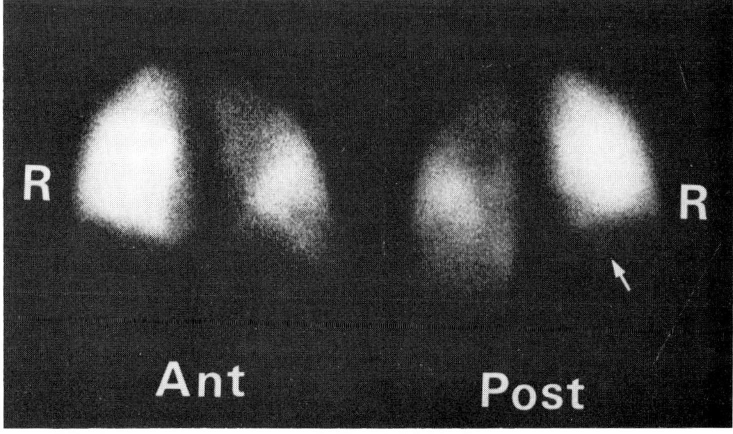

Figure 5–12. Pulmonary emboli, perfusion study. The posterior view of this pulmonary perfusion study best shows the large defects involving the base of the right lung (*arrow*) and the apex and base of the left lung. These perfusion deficits are highly suggestive of pulmonary emboli.

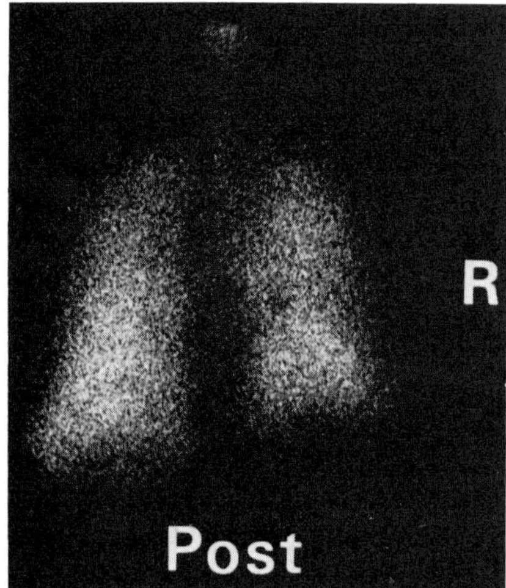

Figure 5–13. Pulmonary emboli, ventilation study. A single-breath xenon ventilation study of the same patient as in Figure 5–12 shows good distribution of the gas throughout both lungs. This characteristic ventilation/perfusion mismatch is highly indicative of underlying pulmonary emboli.

with pneumonia, chronic lung disease, asthma, and tumor; hence, it is important to be able to exclude these diagnostic possibilities on the basis of radiographs.

Quantitative regional lung function studies may also be performed by using a computer. Images are obtained after radioxenon gas in saline solution is intravenously injected. Upon entering the lung, the gas rapidly leaves the blood of the pulmonary capillary bed and enters the alveoli. The initial pattern of xenon distribution therefore represents pulmonary blood flow ($\dot{Q}$), whereas subsequent images obtained during rebreathing represent pulmonary ventilation ($\dot{V}$). These studies can be important in assessing pulmonary perfusion in patients before pneumonectomy or radiation therapy (Figure 5–14).

CARDIAC STUDIES

Applications of nuclear medicine in cardiology represent the area of most rapid growth in radionuclide imaging over the past few years. Diagnostic studies currently available include assessment of myocardial perfusion, evaluation of blood flow through the cardiac chambers and great vessels, blood pool studies of ventricular anatomy and function, and imaging of infarcts.

When thallium-201 (^{201}Tl) is administered intravenously, it distributes to the normal myocardium in a pattern that reflects the myocardial perfusion. An abnormal study therefore shows a focal area of decreased or absent uptake, which may reflect a direct compromise to blood flow, an infarct, or an alteration in the ability of that region of the heart to extract radionuclide efficiently (Figure 5–15). ^{201}Tl has been shown (unfortunately, from a diagnostic point of view) to distribute also to cardiac muscle, which lies distal to a major stenosis of a coronary artery; it is therefore important to subject the patient to strenuous exercise or a "stress test" immediately preceding the administration of tracer in order to appreciate poten-

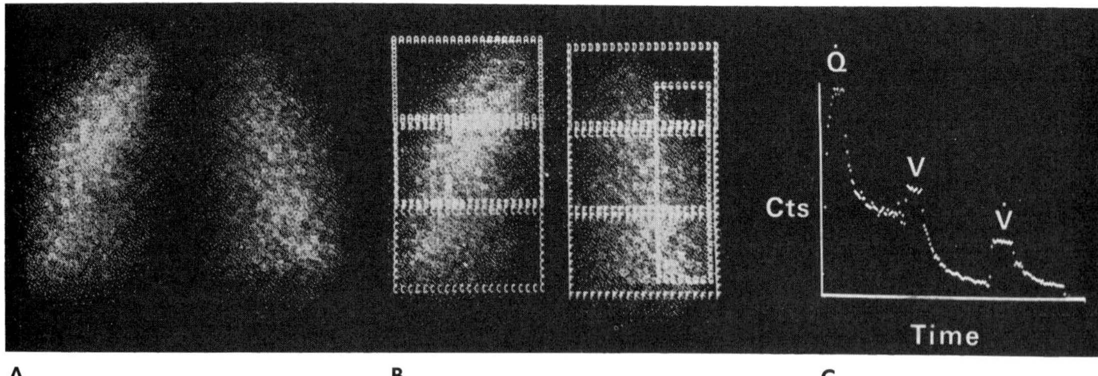

Figure 5–14. Quantitative regional lung function studies. *A*, A posterior image of the lung is seen. *B*, With the use of a computer, regions of interest over the upper, middle, and lower lobes can be defined. *C*, A graph of activity counts versus time in each of these areas can be plotted. Peak activity at perfusion ($\dot{Q}$), volume (V), and ventilation ($\dot{V}$) can be defined, so that ventilation/perfusion ratios can be obtained for any area of the lung.

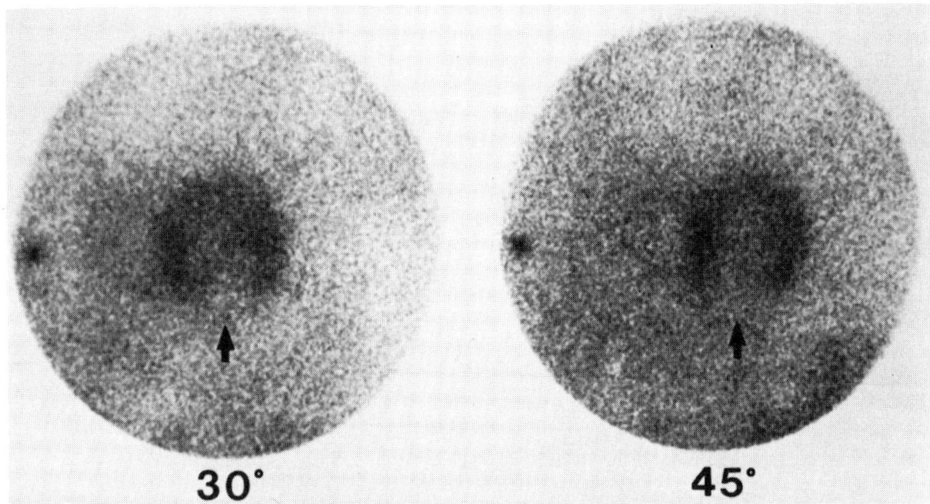

Figure 5–15. Myocardial infarction. In these thallium-201 images of the heart taken in the left anterior oblique projection at 30 degrees and 45 degrees, there is a defect (*arrows*) representing a large apical anterior infarct. (Courtesy of Thomas Hill, M. D., of New England Deaconess Hospital.)

tially abnormal areas of myocardial perfusion. A stress test, when combined with administration of ^{201}Tl, defines myocardial perfusion defects in over 80 per cent of patients with significant coronary artery disease. If a myocardial scan taken at rest is normal and a scan taken after exercise shows areas of diminished activity, there is a likelihood of myocardial ischemia. On the other hand, areas of decreased activity appearing on scans taken both at rest and after exercise suggest actual infarction or scar tissue.

Imaging the path of a ^{99m}Tc-labelled tracer during injection makes possible the assessment of the great vessels or the cardiac blood pool (Figure 5–16). With the use of a computer, rapid blood pool images of the cardiac chambers can be obtained and can be analyzed for evaluation of ventricular function. Blood pool tracers such as ^{99m}Tc-labelled albumin or ^{99m}Tc-labelled red blood cells allow images of many cardiac cycles to be studied; parameters such as ejection fractions, cardiac output, and ventricular asynchrony, dyskinesis, and akinesis can be defined (Figure 5–17).

Differentiation between acute and nonacute myocardial infarction cannot be made by means of any of these studies. It was

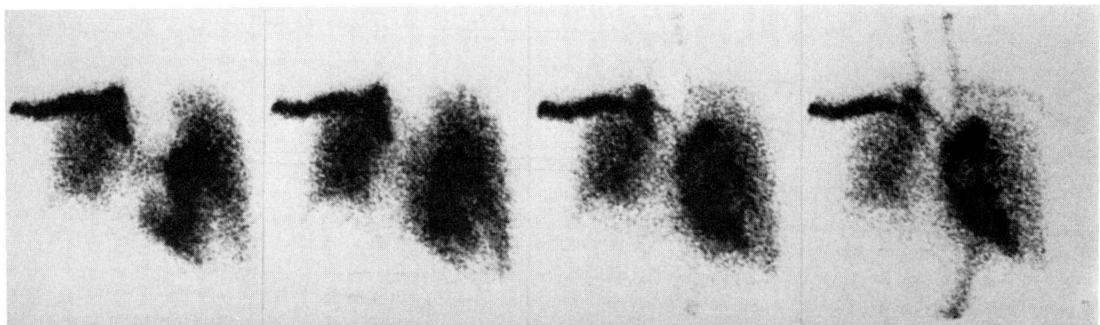

Figure 5–16. Superior vena caval obstruction. Multiple sequential images of the anterior thorax have been obtained at 1-second intervals following the intravenous administration of ^{99m}Tc. Persistent delay of the passage of tracer through the superior vena cava and an underperfused area bordering the aortic arch are seen. These abnormalities were caused by a bronchogenic carcinoma in the right lung that extended inferiorly from the level of the vena cava through the mediastinum.

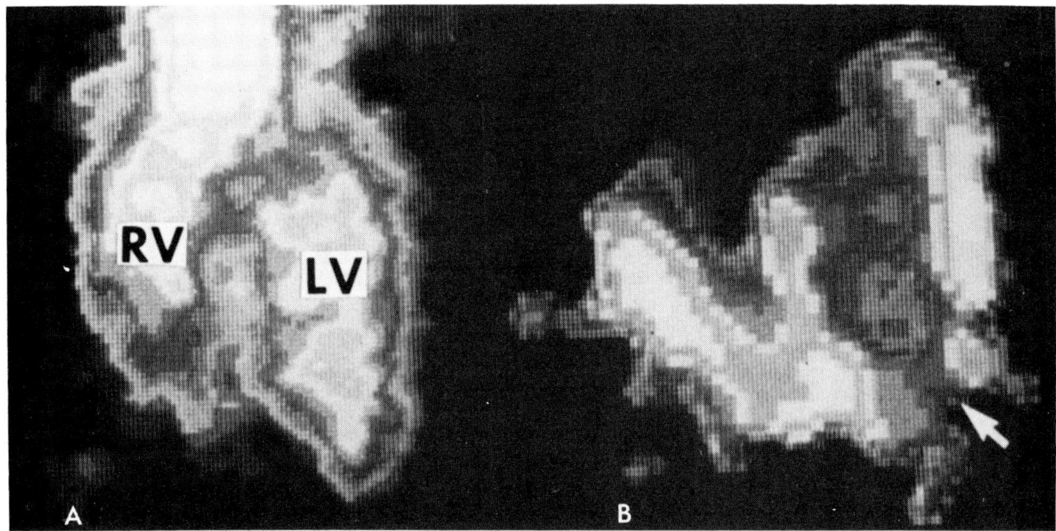

Figure 5–17. Ventricular akinesis. *A*, A computerized representation of a modified left anterior oblique view of the cardiac blood pool is taken during diastole. The right ventricle (RV) and left ventricle (LV) are readily appreciated. The difference between this image and subsequent systolic images allows the depiction of regional ejection fractions. *B*, A computerized representation shows the areas of the heart capable of ejecting blood. The arrow defines a region of apical akinesis where little ejection of blood is taking place. (Courtesy of B. Leonard Holman, M. D., of Peter Bent Brigham Hospital.)

found, however, that some tracers such as ^{99m}Tc-pyrophosphate, which is a bone scanning agent, become sequestered in an acute myocardial infarction within 4 to 8 hours of the insult, with peak activity at 24 hours (Figure 5–18). A scan taken 2 weeks after the infarct is usually normal; thus, infarct scintigraphy provides a method of directly assessing both the presence and the time of onset of myocardial damage. Focal or diffuse myocardial uptake may occur after injury and in conditions such as cardiomyopathy, congestive failure, and ventricular aneurysms.

THYROID IMAGING

The use of radiotracers in evaluating thyroid disease is based on the ability of the

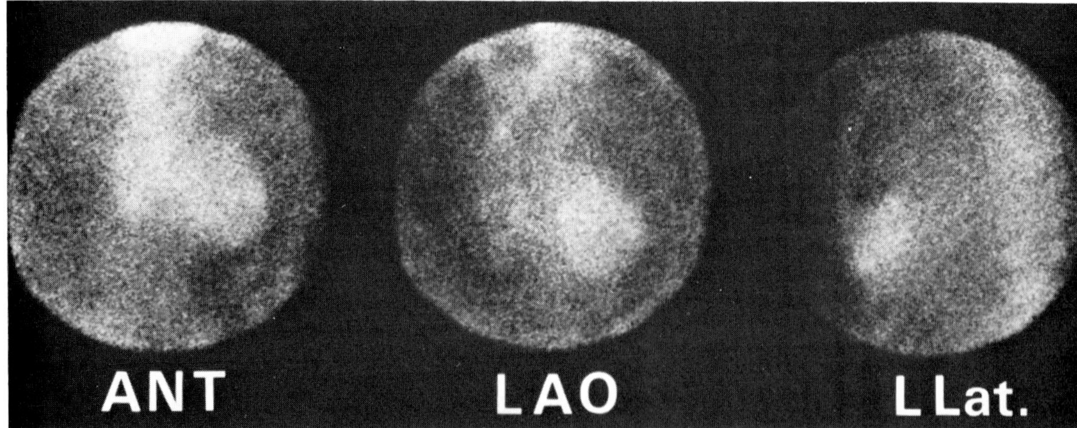

Figure 5–18. Massive myocardial infarction. A ^{99m}Tc-pyrophosphate study of the heart demonstrates diffuse uptake of radionuclide in the anterior, left anterior oblique, and left lateral views. (Courtesy of B. Leonard Holman, M. D., of Peter Bent Brigham Hospital.)

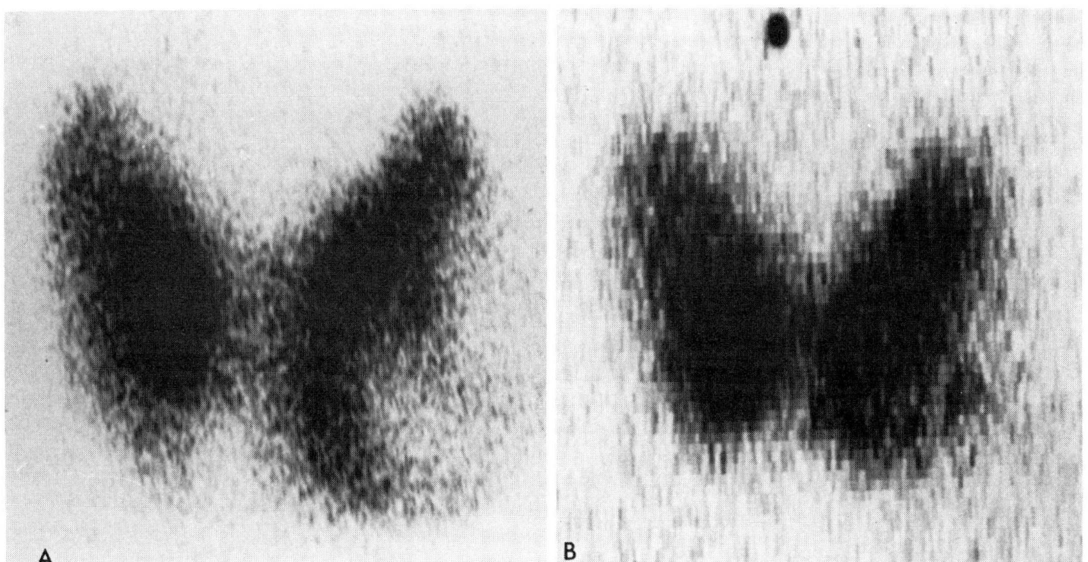

Figure 5–19. Cold thyroid nodule. *A*, A pinhole view of the thyroid gland shows a large cold nodule at the inferior aspect of the patient's left lobe. *B*, A rectilinear scan of the same patient offers less information regarding this area.

thyroid gland to trap anions such as the isotopes of iodine (^{131}I and ^{123}I) and ^{99m}Tc as pertechnetate ($^{99m}TcO_4$). Iodine-133 has become significantly less popular for routine clinical use because of its long physical half-life and emission of beta radiation. The gamma emissions of ^{123}I and $^{99m}TcO_4$ are ideally suited for use with a gamma camera fitted with a pinhole collimator; imaging with the gamma camera and collimator has led to an increase in the sensitivity of thyroid imaging for detecting anatomic abnormalities (Figure 5–19).

The major indications for thyroid imaging include definition of ectopic tissue, particularly in the anterior mediastinum (Figure 5–20). Thyroid imaging in hyperthyroid patients is generally limited to the differentiation between Graves' disease and hyperthyroid states due to toxic nodular goiter or to an autonomous thyroid nodule (Figure 5–21). In hypothyroid patients, particularly in children, the scan may be helpful in defining the only sites of functioning tissue.

There appears to be a significant increase in nodular thyroid disease in patients who received irradiation of the head and neck as children. On surgical exploration of the thyroid gland, approximately one third of these patients with nodules show evidence of malignant change. Experience to date suggests that if a thyroid nodule is clinically palpable

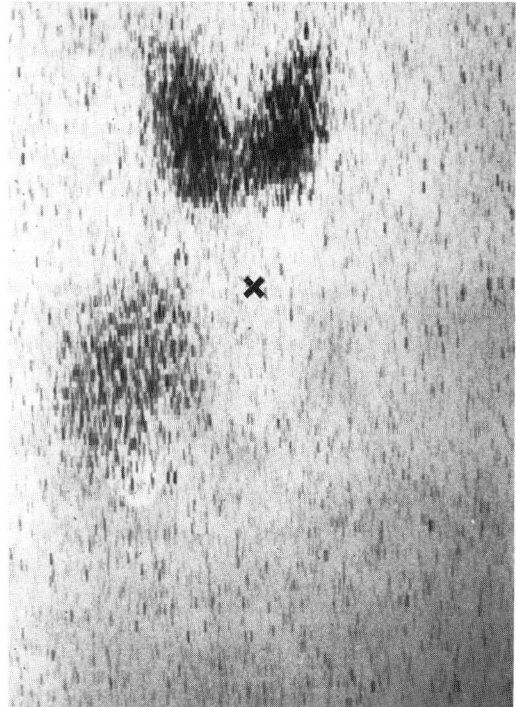

Figure 5–20. Substernal goiter. A rectilinear scan of the thyroid gland and intrathoracic region was performed using ^{131}I. The sternal notch is marked by an x. Note the diffuse uptake inferior to the thyroid gland within the thorax. Subtle linear uptake can be seen connecting this intrathoracic mass to the inferior aspect of the right thoracic lobe.

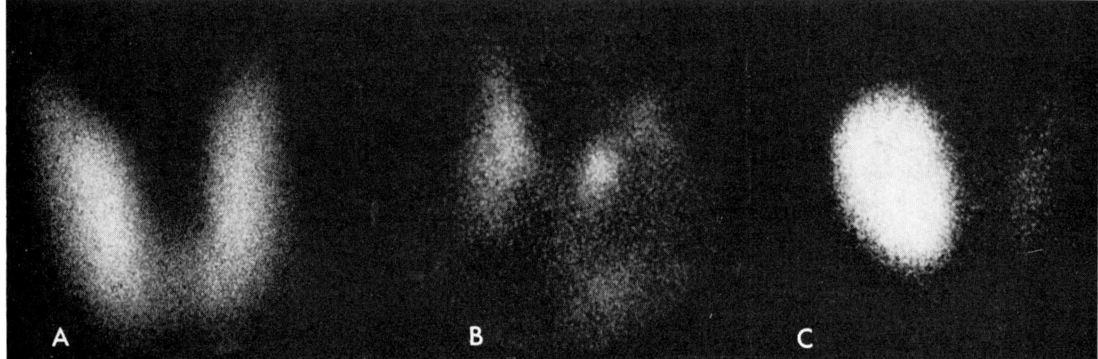

Figure 5–21. Hyperthyroidism, pinhole gamma camera views of three patients. *A*, There is homogeneous and avid uptake indicating an enlarged thyroid gland in this patient with Graves' disease. *B*, In this patient with toxic nodular goiter, there are focal areas of increased and decreased uptake. *C*, An autonomous nodule has also suppressed uptake in the opposite lobe of the thyroid of this patient.

in patients previously exposed to radiation, thyroid imaging is indicated (Figure 5–22).

Metastases from thyroid tumors may appear months or years after resection of the primary malignancy, and thyroid imaging can demonstrate these foci; for this purpose, ^{131}I is the isotope of choice. Because both primary and metastatic lesions of the thyroid are usually moderately well-differentiated, trapping and subsequent localization of the lesions are facilitated. Since there can be significant competition between normal functioning tissue and the relatively small site of tumor metastasis, it is unusual to identify metastases unless the thyroid gland has been surgically or isotopically ablated.

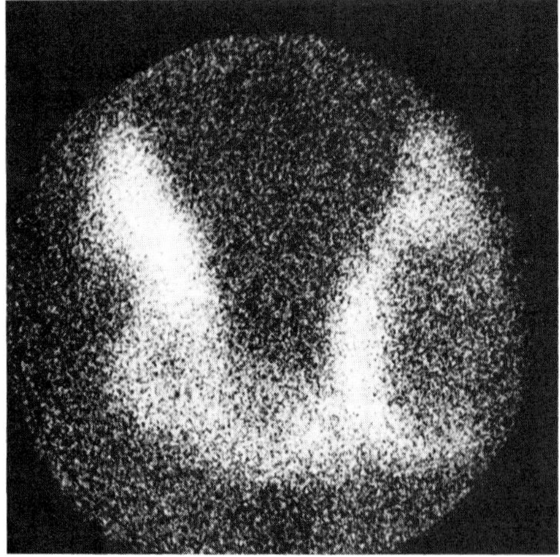

Figure 5–22. Mixed papillary follicular adenocarcinoma. This patient received radiation therapy to the neck. Now the thyroid gland is diffusely involved, and there are multiple focal areas of decreased uptake. The largest of the cold nodules occupies a major portion of the left lobe.

BRAIN IMAGING

Brain imaging used to be a common method for evaluating neurological disease; with the advent of computerized tomographic (CT) scanning, radionuclide studies are less often performed. Certain intracerebral abnormalities, however, are still best investigated using a radionuclide brain scan. These include suspected inflammatory disease, posterior fossa lesions, and subdural hematomas. Radionuclide scans are also used in evaluation of cerebral blood flow and verification of brain death.

In a normal study, the brain appears as a region of decreased activity surrounded by radionuclide circulating in normal structures such as the scalp, skull, and venous sinuses (Figure 5–23).

In diffuse inflammatory disease of the brain, as in encephalitis or meningitis, alterations in the blood-brain barrier can be readily detected using a radionuclide study (Figure 5–24), whereas a CT scan commonly shows little abnormality early in the course of the disease. The CT scan and brain scan are equally sensitive for the identification of brain abscesses. The commonly seen "doughnut sign" on a brain scan represents pericapsular accumulation of radioiso-

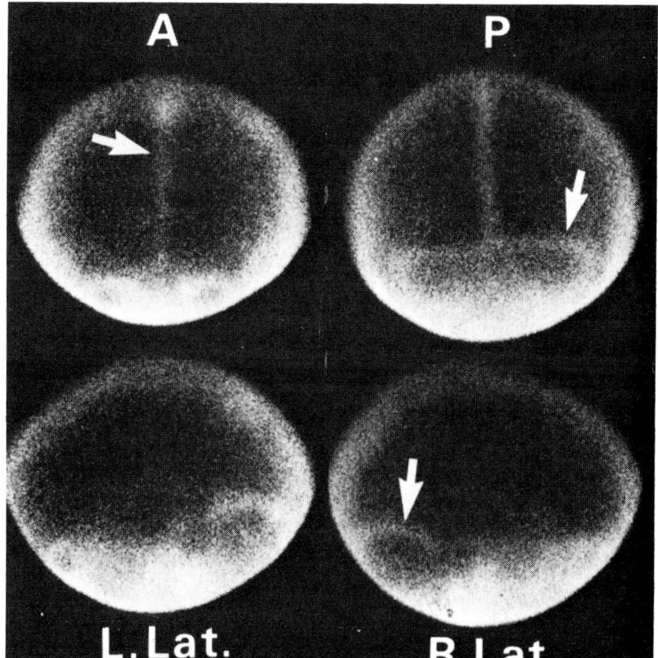

Figure 5–23. Normal brain scan. In this normal four-view radionuclide study of the brain, note that there is no activity within the cerebral or cerebellar hemispheres. The arrows delineate the normal venous sinuses clearly seen on all views.

tope with the central absence of activity (the "hole" of the doughnut) coinciding with the area of necrosis (Figure 5–25). This sign is not specific for abscesses and has also been seen in intracerebral neoplasms and resolving infarcts.

Certain specific lesions arise in the posterior fossa: medulloblastomas and cystic astrocytomas in children and acoustic neuromas, ependymomas, and astrocytomas in adults. These tumors offer a particular challenge to the clinician, since the posterior

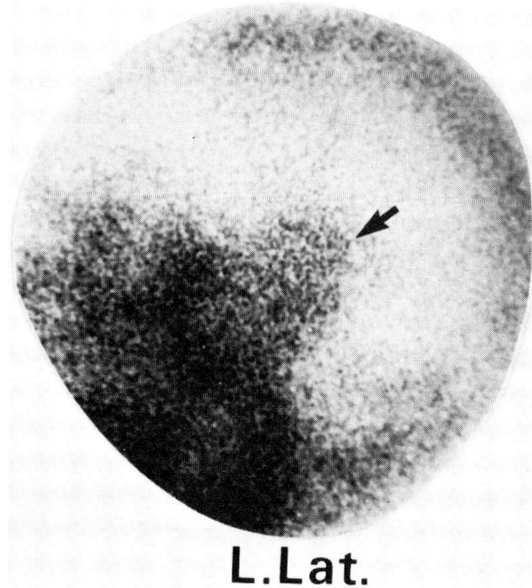

Figure 5–24. Herpes encephalitis. This left lateral image of the brain shows an area of significantly increased uptake in the left temporal lobe (*arrow*).

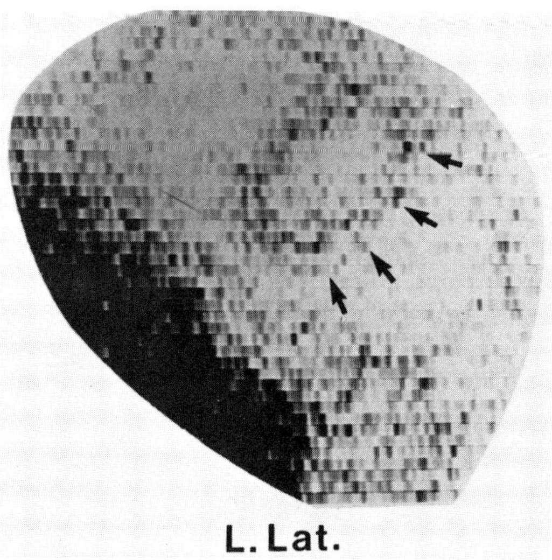

Figure 5–25. Parietal lobe abscess. A circular area of increased activity (*arrows*) with a central "cold" region is seen in this left lateral rectilinear brain scan.

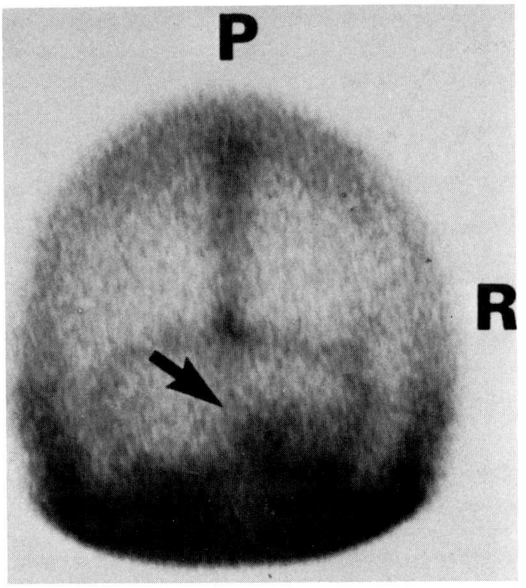

Figure 5–26. Acoustic neuroma. There is a focal area of increased uptake to the right of the midline in the cerebellar hemisphere (*arrow*).

fossa is one of the most difficult regions of the brain to image satisfactorily. If a patient is unable, because of physical limitations, to properly flex the neck for the posterior fossa views taken in a CT examination, the radionuclide brain scan, which affords excellent visualization of this region, can be performed without the need for flexion (Figure 5–26).

CT scanning is the examination of choice for the detection of acute subdural hematomas. When a suspected hematoma is not identified by this procedure, a dynamic cerebral flow study may provide the required diagnostic information. A subdural hematoma appears on a flow study as a concave defect located at the periphery of the cortex (Figure 5–27A). When the hematoma is undergoing resorption, the CT image may be falsely interpreted as normal. It is precisely

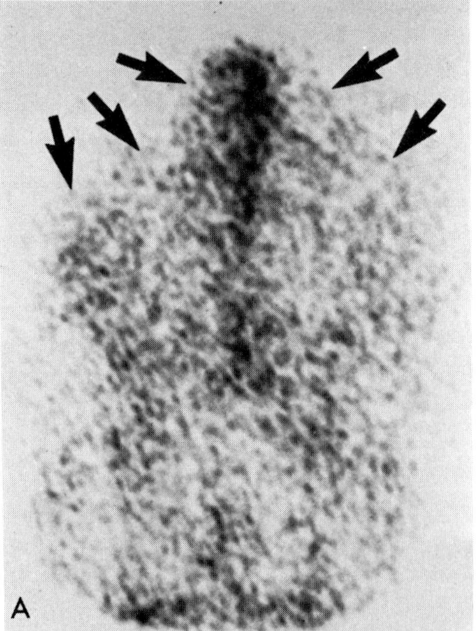

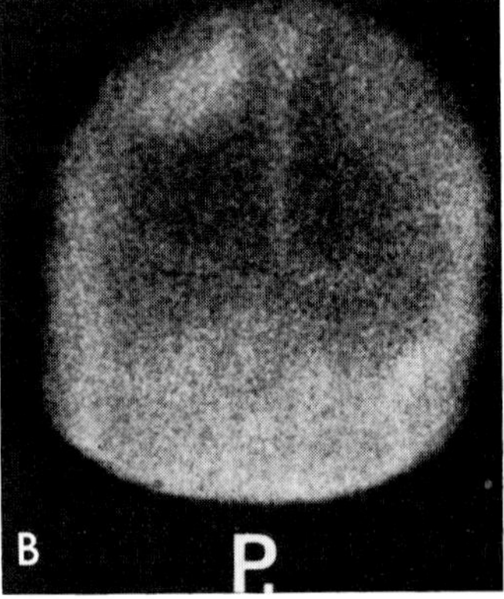

Figure 5–27. Subdural hematoma. *A*, A single 1-second frame from a dynamic cerebral flow study shows bilateral concave defects in the distribution of the middle cerebral artery (*arrows*). *B*, In a posterior static image of the brain of the same patient, there is biparietal uptake in the areas of no perfusion. These images present the classic radionuclide findings of subdural hematoma.

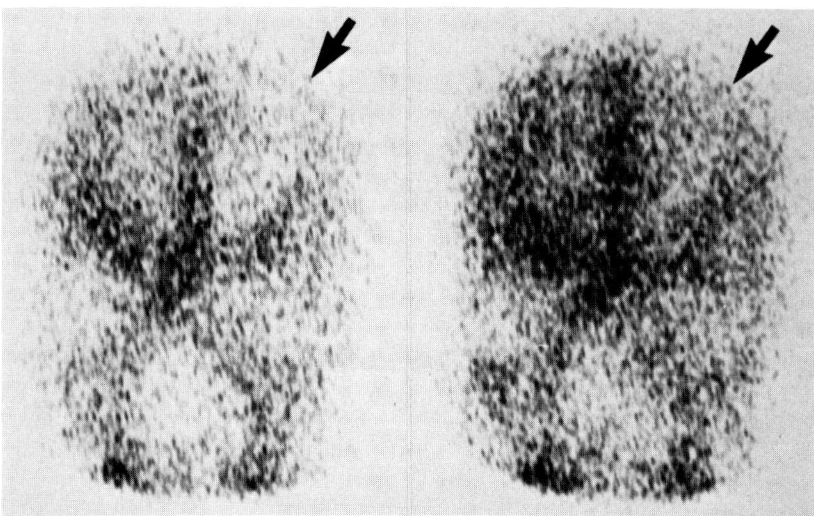

Figure 5–28. Recent occlusion of the left middle cerebral artery. In two sequential images taken at 1-second intervals during an anterior cerebral flow study, there is an area of diminished perfusion overlying the left parietal area (*arrows*). Note that the distribution of the middle cerebral artery on the left shows significantly less activity than its counterpart on the right.

at this time during the reparative process that a static radionuclide image shows marked uptake, which appears as a crescentic focus of activity and is seen approximately ten days after the injury (Figure 5–27B).

A dynamic cerebral flow study, in addition to offering a means of early detection of subdural hematomas, is a noninvasive method of defining the distribution of the common and internal carotid arteries as well as the intracerebral anterior, middle, and posterior cerebral arteries. Changes in blood flow reflect major luminal occlusion. The technique of rapid imaging of the brain during intravenous injection of a bolus of tracer provides useful information in the investigation of suspected infarcts (Figure 5–28) and the substantiation of brain death (Figure 5–29).

The overall sensitivity of radionuclide imaging for primary brain tumors is about 85 per cent. Tumors located in the cerebral hemispheres or the posterior fossa are readily identified by radionuclide brain scanning, whereas those located near the sella turcica and brain stem are best identified by

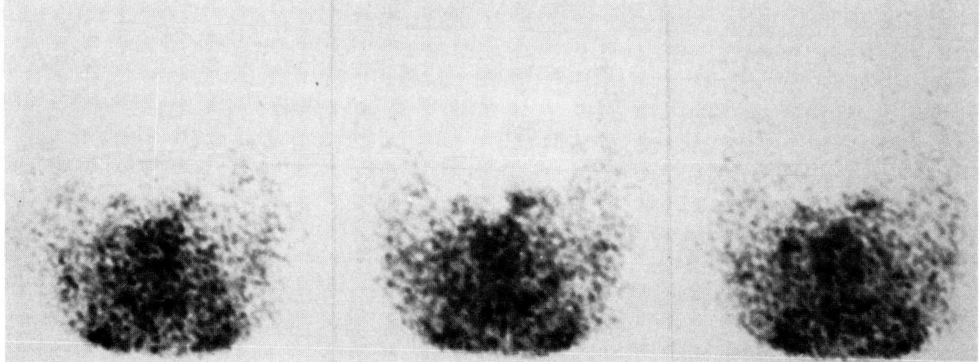

Figure 5–29. Brain death. Three sequential images obtained at 1-second intervals during an anterior dynamic cerebral flow study show no activity within the distribution of the anterior or middle cerebral arteries. The barely perceptible activity over the calvarium is associated with blood flow to the bone and scalp.

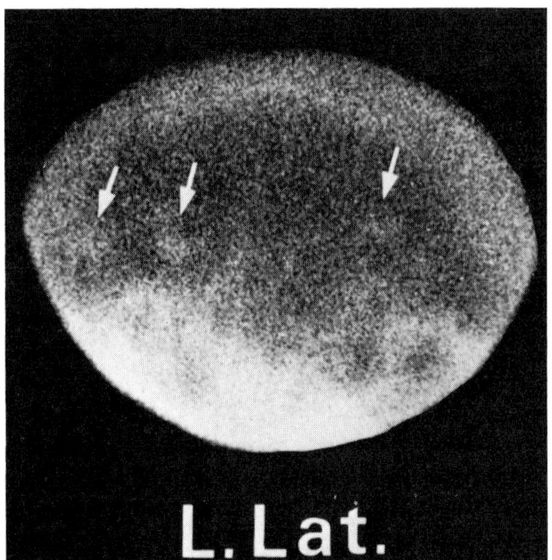

Figure 5–30. Cerebral metastases. This left lateral radionuclide image of the brain shows numerous focal areas of increased uptake within the frontal and parietal lobes (*arrows*).

CT scanning. Cystic or avascular tumors such as low-grade gliomas are not readily identified by tracer techniques but can be detected by CT imaging. The overall sensitivity of radionuclide imaging for detecting a single metastatic lesion approaches 90 per cent (Figure 5–30).

GALLIUM SCANNING

Gallium-67 (^{67}Ga) is the radionuclide most widely used for ascertaining the presence of neoplastic or inflammatory tissue. Experimentation has shown that an abscess as young as 4 hours of age can concentrate ^{67}Ga. Clinically, abscesses five to ten days old sequester adequate activity for identification on a scan. The optimum time for imaging abscesses is 24 to 48 hours after administration of gallium-67. A negative result of a scan taken at 48 hours indicates a low probability that the patient has a drainable collection of pus. A positive result can be seen in diffuse inflammatory lesions and localized collections of pus (the wall of the abscess being the site of greatest gallium deposition). The conditions can usually be differentiated by the pattern seen on the scan (Figure 5–31.)

There are three major indications for the use of ^{67}Ga in the identification of neoplastic sites: the evaluation of patients with lymphoma, the preoperative and postoperative assessment of patients with lung cancer, and the identification of inadequately treated or recurrent tumors.

The sensitivity of gallium-67 imaging for detecting at least one abnormal focus in patients with Hodgkin's disease or histiocytic lymphoma approaches 80 per cent (Figure 5–32). However, in the initial work-up of patients suspected of having lymphoma, a negative result does not exclude the possibility of disease. On the other hand, the demonstration of an abnormal focus strongly suggests tumor, since the false positive rate is less than 5 per cent.

The overall sensitivity of gallium-67 imaging in defining neoplastic foci in the lung approaches 90 per cent. The indications for gallium scanning in suspected bronchogenic carcinoma include: a patient in whom cytologic examination of the sputum is positive for malignancy but other diagnostic studies are normal, and a patient with a hydrothorax in whom standard radiographic procedures are unrevealing and bronchoscopy is contraindicated. Since normal pulmonary tissue does not sequester

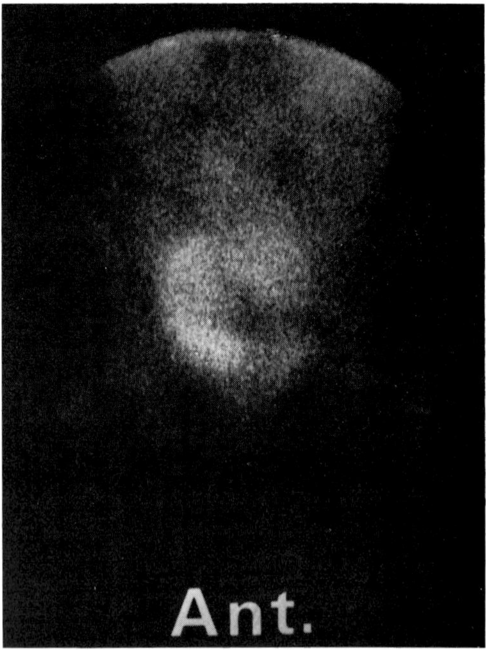

Figure 5–31. Large pelvic abscess undergoing central necrosis. On an anterior ^{67}Ga image of the lower abdomen and pelvis, a circular area of increased uptake with a region of central decreased activity can be seen.

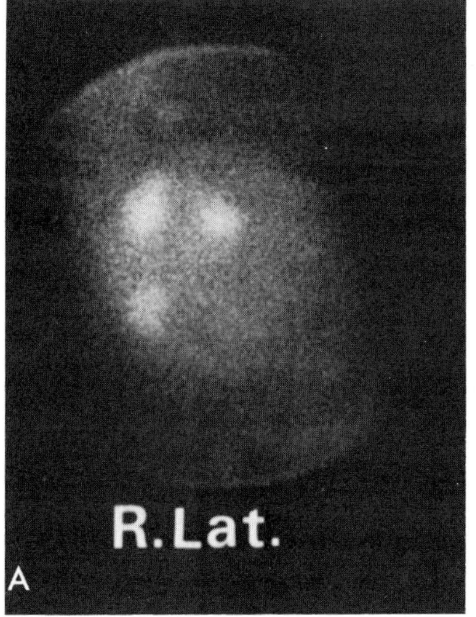

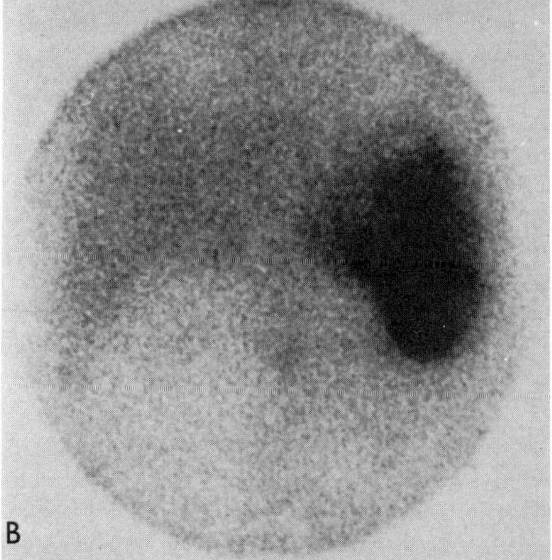

Figure 5–32. Lymphoma involving the liver and spleen. *A*, A right lateral view of the liver taken using ^{67}Ga in a patient with Hodgkin's disease shows three discrete focal areas of increased uptake. *B*, On an anterior view of the abdomen we see avid uptake of ^{67}Ga-citrate through the spleen with only subtle activity distributed to the liver in this patient with histiocytic lymphoma.

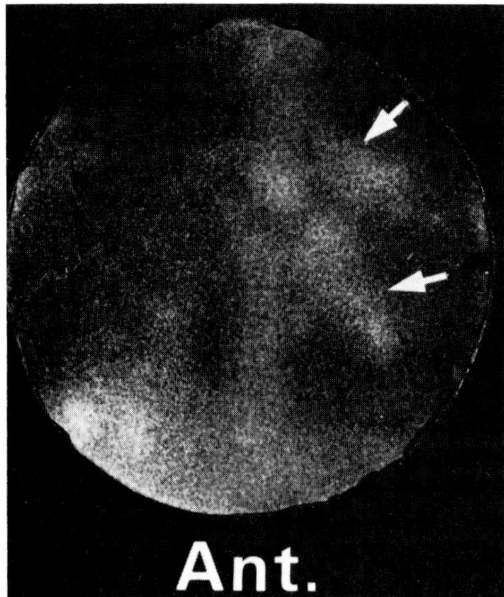

Figure 5–33. Pulmonary involvement by tumor. An anterior view of the thorax obtained on ^{67}Ga imaging shows extensive involvement of the mediastinum, left lung (*arrows*) and left supraclavicular region that was not apparent on standard radiographs.

gallium-67 (although the normal thoracic skeleton may do so), this radionuclide is extremely useful in identifying the extent of pulmonary tumor and defining previously undetected sites (Figure 5–33).

Although the false negative rate for gallium scanning is about 5 per cent, numerous other pulmonary processes can take up the tracer. Positive ^{67}Ga uptake has been seen after lymphography and in pneumonia, sarcoidosis, active tuberculosis, radiation pneumonitis, and tumors. It is therefore essential to take a chest radiograph to exclude the possibility of non-neoplastic conditions.

A gallium scan is useful in observing the effects of tumor therapy (Figure 5–34). Since radiotherapy and chemotherapy decrease the uptake of ^{67}Ga within neoplastic tissue, a normal gallium scan cannot rule out the possibility of microscopic foci of malignancy. However, an abnormal scan is extremely helpful. If a scan taken immediately after therapy is normal, but a scan taken at a later date is abnormal, recurrent malignancy is most likely. The gallium scan frequently

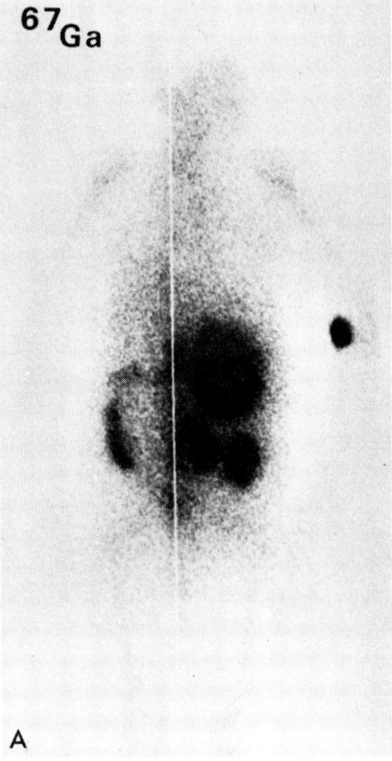

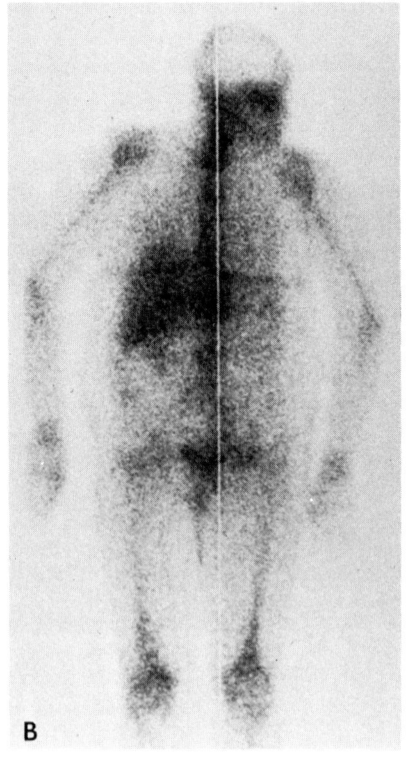

Figure 5–34. Lymphoma. *A*, A total body ^{67}Ga study of a patient with histiocytic lymphoma was taken before treatment. *B*, A study taken after chemotherapy shows normal distribution of radiotracer and supports the clinical impression of remission.

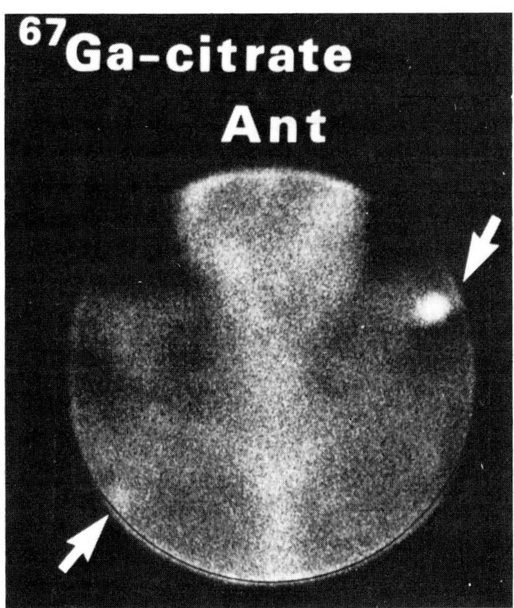

Figure 5–35. This patient with poorly differentiated lymphoma presented one year after therapy with a cutaneous lesion of the left shoulder. Significant gallium uptake can be seen (*upper arrow*). In addition, there is a second, clinically unsuspected focus in the right axilla (*lower arrow*) of this patient with recurrent disease.

provides evidence of sites of recurrent tumor for which there is absolutely no clinical suspicion (Figure 5–35).

The best strategy for the evaluation of tumors appears to be to use standard scintigraphic approaches and then to employ ^{67}Ga scanning as a "second line" procedure. Gallium, however, is the best radioindicator available for localizing inflammatory tissue. In searching for inflammatory foci, a gallium total body image should be strongly considered before more invasive procedures are employed.

ACKNOWLEDGMENTS

My thanks to Deborah Hansen for illustrations, John Buckley for photography, and Nancy Buck for secretarial assistance.

CHAPTER 6

CLINICAL ULTRASONOGRAPHY

Diagnostic ultrasonography includes all medical investigations employing high-frequency sound waves. Strictly speaking, *ultrasound* means nothing more than those high-frequency sound waves above the range of normal human hearing, which is below 20,000 cycles per second, or 20 kilohertz (hertz = cycles per second). It is interesting that Galton's production in 1880 of the first high-frequency sound waves using a whistle device corresponded, at least temporally, with Roentgen's discovery of x-rays. The development and application of ultrasound devices, however, did not advance nearly as rapidly as the development and refinement of x-ray technology. With the appearance of the submarine menace in World War I, a system was needed for the detection of submarines under water. Langevin and others in France developed ultrasound devices for this purpose. Even after this initial interest, ultrasound developed very slowly until another war aided further advancement. The outbreak of World War II brought with it a sudden need for sophisticated sonar devices for use by the military. Rapid development of highly advanced electronic devices to be used in complex sonar installations ensued, and it was from this technology that medical ultrasonography finally emerged.

While attempts had been made to develop medical applications of ultrasound before the second World War (by Dussik, for example, who worked on intracranial imaging), it was not until the postwar period that medical ultrasound truly blossomed. In the late 1940s, Douglas Howry championed the cause for medical ultrasound and with other researchers used surplus war equipment to develop devices capable of body organ imaging using high-frequency sound waves. During the 1950s, great advances were made in the imaging of various organ systems and masses such as the brain, breast, intestines, eyes, and pelvic organs. These early devices required immersion of the organ or patient in a tank of water to achieve adequate imaging, a rather difficult problem for the seriously ill patient. Further development of ultrasound equipment did away with the need for total patient immersion, and devices were developed for ultrasound imaging using what is called a *contact scanner*; now only the end of a moistened cylinder need touch the patient to achieve adequate imaging (Fig. 6–1). While an in-depth discussion of the physics and circuitry of ultrasound is beyond the scope of this text, we will answer five questions that should give some appreciation of how the ultrasonographic image is finally produced.

How and where is the sound made?

What is done with the sound after it has been produced?

How is the image constructed?

This chapter was written with the help of E. Barney Black, M. D.

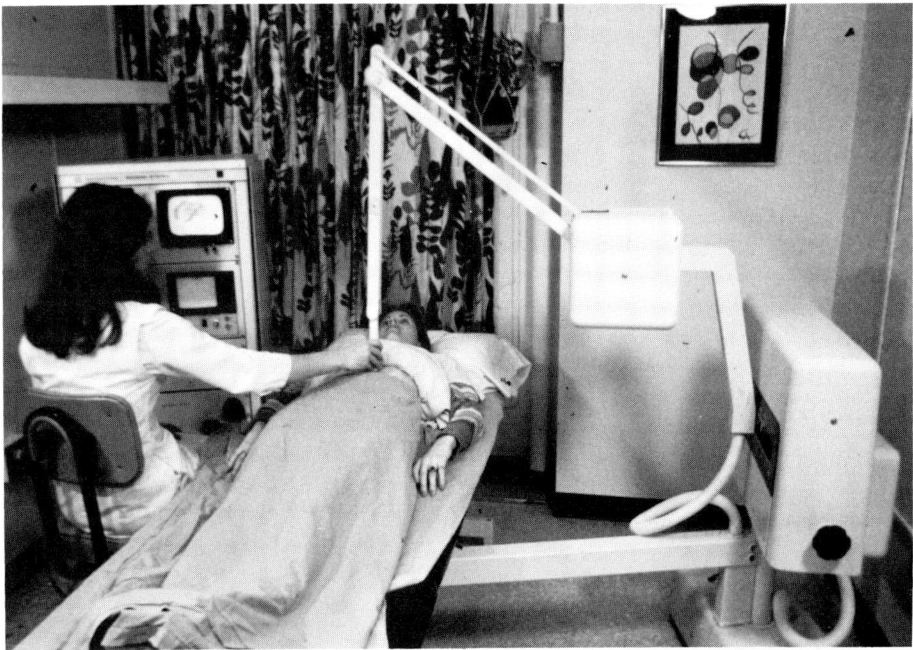

Figure 6–1. Transverse imaging of the abdomen with a B-mode gray scale sector scanner. The technician is guiding the probe (sound source) with her right hand.

What is gray scale?
What is real time?

How and Where Is the Sound Made?

The cylindrical device that comes in contact with the patient during an examination employing ultrasound is termed the *probe* or *transducer* (Fig. 6–2). A transducer is a device that converts one form of energy into another — in this case, electrical energy into mechanical energy (sound). In clinical ultrasonography, the high-frequency sound waves are produced by the ringing of a ceramic material or piezoelectric crystal inside the housing of the probe, which is held in the hand of the examiner. The ringing crystal is really the transducer. In the probe itself, there is a backing substance on the transducer crystal that helps regulate its ringing. There is also an acoustical lens device to direct the sound waves after their production. In one-dimensional examinations such as echocardiography or echoencephalography, the probe may be held free in the examiner's hand. In two-dimensional studies, the probe is attached to an arm or frame that mechanically controls the spatial orientation of the probe to the patient or organ during the examination. This process allows two-dimensional representation on the reading device of acoustic interfaces in the patient.

In 1884, Curie described the phenomena termed the *piezoelectric effect* and the *reverse piezoelectric effect*. In the reverse pi-

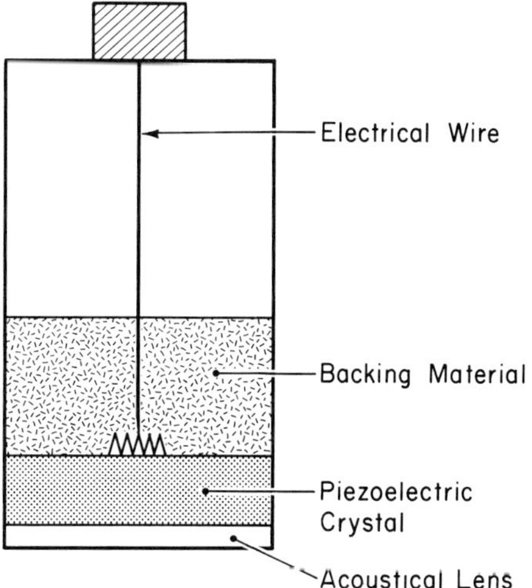

Figure 6–2. Diagram of the probe housing the transducer crystal.

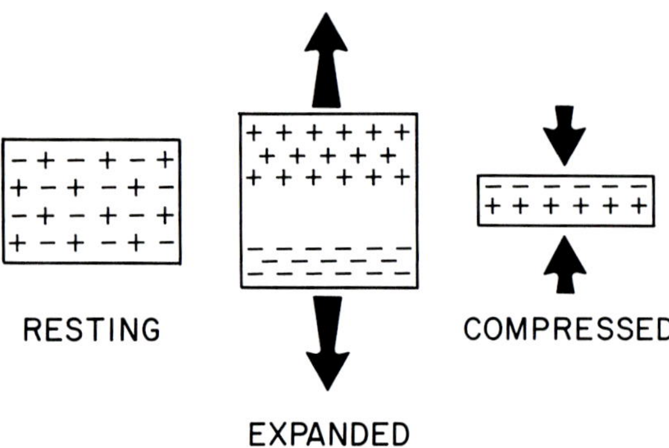

Figure 6–3. Diagram illustrating the changes in crystal configuration from the resting state to application of an electrical potential across the crystal (reverse piezoelectric effect). Conversely, when the resting crystal is stressed, producing a change in its shape, electrical potential is generated across it (piezoelectric effect).

ezoelectric effect, a potential applied across a crystal causes the crystal to change shape (Fig. 6–3). When an electrical potential is applied to a piezoelectric crystal (such as a crystal of barium titanate or lead zirconate, which is used in the ultrasonographic transducer), the crystal becomes excited and vibrates at its natural frequency — as a bell or gong vibrates after being struck. The natural frequency of the crystal is determined by its thickness. This vibrating crystal is the sound source used in diagnostic ultrasound.

What Is Done With the Sound After It Has Been Produced?

The high-frequency sound waves produced by the transducer are focused by a lens device into a more or less pencil-shaped beam as they exit from the probe. This thin beam of sound waves is directed into the patient. Unlike the waves in electromagnetic radiation, sound waves cannot be propagated in a vacuum but must be directed through a molecular medium. The manipulation of high-frequency sound waves and the recording of their echoes are very similar to the interactions that occur during submarine detection using sonar. A sound wave of known velocity is produced and passes uninhibited through a homogeneous medium such as water until it meets a boundary between the homogeneous medium and another substance, where it is reflected back to its source. The reflecting boundary is termed an *acoustic interface,* a boundary between substances of different acoustic impedance. *Acoustic impedance* is defined as the product of the density of the substance multiplied by the speed of sound in that substance. The greater the difference in acoustic impedance of two substances, the greater the amount of sound reflected back from a boundary between them (Fig. 6–4).

Sound waves are reflected from the acoustic interfaces back toward their source and are recorded. In diagnostic ultrasound, the oscillating crystal sound source also acts as the sound receiver. In the *piezoelectric effect* (as opposed to the reverse piezoelectric effect described previously), changes of shape in a piezoelectric crystal cause an electrical potential to be produced across the crystal. This is the mechanism for recording returning echoes in an ultrasound device. In submarine detection work, the interface between water and the hull of the ship provides the reflecting surface. Since the speed of the propagating sound and the length of time it takes the sound to pass to the reflecting interface and return to the sound source are known, it is possible to calculate the distance between the sound source and the reflecting interface (distance = time × speed; in sonar the right side of the equation is known). The distance between the sound source and the submarine is seen on the oscilloscope screen (Fig. 6–5). Deflections from the baseline, representing the distance between the sound source and the reflecting interface, are displayed on the screen. Such a picture is similar to that produced in *echoencephalography* (A-mode scanning of the brain), in which the image produced consists of three deflections from a baseline, the two outer ones representing the skull boundaries and the middle deflection representing the brain midline structures, probably the posterior aspect of the third ventricle (Fig. 6–6). With this image it is possible to determine the location of the expected midline structures, which may be shifted in patients with intracranial mass lesions such as brain tumors or subdural hematomas. This type of ultrasonographic representation is termed *A-mode (amplitude modulation) ultrasound.*

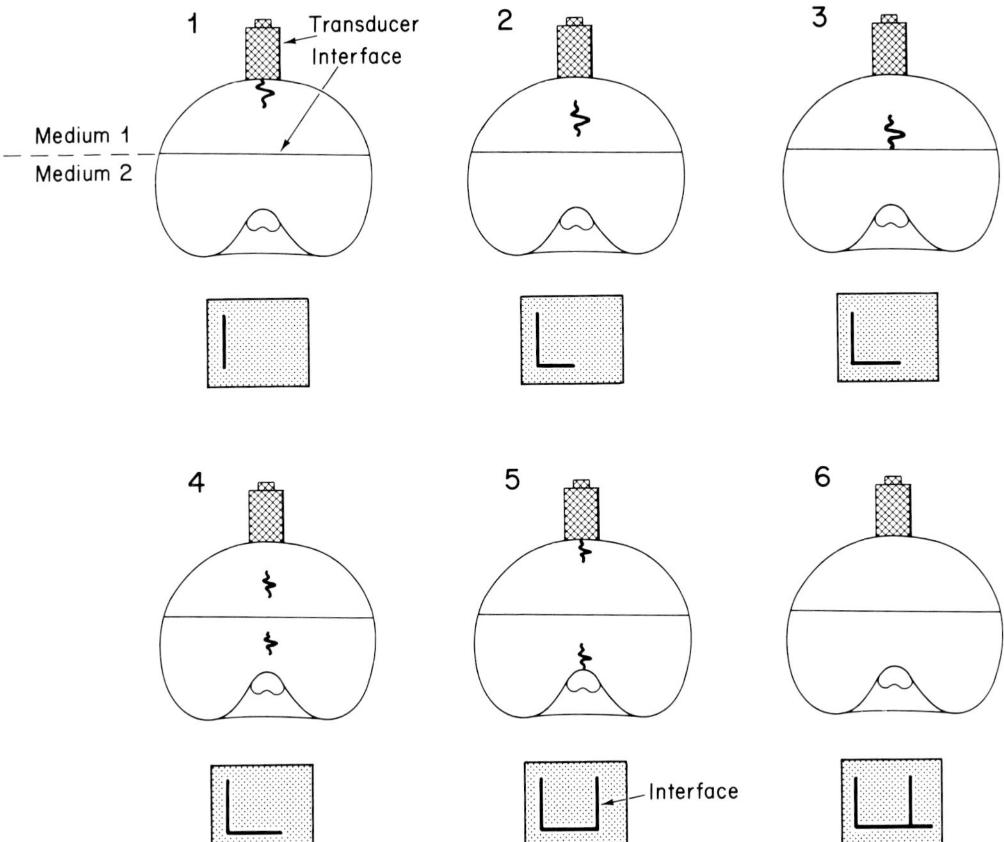

Figure 6–4. Diagrammatic representation of a sound wave travelling across a structure composed of two homogeneous media that differ in density and in velocity of sound transmission. At the interface between the media, a portion of the sound energy is reflected back to the resting transducer crystal, and a portion is transmitted beyond the interface. Corresponding amplitude spikes are depicted along a horizontal axis. The initial spike represents sound reflection at the interface between the transducer and the surface of medium 1. The second spike represents sound reflection from the acoustical interface between medium 1 and medium 2, and the horizontal distance between the first and second spikes is proportional to the distance between the surface of medium 1 and the acoustical interface at medium 2.

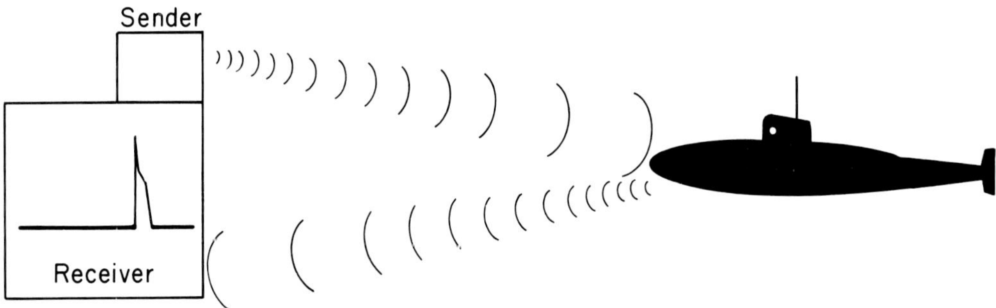

Figure 6–5. Basic concept of the use of sonar by a submarine.

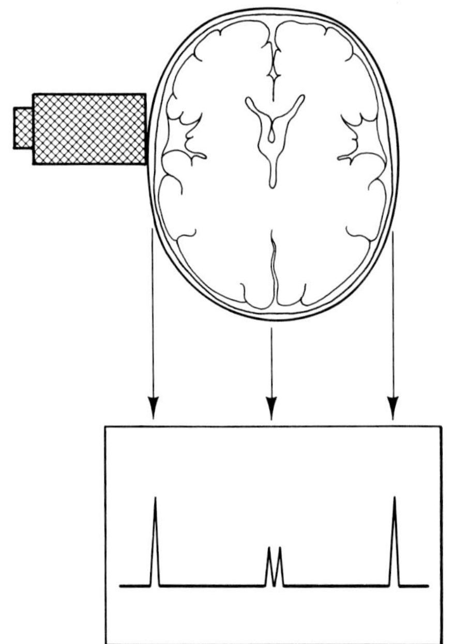

Figure 6–6. Diagram of the basic concept of echoencephalography.

How Is the Image Constructed?

Another form of ultrasonographic representation provides not only distance determination but also two-dimensional representations of reflecting surfaces. This process is termed *B-mode scanning* or *compound scanning.* It is achieved by a two-step modification of A-mode imaging. First, the reflecting interfaces on the oscilloscope screen are represented by a dot rather than a baseline deflection. In A-mode imaging, the intensity of returning echoes is represented by varying heights of baseline deflections seen on the oscilloscope screen. In *B-mode (brightness modulation) scanning,* the brightness of the dot reflects the intensity of the returning echo. Second, instead of imaging the reflecting surfaces in the small space traversed by the thin stationary sound beam, in B-mode scanning a whole plane of reflecting interfaces is imaged by moving the sound source and receiver during imaging, sampling many reflecting interfaces, and recording all the interface dots on the screen as one single image. For example, in imaging a liver with A-mode scanning one would see only deflections from the baseline on the oscilloscope screen; in B-mode representation of the liver, one would see dots on the screen. In *compound scanning,* the B-mode representations are "added together" to produce a two-dimensional image known as a *compound B-scan* (Fig. 6–7).

One area of the body difficult to image in such a manner is the heart. Surrounded by bone and lung (which is a poor sound-transmitting organ), the heart is relatively inaccessible. Investigation of the heart by ultrasound uses a form of ultrasound termed *M-mode (motion) scanning.* This form of ultrasound is nothing more than a dynamic B-mode image. In B-mode imaging the reflecting interfaces are represented by dots rather than spikes or deflections from the baseline on the oscilloscope screen. In M-mode imaging, one dot (representing one reflecting interface) is selected and watched over a period of time (Fig. 6–8). In echocardiography, for example, an image of the reflecting surface of the mitral valve is obtained on the screen and then a dynamic image is obtained by watching the "to-and-fro" action of the valve surface; it is thus possible to determine the extent and speed of motion of the valvular structure. In addition, M-mode ultrasound allows one to evaluate the contractility of part of the myocardium by watching the heart muscle contract during the cardiac cycle. Since M-mode imaging can give representation of all the reflecting surfaces within the heart, from pericardium to pericardium, it is possible to evaluate chamber size and discover abnormalities such as pericardial effusions by looking for separation between the epicardial surface and the overlying pericardium.

What Is Gray Scale?

Thus far it must appear that ultrasound achieves nothing more than delineation of boundaries of organs or the motion of those boundaries. There is, however, a newer refinement of ultrasound, termed *gray scale,* which provides us with a representation of organ texture. Each organ has its own internal reflecting surfaces in addition to the reflecting surface of its outer margin; for example, the liver contains thousands of bile ducts, lymphatics, veins, and arteries that are different from the internal reflecting surfaces of the kidney, which has a renal pelvis, a different vascular pattern, lymphatics, and nephrons. Gray scale imaging provides

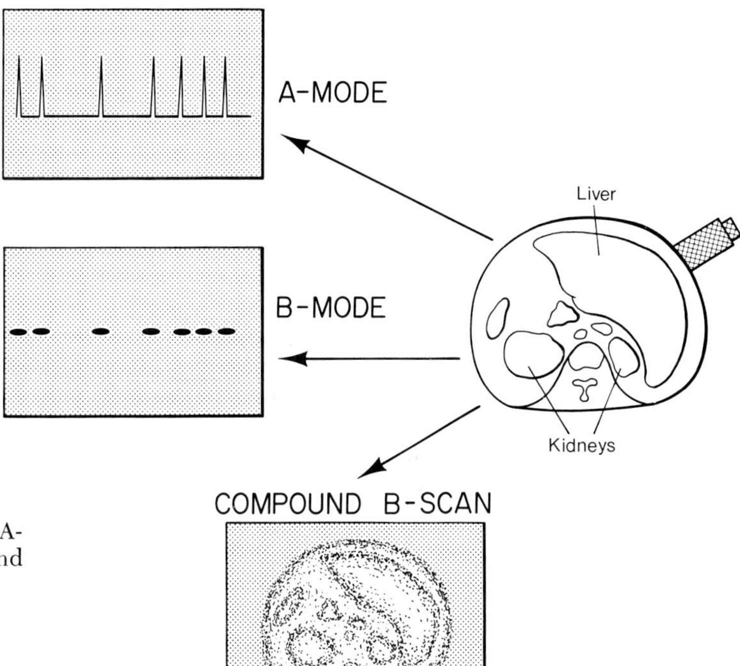

Figure 6–7. Illustration of A-mode, B-mode, and compound B-scan images of the abdomen.

us with a means of representing the spectrum of echoes arising from within the substance of the organ, not just from its surface. Variations between the internal textures of various organs are displayed on a television screen in varying shades of gray; hence the term *gray scale.* This system allows detection and evaluation of lesions arising within the individual organ; for example, one can demonstrate intrahepatic mass lesions such as abscesses, metastases, or cysts.

What Is Real Time?

Real time imaging is like fluoroscopy in that it produces an instantaneous image of the tissues in the beam and in motion. It allows rapid evaluation, especially of regions where multiple planes are needed to explore a complex process. For example, real time imaging is extremely useful in the evaluation of fetal heart motion in cases of suspected fetal death, in the examination of the gallbladder, for the rapid assessment of the size of the abdominal aorta, for the demonstration of pelvic anatomy in diagnosing obstetrical and gynecological problems, and in the evaluation of cardiac anatomy, particularly with respect to congenital heart disease. The difference between real time imaging and B-mode compound scanning is in the size of the sound beam. Whereas in B-mode scanning the beam is pencil-shaped, in real time imaging a larger sound beam is used. A larger beam can be achieved in three ways: by having a *linear array* of crystals that produce a broad ultrasonic beam with a rectangular configuration, by using a group of crystals (*phased array*) with

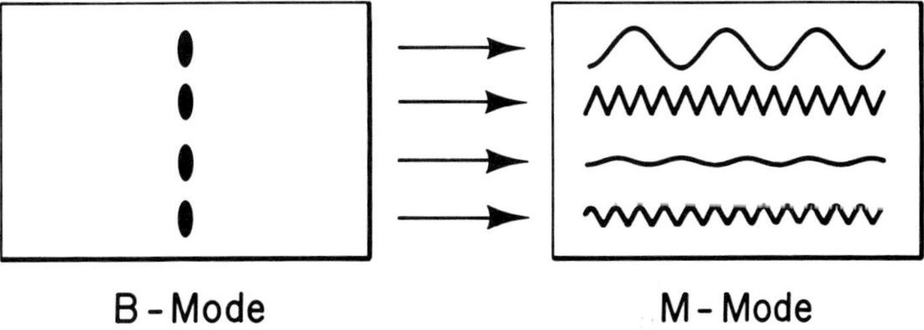

Figure 6–8. Relationship between B-mode and M-mode imaging. In this case, four reflecting surfaces are imaged with a B-mode scanner. A strip recorder images the motion of these reflecting surfaces with time. In this way, cardiac valvular motion can be evaluated.

the beam sweeping sequentially along them, or by causing a single crystal to oscillate continually to produce a fanlike distribution of sound waves (*mechanical sector scanner*).

CLINICAL APPLICATIONS OF ULTRASOUND

In the assessment of mass lesions within an organ, ultrasound provides one specific and useful function. It can determine whether a space-occupying lesion is cystic or solid in nature. This differentiation is extremely important in the evaluation of masses in the kidney—for example, if a small mass seen on intravenous pyelography fails to demonstrate the classic radiographic criteria of a renal cyst. Normally, angiographic evaluation of the mass would be done, but ultrasound is able to demonstrate whether the mass is fluid-filled or not. Many radiologists believe that if ultrasonographic examination indicates a cyst is fluid-filled, angiography is not necessary. A fluid-containing cyst is normally seen as a well-defined sonolucency within the parent organ when imaged ultrasonographically. The lesion has no demonstrable internal echoes and shows a well-defined posterior wall. There is also good sound transmission through the cyst, and strong echoes can be found arising from behind the cystic lesion itself. If the mass seen on an intravenous pyelogram is a solid mass, ultrasonographically it has poorly defined borders and multiple internal echoes and transmits sound poorly (Fig. 6–9).

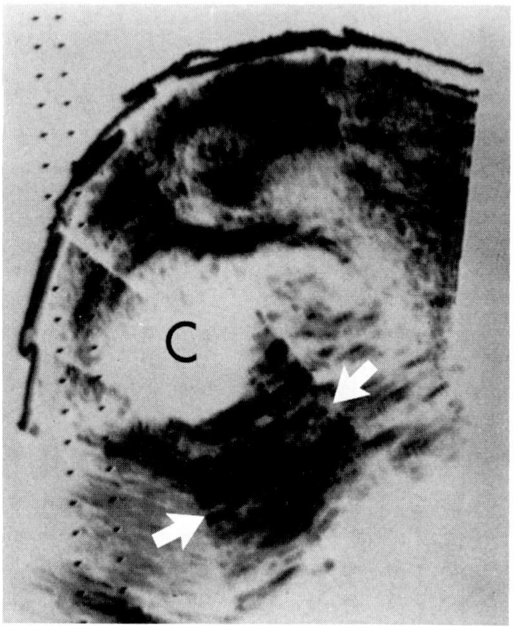

Figure 6–9. Characteristic echo pattern of a cyst (C) filled with an acoustically homogeneous fluid. The typical features include an absence of echoes arising from within the structure, good sound transmission through it with strong echoes behind (*arrows*), and sharp margination of the structure.

Before a discussion of the clinical applications of ultrasound, a few words should be said regarding its safety. Early applications of ultrasound for military purposes quickly showed some deleterious effects. During the early submarine searches employing ultrasound, it was noted that dead fish floated in the wake of the searching vessels, apparently killed by exposure to high-frequency sound waves. Despite these observations and despite the fact that high-frequency sounds are used in industrial cleaning to fragment unwanted substances, there is no good evidence to date that high-frequency sound at the energy levels used in diagnostic ultrasonography causes any appreciable or significant somatic or genetic damage. The safety of ultrasound is particularly advantageous in application to obstetrical and gynecological problems. Solving medical problems in the gravid patient or the patient of child-bearing age without the use of ionizing radiation is obviously of tremendous significance. This point should be kept in mind when we discuss the spectrum of clinical applications of ultrasound and also with respect to the use of x-rays and radioisotopes for the diagnosis of many of these problems.

Head and Neck

The head was one of the first areas investigated by the early ultrasonographers. It was possible to image intracranial midline structures, and some investigators showed the effect of intracranial space-occupying lesions by demonstrating midline shift. Echoencephalography, however, can miss bilateral masses such as bilateral subdural hematomas, since they produce no demonstrable midline shift. Recently, computerized tomography (CT scanning) has been used to evaluate patients in whom intracranial masses are suspected, because CT scanning delineates not only midline structures but also ventricular anatomy and intracranial masses.

Ultrasonic evaluation of thyroid nodules to determine whether they are cystic or solid is another indication for ultrasonography of the head and neck. This can be done easily when the masses are greater than 1 cm in diameter. Multiple transverse and longitudinal sonographic images of the thyroid and any co-existing mass lesion are made, and consistency of the thyroid tissue can be determined.

Heart

Evaluation of the heart using ultrasound yields a wide variety of data regarding cardiac anatomy, valvular mobility, myocardial contractility, and the presence of pericardial effusions. Imaging techniques employing ultrasound and gating devices allow determination of cardiac chamber contour and size during various phases of the cardiac cycle. In addition, M-mode studies of the heart also provide visualization of the valvular excursion during systole and diastole. The excursion of the mitral valve and its speed of closure were studied by the early echocardiographers. With echocardiography (ultrasonic examination of the heart), other parameters of cardiac function can also be evaluated such as ejection fraction, stroke volume, and septal and leaflet motion. Real time imaging is particularly applicable to the investigation of cardiac abnormalities.

Breast

Much interest has been given to applying ultrasonic examination of the breast, particularly in evaluating well-circumscribed solitary breast masses greater than 1 cm in diameter. Under certain circumstances, it is possible to make a determination of the nature of the mass as cystic or solid.

Abdomen

There is a wide spectrum of applications for ultrasound in the abdomen, and virtually all intra-abdominal organs lend themselves to ultrasonic investigation. Before the discussion of the applications of ultrasound to individual intra-abdominal organs, mention should be made of the image display conventions used in ultrasound. The pictorial display of echoes obtained in ultrasonographic examination is called a *sonogram*. When transverse images of the body are obtained they are displayed as though the examiner were viewing the cut section from below. In this way (with the patient supine), the patient's right side is imaged on the left of the screen. The transverse images in this chapter are displayed in this manner. In longitudinal views of the supine patient, the patient's head is to the left of the image.

The liver, being a relatively homogeneous organ, is easily evaluated ultrasonographically. In some patients, however, evaluation of the liver is hindered because the organ is located high in the right upper quadrant and is surrounded by the rib cage as well as by air-filled lung. In such a location, the liver can at times be acoustically inaccessible to ultrasound. Nevertheless, in most people it is possible to image the liver, and ultrasound has been used as an adjunct to radionuclide scanning. Defects in the liver seen on a radioisotopic liver scan should be assessed further by ultrasound. Finding a benign hepatic cyst rather than a solid hepatic neoplasm has markedly different prognostic implications, and differentiation between these two lesions is frequently possible with ultrasound. In routine liver evaluation, a series of longitudinal and transverse sonograms is usually obtained (Fig. 6–10). By such sectional evaluation of the liver, variations in internal texture and the presence of contour margins caused by internal mass lesions can be readily appreciated (Figs. 6–11, 6–12, and 6–13). Ultrasonographic imaging of the liver documents the presence of a mass lesion; often supplies information to determine whether the lesion is cystic (benign cyst) or solid (hepatic neoplasm or metastasis); and helps with the diagnostic investigation of demonstrated hepatic masses.

In recent years, ultrasonographically guided percutaneous biopsies have become widely accepted. Solitary hepatic, pancreatic, and other masses can be accurately localized with ultrasound, and the passage of a biopsy needle or an aspiration needle into

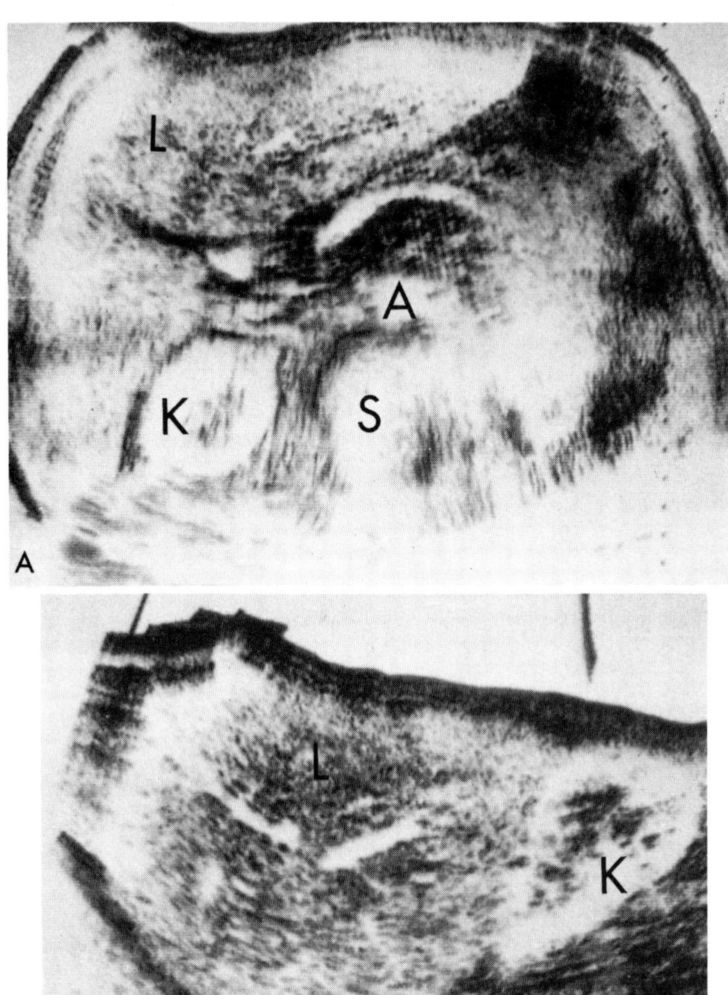

Figure 6–10. *A*, Transverse image of the midabdomen showing a cross-section of the liver (L). In the same section, views of the kidney (K), aorta (A), and spine (S) are seen. The linear sonolucent structure crossing the midline above the aorta is the splenic vein. *B*, Longitudinal views of the liver (L) as seen on a section 8 cm to the right of the midline. Below the liver edge is the right kidney (K). This examination was part of an evaluation of a palpable right lower quadrant mass that proved to be an anterior right kidney.

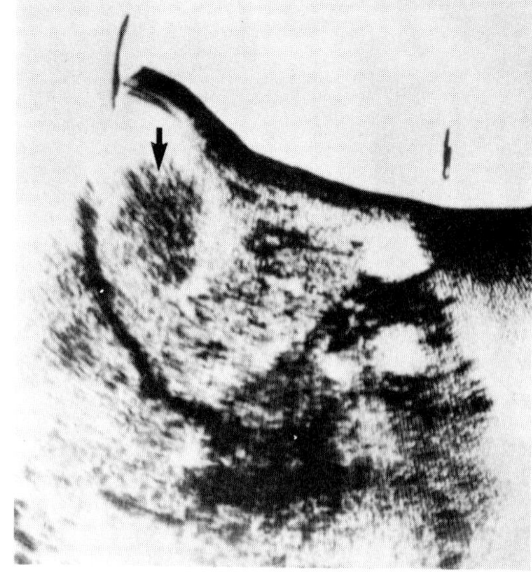

Figure 6–11. Longitudinal image of the liver 8 cm to the right of midline showing an echogenic tumor mass (*arrow*) surrounded by a sonolucent rim. This image was obtained with the patient supine. The patient's head is to the left of the image and the feet are to the right. Compare the texture of the liver to that shown in Figure 6–10B.

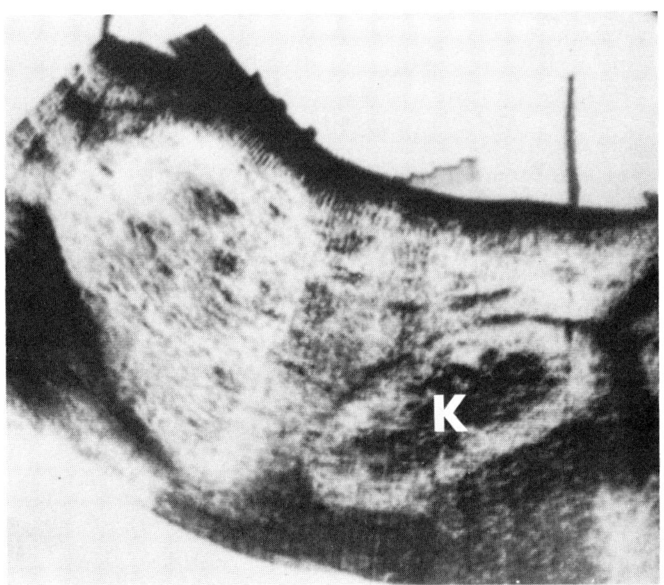

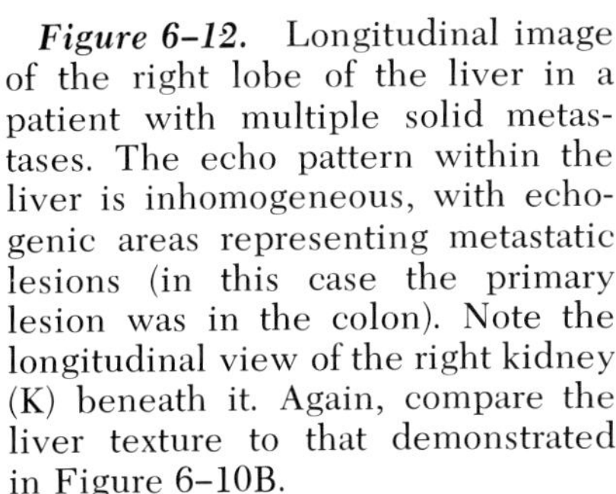
Figure 6–12. Longitudinal image of the right lobe of the liver in a patient with multiple solid metastases. The echo pattern within the liver is inhomogeneous, with echogenic areas representing metastatic lesions (in this case the primary lesion was in the colon). Note the longitudinal view of the right kidney (K) beneath it. Again, compare the liver texture to that demonstrated in Figure 6–10B.

the mass is facilitated by ultrasonographic guidance. Using ultrasound and a *biopsy transducer,* it is possible to "follow" the passage of the biopsy needle into the lesion. Percutaneous aspiration of intra-abdominal masses using ultrasound has become common in many radiology departments; biopsy of small hepatic and pancreatic masses can be performed using ultrasound guidance with an approach through the anterior abdominal wall.

Brief mention should be made of the application of ultrasound to evaluation of the spleen. With ultrasonographic examination, a defect seen on radioisotopic spleen scan can at times be easily evaluated and filling defects caused by fluid collections such as a splenic hematoma or cyst can be readily appreciated. Evaluation of the splenic area in patients who have suffered left upper quadrant injury can also be rewarding and can help to demonstrate the presence of hematomas or fluid collections in or around the spleen. Perisplenic fluid collections can at times be most accurately evaluated by ultrasound, since radionuclide spleen scans may

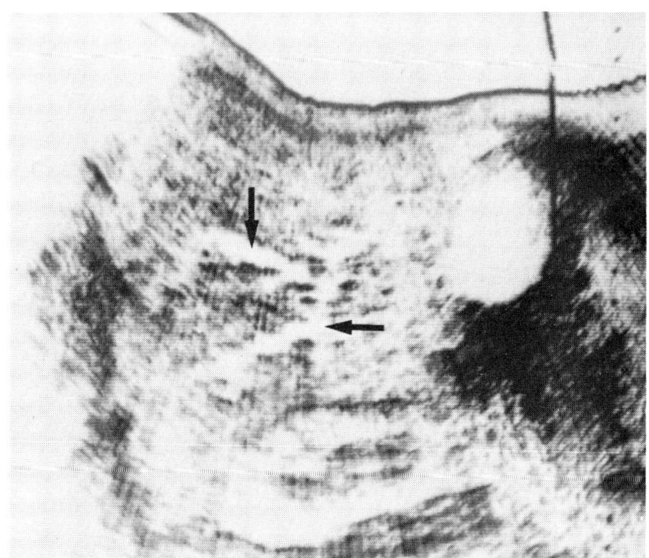

Figure 6–13. Longitudinal image of the liver in a patient with dilated intrahepatic bile ducts resulting from common duct obstruction. The dilated bile ducts appear as a network of multiple branching sonolucent structures within the liver (*arrows*). Frequent branching distinguishes bile ducts from blood vessels.

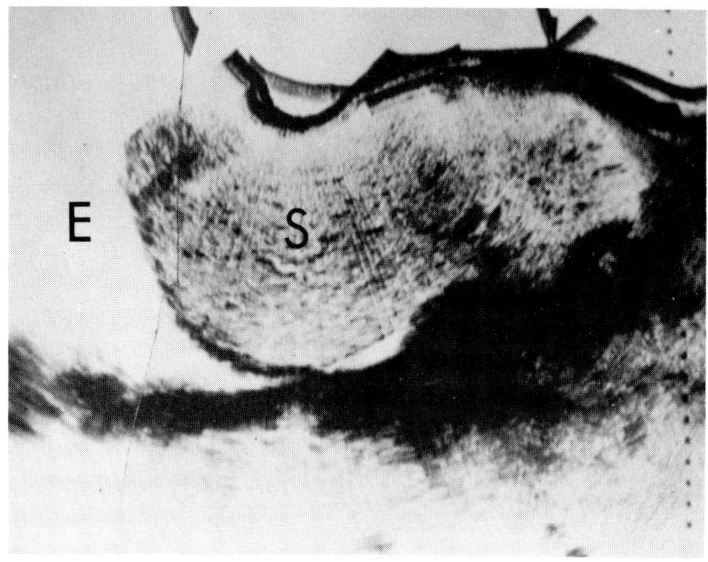

Figure 6–14. Longitudinal image of an enlarged spleen (S) in a patient with myelofibrosis. This image is obtained as a longitudinal view of the left side of the abdomen with the patient lying supine. The upper pole of the spleen is to the left of the image. The sonolucent area above the spleen represents a large left pleural effusion (E). The left hemidiaphragm is imaged as a thin echogenic structure between the effusion and the upper pole of the spleen. The linear array of dots on the right side of the image is used for measuring. The distance between the dots is proportional to 1 cm.

not show fluid collections that lie outside the spleen itself. Ultrasound may also be useful in the evaluation of splenic size and location (Fig. 6–14). Ultrasonographic examination has great importance in the evaluation of the splenic bed after splenectomy, particularly in the search for a subphrenic abscess. Gallium scanning coupled with ultrasound is an extremely useful method of evaluating suspected abscesses, and aspiration of pus collections can also be aided by ultrasound. Ultrasound can also be used in the evaluation of patients with increasing abdominal girth and suspected ascites (Fig. 6–15).

The gallbladder is another organ easily imaged by ultrasound. Ultrasound can be extremely helpful in the evaluation of a patient with suspected gallstones whose gallbladder fails to opacify during oral cholecystography or intravenous cholangiography. It is possible not only to see the gallbladder and to observe its response to a fatty meal but also to evaluate the internal acoustic characteristics of the organ, particularly with respect to the dem-

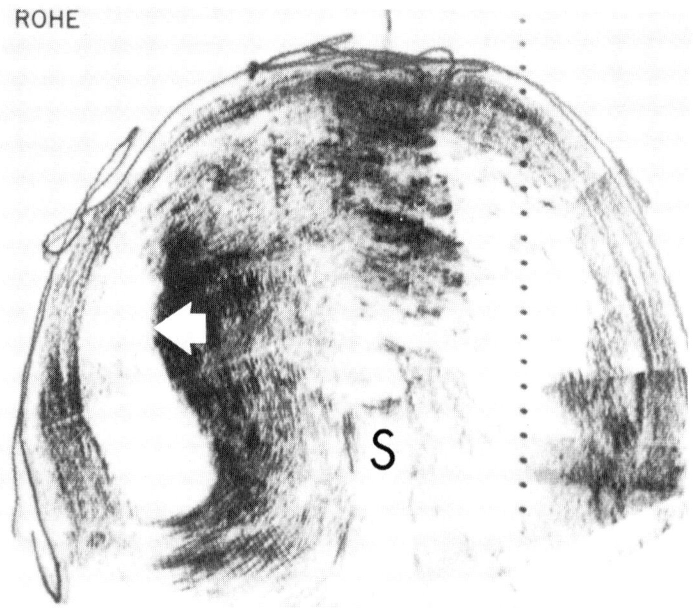

Figure 6–15. In this image the patient is supine. The spine (S) is seen posteriorly. Transverse image of the abdomen with a collection of fluid (ascites) adjacent to the lateral flank (*arrow*). The ascites appears sonolucent because it is composed of an acoustically homogeneous fluid medium. The central echogenic area represents bowel that is floating centrally because of the ascites.

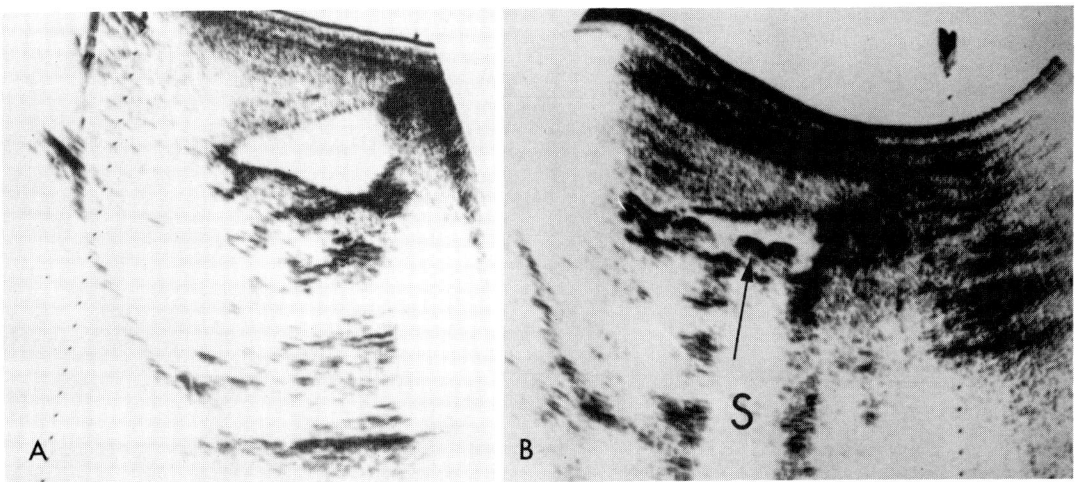

Figure 6–16. A, Longitudinal image of the normal gallbladder obtained with the patient lying supine. The patient is scanned 8 cm to the right of the midline. The gallbladder is seen as a pear-shaped sonolucent structure in the central portion of the image. Since bile is an acoustically homogeneous medium, no echoes arise from within it. *B*, A gallbladder containing three gallstones. The gallstones surrounded by bile are strongly reflective interfaces. The characteristic echo pattern includes a strong echo from the surfaces of the gallstones (*arrow*) and the "acoustical shadow" (S) behind the gallstone in the direction of the sound beam. This pattern is virtually diagnostic of gallstones.

onstration of gallstones. It is suggested that the evaluation of the nonvisualized gallbladder during cholecystography should include ultrasound (Fig. 6–16).

The pancreas has proven relatively inaccessible to evaluation by conventional radiographic techniques. Although it is, of course, possible to gather information using special techniques such as angiography or pancreatic duct cannulation, ultrasonographic examination can be extremely helpful in demonstrating pancreatic masses and evidence of peripancreatic disease (Figs. 6–17, 6–18, 6–19, and 6–20). Also, as mentioned

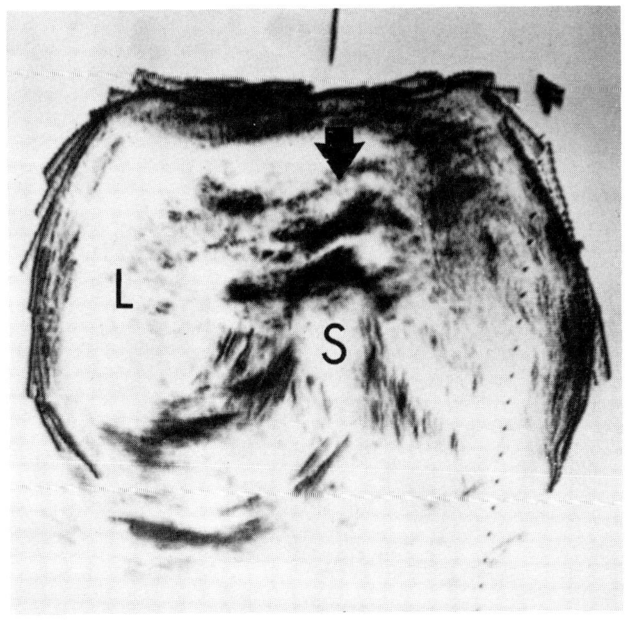

Figure 6–17. Transverse image of the abdomen at the level of the pancreas and liver (L). The normal pancreas (*arrow*) is seen arching across the midline. The spine (S) is well demonstrated. The round, sonolucent structure just above it is the aorta, from which the right renal artery is seen to arise and pass to the patient's right.

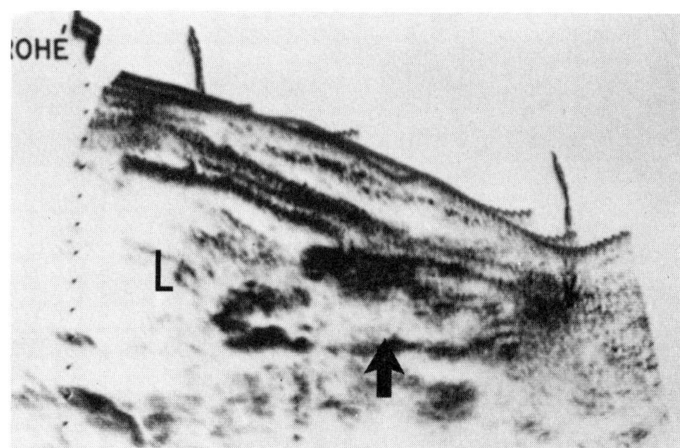

Figure 6–18. Longitudinal view of the abdomen 2 cm to the right of the midline and passing through the pancreatic head (*arrow*). The patient's head is to the left. The two vertical linear densities extending from the anterior abdominal wall superiorly mark from left to right the level of the xiphoid and umbilicus respectively. The liver (L) is again seen to the left.

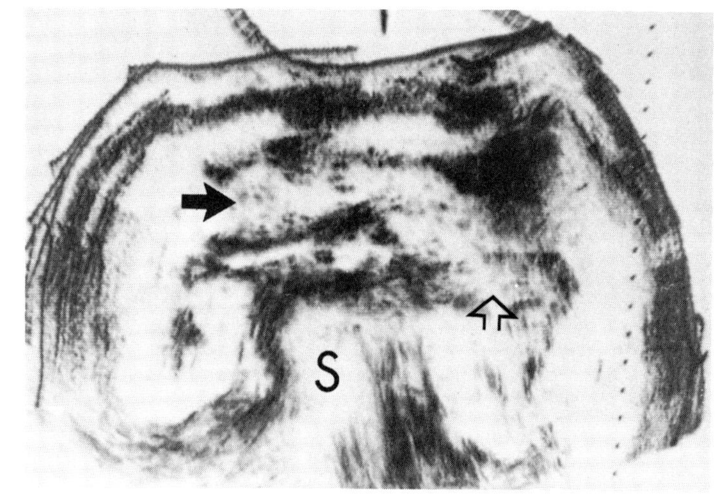

Figure 6–19. Transverse section of the abdomen at the level of the pancreas in a patient with a history of alcoholism and epigastric pain. The pancreas is enlarged in the region of the head (*solid arrow*), body, and tail (*hollow arrow*). The spine (S) is well seen. The enlarged spleen is seen on the left side of the abdomen. The pancreas is hypoechoic (it gives off few echoes) and enlarged, indicating generalized edema of the gland. In this case, the diagnosis was acute pancreatitis. The distinction between pancreatitis and pancreatic carcinoma cannot be made on the basis of the ultrasound image alone. Compare the pancreas in this image to that shown in Figure 6–17.

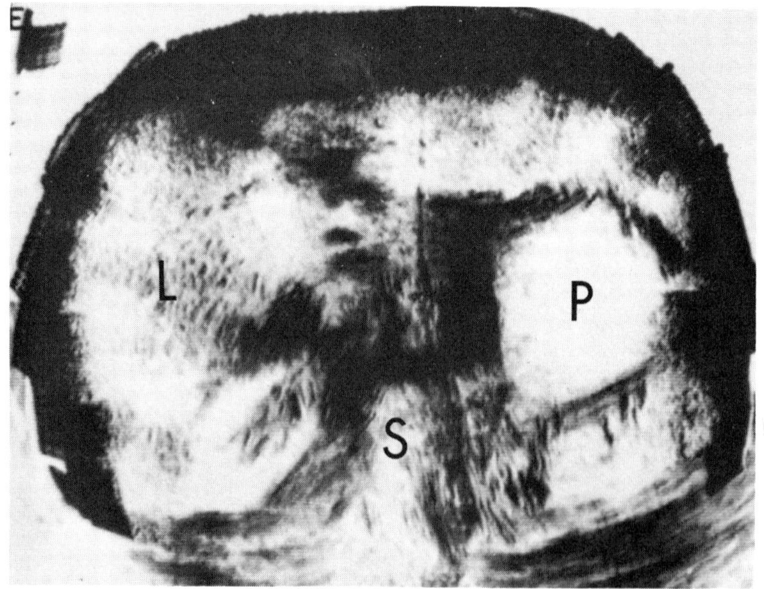

Figure 6–20. Transverse image of the abdomen at the level of a palpable left upper quadrant mass. The patient had a long history of alcoholism. A pseudocyst (P) arising from the tail of the pancreas is seen on the patient's left. Note that this mass appears similar to any cystic structure. The relationship of the cystic mass to the pancreas suggests the diagnosis of a pancreatic pseudocyst, which was confirmed at operation. The liver (L) and spine (S) are also seen.

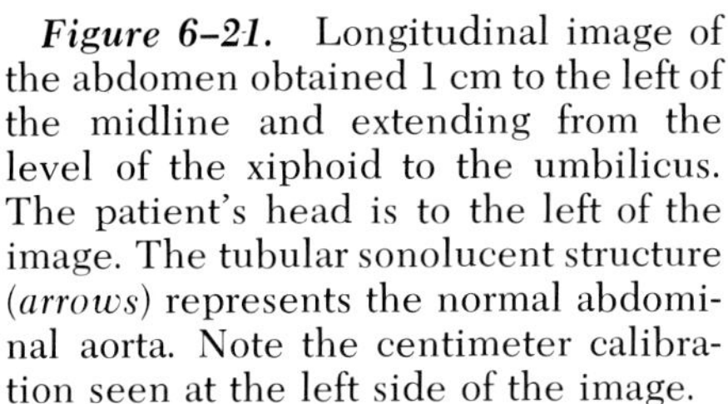

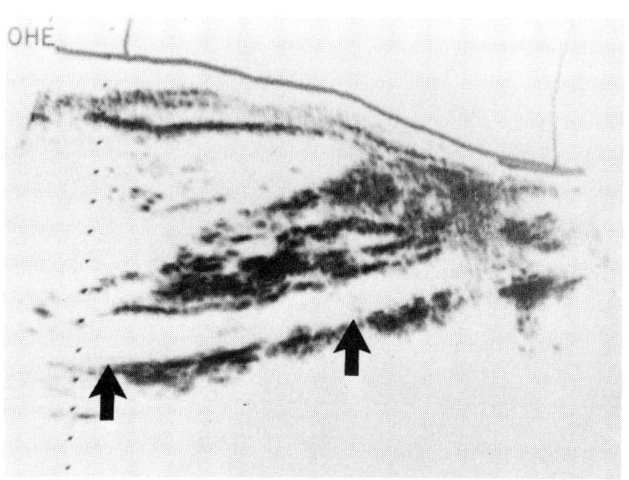

Figure 6–21. Longitudinal image of the abdomen obtained 1 cm to the left of the midline and extending from the level of the xiphoid to the umbilicus. The patient's head is to the left of the image. The tubular sonolucent structure (*arrows*) represents the normal abdominal aorta. Note the centimeter calibration seen at the left side of the image.

earlier, the pancreas is one of the organs for which biopsy using percutaneously introduced biopsy needles guided by ultrasound has been successful. Such evaluation may obviate the need for angiography or surgery.

Noninvasive examination of abdominal organs includes ultrasonographic evaluation of the aorta (Figs. 6–21 and 6–22). A patient with a pulsatile abdominal mass may present a clinical dilemma to his physician (Fig. 6–23). Does the patient have an aneurysm or not? Is there an abdominal mass situated over a normal aorta mimicking a pulsatile mass? Is the "mass" simply a prominent aorta in a patient with a marked lumbar kyphosis? These problems can frequently be solved by ultrasound instead of abdominal angiography. After the diagnosis of an abdominal aortic aneurysm is made, ultrasonographic evaluation is still useful. If the size of the aneurysm is such that the patient is not considered a candidate for operation, the aorta may be sequentially evaluated by ultrasound to determine progressive changes in aortic size without repeated angiographic procedures. Ultrasound has yet another advantage over

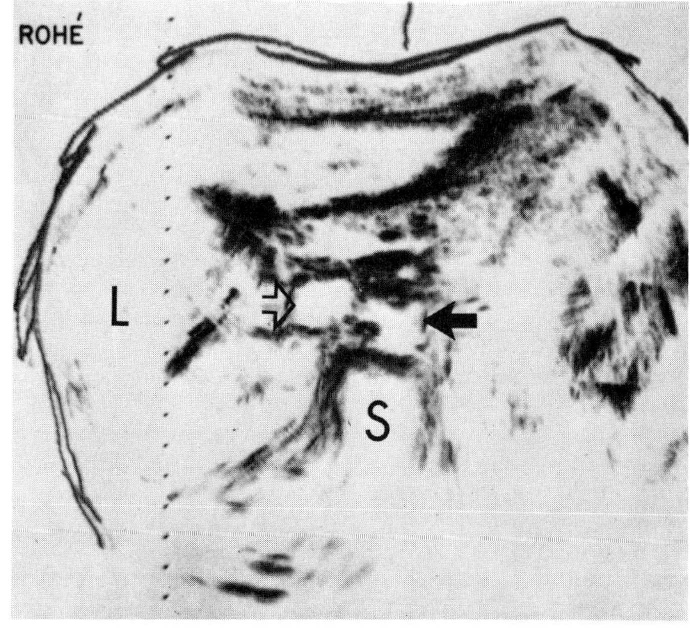

Figure 6–22. This is a transverse image of the abdomen at the level of the liver (L), demonstrating the aorta (*solid arrow*) and inferior vena cava (*hollow arrow*) ventral to the spine (S). The sonolucent structure seen ventral to the aorta is the splenic vein crossing the midline.

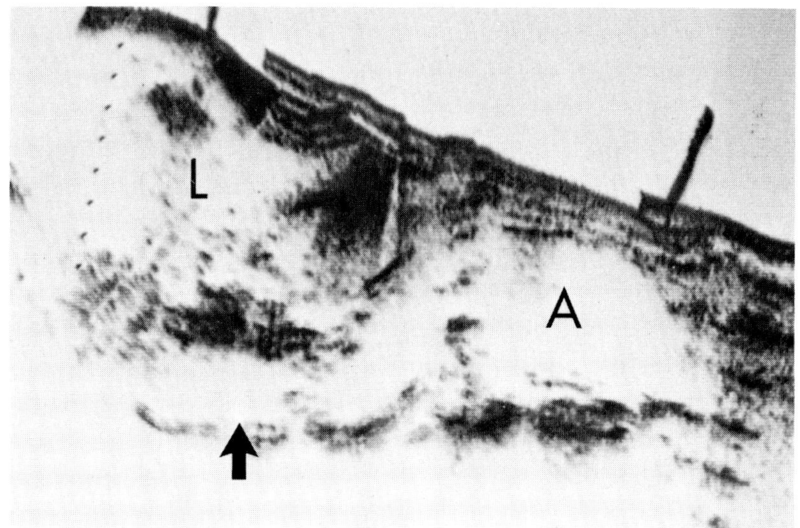

Figure 6–23. A longitudinal image of the abdomen in a plane 1 cm to the left of the midline and extending from the xiphoid to the umbilicus in a patient with a pulsatile abdominal mass. The abdominal aorta is imaged along its longitudinal axis, and an abdominal aortic aneurysm (A) corresponding to the pulsatile mass is demonstrated. Compare the configuration of the abdominal aorta in this image to that in Figure 6–21. The more normal appearing abdominal aorta (*arrow*) is seen proximal to the aneurysm on this image. The liver (L) is seen on the left of the image.

angiography in the evaluation of abdominal aortic aneurysms. Angiography is accurate in evaluating the dimensions of the aortic lumen, but the presence of clot within the aneurysm can at times cause one to underestimate aortic diameter. Using ultrasound, one can distinguish between blood-carrying portions of the aorta and a thrombus. Therefore, with ultrasound one can obtain an accurate measurement of the size of the aneurysm as well as the dimensions of the blood-containing part of the aortic lumen. One advantage of angiography over ultrasound in the evaluation of the abdominal aorta is that angiography also allows one to assess the extent of the aneurysmal involvement of the renal arteries, iliac arteries, and other branches arising from the aorta.

Like the pancreas, the retroperitoneum is generally a somewhat inaccessible area for conventional radiographic techniques, and unless a retroperitoneal mass erodes adjacent bones or displaces a kidney, ureter, or overlying loops of bowel, it can go unnoticed. Ultrasound has made easy investigation of the retroperitoneum possible; for example, retroperitoneal lymph node enlargement may be evaluated by ultrasound without the use of lymphographic contrast agents. In addition, retroperitoneal tumors may be easily seen and their response to therapy may be followed without using such techniques as retroperitoneal CO_2 injections, lymphangiography, and repeated abdominal angiography.

Ultrasound is a useful method of investigation for the assessment of lesions in or about the kidneys. With the patient in a prone position, longitudinal and transverse sonographic images of the kidneys may be obtained (Figs. 6–24 and 6–25). In cross-section, the kidneys are paramedian and posterior, appearing ultrasonographically as two doughnuts. The cortices are relatively sonolucent (echo-free), and the center of each kidney is shown by a dense clump of echoes, representing the renal collecting systems. Much information can be gathered from ultrasound studies of the kidneys and renal tract:

1. *Renal size.* Size of the kidneys may be determined accurately without the need for urographic contrast agents.

2. *Renal location.* Location of the kidneys may be documented using ultrasound; this is particularly useful in planning x-ray therapy for a renal tumor.

3. *Renal non-function.* In a patient who exhibits one functioning kidney on intravenous pyelography, the non-functioning renal bed may be evaluated ultrasonogra-

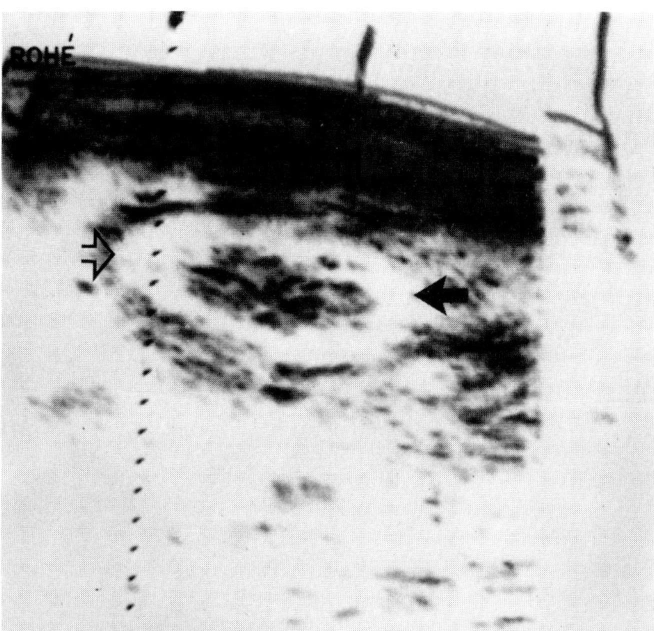

Figure 6–24. Longitudinal image of a kidney with the patient lying prone. The patient's head is to the left of the image. The upper pole is demarcated (*hollow arrow*) as is the lower pole (*solid arrow*). The central collecting structures are imaged as dense echogenic structures arising from the central portion of the kidney. Around the collecting system a less echogenic rim is seen, representing the normal renal parenchyma.

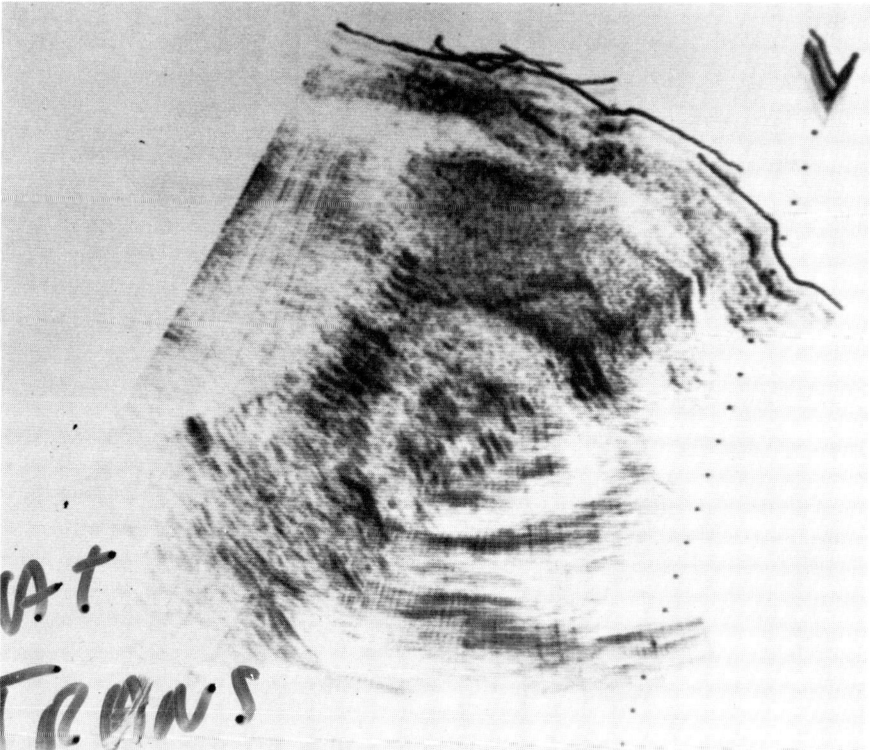

Figure 6–25. This is a transverse image of a kidney. The dense central echoes can be seen arising from the renal collecting system. The more sonolucent renal parenchyma surrounds the central dense collections. This "doughnut" shape is typical of a transverse image made through a kidney.

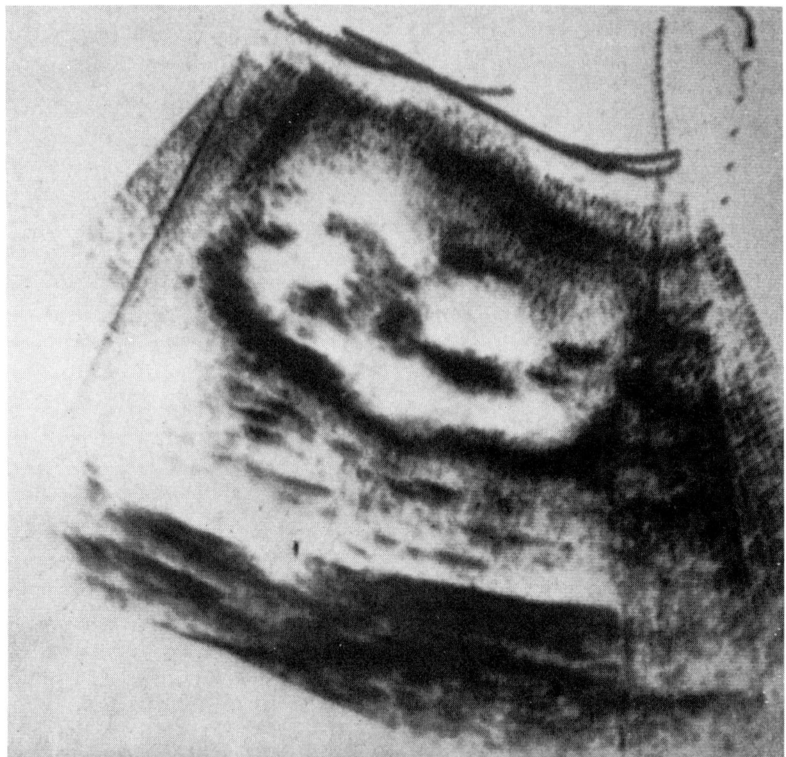

Figure 6–26. Longitudinal image of a hydronephrotic kidney. Multiple cystic areas within the central collecting system of the kidney are noted. These correspond to dilated calyces. Compare the appearance of the collecting system on this longitudinal image to that seen in Figure 6–24, in which the central collection is dense and homogeneous.

phically, and the possibilities of renal agenesis, tumor replacement, or hydronephrosis may be assessed. In agenesis, no renal tissue is identified; in mass replacement of the kidney, a retroperitoneal tumor will become apparent; in hydronephrosis, the dilated collecting systems can be easily seen without the need for studies using retrograde injection of contrast agents (Fig. 6–26).

4. *Renal mass evaluation.* If a solitary renal mass is seen on intravenous pyelography, the mass should be evaluated using ultrasound, by which cystic and solid masses may be easily distinguished. Solid masses require angiographic evaluation, whereas cystic lesions require only percutaneous puncture and aspiration, which can be done easily using ultrasonographic guidance (Figs. 6–27, 6–28, and 6–29).

5. *Renal biopsy.* Renal localization can also be performed ultrasonographically to guide the needle during percutaneous renal biopsy.

6. *Bladder evaluation.* A urine-filled bladder is easily seen ultrasonographically. Since it is a homogeneous structure when filled with urine, the exact dimensions and contours of the bladder may be mapped using ultrasound. Thus, it is possible not only to see alterations in bladder configuration caused by contiguous masses but also to estimate urine volume before and after voiding. Such measurements provide a simple method of estimating post-void residual urine volume, obviating the need for bladder catheterization and reducing the risk of subsequent urinary tract infections.

Pelvic Structures

Pelvic masses, postmenopausal bleeding, third trimester bleeding, "size for dates" problems, questions of fetal age, multiple and ectopic pregnancies, and missed abortions are problems that can be dealt with using ultrasonographic examination. If a

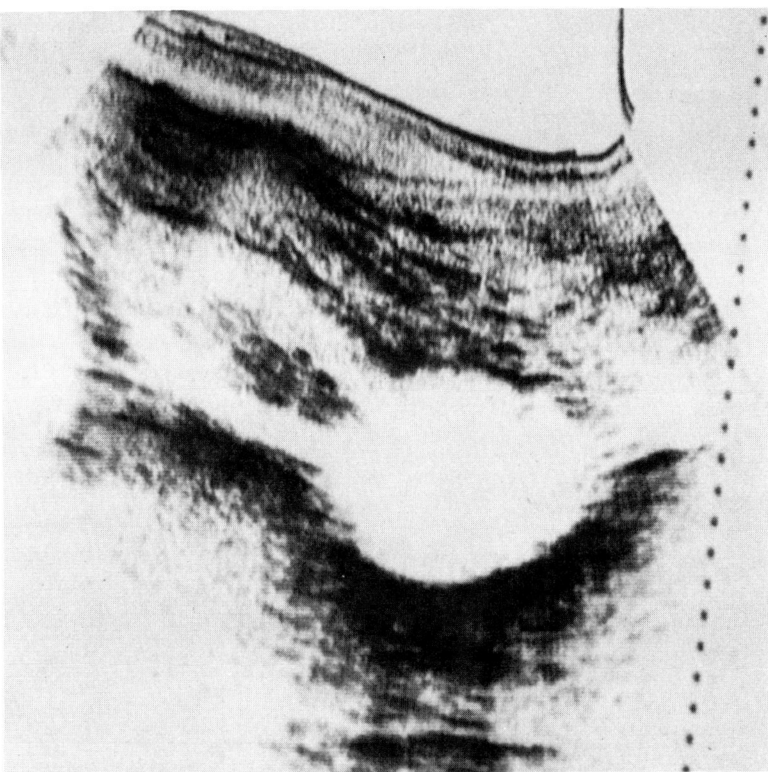

Figure 6–27. This is a longitudinal image of a kidney that, when evaluated by intravenous pyelography, demonstrated a mass arising from the lower pole. This longitudinal image shows a sonolucent mass arising from its lower pole, representing a simple renal cyst.

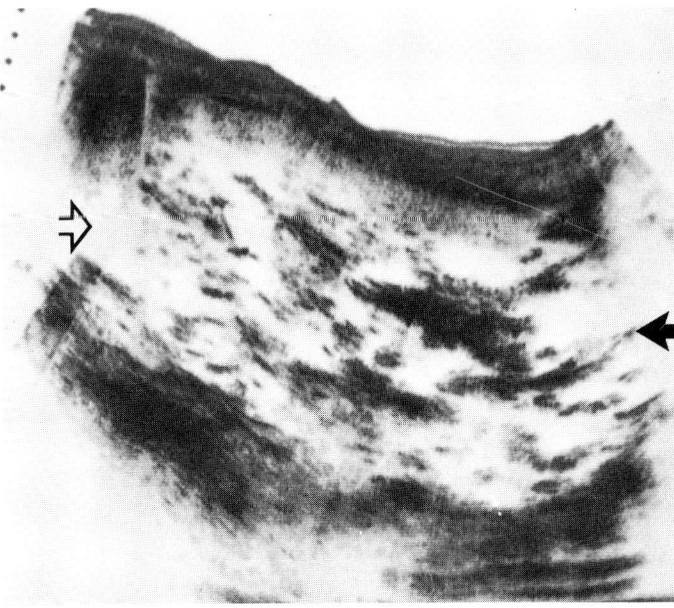

Figure 6–28. A polycystic kidney demonstrated in a longitudinal image. Note the enlargement of the kidney: See the centimeter calibrations in the left upper corner of this image. There are multiple cystic spaces throughout the kidney, representing the numerous cysts seen in polycystic kidney disease. The upper pole (*hollow arrow*) and lower pole (*solid arrow*) of the kidney are visible.

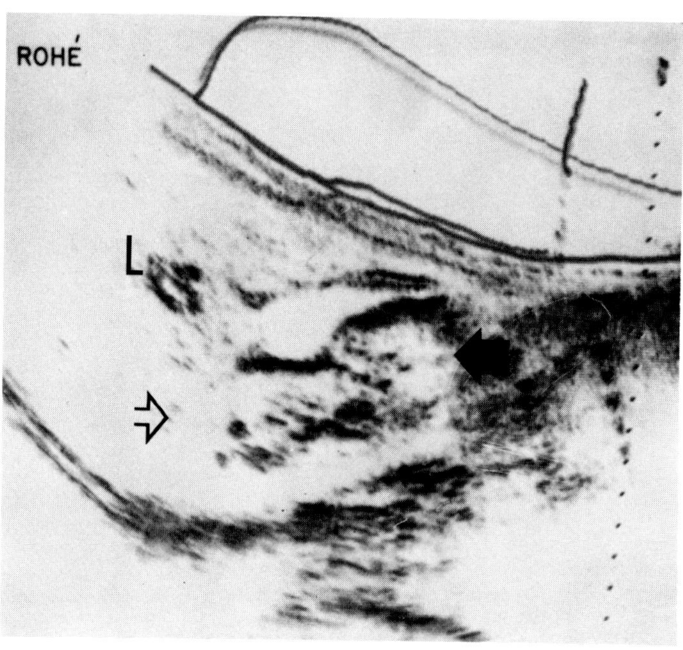

Figure 6–29. A longitudinal image of the right kidney obtained with the patient supine. Imaging is obtained through the liver. A mass arises from the lower pole of the right kidney (*solid arrow*). Echoes from within this mass indicate that it is solid and contains multiple acoustic interfaces. The mass is seen to deform the gallbladder, which is the pear-shaped sonolucent structure lying ventrally. Compare the appearance of the lower pole renal mass to that imaged in Figure 6–27. At operation, the solid lower pole renal mass was found to be a hypernephroma. In this image, the upper pole of the kidney is demarcated (*hollow arrow*).

woman has a suspected pathologic pelvic condition and cannot be examined because of obesity or some other reason, ultrasound can be used.

With a full bladder, the patient is positioned supine, and initially a series of longitudinal sonograms is obtained. The first image is in the midline plane and extends from the umbilicus down to the pubic symphysis (Fig. 6–30). Subsequently, a series of longitudinal images is constructed at 1-cm intervals both to the left and to the right of the midline. The examination plane is then rotated 90 degrees, and a series of transverse images is obtained through the pelvis and extending from the pubic symphysis up to the umbilicus (Fig. 6–31). In the evaluation of these pelvic images, the urinary bladder is first identified anteriorly, deep in the pelvis, usually appearing oval in shape

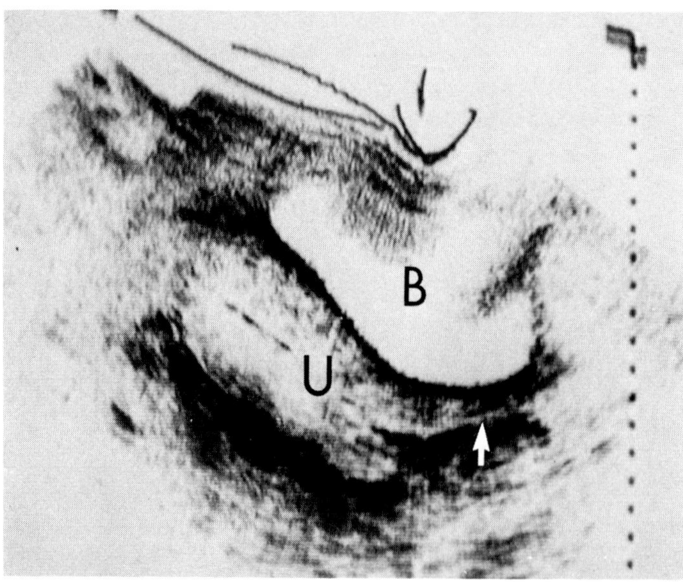

Figure 6–30. The normal female pelvis seen in a longitudinal image. The patient's head is to the left. The sonolucent structure seen anterior in the pelvis is the urinary bladder (B), which for pelvic examination must be full. The full bladder provides a homogeneous acoustical "window" for imaging the deep pelvic structures. The normal vagina (*arrow*), cervix, and uterus (U) are seen behind the fluid-filled urinary bladder.

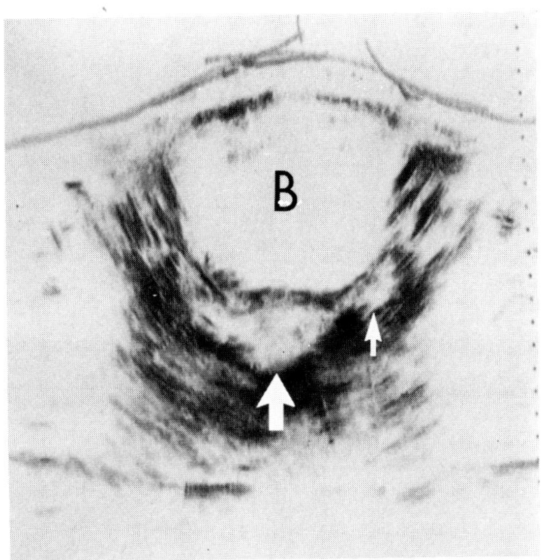

Figure 6–31. Transverse image of the normal female pelvis. In this image, the patient is supine. The uterus (*large arrow*) is seen as a midline structure behind the urinary bladder (B). The left ovary (*small arrow*) is seen adjacent to the lateral margin of the uterus.

and recognizable because sound waves pass through it so easily. Behind the bladder is a relatively homogeneous pear-shaped structure, the uterus, which may give off central linear echoes arising from the uterine cavity. Portions of the air-filled and stool-filled rectum may be seen behind the uterus. The ovaries may be seen lateral to the uterus, but their appearance is variable. Once the normal structures are identified, it is possible to tailor the examination to the individual patient.

Pelvic Mass Evaluation

In patients with a known or suspected pelvic mass, it is possible with ultrasound not only to confirm the presence of a mass but also to obtain significant information regarding its nature and origin. Once the mass is seen ultrasonographically, its texture can be determined with great accuracy. The differentiation of an ovarian mass, a cyst arising from the ovary or fallopian tube, and a uterine mass can be made with ultrasound (Figs. 6–32, 6–33, and 6–34).

Obstetrical Problems

It is easy to visualize the placenta using ultrasound and thereby to evaluate possible causes of late gestational bleeding, such as abruptio placenta or placenta previa. A few words of caution with regard to the diagnosis of placenta previa: The relationship between the placenta and the uterus is a dynamic one that changes as gestation proceeds. Thus, the diagnosis of placenta

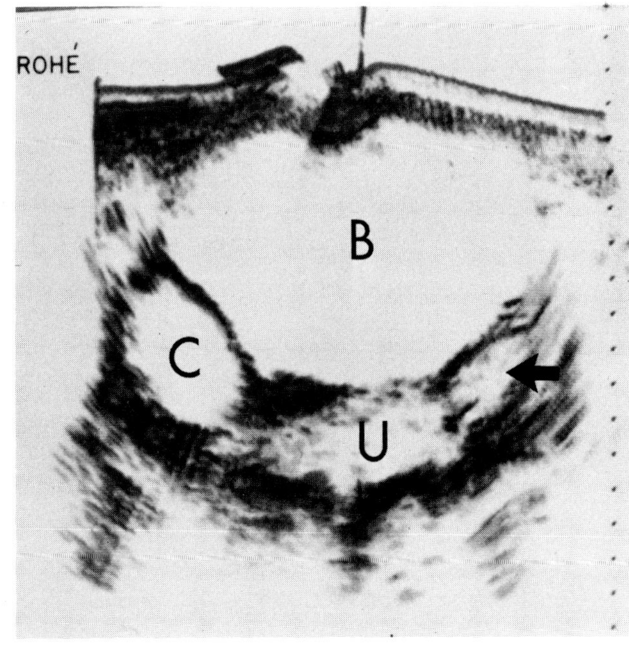

Figure 6–32. This is a transverse image of pelvic structures obtained in the supine position in a young female patient with right pelvic pain. There is a cystic mass 4 cm in diameter in the right adnexa, representing an ovarian cyst (C). Note the bladder (B), the normal uterus (U) in the midline, and the normal left ovary (*arrow*). Remember: In the imaging convention used in ultrasound, one views the patient from the feet in transverse images; therefore, the patient's right appears to the left of the image.

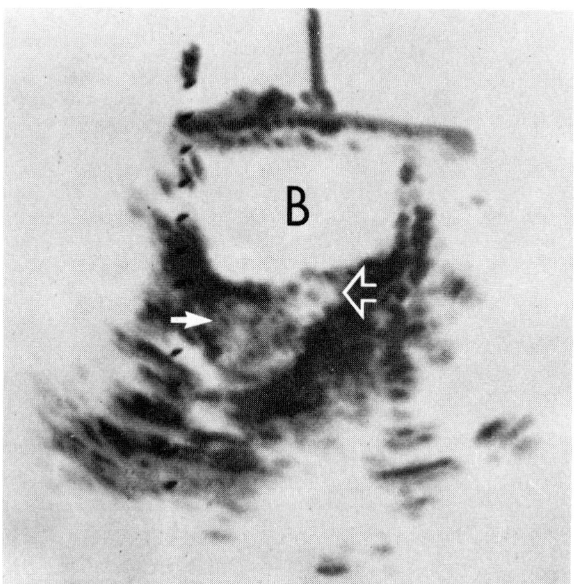

Figure 6–33. Transverse image of the pelvis of a 9-year-old female who presented with precocious puberty. An adequate physical examination could not be performed because of the patient's age. On transverse image of the pelvis there is a mass 2.4 cm in diameter (*small arrow*) in the right adnexal area, adjacent to the uterus (*open arrow*). Note that this mass contains numerous internal echoes, indicating that it is solid. At operation, a hormonally active granulosa cell tumor of the right ovary was removed. Note the sonolucent bladder (B).

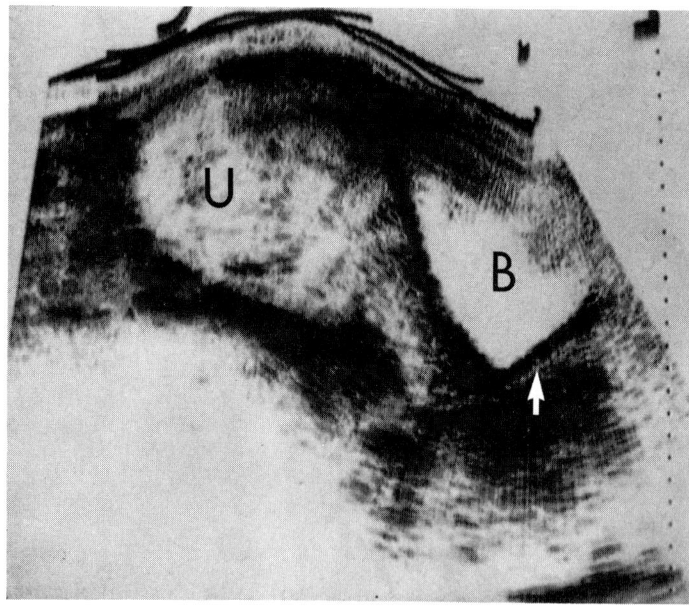

Figure 6–34. This is a midline sonogram of the pelvis of a perimenopausal woman who presented with a lower abdominal mass. The patient is supine, and her head is to the left. The bladder (B) is easily seen deep in the pelvis. Above the bladder is a large, solid mass inseparable from the cervix and vagina (*arrow*), representing a uterus enlarged by fibroids (U).

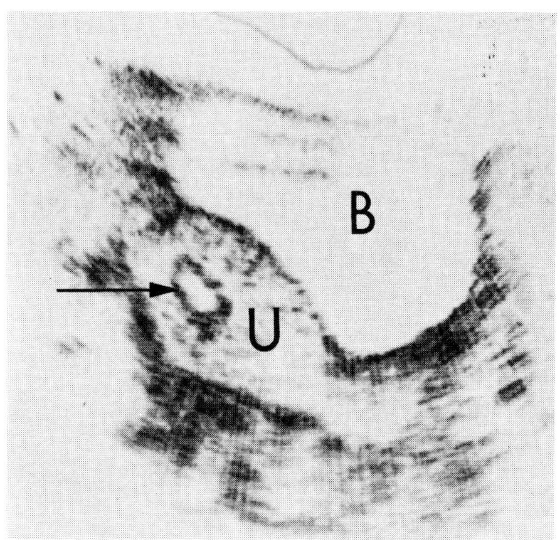

Figure 6–35. Longitudinal sonogram through the pelvis of a female in the first trimester of pregnancy. The patient is supine, with the head to the left of the image. The sonolucent bladder (B) is easily visualized deep in the pelvis. Behind it, the somewhat enlarged uterus (U) is seen. Within the uterus is a ring-like structure (*arrow*) representing the gestational sac. The sac is first seen at about five weeks of gestation. It enlarges progressively during the first trimester of pregnancy. The fetal head is first visualized at approximately twelve weeks.

previa is valid only for the period of time shortly after the diagnosis is made, since the placenta may "migrate" away from the internal os as the uterus enlarges.

With ultrasound, it is possible to document pregnancy (Fig. 6–35) and to predict with some accuracy the age of the fetus by performing biparietal diameter measurements of the fetal skull (Fig. 6–36). Other measurements such as crown-rump lengths have also been used to estimate fetal age.

The problem of failure of the uterus to enlarge coupled with the possibility of fetal death may also be studied using ultrasound. The diagnosis of a hydatidiform mole can be made with certainty using ultrasound because of its characteristic appearance. Fetal death can be confirmed by ultrasound, by

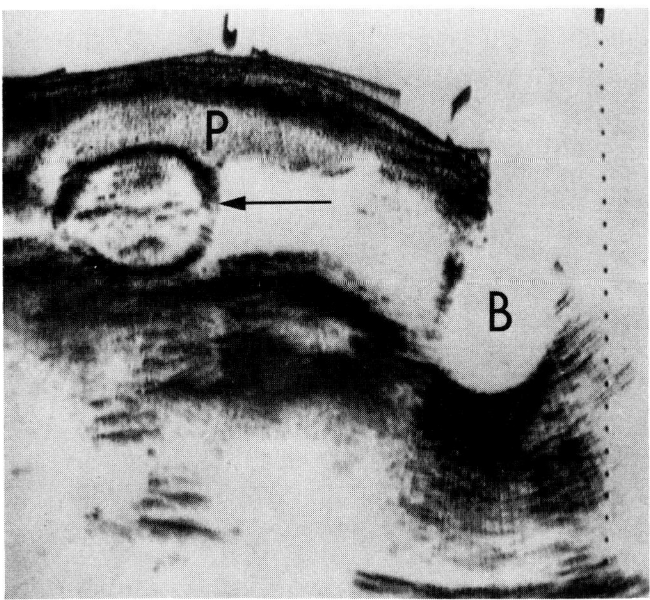

Figure 6–36. Longitudinal image of the uterus in a 22.4 week pregnancy. The patient is imaged supine, with her head to the left. The sonolucent bladder (B) is easily seen deep in the pelvis. The enlarged uterus is seen above it. The fetal skull (*arrow*) is imaged as a ring of high-level echoes in the uterus. The placenta (P) with its characteristic echo pattern is seen along the ventral margin of the uterus. The remainder of the fetal body does not lie within the plane of this section.

demonstrating deformity of the fetal head, absence of expected fetal growth on sequential examinations, or absence of fetal heartbeat on M-mode evaluation.

Ultrasound may be used for the evaluation of patients with pelvic fluid collections or pelvic inflammatory disease. It is possible to image loculated pelvic fluid collections or loculated inflammatory masses with ultrasound; not only can a fluid collection be seen, but ultrasound may also be used to help in the percutaneous aspiration of the collection, either through the anterior abdominal wall or through the vaginal vault. The technique of percutaneous biopsy under ultrasound guidance can obviate the need for surgical intervention.

CHAPTER 7

OTHER AVAILABLE TECHNIQUES

Although many people consider the field of diagnostic radiology to encompass only techniques that use x-rays, it is obvious that the use of both radionuclides and ultrasound has become an integral part of a modern radiology department. Other imaging techniques also have specific applications in diagnostic radiology, and they will be discussed briefly in this chapter. Some of these newer techniques, such as computerized tomography (CT scanning) and xeroradiography, employ x-rays as the energy source but have an imaging system different from that of radiography, and others, like thermography, electrostatic imaging, and holography, use a different energy source and a different imaging system. Many radiology departments have CT scanners (either a head scanner or a whole-body scanner) and xeroradiographic units, and some have thermographic units. Few departments, however, have electrostatic imaging devices, and the radiological applications of medical holography are still experimental.

Because it has such a wide variety of applications, CT scanning may seem to be the only alternative worth mentioning. This procedure, however, is still in its infancy. Xeroradiography and thermography are now well-established, and specific if somewhat specialized indications are accepted for performing these techniques. We will not, however, consider CT scanning in great depth, for several reasons. First, we have probably almost reached the limitations of the imaging technique and have found that it is not as precise as was initially hoped. Second and more important, the United States government is becoming involved in the placement of expensive medical equipment and is limiting the number of CT scanners placed in any particular area. Third, the radiation dose used in computerized tomography is too high for it to be used as a routine screening procedure. Fourth, as with any new development in a technical field, CT scanning was regarded initially with skepticism, and this was followed by great enthusiasm; now, however, we are in the process of assessing the place of CT scanning in modern imaging. CT scanning offers a magnificent new way of looking at the brain and certain "hidden" parts of the body, but it should be considered an adjunct to other modes of imaging rather than a replacement for them.

The reactions to the development of xeroradiography and thermography were similar. Xeroradiography was hailed as a breakthrough when first introduced because it produces clear, precise soft-tissue images. Its use was advocated for every sort of radiographic procedure from barium studies to arthrography as well as mammography and examination of soft-tissue lesions. Some physicians still use xeroradiography extensively, but drawbacks of the procedure have become apparent. One drawback, the most important one for the patient, is that xeroradiography requires a higher dose of radiation than a plain radiograph of the same area. Another drawback is that the processing time is rather longer than that in radiography and the processing system is more complex and thus more liable to breakdown. Third, xeroradiography is more expensive. The only indications for this technique should be better definition of soft-tissue tumors, particularly in mammography. Thermography was also hailed initially as a magnificent method of diagnosing all sorts of disorders, from backache to migraine, but use of the procedure has slowly become limited to two specific clinical applications, in the diagnosis of breast disease and of peripheral vascular disease.

COMPUTERIZED TOMOGRAPHY

The use of computerized tomography in neuroradiology is discussed in Chapter 4. The same principle of cross-sectional imaging can be used elsewhere in the body, and as CT scanning has become more sophisticated, whole-body scanners have been developed that can scan the head and the body at much faster rates, often producing more detailed and better images.

The CT scanner consists of a large doughnut-shaped detector connected to a highly specialized computerized imaging system. The patient is positioned so that the area of the body in which a pathologic condition is suspected lies in the "hole" of the doughnut. Mounted in the doughnut are one or more x-ray tubes, each of which rotates around the patient and emits an x-ray beam. An extremely sensitive detection device is mounted opposite the x-ray tube and moves with the tube in order to receive the information generated by the x-ray beam as it passes through the body. The information received relates to the differing radiation absorption coefficients of different tissues, and often 40,000 readings taken in 90 or 180 separate images constitute each "slice," which may take five seconds to four minutes to perform, depending on the sophistication of the machine. Although originally the slices were 13 mm or thicker, the more recently developed CT scanners are capable of imaging slices of only 3 to 6 mm. This information is then passed on to the computer, which generates an image. The image may be recorded in a number of different ways: on a digital print-out, on a cathode-ray tube or television screen, on a Polaroid picture, or even on a radiograph. Recently, a controversial decision was made to present the image as one would see it if one were standing at the patient's feet, so that the patient's left side is on the right.

The major advantage of the CT scanner is that it provides an image in the transverse, or axial, plane (hence, it is also called *CAT* [computerized axial tomography] scanning). Each "slice" of the body delineates the spatial relationships of the organs and demonstrates whatever pathologic condition may be present. Another advantage is that CT scanning is a largely noninvasive technique that will not inconvenience the patient to any great extent. The major drawbacks of the system are the great expense of the scanner and the radiation dose the patient receives during a series of scans.

CT scans can differentiate easily among air, fat, soft tissue, and bone. Tumors of differing densities can be visualized. Using water-soluble contrast agents allows vascular and avascular structures to be distinguished and the kidneys and urinary tract to be seen. Distortion and infiltration of soft tissue planes are easily seen in the retroperitoneum and pelvis. Calcifications, such as those seen in tumors, thrombi, and lymph nodes, can be identified. It may therefore be argued that any clinical suspicion is an indication for CT scanning. Since radiation dosage will soon be limited by national legislation, and since many states already have laws concerning the use and abuse of the CT scanner, it is wise for the medical profession to limit the use of CT scanning to those situations for which it has already proved valuable. CT scanning is just another form of imaging, and it should be used in conjunction with the more conventional radiographic techniques discussed in the first six chapters of this book. Often, computerized tomography can provide more information about a lesion than can be gained from routine radiological, radionuclide, or ultrasonic techniques. CT scanning appears to have particular value in demonstrating the full *extent* of a lesion and the degree of involvement of surrounding tissues. The spatial relationships between the lesion and its environment become apparent on a CT scan, which may help the surgeon or the radiotherapist in choosing an approach to therapy.

The indications for CT scanning of the brain are discussed in Chapter 4. Indications for whole-body scanning include the following.

Retroperitoneal lesions. Both tumors and benign lesions may be evaluated with CT scanning (Fig. 7–1). Some particular indications should be considered.

1. To evaluate the *extent* of any retroperitoneal lesions.
2. To study the *extent* and involvement of lymph nodes, as in lymphoma.
3. To investigate lesions of the pancreas, although it has not proven quite as useful in this area as many physicians had hoped.
4. To investigate renal and adrenal lesions, particularly with respect to their *extent* as well as the involvement and displacement of surrounding structures.
5. To demonstrate masses in the liver, both primary and metastatic.

Lesions in the neck and the base of the skull. CT scanning should be used in this area (Fig. 7–2) for the following purposes.

1. To investigate the *extent* of tumors in the paranasal sinuses.
2. To investigate lesions of the orbit, including tumors, fractures, hematomas, and fluid.
3. To investigate thyroid and parathyroid masses, although perhaps radionuclide scanning can provide more information.
4. To investigate the *extent* of pharyngeal and laryngeal tumors.

Mediastinal lesions. CT scanning can be used to evaluate mediastinal lesions, particularly congenital cysts and arteriovenous malformations. The *extent* of lymphomatous and other tumors as well as metastatic spread directly from a bronchogenic or other malignancy may also be investigated.

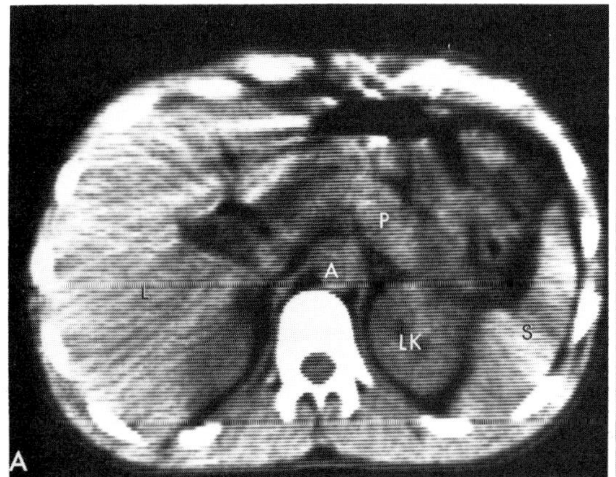

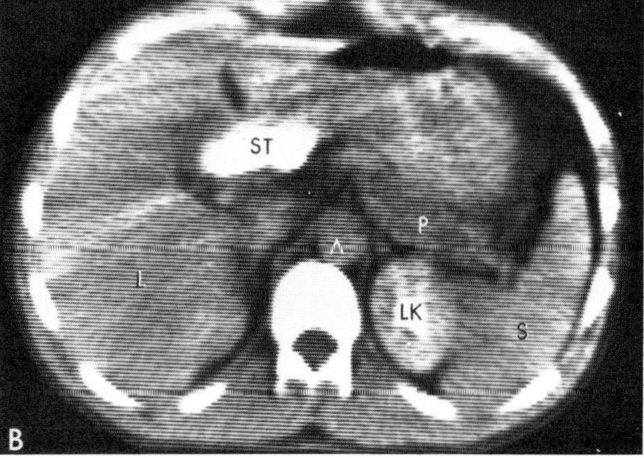

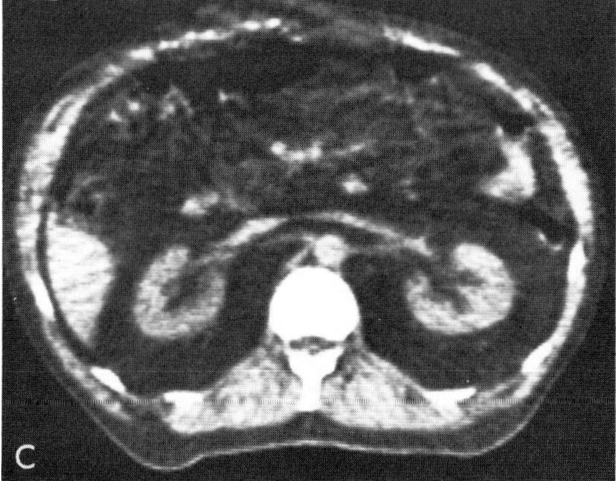

Figure 7–1. Normal CT scans of retroperitoneum. *A*, Nonenhanced scan. *B*, Scan of the same patient enhanced with contrast. *C*, A more caudal scan of a different patient. Note that the liver (L) and spleen (S) are easily identified. The left kidney (LK) is best seen with contrast enhancement. The stomach (ST) is clearly seen with Gastrografin. The pancreas (P) and aorta (A) can also be identified. In the scan of the second patient (*C*), the excessive amounts of fat clearly outline the kidneys and their vasculature.

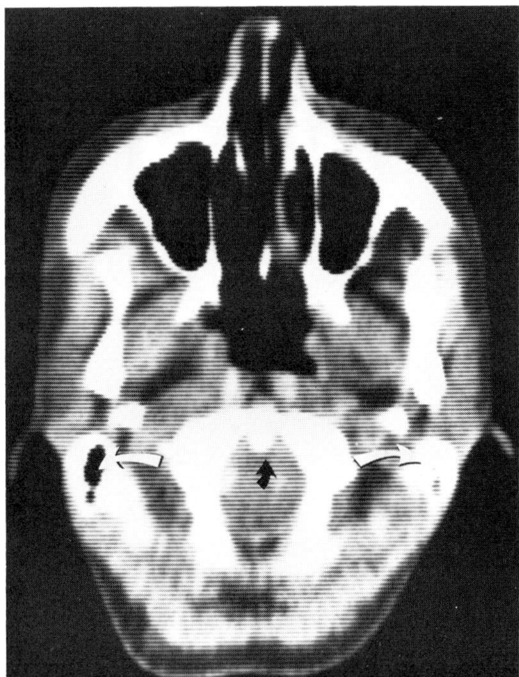

Figure 7–2. Normal CT scan of the base of the skull. Note the air-filled maxillary antra, nasopharynx, and nose. The arch of the atlas with the odontoid (*black arrow*) is clearly seen. The mastoids with some air cells can be seen (*white arrows*).

LESIONS INVOLVING THE SKELETON. CT scanning is particularly helpful in determining the *extent* of involvement of both osseous and soft-tissue components (Fig. 7–3A).

1. To assess the *extent* of osseous involvement in widespread pelvic lesions such as metastases.
2. To demonstrate the *extent* of osseous involvement in lesions of the ribs and vertebral column.
3. To assess the *extent* of fracture and displacement of fragments, particularly in trauma to the pelvis and hips, as well as to the shoulder.
4. To show congenital lesions and fractures of the spine (Fig. 7–3B), particularly of the cervical region.

XERORADIOGRAPHY

Xeroradiography is a different method of processing and producing an image using an emerging x-ray beam similar to that used in conventional radiography. An ordinary x-ray tube is used, and the patient is positioned in the normal way, but the x-ray beam strikes an electrostatically charged plate instead of a film. This plate is given a charge in such a

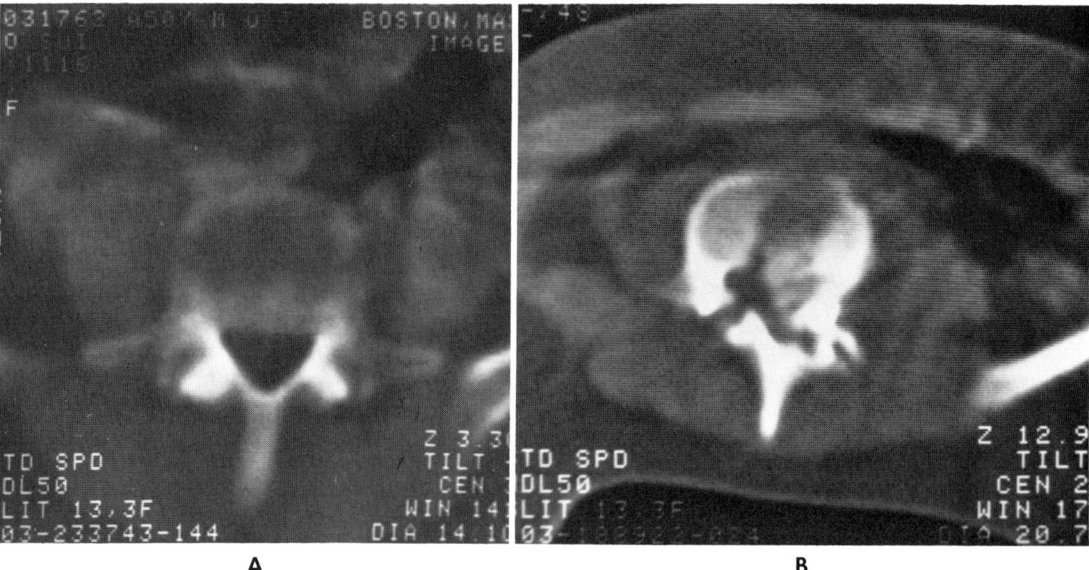

Figure 7–3. CT scans of the spine. *A*, normal lumbar vertebra. Note how clearly the normal anatomy can be seen. *B*, Scan of a young adult involved in an automobile accident. An explosive injury of the body and both pedicles of L4 can be seen, and marked deformity of the normally triangular spinal canal is well illustrated.

way that x-rays will dissipate the electrostatic charge in a manner directly proportional to the number of photons (or amount of energy) in the x-ray beam as it strikes the plate. Thus, a non-attenuated beam going through air will dissipate most of the charge, but a beam of low energy that has gone through bone or metal will remove little of the charge. The plate is then placed in a special processer and a blue powder is spread on it that adheres to the parts still containing a charge. The amount of powder that adheres is in direct proportion to the amount of charge remaining on the plate. A contact print is then made. The final image may be produced either on photographic paper, which is most frequently used, or on translucent film. There are two "modes" of xeroradiographic processing, a *positive mode* and a *negative mode*. In the positive mode the air appears blue and the bone white, and in the negative mode, the bone appears blue and the air white. Choice of mode is a matter of preference, much as it is for radiographs.

Since xeroradiography is only a different method of processing and presenting the radiographic information, it may obviously be used for most situations outlined in previous chapters. In fact, a few radiology departments use xeroradiography for much of their imaging. One major drawback to xeroradiography is that the amount of radiation required to discharge each plate is 1.5 to 2 times that used for a similar conventional radiograph. (The Xerox Corporation, developer of xeroradiography, has been working on this problem and has announced a new system that requires less radiation.) Another drawback is that the processing techniques are not infallible and problems have been experienced with the charging of the plates, the adherence of the powder, and jamming of plates in the processer. Some of these problems are familiar to those of us who use conventional radiographic processing equipment, although the overall technical failure rate for conventional radiography is lower than that for xeroradiography.

What, then, are the advantages of xeroradiography over conventional radiography? Xeroradiography provides better detail in soft-tissue images and increased enhancement of edges. This allows differentiation between the various soft-tissue planes, particularly in the extremities, and shows more detail in the breast. Xeroradiography can also be used for some procedures using contrast agents when visualization is difficult, such as in gallbladder studies, arthrography, and peripheral vascular procedures. Because it requires a higher radiation dose, however, few radiology departments use xeroradiography routinely except in two situations.

MAMMOGRAPHIC XERORADIOGRAPHY. Xeroradiography provides clear images of the breast in which the stroma, vessels, skin, and subcutaneous tissue can be easily seen (Fig. 7–4A). With the improved edge enhancement, tumors become more readily visible and calcifications (both benign and malignant) stand out clearly (Fig. 7–4B). In spite of the high radiation dose involved, the improved rate of diagnosis of breast cancers with xeroradiography justifies its use, although not as a routine screening procedure in women under 50.

SOFT-TISSUE XERORADIOGRAPHY. Xeroradiography is useful in looking at lesions of the muscles and underlying skeleton, where the periosteal margin of the bone and trabecular pattern can be clearly visualized and any distortion of the muscle planes or the subcutaneous tissues can be clearly seen. The indications for soft-tissue xeroradiography include muscle tumors, trauma, infections, and periosteal lesions.

THERMOGRAPHY

Aerial photographs taken with an infrared camera and special film make it possible to discern different crops or types of trees on the ground. A similar technique may be used to take pictures of the human body in order to discern different temperatures in the tissues. This is called *thermography*. Two particular uses for this procedure have become apparent. Thermography may serve as a screening technique in breast cancer and as part of an investigation of peripheral vascular disease. The system uses thermal radiations and special film, so there is no radiation danger. Unfortunately, this technique has never lived up to its initial promise because it has a high rate of false positive and false negative results. Although

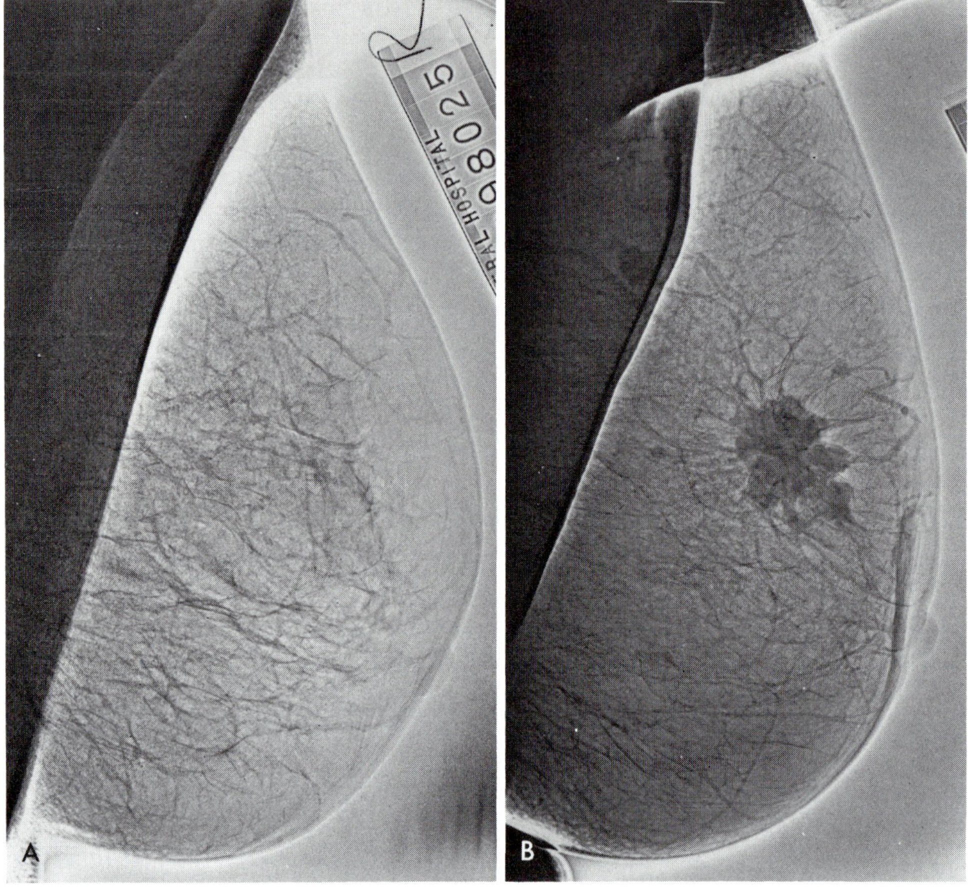

Figure 7–4. Two lateral xeroradiographs in a fatty-replaced breast. *A*, Normal breast. *B*, Infiltrating carcinoma of the breast. There is no underlying glandular tissue. Both patients were in their fifties. The normal xeroradiograph (*A*) shows the nipple and skin as well as the stroma and vasculature of the normal breast. The abnormal xeroradiograph (*B*) shows a large mass with a number of small satellite masses. On biopsy this was found to be a ductal carcinoma.

many departments have thermographic units, they are little used today.

Breast disease. Most superficial breast cancers are surrounded by an area of hyperemia that causes the overlying skin temperature to be somewhat higher than the surrounding tissues, and a thermogram is able to identify this alteration in pattern (Fig. 7–5). Not all breast cancers, however, are superficial, and a thermogram of a breast with a deeper cancer would produce false negative results. Lesions other than cancer, such as abscesses, mastitis, and fibrocystic disease of the breast, may also produce higher temperatures than normal, and thermography then gives false positive results. When all the forms of mammographic investigation are considered, thermography is too inaccurate to be used alone as a screening device for breast cancer, except in unusual circumstances, such as in hospitals with inadequate radiological coverage or in regions where breast screening of the entire population has been considered prudent.

Peripheral vascular disease. A thermogram is capable of differentiating between areas with good blood supply and those with poor blood supply, thus aiding the surgeon in decisions about operative approach. Indications for thermography in this situation include: Raynaud's phenomenon in the arm, atheroma, arteriosclerosis, and

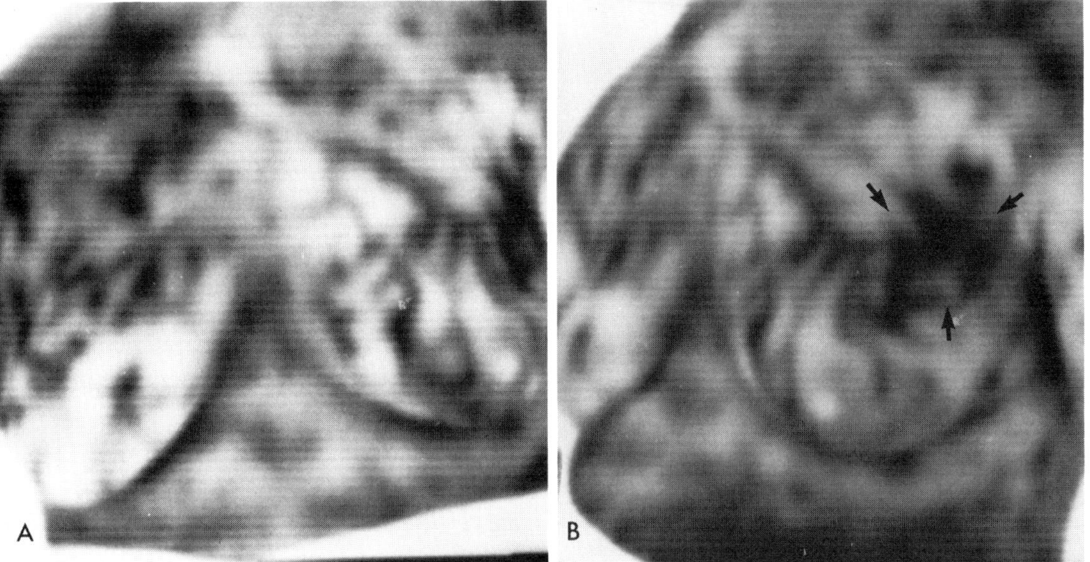

Figure 7–5. Thermogram. The temperature range is from cold (white) to hot (black). *A*, The right breast is normal. *B*, The left breast has a "hot spot," an area of increased density (*arrows*) in the axillary tail of the breast. On biopsy this proved to be fibroadenomatosis.

Buerger's disease in the lower limb, and lesions involving the external carotid arteries in the face, such as temporal arteritis. Thermography may also be part of continuing investigation and follow-up of patients with resutured amputations or extensive burns. Many modern vascular surgeons use thermography not only because there is no radiation hazard with frequent use, but also because the procedure is painless and easy to perform and often provides information that is otherwise unobtainable.

ELECTROSTATIC IMAGING

If one is able to use an x-ray beam to penetrate the body, it should be theoretically possible to use other sources of energy, preferably sources that involve less radiation hazard. One such source of energy, ultrasound, is discussed in Chapter 6. There is another nonhazardous method of imaging that is currently available although still relatively unknown. An electron beam was first used some 60 years ago by Japanese researchers, who found that the radiation dose is slight (some 5 to 10 per cent of that in an equivalent x-ray beam), the beam is more easily controlled, and the images produced have much finer detail. This procedure is called *electrostatic imaging.* As the electron beam passes through the patient, it is absorbed proportionately to the density of the part it strikes. The emerging beam strikes an electrostatically charged vacuum-packed plate which is covered with powder similar to that used in xeroradiography. Where the beam hits the plate with a great deal of energy much of the charge is lost, and where the beam fails to hit the plate at all, no charge is lost. The image produced varies from white to black with a wide spectrum of grays. Once the image is formed it must be transferred from the plate into some permanent form, such as a translucent film similar to a radiograph. This last stage has proved the most difficult, in that the vacuum is easily lost and the plates frequently spontaneously discharge themselves. Should the transfer process succeed, however, a clear image with particularly good edge enhancement is produced (Fig. 7–6). *Edge enhancement* means that the edges of each tissue plane are more clearly delineated, as they are in xeroradiography. A good example of edge enhancement is the separation of the various muscle bundle planes in the arm or leg.

There is little radiation involved in elec-

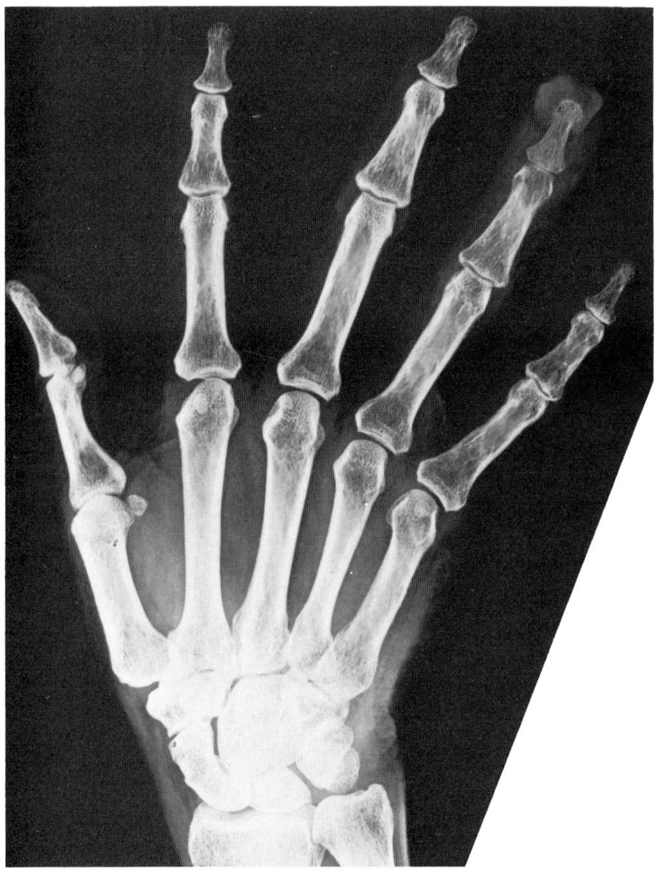

Figure 7–6. Electrostatic image of a normal hand. Note the abnormality in the nail of the ring finger.

trostatic imaging, and if the system can be made to function successfully, it can be used for many diagnostic purposes. In spite of the present technical problems, the advantages of low radiation and increased edge enhancement make electrostatic imaging useful for taking pictures of the chest, particularly the lung fields, evaluating peripheral soft-tissue lesions, and examining the breast.

It is difficult to foretell the future of electrostatic imaging. Since the radiation dose involved is negligible, if the technical difficulties can be surmounted, it is conceivable that the procedure will replace conventional diagnostic radiography. The technical difficulties are apparently so great, however, that it is impossible to run an efficient radiology department using only this form of imaging.

HOLOGRAPHY

Holography is a type of photography largely dependent on laser beams and has the unique property of creating three-dimensional images. A holographic chest radiograph is extraordinary in that the image gives one a spatial perception of the chest contents and demonstrates, for example, the intrapulmonary vessels spreading evenly from the hilar shadows, an effect difficult if not impossible for even an experienced radiologist to visualize from a plain chest radiograph. It is impossible to predict what the future of radiographic holography holds, but it is easy to conceive of many useful applications for three-dimensional radiography, such as investigation of pelvic fractures, identification of intracranial calcification, and location of abdominal tumors.

CHAPTER 8

THE CHEST

We have mentioned previously that 60 per cent of all x-rays taken are chest radiographs, and a careful assessment of each is essential. We suggest a system in Chapter 2, but it is important to establish a system of one's own when viewing chest x-rays. In our system, assessment begins below the diaphragm and then proceeds to the heart, hila, mediastinum, lung fields, bones, and soft tissues. In this chapter we look at patients who present with a number of classic symptoms referable to the chest, although we will begin with some of the findings that may become evident on a routine chest x-ray.

ASYMPTOMATIC ABNORMALITIES SEEN ON ROUTINE CHEST FILMS

Many people have a routine chest film taken every year or so, and although the vast majority are normal, a number of conditions begin asymptomatically. It is possible to detect these disorders earlier on a routine film, before the patient develops symptoms. A number of congenital abnormalities may also be discovered on a routine chest radiograph, most of which have no clinical importance. Some congenital anomalies, however, are of extreme importance to both patient and physician.

Case C1

Aloysius Golightly, age 24, came to the emergency room complain- of severe cramping abdominal pain associated with diarrhea. On examination, he was found to be febrile and in great discomfort, with pain and guarding in his left lower abdomen. The surgeon made a diagnosis of possible ulcerative colitis with or without perforation and admitted the patient. As is usual in this hospital, a routine chest x-ray (Fig. 8–1) as well as an abdominal film was obtained. What does the x-ray show?

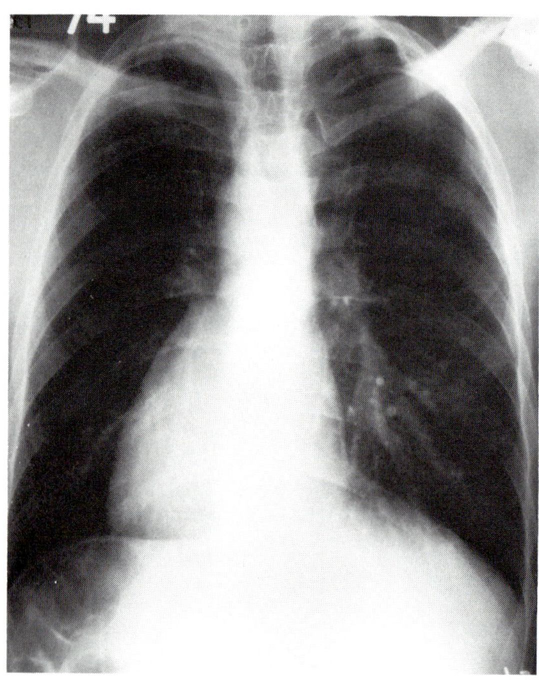

Figure 8–1. Dextrocardia. In this PA chest film, there is a "mirror image" effect, with the heart lying in the right hemithorax, the liver on the left, and the splenic flexure and gastric air bubble under the *right* hemidiaphragm.

This is a typical example of dextrocardia and, of course, also an example of situs inversus, as the KUB confirmed. The patient's liver was on the left, the spleen was on the right, and the cause of his abdominal pain was a ruptured appendix on the left side, which was successfully removed. If the surgical resident had examined this patient more carefully, the apex heartbeat would have been heard on the right side rather than the left.

Other congenital abnormalities such as accessory lobes or fissures can be found on routine chest radiography. The most common accessory lobe is in the right apical region and is known as the *azygos lobe* (Fig. 8–2); it occurs in about 2 per cent of the population and is without clinical significance. Accessory fissures are those found in addition to the major or oblique fissures, which are only seen on the lateral view, and the minor or horizontal fissure, which may be seen on both lateral and PA views in about 60 per cent of patients. Accessory fissures represent subsegmental pleural reflections between various segments or lobes of the lung and occur in about 5 per cent of the population. They, too, are without significance, although often their presence provides additional information with respect to changes of volume in adjacent pulmonary segments.

Many congenital cardiac anomalies first become apparent on routine chest radiographs. While many are not important, significant anomalies are usually detected when the patient complains of certain symptoms.

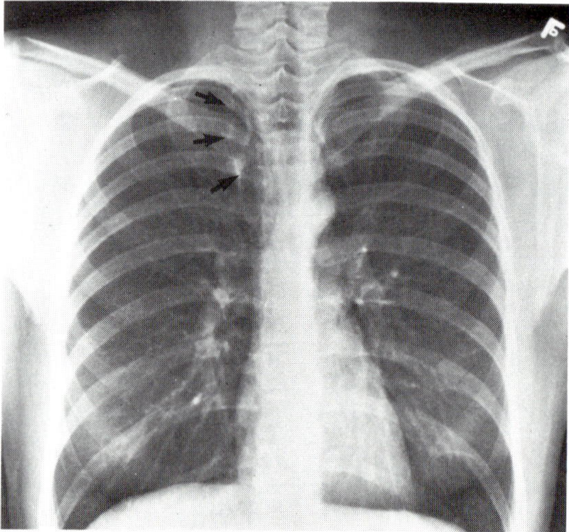

Figure 8–2. Azygos lobe. An almost vertical line can be seen at the apex of the right lung (*arrows*). This represents a fissure running between the normal right upper lobe and the accessory azygos lobe.

Case C2

Mulliwallida Gullabjam was an Indian male who had a routine chest x-ray for immigration purposes (Fig. 8–3). He was totally asymptomatic. What does the film show?

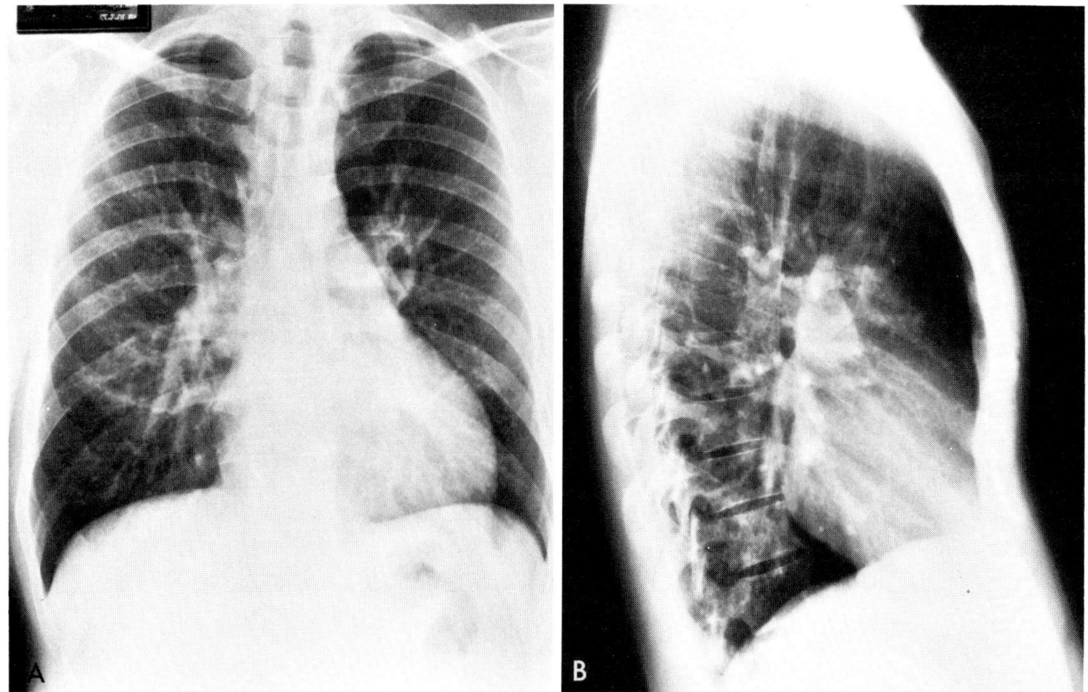

Figure 8–3. Atrial septal defect, PA view (*A*) and lateral view (*B*). This 56-year-old patient has left ventricular enlargement as well as prominent pulmonary vasculature. Note also an azygos lobe. The left ventricular enlargement was caused by hypertension.

The appearances on this x-ray are typical of an uncomplicated left to right shunt, and in an asymptomatic patient of this age, an atrial septal defect must be considered. Many septal defects are discovered on routine chest films. Radiographic differentiation between atrial and ventricular septal defects may be quite difficult. In an atrial septal defect, there is usually no enlargement of the left atrium, whereas a ventricular septal defect or a patent ductus will be associated with left-sided chamber enlargement. Changes in pulmonary vasculature occur only if the shunt is large enough to increase pulmonary blood flow to at least two and one half times normal. It is essential to perform angiocardiography on those patients in whom other defects are suspected and in whom surgical closure of the shunt is considered necessary.

Case C3

Hermione Sidebotham, age 45, was a rather stoutish lady who recently changed jobs to become a supervisor in a new rubber goods factory at the edge of town. The factory requested that she have an annual physical examination, and the examining doctor thought that apart from obesity, Mrs. Sidebotham was in good shape for her age.

A routine chest x-ray was taken (Fig. 8–4). What does it show?

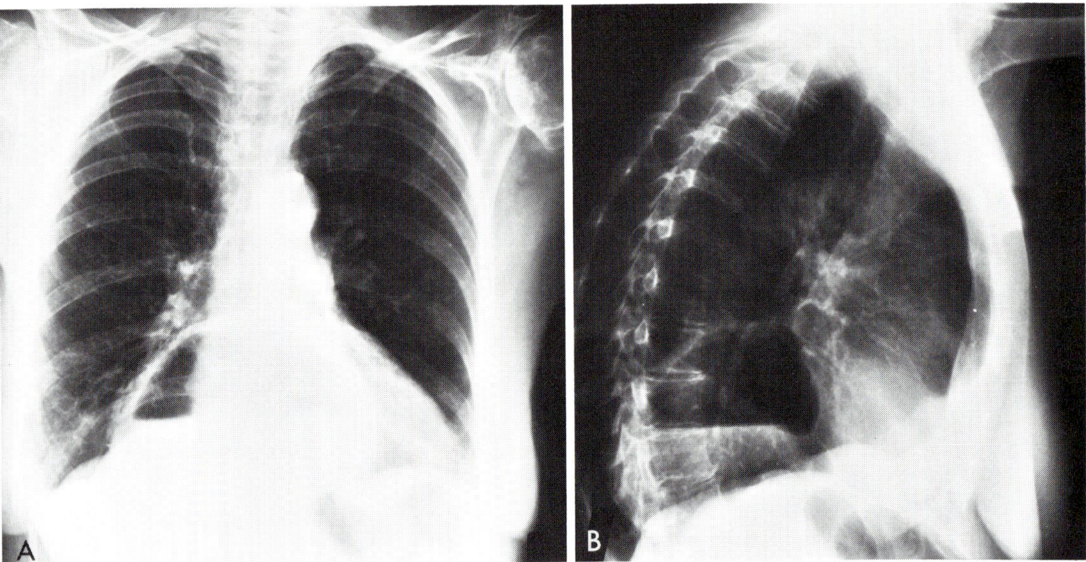

Figure 8–4. Hiatus hernia, PA view (*A*) and lateral view (*B*). There is a large "mass" overlying the heart on the PA view and lying behind the heart on the lateral view. Note the obvious air-fluid level.

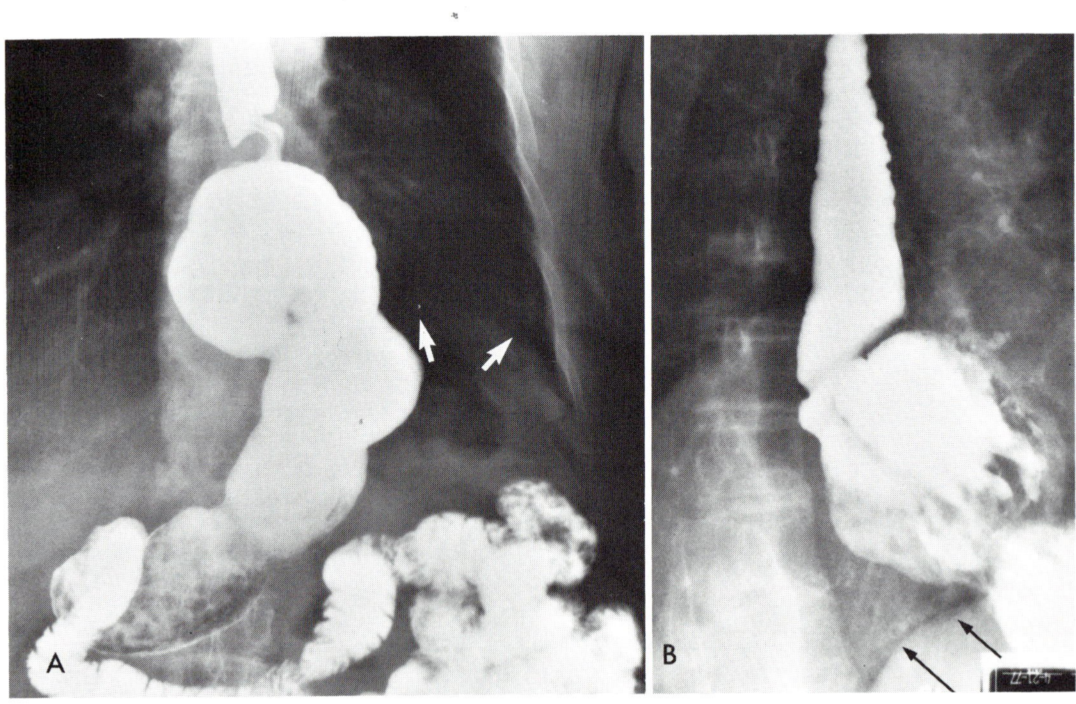

Figure 8–5. Hiatus hernia demonstrated by barium swallow, PA view (*A*) and oblique view (*B*). The esophagogastric junction and most of the gastric fundus lie above the left hemidiaphragm (*arrows*).

A "mass" is seen behind the heart on both views and contains an air-fluid level. Not every hiatus hernia is this large or has an air-fluid level but if this disorder is suspected, a barium swallow study will confirm the diagnosis (Fig. 8–5). Many patients with hiatus hernias are relatively asymptomatic, although careful questioning elicits a history of discomfort or regurgitation on bending down. There is a definite relationship between obesity and the presence of a hiatus hernia.

Many other hernias and related abnormalities may be found on routine chest x-rays and have no clinical importance. Congenital anterior diaphragmatic hernias (Morgagni hernias), for instance, are often quite small. They may be associated with congenital intestinal abnormalities such as malrotation of the gut. Sometimes a Morgagni hernia is difficult to differentiate from an anterior mediastinal mass or pericardial cyst. On an erect film taken after diagnostic pneumoperitoneography is performed, air should be seen to "track up" into the Morgagni hernia. A congenital posterior hernia through the foramen of Bochdalek may be very large and may contain stomach or intestine; such a hernia may be large enough to cause dyspnea in the neonate, but it is usually asymptomatic in adults and older children.

Sometimes other diaphragmatic anomalies may be seen, particularly irregularities of the diaphragmatic surface. Elevation of one hemidiaphragm is known as *eventration* if it is caused by a congenital or acquired weakness of the diaphragmatic muscle. Eventration is usually of no significance, although occasionally it must be differentiated from elevation caused by a pathologically enlarged liver, from a large lower zone pulmonary mass, or from paralysis of the diaphragm.

Case C4

Chollomondly Knickerbocker was a heavy smoker about 50 years old who went to his family practitioner to have an annual physical examination. He appeared to be normal and a routine chest x-ray was taken that showed an elevated left hemidiaphragm (Fig. 8–6). Knowing the patient's history of smoking, the physician considered the possibility that a small underlying peripheral cancer might be causing paralysis of the diaphragm, and he sent Mr. Knickerbocker to a nearby x-ray department. What would you do?

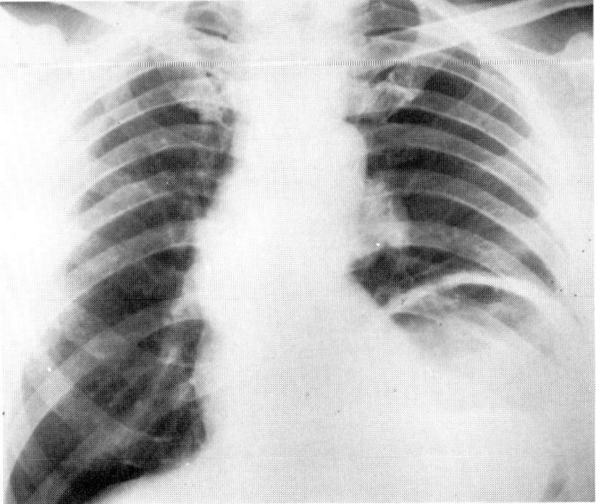

Figure 8–6. Eventration of the hemidiaphragm. There is marked elevation of the left hemidiaphragm with distortion of the left hilum. However, the hemidiaphragm moved freely on fluoroscopy, and comparison with a film taken ten years previously showed that there had been no change.

The patient underwent fluoroscopy. Since the diaphragm moved freely with respiration, the radiologist diagnosed the abnormality as eventration of the diaphragm and of no significance. The patient belatedly remembered that ten years previously he had been through the same procedure. Comparison of previous and current films showed that there had been no change.

Congenital weakness of the diaphragm often allows the liver to become displaced up into the thorax. Possibly because the liver is pushing the right diaphragm up and the apex of the heart is lying on the left diaphragm, eventration of the diaphragm is far more common on the right than on the left.

So far we have considered only congenital lesions and acquired lesions of little clinical significance. It is obvious, however, that not all routine chest x-rays are straightforward or show benign abnormalities.

Case C5

Bartholomew Wade, 60-year-old senior executive for a large international industrial corporation, went to the company's medical department for a routine physical examination shortly following his return to the United States after many years in the Australian office. On examination, the company physician found that although Mr. Wade had smoked heavily for years, he appeared well, and a routine CXR was performed (Fig. 8–7).

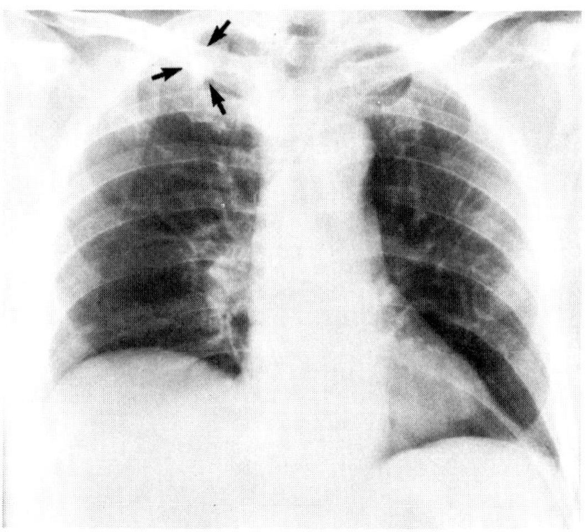

Figure 8–7. Mass in the apex. On the PA view, there is a round "coin" lesion lying behind the clavicle (*arrows*). Note the elevation of the right hemidiaphragm, which was due to eventration.

Here is a very common radiological problem: a 60-year-old man, apparently with no symptoms of disease, whose chest film shows a solitary lung mass. The differential diagnosis includes many conditions, the most important of which are early carcinoma (usually bronchogenic), hamartoma, an old tuberculous focus, and metastasis from a distant primary lesion. Undoubtedly, the most useful thing the radiologist can have at a time like this is a previous film for comparison. Films for this patient, however, were in Australia and not immediately available.

What would you do now? It is first necessary to exclude the possibility of film artifacts or external lesions. Careful examination of the patient's skin is required, to look

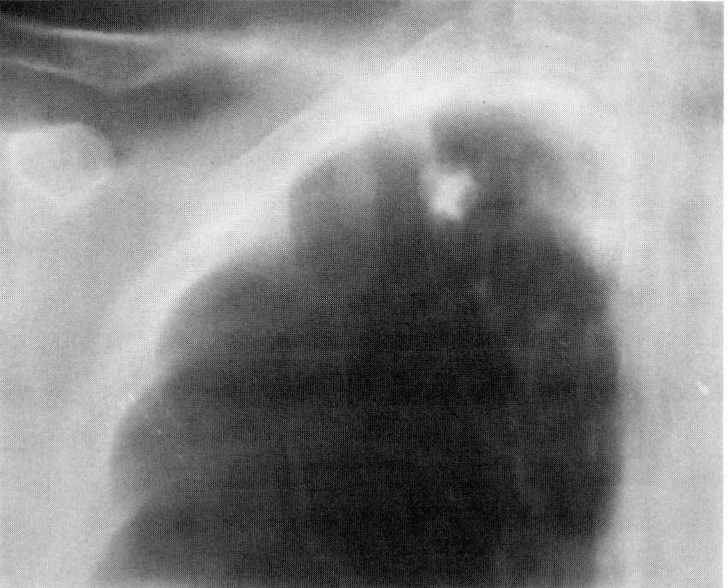

Figure 8–8. Mass seen on a tomogram. The mass is shown to be densely calcified and well circumscribed, without any abnormal vasculature or pleural reaction. These are all important clues that lead us to the diagnosis of benign calcified granuloma.

for sessile polyps, warts, and other skin lesions. If the "mass" is in the lower lung fields, another film should be taken using metallic nipple markers to exclude nipple shadows, which may have looked on the first film like pulmonary tumors. In any case, the presence and location of the mass should be confirmed; this is done by taking a second series of films. The patient may undergo fluoroscopy, at which time he breathes in and out slowly while the radiologist observes the mass. Its association with pulmonary vessels and bronchi is noted. Rotating the patient allows the approximate location of the mass to be identified. The presence or absence of calcification also can be assessed by fluoroscopy, but tomography is often necessary to confirm its presence (Fig. 8–8). Tomography also enables the radiologist to look at the margins of the mass and to observe its relationship to bronchi, blood vessels, and pleura.

All these signs are helpful in differentiating between benign and malignant pulmonary masses. In this case, calcification was found within the lesion at fluoroscopy and was confirmed by tomography. The mass was found to be well-circumscribed, without apparent attachment to surrounding vessels or bronchi, and with no connection to the pleura. When questioned, the patient admitted to having had tuberculosis forty years before, and when previous films were obtained from Australia, the mass was found to have been present ten years before and to be unchanged. Thus, it was a benign granulomatous mass with central calcification.

One might think that the case could rest with this diagnosis. Most radiologists, however, have seen what appears to be a totally benign mass that may have been unchanged for years start to grow rapidly, ultimately causing death. Whether this lesion is a carcinoma to begin with or a so-called *scar carcinoma* (malignant change occurring in an old tuberculous scar, a relatively common occurrence) is impossible to decide.

If Mr. Wade were your patient, what would you do now? Most physicians would judge the situation. Previous films show no change in the mass over ten years. There is tomographic proof of calcification. Both clues are strong signs that the lesion is benign. In view of the patient's age and smoking history, however, it would be reasonable to take a routine chest x-ray yearly, as long as he remains asymptomatic.

There are many variations of this situation, but only two will be considered here. If the patient had no previous films for comparison but calcification were seen on tomography, the consensus would still be that this was a benign lesion. A routine chest radiograph would be performed after six months, and if there was still no change, perhaps routine yearly films would be done if the patient were over 50. If there were no previous films and the mass did not contain any calcification, the diagnostic approach would be different. Ten years ago, this would have been a serious problem because metal bronchoscopy tubes then in use could not have reached the lung periphery. If there was any suspicion of malignancy, a thoracotomy would have been performed. With the new fiberoptic bronchoscopy tubes and the various simple percutaneous biopsy techniques that are now available, it is relatively easy to perform a biopsy on a peripheral lung lesion. These procedures are usually done on an outpatient basis under fluoroscopic guidance, and they have far lower morbidity and mortality rates than thoracotomy.

Case C6

Adelaide Witherspoon was a 23-year-old female who came to the local emergency room at midnight complaining of fatigue. A chronic hypochondriac, Miss Witherspoon was well known to the emergency room staff, because she would appear every week for a chat and a cup of tea. This particular night there had been a rather bad accident, and everyone was too busy treating the victims to listen to Miss Witherspoon's complaints. She was sent down to x-ray to while away an hour or two having a routine chest x-ray (Fig. 8–9). What does it show?

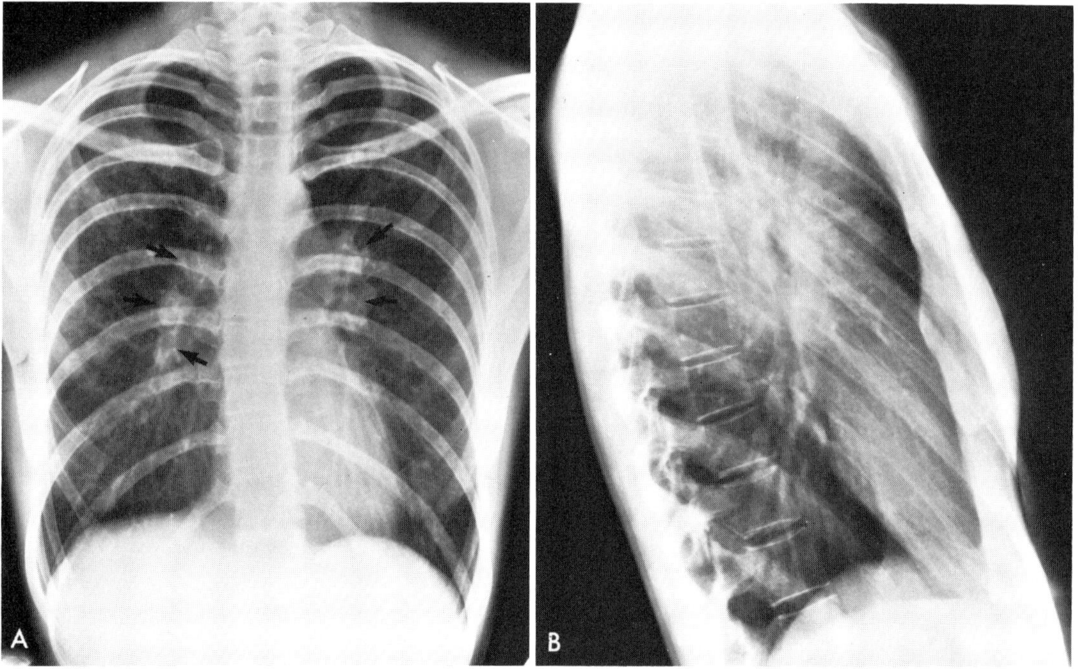

Figure 8–9. Sarcoidosis, AP view (*A*) and lateral view (*B*). There is bilateral hilar node enlargement (*arrows*) as well as a generalized increase in the lung markings. The mediastinum does not appear widened. These appearances are more typical of sarcoidosis than of lymphoma.

This is another common situation, and it usually involves young patients. Although the clinical presentation is often associated with symptoms, the condition is occasionally asymptomatic. The distribution of the enlarged hilar and mediastinal nodes on this film suggests that the patient has sarcoidosis, although various forms of lymphoma may also be associated with a mediastinal mass in an asymptomatic patient. The differential diagnosis between these two conditions is considered later in this chapter.

Enlarged hilar and mediastinal nodes are not infrequently found on routine chest radiographs, and the approach is to obtain previous films for comparison. Alterations in the lung fields should be sought, and the patient should be examined for other evidence of disease such as splenic calcifications, which can occur in granulomatous diseases. Tomography may be helpful in confirming the exact distribution of the nodes and in looking for any evidence of bronchial narrowing, carinal widening or active tuberculosis. Should there still be any doubt about the diagnosis, a biopsy should be performed, usually by mediastinoscopy. Sarcoidosis and lymphoma are often detected relatively early in patients whose only real complaint is fatigue or malaise.

Case C7

Serendipidy Smith, age 35, came to the local hospital complaining of fatigue. He was carefully examined before being sent to x-ray, but apart from being lethargic he appeared quite normal. A routine chest x-ray was ordered (Fig. 8–10). What does it show?

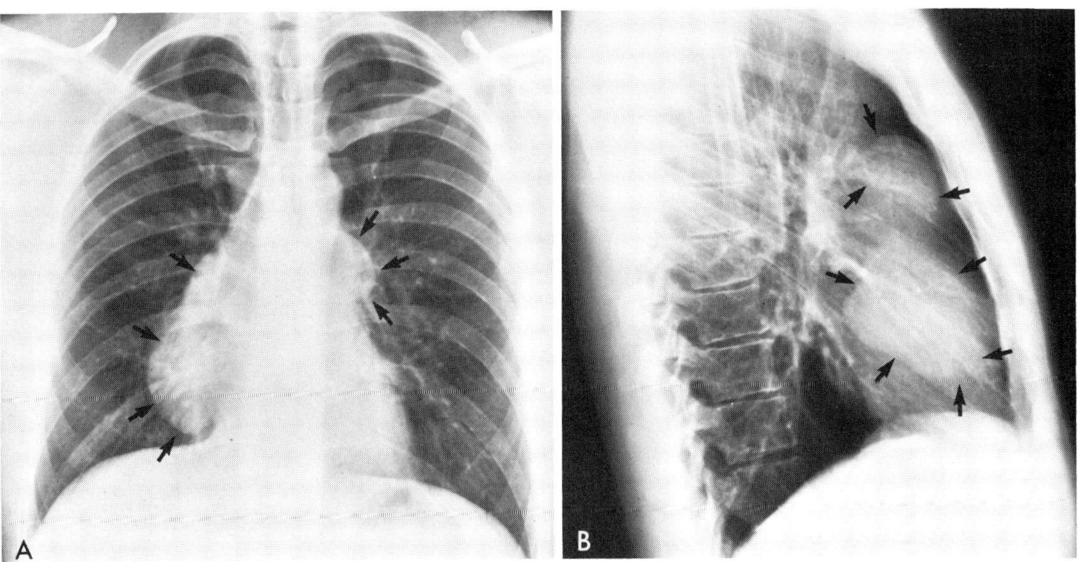

Figure 8–10. Thymoma. *A*, On the AP view, a large lobulated anterior mediastinal mass can be seen, apparently enlarging both sides of the cardiac shadow (*arrows*). *B*, On the lateral view, the mass can be seen to lie above and alongside the heart (*arrows*).

Here again is an unsuspected finding — a large anterior mediastinal mass in a relatively asymptomatic patient. Fluoroscopy and tomography may be performed but are usually unnecessary because the two routine views of the chest provide enough information about the mass. At operation, this patient was found to have a thymoma. He also had myasthenia gravis.

Differential diagnosis of mediastinal masses depends on their anatomical position (Table 8–1). A mass in the anterior part of the mediastinum may be diagnosed as one of the "four Ts": thyroid, teratoma, thymoma, or "terrible" lymphoma. Posterior mediastinal masses may be neurogenic masses, pulmonary duplications, or carcinoma of the lung or pleura. The radiological

TABLE 8–1. Possible Causes of Mediastinal Masses

LOCATION OF MASS	POSSIBLE CAUSES
Anterior mediastinum	Tumor of thymus Tumor of thyroid Teratoma Pericardial cyst Lymphoma Morgagni hernia
Middle mediastinum	Lymphoma Bronchogenic cyst Sarcoidosis Bronchogenic carcinoma Hiatal hernia
Posterior mediastinum	Neural lesion (neurofibroma, ganglioneuroma) Neurenteric cyst Esophageal lesion (diverticulum, achalasia) Bochdalek hernia
Anterior, middle, or posterior mediastinum	Abscess or infection Aortic aneurysm Hematoma Mesenchymal tumor (myoma, lipoma, fibroma, hemangioma, lymphangioma) Hernia

approach to a mediastinal tumor depends on its location and may include angiography or CT scanning to help delineate its boundaries and extent. Myelography is also useful in the investigation of neurogenic lesions, and radioisotopic scanning is helpful in the investigation of thyroid tumors.

DYSPNEA

Many conditions involving the lungs, heart, and mediastinum produce breathlessness without other symptoms, and "dyspnea on exertion" is a common complaint. After a thorough clinical examination that includes listening to the lung fields, watching the patient breathe, noting the color of the skin and nail beds, listening to the heart, and looking for clubbing, the patient is sent to the radiology department for a chest radiograph. For many dyspneic patients, the radiologist will be able to make a diagnosis or at least to suggest several. There are four common groups of conditions for which "dyspnea on exertion" is the predominant complaint.

Pulmonary Edema and Congestive Heart Failure

In interstitial pulmonary edema, the margins of the vessels appear blurred on a radiograph, and some vessels seem to end and

Case C8

Uri A. Drywell, age 48, had chronic glomerulonephritis and developed renal failure. He was scheduled for dialysis treatment 3 times a week, but because he lived far out of town, Mr. Drywell sometimes missed a session. One week he missed a Wednesday session because of snow, and on Friday when he was able to reach the hospital, he complained of shortness of breath. Chest x-rays were taken just before and shortly after dialysis. The change in the lung fields is remarkable (Fig. 8–11).

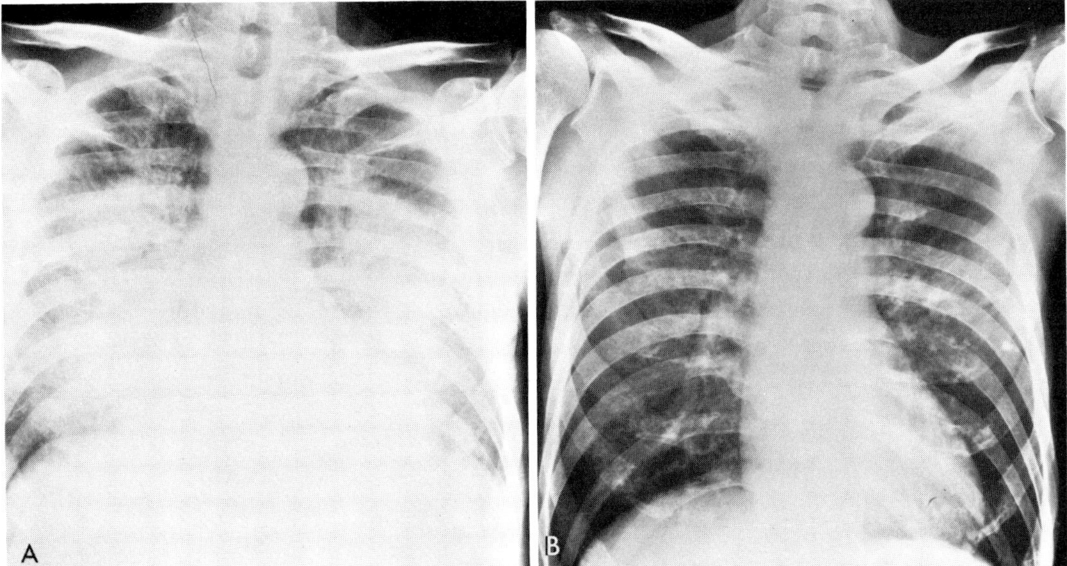

Figure 8–11. Pulmonary edema with clearing. *A*, The predialysis film shows the classic butterfly distribution of pulmonary edema spreading out from both hilar areas with obliteration of most of the pulmonary markings. *B*, The postdialysis film shows almost total resolution of pulmonary edema.

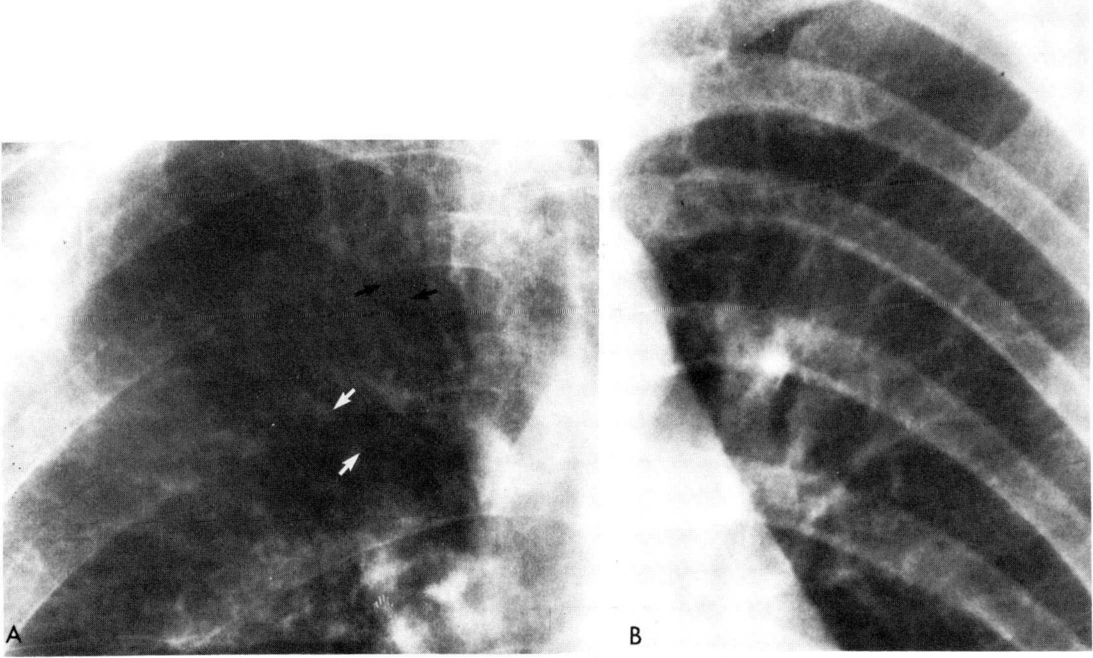

Figure 8–12. Interstitial pulmonary edema. *A*, Close-up view of pulmonary vessels. The vessel margins are blurred, and some vessels apparently come to an abrupt halt, only to begin again (*arrows*). See the text and Figure 8–13 for an explanation of this radiographic finding, which occurs in any interstitial disease as well as in interstitial pulmonary edema. *B*, Film of a normal patient for comparison.

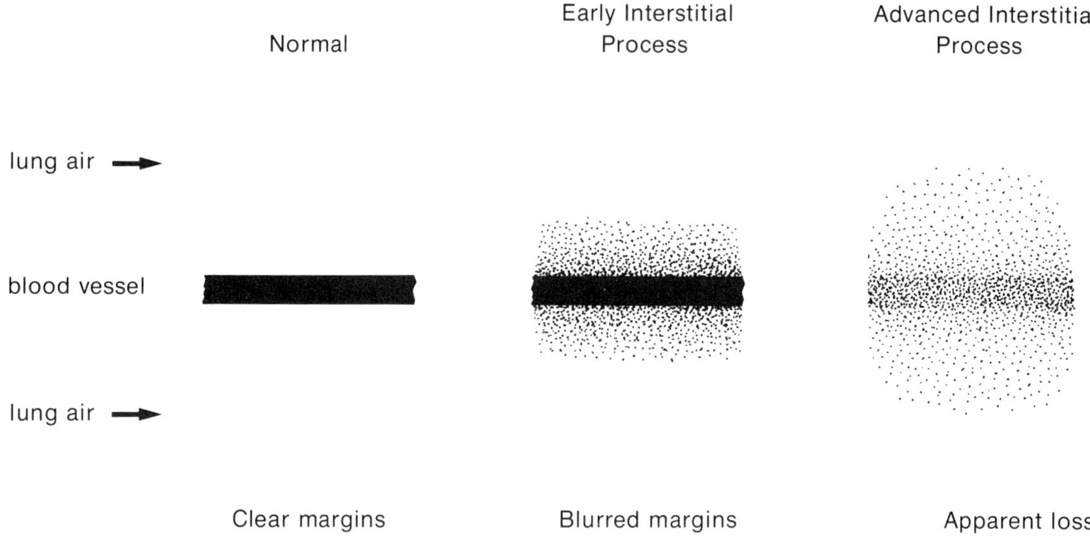

Figure 8–13. Interstitial pulmonary edema. Representation of the loss of vessel margins seen on an x-ray.

start up again (Fig. 8–12). Blurring of the vessel margins is caused by interstitial fluid in this disorder but may also be seen in infiltrative conditions and pulmonary fibrosis. The explanation is simple: Normally, the interface between the air (which appears black) and the blood vessel (which appears white) is clearcut. In pulmonary edema, fluid surrounds the vessel, so one would see air / fluid / vessel / fluid / air (Fig. 8–13). On a radiograph, this would appear as black / dark to light gray / white / light to dark gray / black; thus the vessel margins are blurred or totally lost on an x-ray. Pulmonary edema is usually widespread, involving both the lung fields (Fig. 8–14), and it is frequently concentrated close to the heart and hilar regions. Al-

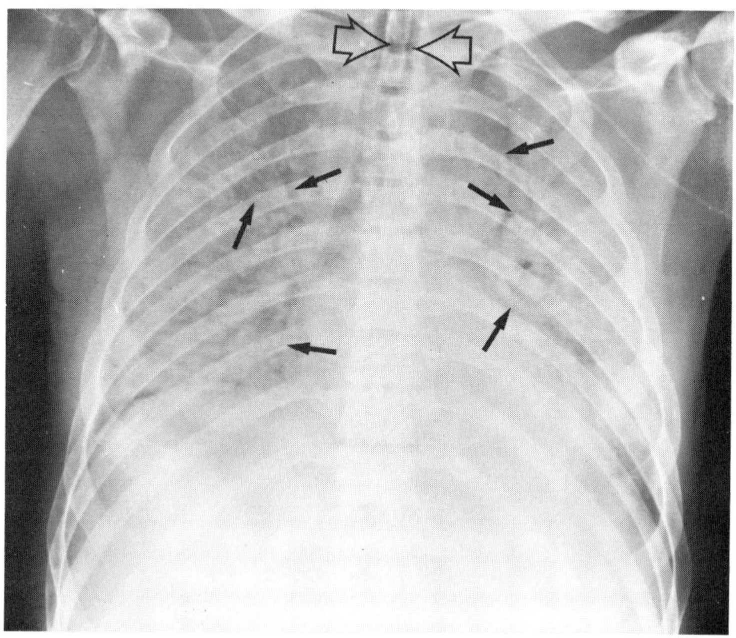

Figure 8–14. Widespread pulmonary edema. There is almost total loss of lung markings, although some bronchi now stand out as black lines (*arrows*) from the generalized opacification of the lung fields – the "air bronchogram" sign, which occurs in any condition in which there are patent airways surrounded by opacified lung, e.g. pneumonia. This patient had had a myocardial infarct and in spite of active treatment and a tracheostomy (*hollow arrows*), he succumbed 5 days later.

though nearly always bilateral in distribution, pulmonary edema may be unilateral or patchy. These more unusual patterns of pulmonary edema may result if a sick patient lies mainly on one side, or if a patient has severe chronic lung disease that prevents the lungs from filling up uniformly with fluid. Thus, one may see unilateral opacification and pulmonary edema that appear as blotchy opacities extending throughout the lung fields and resembling metastases.

Case C9

Eugenia Pickle, age 72, hated doctors and had never been to one. Now, however, she was unable to climb the 23 flights of stairs to her apartment without stopping five or six times to catch her breath, so she went to the local hospital's clinic. On examination, she was noted to be mentally very alert, and she denied having any symptoms other than dyspnea. Rales were heard on auscultation, and her neck veins were engorged. Her heart was enlarged, with a marked left ventricular impulse. Blood pressure was 180/120. An EKG showed left ventricular strain. A chest x-ray was taken (Fig. 8–15). What does it show?

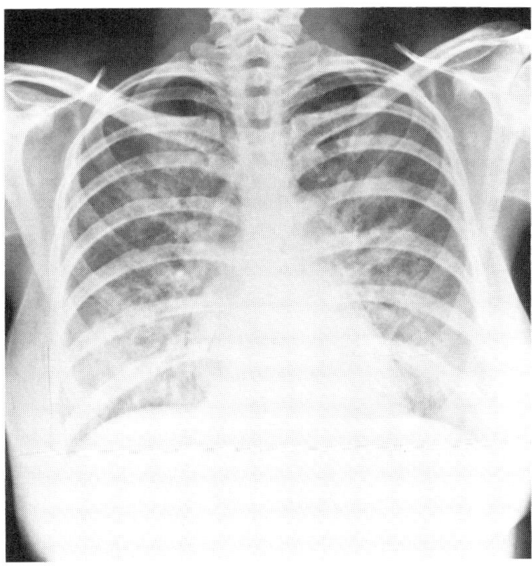

Figure 8–15. Acute pulmonary edema. There is an ill-defined haze throughout both lung fields which is patchy in some places. Most of the pulmonary vessels are obscured. These are typical findings in interstitial pulmonary edema.

The classic radiological findings in congestive heart failure (CHF) include enlargement of the heart and pulmonary edema, which can be seen as a "haze" arising from the hilar regions and spreading throughout the lung fields. Some horizontal lines may be seen at the bases; these represent fluid in the interlobar septa and are known as *Kerley B lines* (Fig. 8–16). They are characteristic of congestive heart failure and left ventricular failure but are also seen in mitral stenosis, various infiltrative diseases, chronic fibrosis, and lymphangitic spread of tumors. Kerley B lines are often an early sign of left-sided heart failure and are best seen on an upright PA view of the chest. *Kerley A lines*, which may also occur in these disorders, are unbranching lines that run toward the hila in the perihilar regions of the lung fields; they are only rarely seen.

Apart from the clinical findings of dysp-

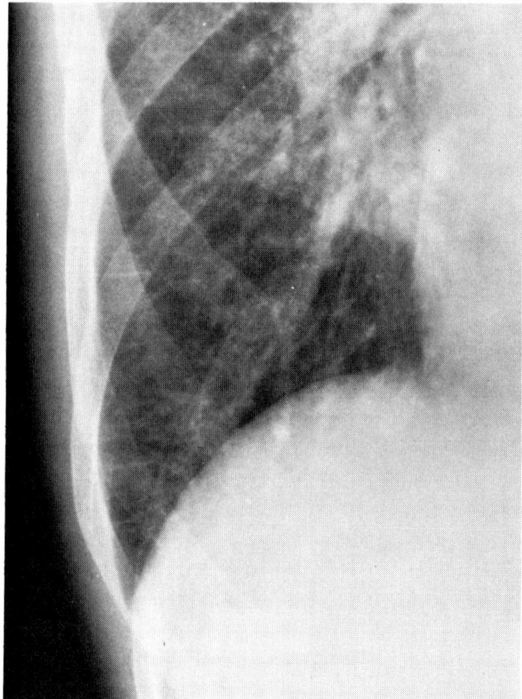

Figure 8–16. Kerley B lines, close-up of right costophrenic angle. Many horizontal lines can be seen at the base in this patient with mitral valvular disease who has chronic congestive cardiac failure. These Kerley B lines are a characteristic finding in patients with CHF, LVF, and mitral stenosis.

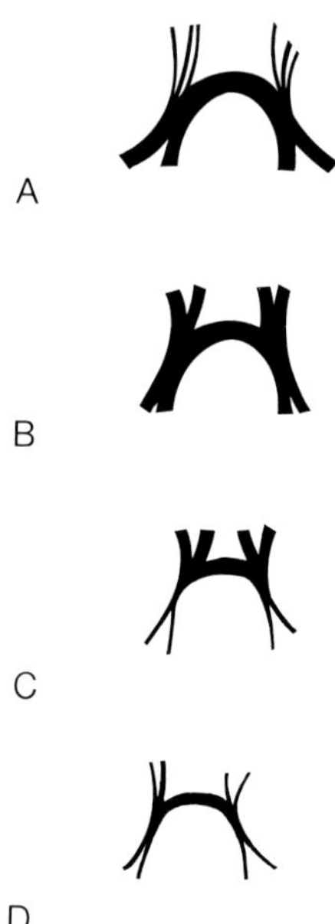

Figure 8–18. Diagram of pulmonary vascular redistribution. *A*, In the normal state, the lower zone veins are larger than those in the upper zones. *B*, The vessels in the upper zones are the same size as those in the lower zones (Grade I). *C*, The upper zone vessels are now larger (Grade II). *D*, In chronic pulmonary hypertension the upper zone veins once again revert to normal and appear to be the same size as those in the lower zones (Grade III).

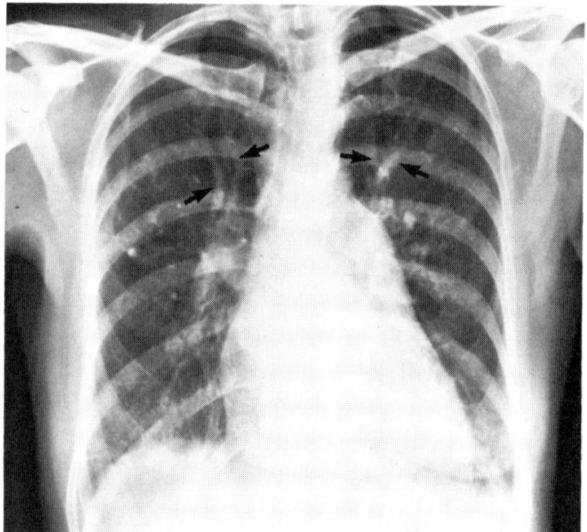

Figure 8–17. Pulmonary vascular redistribution. In this 44-year-old patient with known mitral stenosis, note the left atrial enlargement, prominence of the left atrial appendage, and the engorged pulmonary veins in the upper zones (*arrows*). By comparison, the lower zone veins are narrower. This is Grade II redistribution.

nea and widespread rales, what other radiological features of left-sided heart failure or left ventricular failure (LVF) might one expect to see? An enlarged left ventricle is almost always present, and a phenomenon known as *pulmonary vascular redistribution* occurs. This is extremely helpful in the early diagnosis of left ventricular failure (Fig. 8–17). Pulmonary vascular redistribution, in which the vessels of the upper zones become larger than those in the lower zones, is caused by an increasing left atrial pressure and occurs in three stages (Fig. 8–18). The combination of pulmonary edema, congestive cardiac failure, and vascular redistribution is very common (Figs. 8–19 and 8–20). In chronic redistribution such as occurs in pulmonary hypertension, it is possible for the peripheral pulmonary vasculature to revert to an almost normal pattern, albeit with engorged central pulmonary vessels.

As congestive cardiac failure progresses,

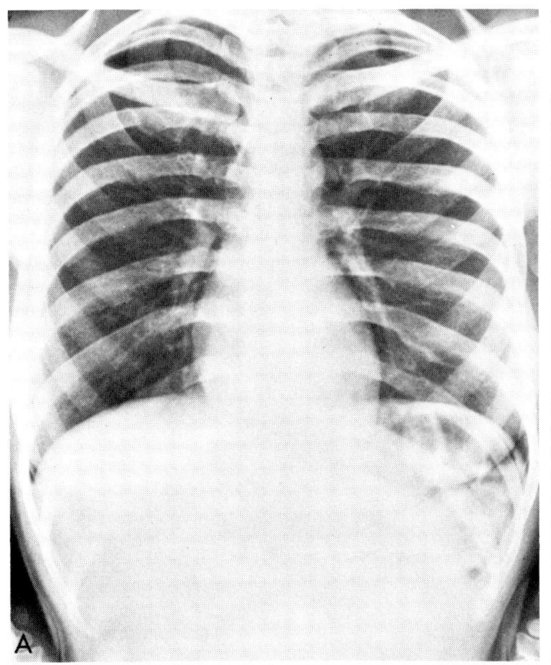

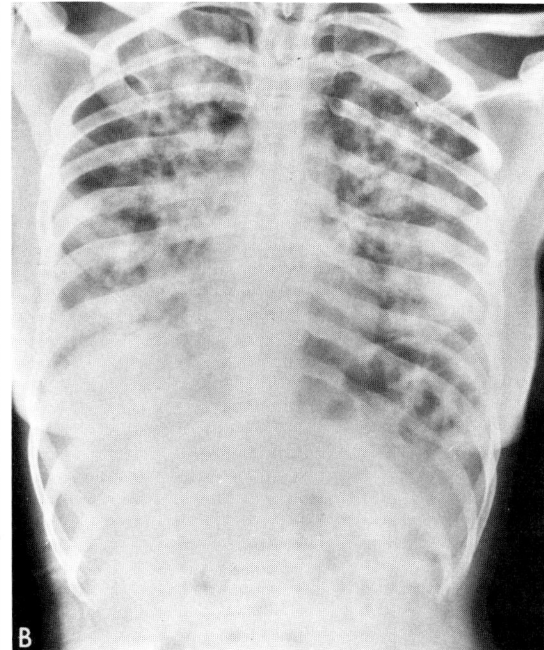

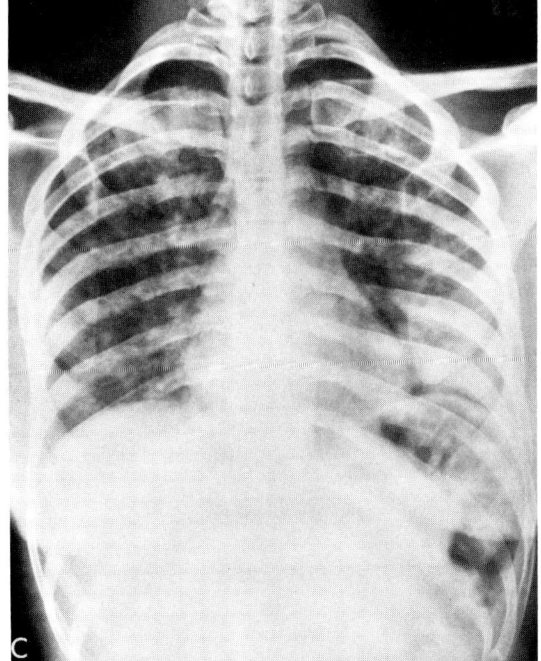

Figure 8–19. Pulmonary edema in anaphylactic reaction, PA view. *A*, The first film is normal. The patient had a surgical procedure and received 4 pints of blood following which she became febrile, developed hives and acute respiratory distress. *B*, At this time the second film was taken, which shows diffuse ill-defined opacities throughout both lung fields with obliteration of the normal lung markings. The patient was started on diuretics and steroids. *C*, Within 24 hours, there was significant clearing of the pulmonary edema.

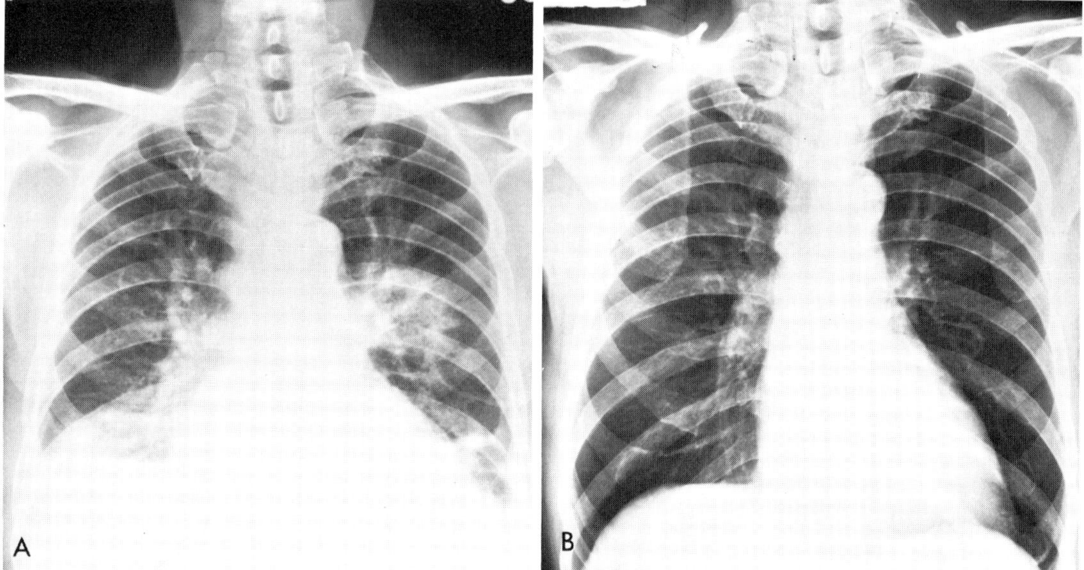

Figure 8–20. Pulmonary edema and response to treatment. This 62-year-old male patient was diagnosed as having hypertensive cardiovascular disease. On a trip to Europe he developed progressive dyspnea and ankle edema. *A*, The initial film shows blunting of both costophrenic angles due to small bilateral pleural effusions. There is pulmonary vascular redistribution and cardiac enlargement. The pulmonary vasculature appears blurred and a number of poorly defined densities are present. The differential diagnosis of the densities would include metastases, pulmonary infarcts, pulmonary edema or patches of pneumonia. *B*, The second film, taken after one week of therapy with digitalis and diuretics, shows clear lung fields and a decrease in the heart size.

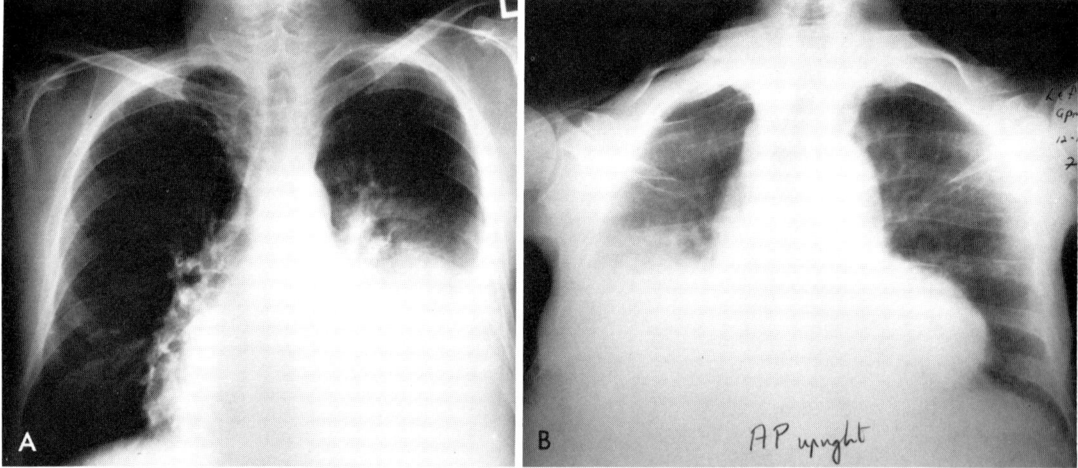

Figure 8–21. Pleural effusions. *A*, This 62-year-old man had recurrent attacks of congestive heart failure following a severe myocardial infarct. This portable film shows a large left sided pleural effusion with a meniscus and fluid running up into the axillary region. *B*, This 69-year-old woman with a long history of hypertension recently had a myocardial infarction. She went into heart failure with a large right-sided effusion. Note that although this film is labelled "upright," it is really an apical lordotic view. Also note the exaggerated cardiac enlargement, which is due to the AP projection.

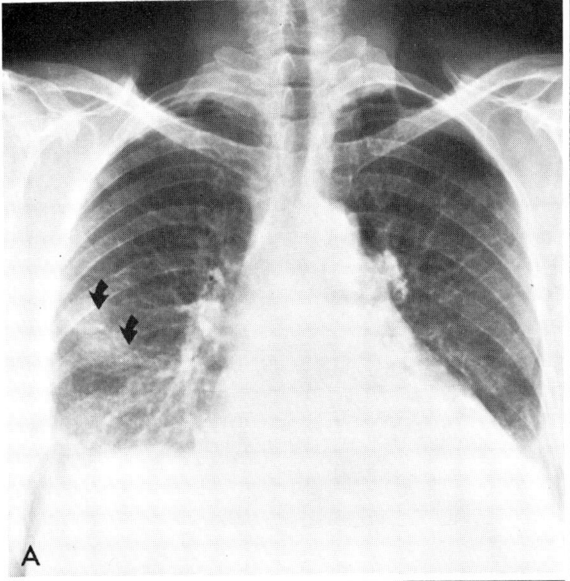

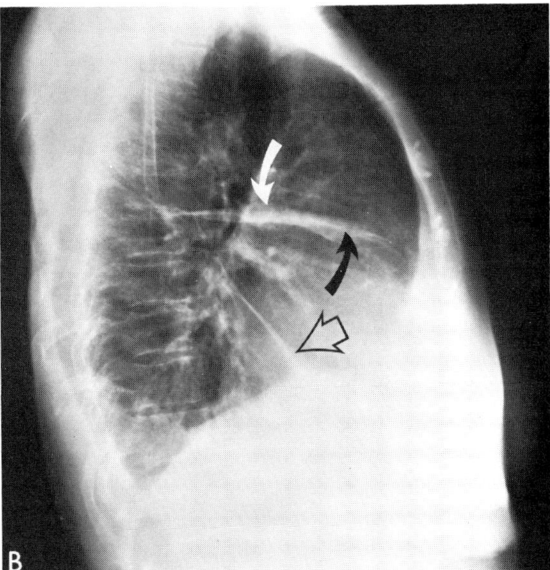

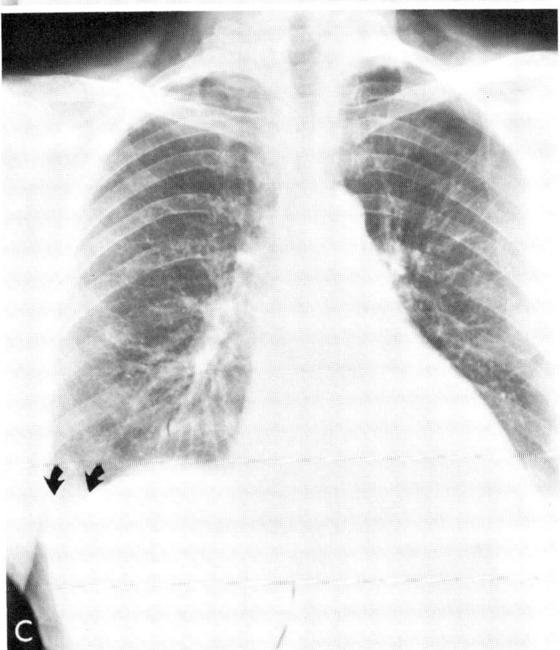

Figure 8–22. Interlobar effusion appearing as a "pseudotumor." All three films show an enlarged heart, blunting of the right costophrenic angle, and some blurring of the lung markings, suggesting pulmonary edema. *A*, The PA view shows two poorly defined masses in the right midzone (*arrows*). *B*, On the lateral view, fluid can be seen in both the major oblique (*hollow arrow*) and the minor horizontal fissure (*curved arrows*). Thus, these "masses" are caused by loculated fluid. *C*, A film taken six days later, after diuresis, confirms this was fluid, although the small right basal pleural effusion remains (*arrows*).

another complication ensues. Because the left side of the heart is failing more rapidly than the right, fluid accumulates, initially as pulmonary edema and secondarily as pleural effusions. In chronic CHF, pleural effusions are common (Fig. 8–21) and usually easy to diagnose from their position (at the bases) and shape (they have menisci). Effusions are more common and often larger on the right than on the left side, but they can have unusual appearances. An effusion may become loculated in a fissure and may appear as a "mass lesion," particularly in the middle lobe fissure on the right; this appearance is known as a *pseudotumor* (Fig. 8–22), another reason for taking more than one view of the chest. On occasion, the fluid will accumulate at one base in the shape of the diaphragm and will not have a normal meniscus (Fig. 8–23A); these fluid collections are known as *subpulmonic effusions.*

What would you do for a patient whose chest film showed subpulmonic effusions?

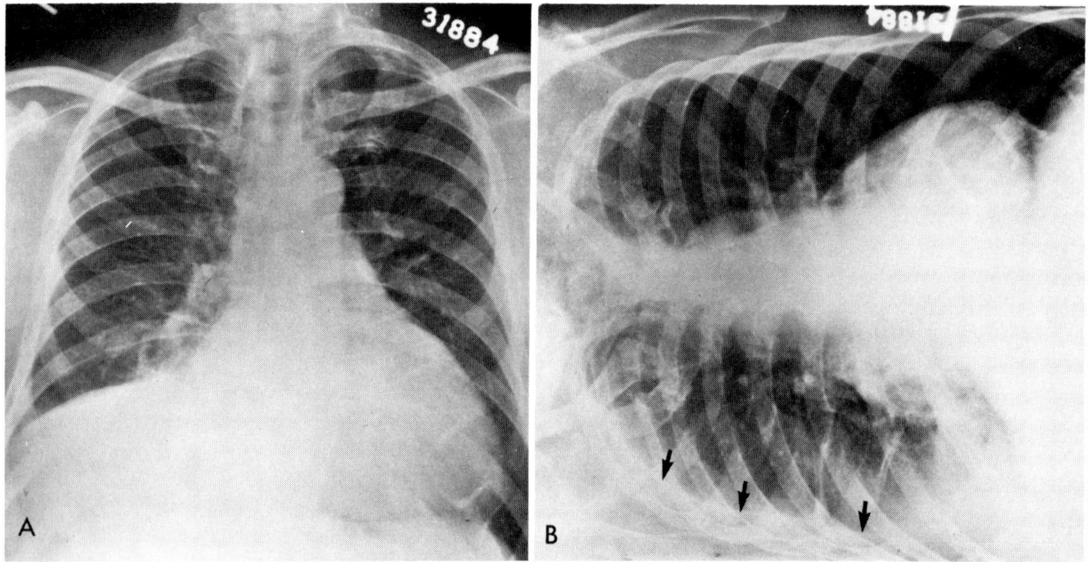

Figure 8–23. Subpulmonic effusion. *A*, On the PA film, there is enlargement of the heart and increased pulmonary vascular markings. The right diaphragm appears elevated. *B*, On the decubitus view, this is shown to be due to a large effusion (*arrows*), which layers out.

This patient seems to have an elevated right hemidiaphragm. The first stage of treatment is to take a decubitus view of the chest (Fig. 8–23B). The fluid should "layer out" on the decubitus view, and should be seen on fluoroscopy to splash around as the patient breathes. Following removal of the fluid by a chest tap, a chest x-ray is useful in looking for a pneumothorax, should one be suspected clinically. Small pneumothoraces that occur with removal of pleural fluid are common, however, and without significance.

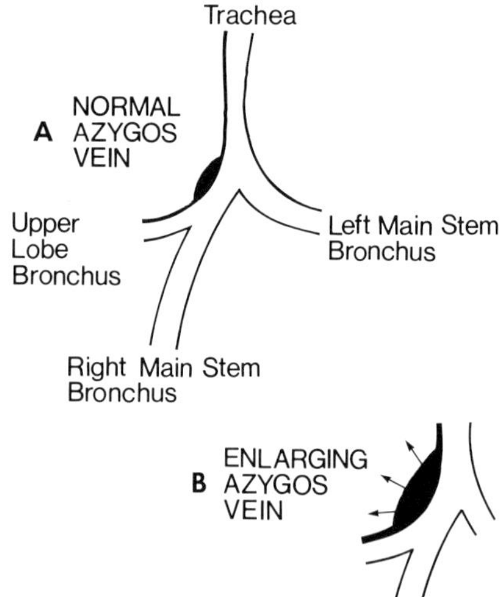

Figure 8–24. Drawing of azygos vein. *A*, The azygos vein lies in the curve between the trachea and the right main stem upper lobe bronchus. It appears as an oval shadow that in normal people is never wider than 4 mm. *B*, When the azygos vein enlarges its shadow enlarges up and to the left.

So far we have been discussing the changes seen in left-sided heart failure and congestive heart failure, which usually involves left ventricular failure. Right-sided ventricular failure (RVF) has a more subtle appearance on the chest radiograph. Often in true RVF, which is rare, the only radiographic finding of note is engorgement of the azygos vein, although dilatation of the right atrium, right ventricle, and superior vena cava may also be seen.

The azygos vein can be seen in the soft-tissue shoulder at the junction where the trachea divides at the carina and the right main stem bronchus branches off (Fig. 8–24A). On a normal erect PA chest film, the azygos vein either is invisible or measures less than 4 mm across its greatest width. The vein enlarges, in the direction indicated in Figure 8–24B *(arrows)*, in patients with RVF and CHF (Case C9 and Fig. 8–15). In patients with pure right heart failure or in combined right and left heart failure, the azygos vein may be as wide as 12 to 14 mm (Fig. 8–25).

With these structural relationships in mind, what would one expect to happen to the azygos vein of a normal person when he

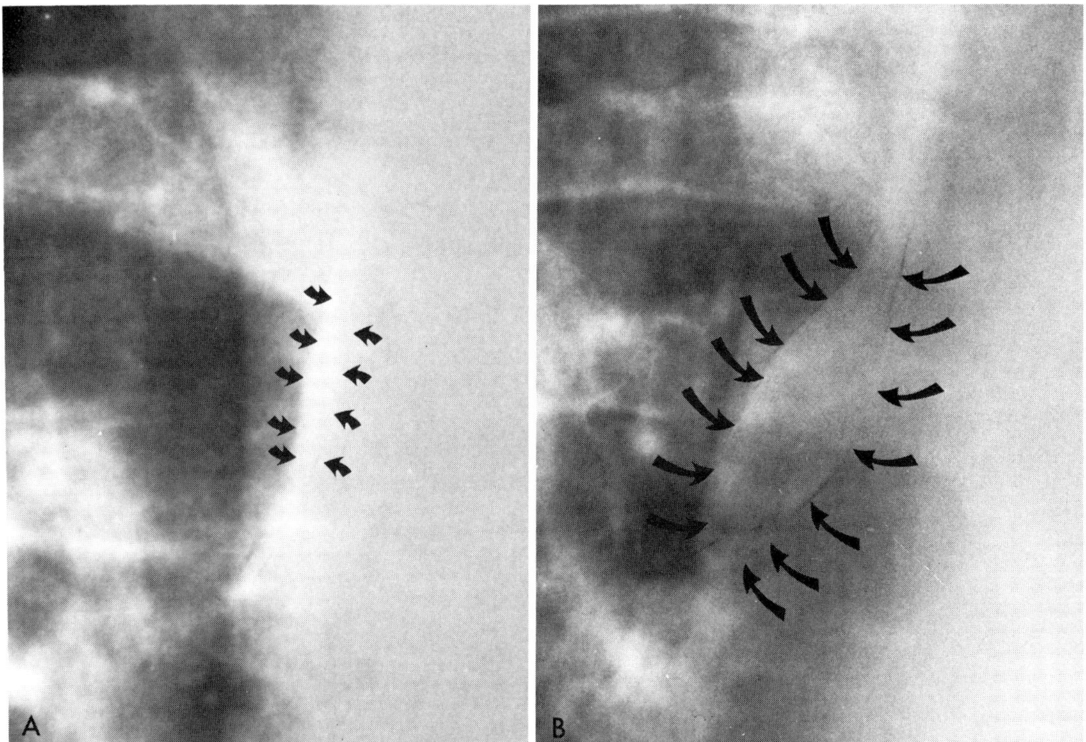

Figure 8–25. Azygos vein. *A*, The azygos vein sits in the shoulder of the trachea and the right upper lobe bronchus. In the normal person it can scarcely be appreciated (*arrows*). *B*, When the azygos enlarges, it becomes much more obvious (*arrows*).

lies supine? The vein enlarges. This is frequently seen during tomography of the mediastinum; a physiologically (normally) engorged azygos vein should not be mistaken for an enlarged mediastinal lymph node. The size of the vein can be reduced in a normal supine person if he holds his breath, closes his glottis, and attempts to force air out of his lungs *(Valsalva maneuver).*

Chronic Pulmonary Diseases

An even more common cause of dyspnea on exertion than CHF is chronic obstructive pulmonary disease, which is a general category including chronic bronchitis, emphysema, bronchiectasis, asthma, and pulmonary fibrosis. Many people invite the risk of lung disease by smoking cigarettes, but there is also a group of patients who develop severe lung disease because of occupational exposure to particles or dust in the atmosphere. Many types of chronic lung disease are of unknown etiology, and the radiologist will frequently use the term *chronic lung disease* or *chronic obstructive pulmonary disease* (COPD) to refer to this whole spectrum of diseases.

Case C10

Alviol R. Gaspernak, age 56, was in extreme respiratory distress after walking up one flight of stairs to his doctor's office. On examination he was found to be breathing with the accessory respiratory muscles (cervical, intercostal, and abdominal). His chest was barrel-shaped and sounded hyperresonant on percussion, and the breath sounds were distant on auscultation. A chest radiograph was taken (Fig. 8–26). What does it show?

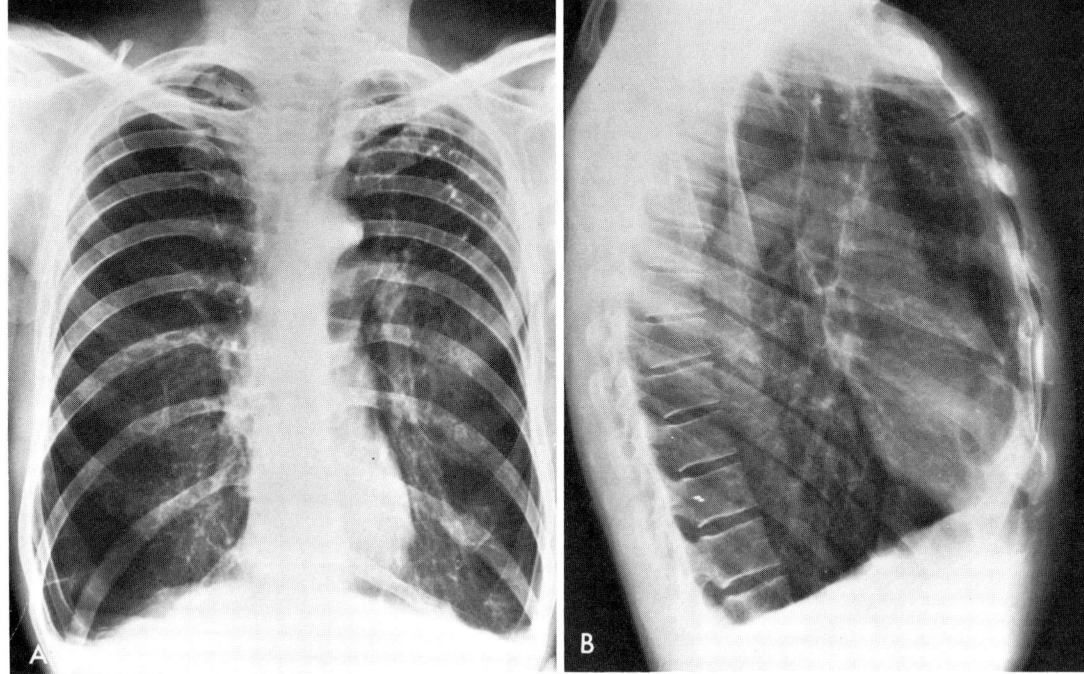

Figure 8–26. Emphysema, PA view (*A*) and lateral view (*B*). Note the marked distortion of the pulmonary parenchyma, with bullae and with hyperinflation of the lungs (low flat diaphragms, sternum pushed forward with large retrosternal air space seen on the lateral, and distortion of the hila). Old fibrocalcific changes from previous tuberculosis are present in the left apex.

The classic signs of emphysema are lungs of large volume with the sternum pushed forward and enlargement of the retrosternal air space. The diaphragms are low and flat, the ribs appear somewhat more horizontal than normal, and the heart is long and thin. The pulmonary vessels are splayed and separated from each other, and the hilar vessels have a more vertical configuration.

Emphysema may be localized or generalized. It may be associated with blebs and bullae in the apices or the lower zones (which is suggestive of alpha$_1$-antitrypsin deficiency). Emphysema may spare one

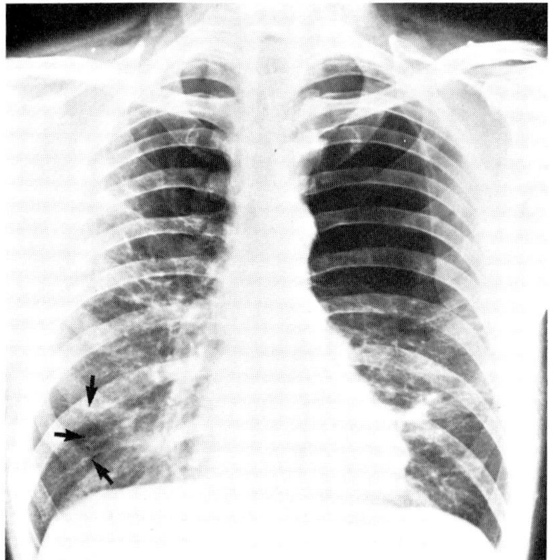

Figure 8–27. Bullous emphysema with marker vessels. This man of 59 has obvious bullae in both upper zones. There is crowding of the lung parenchyma, except in the right lower zone where there are normal "marker vessels" (*arrows*).

segment or lobe of the lung, allowing comparison of the normal vasculature in that part with the abnormal vascular patterns throughout the rest of the hyperinflated lung fields. The normal vessels are known as "marker vessels" (Fig. 8–27).

Chronic bronchitis is a difficult diagnosis to make on the plain film, although occasionally one can see signs such as an increase in the peribronchial markings or thickening of the bronchial walls. Many patients with bronchitis also have emphysema, and the term chronic lung disease is frequently used to describe the combination. The definitive diagnosis depends mainly on the results of pulmonary function tests and bronchography.

Case C11

When Maudy Longtooth, age 65, was a child, she developed severe pneumonia following a bad attack of measles. Since that time she noticed a gradually increasing shortness of breath, and in the winter she produced copious amounts of yellowish sputum. A series of x-rays taken over a number of years were available and have shown little change (Fig. 8–28).

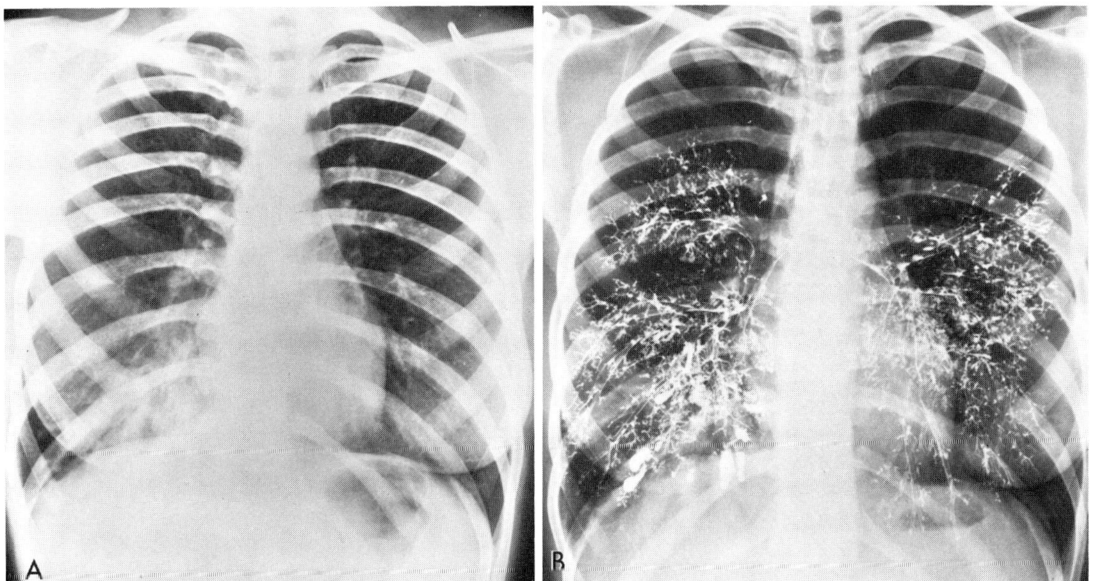

Figure 8–28. Bronchiectasis. *A*, The plain film shows a mottled density at the right base. The remainder of the lung fields are normal. *B*, The bronchogram demonstrates saccular bronchiectasis at the right base. Note the more normal bronchial pattern in the left midzone and lower zones.

The radiological signs of bronchiectasis on plain films are few, although occasionally, multiple rounded lucencies may be seen in one segment or lobe. The lucencies may have air-fluid levels in them, and bronchial wall thickening may also be visible. The investigation of choice for the diagnosis of bronchiectasis is the *bronchogram*. Various forms of bronchiectasis have been described, including cystic, cylindrical, saccular, and fusiform (Fig. 8–29). Using bronchography, it is possible to demonstrate enlargement of the mucous glands on the main bronchial walls, which is seen in chronic bronchitis, as well as to show spasm in some of the smaller bronchi. Obstruction of the bronchi by mucous plugs may occur in bronchitis and on occasion in infected bronchiectasis.

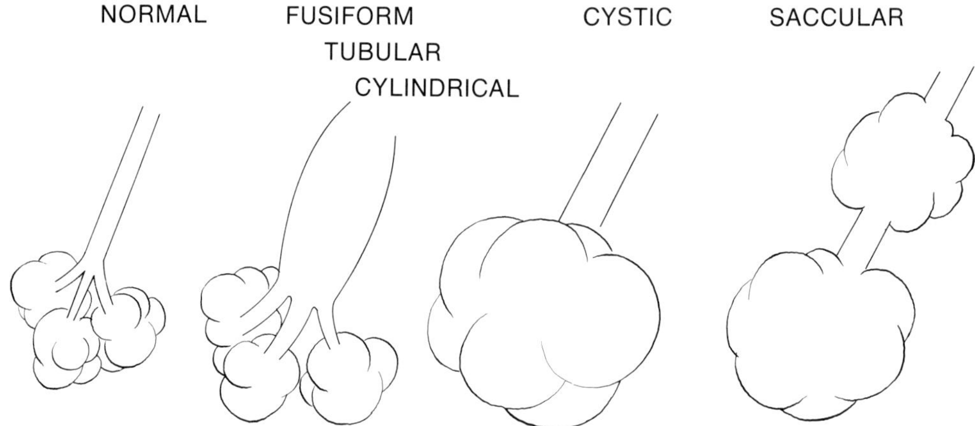

Figure 8–29. Diagram showing the different types of bronchiectasis.

Pulmonary Fibrosis and Pneumoconiosis

Case C12

Porphry Petrovich, a 52-year-old industrial plumber, went to the emergency room of the local hospital complaining of dyspnea. He had been experiencing increasing shortness of breath over the last few years but had not bothered to go to his physician. The emergency room physician found no clinical signs of importance apart from mild dyspnea, and a chest x-ray was taken (Fig. 8–30). What classic findings does it show?

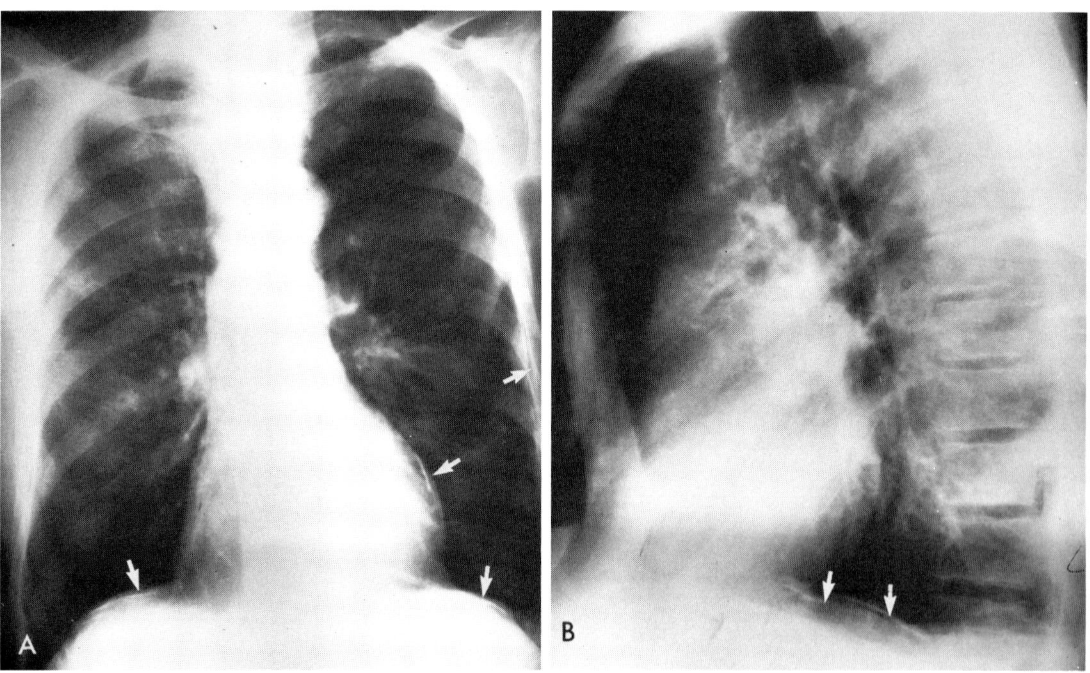

Figure 8–30. Asbestosis, PA view (*A*) and lateral view (*B*). Note the distortion of the pulmonary parenchyma with evidence of hyperinflation of the lung fields (low hemidiaphragm and large retrosternal space) as well as pleural calcifications (*arrows*). These are the typical findings of asbestosis.

Pleural calcification occurs as a result of old healed tuberculosis, old empyema, or hemothorax and in one industrial disease, asbestosis. Mr. Petrovich had spent his life encasing pipes with asbestos; although he was warned about the hazards of his occupation, he had never taken any precautions against inhaling the dust. Patients with asbestosis have a greater than normal incidence of pulmonary tuberculosis and lung cancer. They are also particularly prone to develop malignant mesothelioma of the pleura and peritoneum.

Of the many types of industrial diseases, *pneumoconioses* are a particularly important group. They include exposure to other forms of dust, both organic and inorganic, exposure to various fungi, and hypersensitivity reactions to vegetable irritants. Silicosis (in which eggshell calcification of the hilar nodes may occur), berylliosis, siderosis, talcosis, anthracosis, and asbestosis are examples of pneumoconioses resulting from inhalation of various dusts. Farmer's lung, pigeon-breeder's lung, and bagassosis (due to inhalation of sugar cane dust) are examples of hypersensitivity reaction. The radiological findings in this group of conditions include emphysema, nodular patterns, and pulmonary fibrosis. These findings occur in different combinations and to various degrees. If the dust is inhaled over a long period of time, pulmonary fibrosis becomes the predominant complication. Progressive massive fibrosis often develops, and respiratory death occurs. Other direct and indirect irritants to the lung include excess oxygen, hydrocarbons, and other noxious vapors, smoke, and radiation.

There is yet another group of diseases that cause pulmonary fibrosis and have a similar radiographic picture in the early stages. Many of these interstitial lung disorders are of unknown etiology. The physiological deficit that results has been termed *alveolar-capillary block.* The best known example is the Hamman-Rich syndrome, and the classic radiological appearance is a fine reticular pattern of fibrosis with or without discrete nodules (Fig. 8–31).

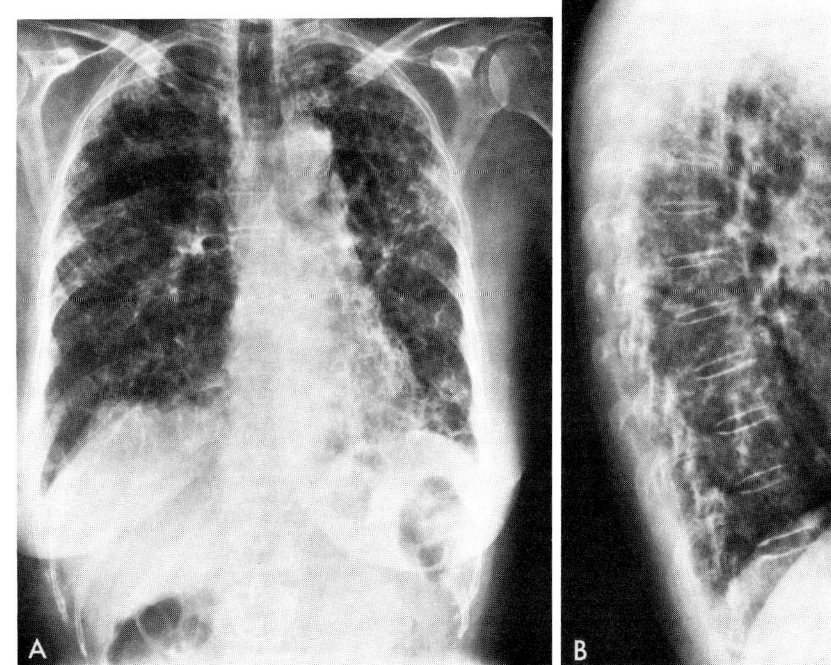

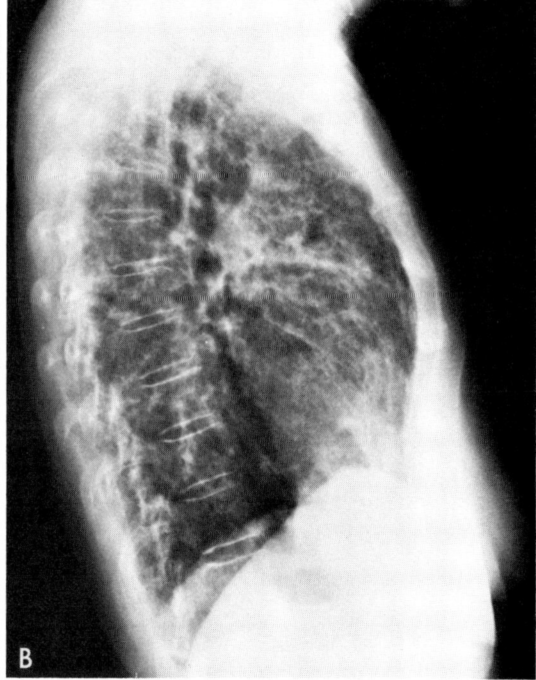

Figure 8–31. Interstitial fibrosis, PA view (*A*) and lateral view (*B*). There is marked distortion of the lung fields with extensive bilateral "honeycombing." There is loss of volume on the left with mediastinal shift. The cause of interstitial pulmonary fibrosis in this 67-year-old female patient was unknown.

Case C13

Rufus T. Firefly, aged 74, came to the hospital to visit his mother. The house officer reassured him about her, but noted that Mr. Firefly was extremely short of breath. Mr. Firefly thought his dyspnea was normal at his age, but he agreed to have a chest x-ray (Fig. 8–32). What does it show?

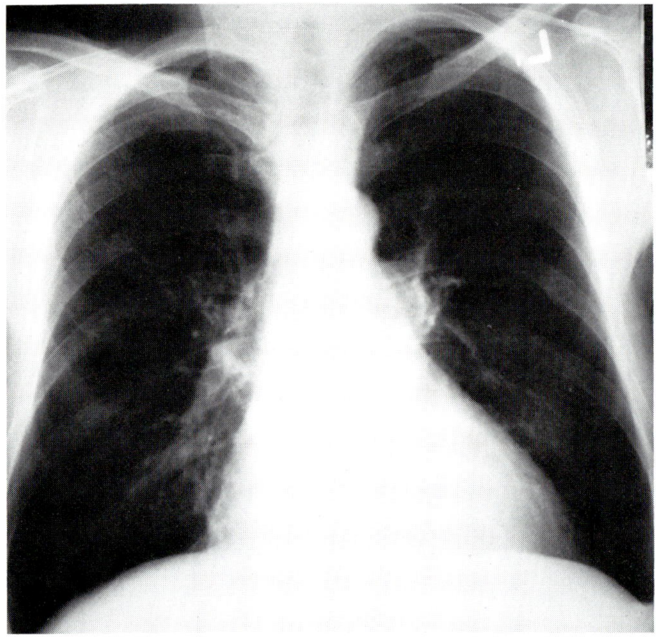

Figure 8–32. "Normal" PA chest x-ray. There is a slight increase in the heart size, but it is probably within normal limits for a man of 74.

The radiographic appearance of chronic lung disease may be very misleading, and it is not uncommon to find a severely dyspneic patient with a relatively normal chest radiograph, as in this case. It is common, however, to spot some distortion of the peripheral pulmonary parenchyma in most people over 25, particularly heavy smokers. Correct diagnosis of chronic lung disease depends on pulmonary function tests, although a chest radiograph helps to exclude the possibility of infections and tumors and provides a simple method of following the progression of the disease. As the lung disease worsens, the radiographic changes become more obvious. Two common patterns become apparent, although the average patient with chronic lung disease exhibits a combination. A fine reticular pattern is suggestive of pulmonary fibrosis and is often best seen in the lower zones and at the bases. The term *reticular* implies a netlike structure and refers to the interstitial fibrosis occurring in the lung fields. A nodular pattern also occurs, the nodules probably representing small intrapulmonary lymph nodes as well as localized areas of fibrosis. The more common mixture of both is referred to as a *reticulonodular pattern* (Fig. 8–33). It is important to remember that many patients with COPD are elderly and have arteriosclerotic heart disease as well. Often, a small infection such as bronchitis causes congestive heart failure. The combination of heart and lung disease is known as *cor pulmonale* (Fig. 8–34).

In this significant group of chronic pulmonary diseases, there are a number of other specific conditions that lead to widespread fibrosis with centrilobular emphysema. The

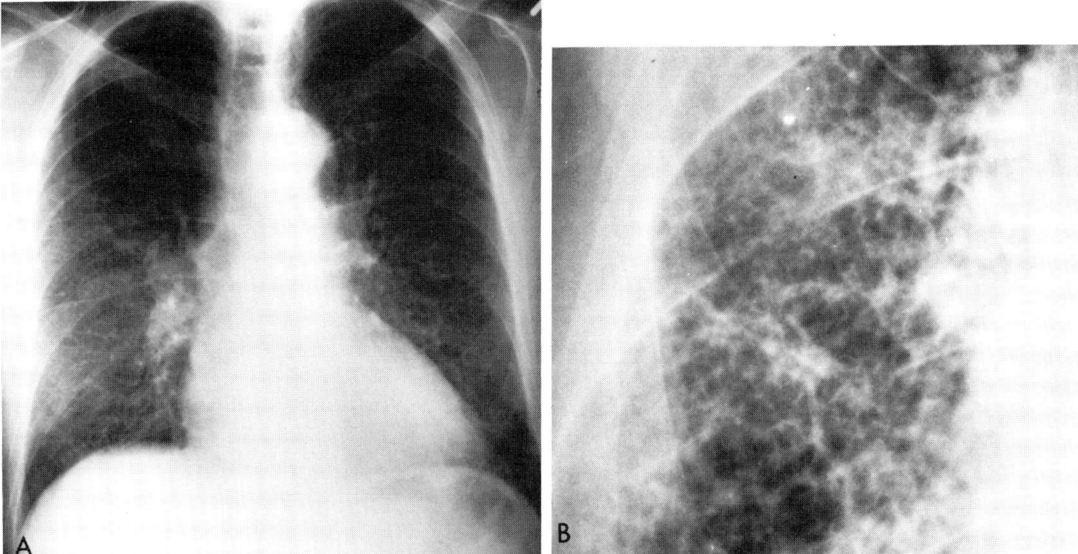

Figure 8–33. Reticulonodular pattern. *A*, PA chest film. *B*, Close-up view of a different patient. The first patient (*A*) shows the early changes, whereas the second patient has pneumoconiosis with severe pulmonary parenchymal disease. The interstitial fibrosis can be seen as a network of fine lines most marked at the bases. The nodules are best seen in the periphery, but are often more obvious in the midzones.

resultant radiological pattern is referred to as *honeycomb lung* (see Figure 8–31).

Thus far our discussion has been concerned with causes of dyspnea on exertion in older people. There is, however, a group of conditions that occur in younger patients, ages 20 through 40, usually with insidious onset of dyspnea. Those conditions may, in fact, be detected on a routine chest radiograph, as discussed earlier.

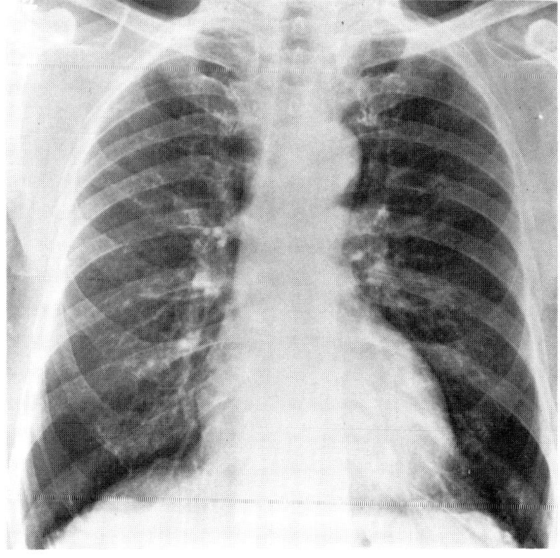

Figure 8–34. Cor pulmonale. This 65-year-old male patient has a history of hypertension and dyspnea. He has had recurrent bouts of congestive cardiac failure; after digitalization, there was improvement in the heart failure. The PA chest x-ray reveals cardiomegaly with chronic redistribution and enlarged hilar vessels, but the peripheral vessels are either normal or smaller than normal.

Case C14 Matilda Netherwood, age 26, presented at the hospital clinic with lethargy, fatigue, and dyspnea. On examination, lymphadenopathy was obvious. A chest x-ray was taken (Fig. 8–35). What does it show?

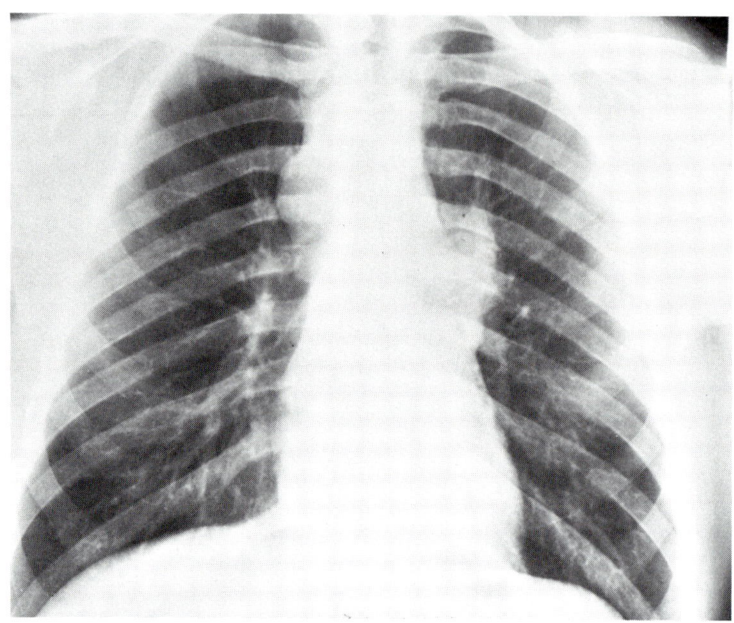

Figure 8–35. Hodgkin's disease. There are noticeably enlarged left hilar and right anterior mediastinal nodes. This PA chest radiograph is otherwise normal.

If this film is compared with that of Adelaide Witherspoon (Fig. 8–9), who had sarcoidosis, it can be seen that in Miss Netherwood the mediastinal nodes are more involved than the hilar nodes. This pattern of involvement is generally seen in lymphomas, particularly Hodgkin's disease. Lymphoma radiographically appears to originate in the mediastinum and then spread to the hilar regions, while often simultaneously being associated with peripheral lymphadenopathy and hepatosplenomegaly. Involvement of the lung parenchyma occurs in about 20 per cent of cases, although it is usually a late manifestation and often follows radiation therapy of the central mediastinum. Lymphoma may progress slowly or rapidly and may be associated with lymphatic spread, actual pulmonary infiltrations, or pulmonary nodules (Fig. 8–36).

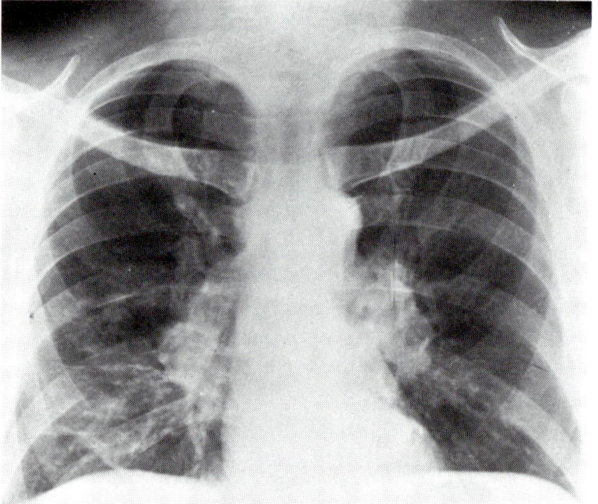

Figure 8–36. Hodgkin's disease. Large hilar nodal masses are noted in this young man with known Hodgkin's disease. There are also a number of opacities in the right lower zone, representing areas of lymphomatous infiltration of the lung parenchyma. After chemotherapy, the nodes and the pulmonary infiltrates regressed. The patient was still alive five years after this film was taken.

Lymphoma involves nodes all over the body; in fact, almost any tissue or organ can be affected. For instance, in the abdomen, retroperitoneal masses may occur, obliterating the psoas shadows and often displacing the ureters. Gastrointestinal involvement occurs in 5 per cent of patients, most commonly in the stomach or small intestine, where infiltration or discrete masses can occur. Osseous involvement ultimately occurs in 10 to 15 per cent of patients, and although almost any bone in the body may be involved, one of the classic findings in lymphoma is a dense white "ivory" vertebra. The investigation of choice for a suspected lymphoma is a *lymphogram*, which allows assessment of the degree to which subdiaphragmatic lymph nodes are involved. This information helps to determine the stage of the disease, which is necessary for planning individual treatment.

Differentiating between Hodgkin's disease and sarcoidosis using the radiographic pattern of mediastinal and hilar lymph node involvement may be difficult. Usually, sarcoidosis is bilateral and begins and remains primarily in the hilar nodes, whereas Hodgkin's disease predominantly involves the mediastinum.

Case C15

Juniper Figpot, age 27, came to her doctor with increasing dyspnea, inflamed eyes, and unusual skin lesions. On examination she had iridocyclitis, erythema nodosum, and multiple rales and rhonchi. A chest x-ray was taken (Fig. 8–37).

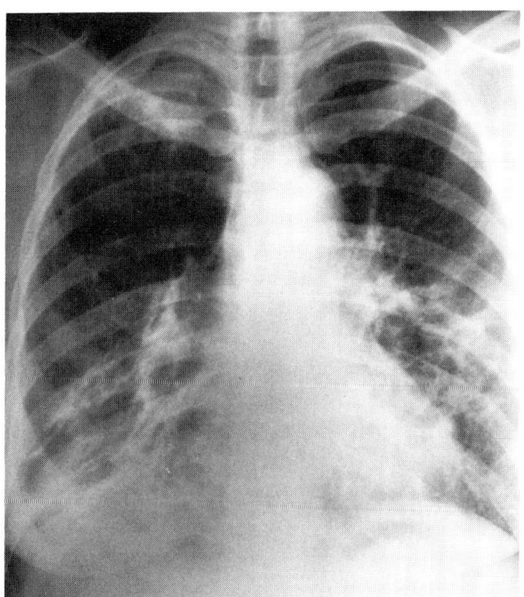

Figure 8–37. Sarcoidosis. This young black female had a five-year history of sarcoidosis with increasing dyspnea. The PA chest radiograph shows progressive pulmonary fibrosis involving the lower lobes predominantly. Note the distorted hila with enlarged nodes.

Compare this radiograph with the previous examples of lymphoma. Bilateral hilar and mediastinal lymph node involvement can be seen, but there is also evidence of lung disease, mainly in the lower zones. This radiographic picture is similar to that of diffuse pulmonary fibrosis from any cause and may be confusing, because in the later stages of sarcoidosis, lymphadenopathy may regress so that the sole radiographic appearance is that of residual pulmonary fibrosis. It is important to remember that the pulmonary fibrosis of sarcoidosis may regress partially or totally with steroid therapy or may progress until it causes death. Bone lesions occur in about 4 per cent of patients with

TABLE 8–2. Classification of Congenital Heart Disease According to Pulmonary Vascular Pattern.*

PULMONARY VASCULAR PATTERN	POSSIBLE DIAGNOSES
Increased pulmonary vascularity without cyanosis	Atrial septal defect Ventricular septal defect Patent ductus arteriosus Miscellaneous left-to-right shunts
Increased pulmonary vascularity with cyanosis	Total anomalous pulmonary venous return Persistent truncus arteriosus Transposition of the great vessels Single ventricle
Decreased pulmonary vascularity	Tetralogy of Fallot Ebstein's anomaly Congenital tricuspid insufficiency Pulmonary stenosis Pulmonary insufficiency
Normal pulmonary vascularity (unless failure occurs)	Aortic stenosis Aortic insufficiency Coarctation of the aorta Congenital mitral stenosis Cor triatriatum Congenital mitral insufficiency Endomyocardial disease

*After Swischuk 1970.

sarcoid; they have a characteristic punched-out appearance and are most often seen in the distal ends of the middle phalanges. Sarcoid is another example of multisystem disease that may involve the eyes, nervous system, skin, joints, gastrointestinal tract, genitourinary tract, lungs, and lymph nodes. Another feature in sarcoidosis seen on radiographs is the occurrence of calcified granulomas in the liver and spleen.

Congenital and Acquired Heart Lesions

A fourth group of conditions may cause a patient to present to the physician with dyspnea on exertion: congenital and acquired heart lesions. Since textbooks have been devoted to this subject, it is obviously impossible and unnecessary to cover the subject adequately in a brief summary. Table 8–2 lists pulmonary vascular patterns and possible diagnoses for the more significant congenital heart diseases. Three disorders will be discussed here.

Careful analysis of every patient's radiograph is essential, especially when heart disease is suspected. Evaluate the pulmonary vasculature to see if it is increased or decreased, look at the heart size, determine whether any chambers are enlarged, check the location and size of the aorta, and assess the size of the main pulmonary outflow tract.

Case C16

Carnelian Fawcett, age 22, came to his physician complaining of mild shortness of breath. On examination, blood pressure in his arms and legs was found to be different. What would one expect a chest x-ray to show (Fig. 8–38)?

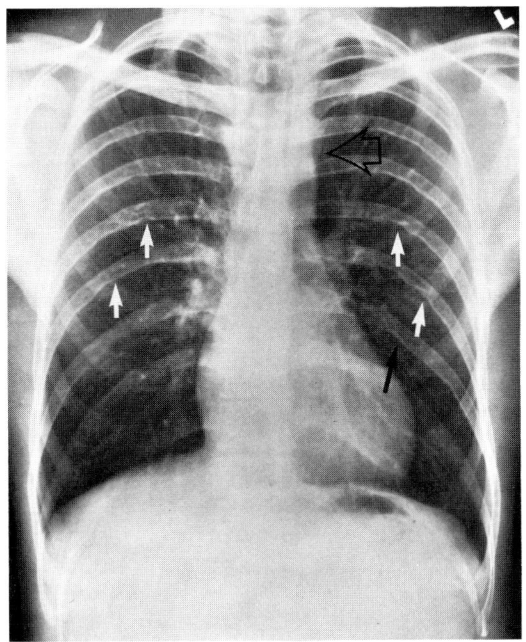

Figure 8–38. Coarctation of the aorta. The heart appears normal. The descending aorta has an indentation just below the aortic knob (*hollow arrow*). The most characteristic finding on this film is the notching of the inferior surfaces of many ribs (*small arrows*), which results from the large collateral blood flow through the intercostal arteries.

Coarctation of the aorta is one of the more subtle congenital heart disorders, clinically and radiologically. The tetralogy of Fallot, however, is more dramatic and has relatively characteristic radiographic findings (Fig. 8–39). This disorder consists of pulmonary stenosis, ventricular septal defect, overriding aorta, and right ventricular hypertrophy.

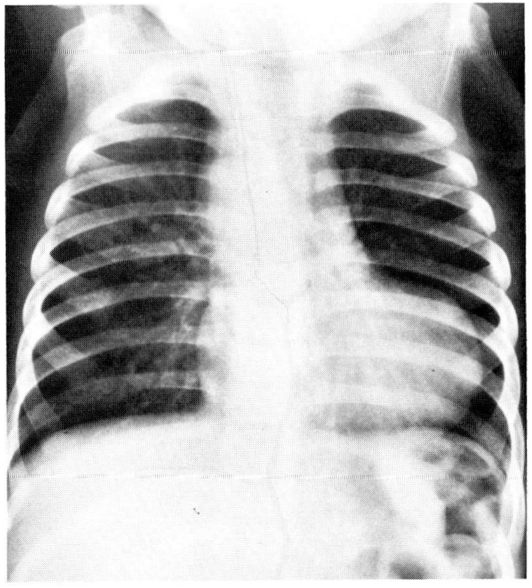

Figure 8–39. Tetralogy of Fallot. The chest radiograph in this cyanotic 11-month-old child shows the characteristic "boot-shaped" heart (coeur en sabot), with enlargement of the apex to the left. There is a right-sided aorta, and the pulmonary markings are diminished.

Case C17

When Violet Whisper, age 19, was 2 years old, she was found to have a cardiac murmur, cyanosis, and clubbing. Recently, she experienced intense chest pain while training to run in the Boston Marathon. She was unable to qualify, however, because of severe dyspnea and exercise intolerance. She was referred by her trainer for a cardiac consultation. Her chest radiograph shows the typical changes associated with a transposition of the great vessels (Fig. 8–40).

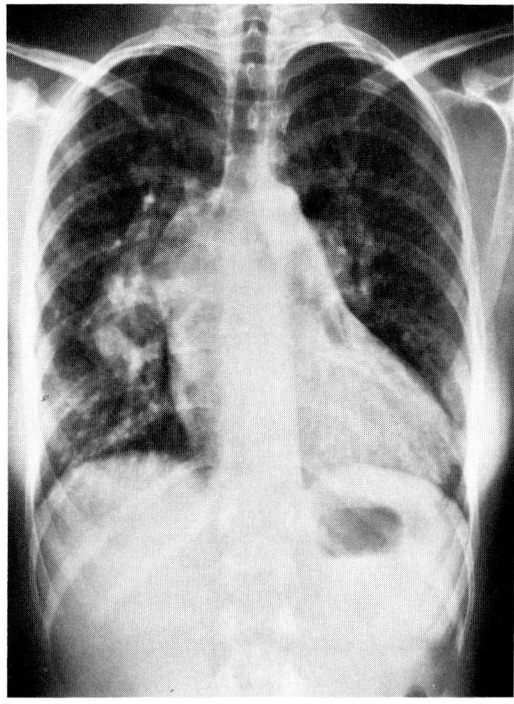

Figure 8–40. Transposition with a left-to-right shunt. There is biventricular enlargement with severely engorged pulmonary arteries, plethoric pulmonary vasculature, and an abnormal configuration in the upper right hilar region. The aortic arch is difficult to identify.

The pulmonary artery arose from a posterior ventricle. There was an associated ventricular septal defect, with the aorta arising astride the defect, and the aorta itself was found to be hypoplastic. The term *corrected transposition* refers to a transposition of the left and right sides of the heart, in which venous blood flows through the embryological left heart into the lungs, returns to the embryological right heart, and flows out the aorta. It does not cause cyanosis.

The findings of angiocardiographic examination are diagnostic in nearly all cases of congenital heart disease. In the radiographic assessment of this disorder, the presence or absence of cyanosis is an important fact that the radiologist must know in order to interpret the film findings adequately. It is also necessary to know if a shunt is suspected. This information is used to determine whether the malformation is predominantly in the left or right heart. If a shunt is present, the radiologist must know its level (atrial or ventricular) and the direction of blood flow (right to left or left to right). A plain chest radiograph allows assessment of pulmonary vasculature as well as chamber size and involvement. Angiocardiography demonstrates specific anatomical abnormalities.

Case C18

Dorothea Lovebind, age 44, presented with increasing dyspnea and fatigue. The doctor found that her heart was enlarged. She had had rheumatic heart disease as a child. A chest radiograph was taken (Fig. 8–41).

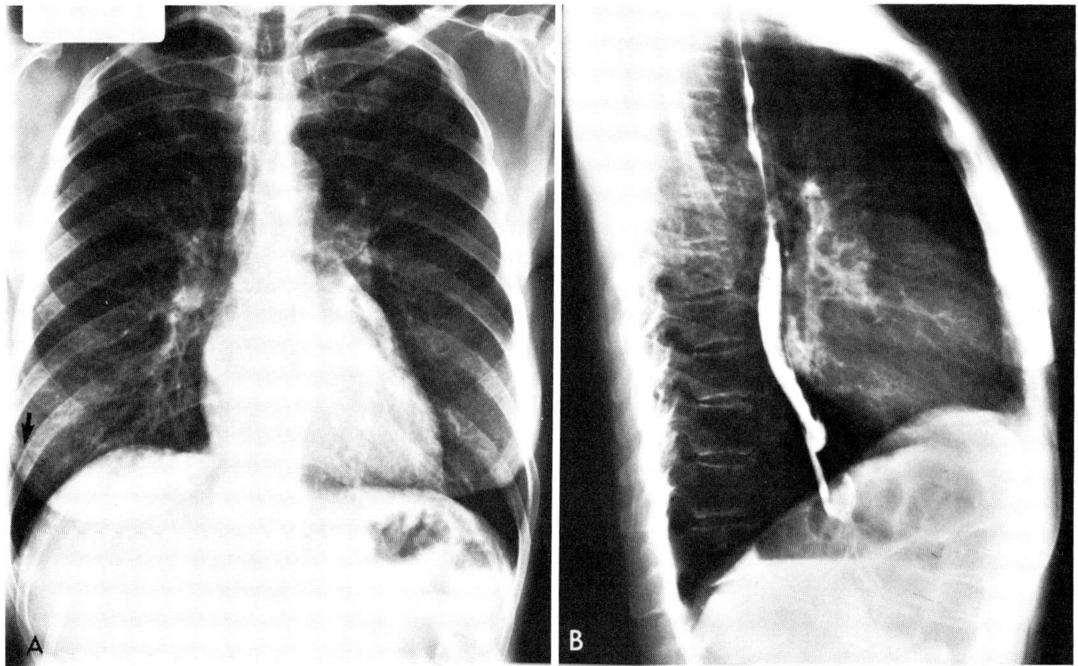

Figure 8–41. Mitral stenosis, PA view (*A*) and lateral view with barium (*B*). There is enlargement of the left atrium with prominence of the pulmonary vasculature. Note that the left main stem bronchus is elevated and that the barium is indented on the lateral view. Kerley B lines are also present (*arrow*).

Acquired valvular disease has become rare, mainly as a result of the use of penicillin in the treatment of rheumatic fever. Patients with the sequelae of rheumatic fever are still seen.

The classic changes of mitral stenosis are an enlarged left atrium, producing a double shadow behind the heart, with elevation of the left main stem bronchus. Main pulmonary vessels are prominent, with pulmonary vascular redistribution and Kerley B lines at the bases. In long-standing cases of mitral stenosis, small rounded densities occur in the lower lung fields. They are caused by

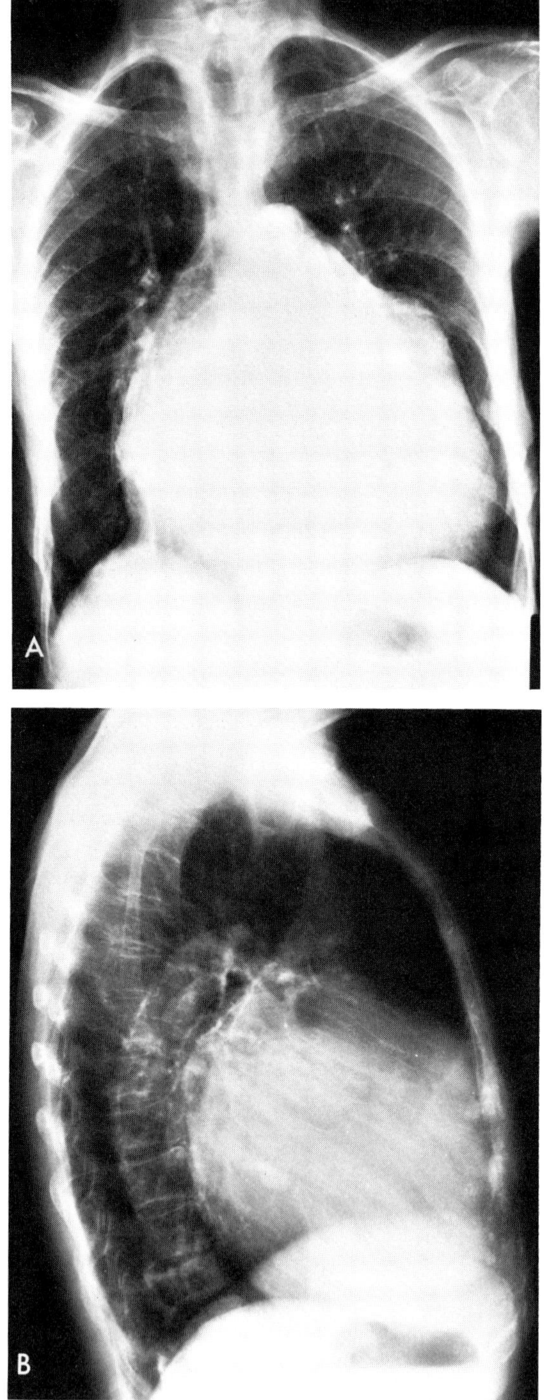

Figure 8–42. Mitral regurgitation, PA view (*A*) and lateral view (*B*). This 79-year-old male patient has a history of rheumatic heart disease, known mitral stenosis, and mitral regurgitation. The left atrium is huge.

hemosiderosis, and they may calcify or ossify. Right ventricular enlargement is also seen and is associated with a normal-sized left ventricle and a small aortic knob.

Mitral incompetence or mitral regurgitation is associated with an enlarged left ventricle and a huge left atrium, but rarely with any sign of pulmonary vascular redistribution (Fig. 8–42). Pure mitral regurgitation is not common, and most patients have a combination of mitral stenosis and regurgitation.

Case C19

Ethan Allen Cole-Lapse, age 48, is a lawyer who went to a physician after he had a syncopal episode that apparently resulted from lugging boulders from a local quarry to his back yard to embellish his wife's rock garden. On being questioned, Mr. Cole-Lapse said that up to that time, his health had been excellent. Physical examination revealed a crescendo-decrescendo systolic murmur best heard over the aortic area but transmitted into the neck. The EKG showed typical changes of left ventricular enlargement. A chest x-ray was taken (Fig. 8–43). What does it show?

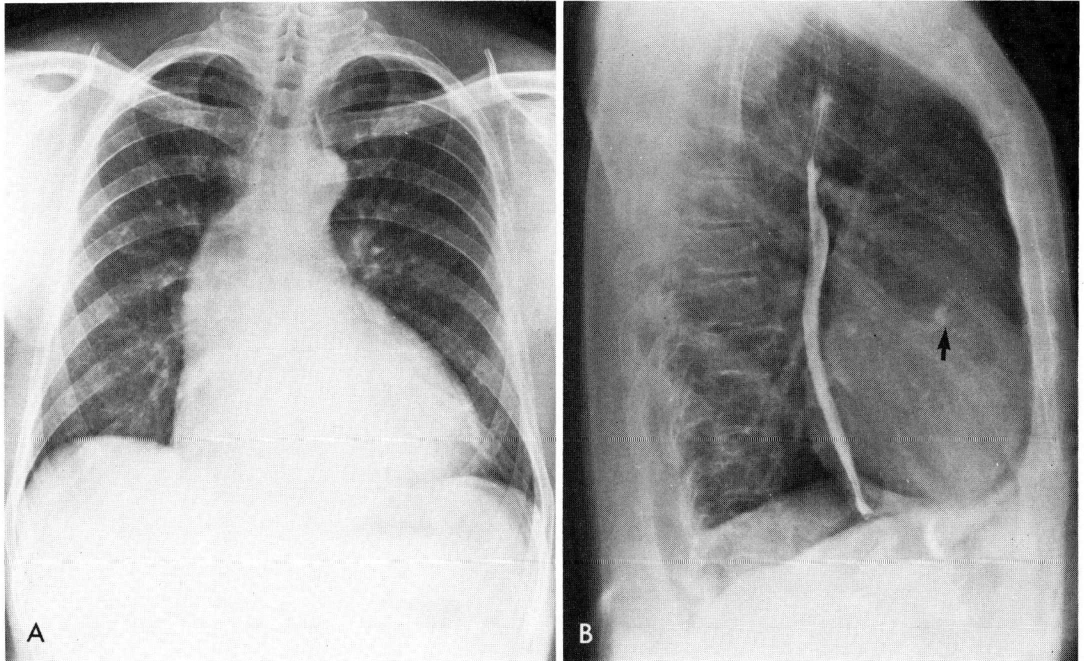

Figure 8–43. Aortic stenosis, PA view (*A*) and lateral view (*B*). There is pronounced cardiac enlargement with unfolding and dilatation of the ascending aorta. Enlargement of the left ventricle and the left atrium is apparent. Calcification can be seen in the region of the aortic valve (*arrow*).

Calcification in the aortic valve and annulus is seen in 85 per cent of patients with aortic stenosis. Most patients with this disorder have few radiographic signs, although some present with heart failure. Aortic insufficiency due to rheumatic fever may also be difficult to diagnose radiographically, but solitary left ventricular enlargement should make the radiologist suspicious of aortic regurgitation.

DYSPNEA AND CHEST PAIN

Some conditions cause dyspnea with pain of one sort or another. They include pneumonia, pulmonary embolus, and bronchogenic carcinoma. In all three conditions, pain results largely from pleural involvement. If a cancerous growth is situated centrally in the lung fields it may be "silent" and may be discovered only on a routine chest x-ray.

Case C20

Dionysius Doolightly, age 24, was riding his bicycle along a country road when a sharp stabbing pain in his chest caused him to lose his balance and fall into a patch of buttercups. When he stood up again, he noticed he was becoming increasingly breathless, so he asked a passing motorist to drive him to the local hospital. A chest x-ray was taken (Fig. 8–44). What does it show?

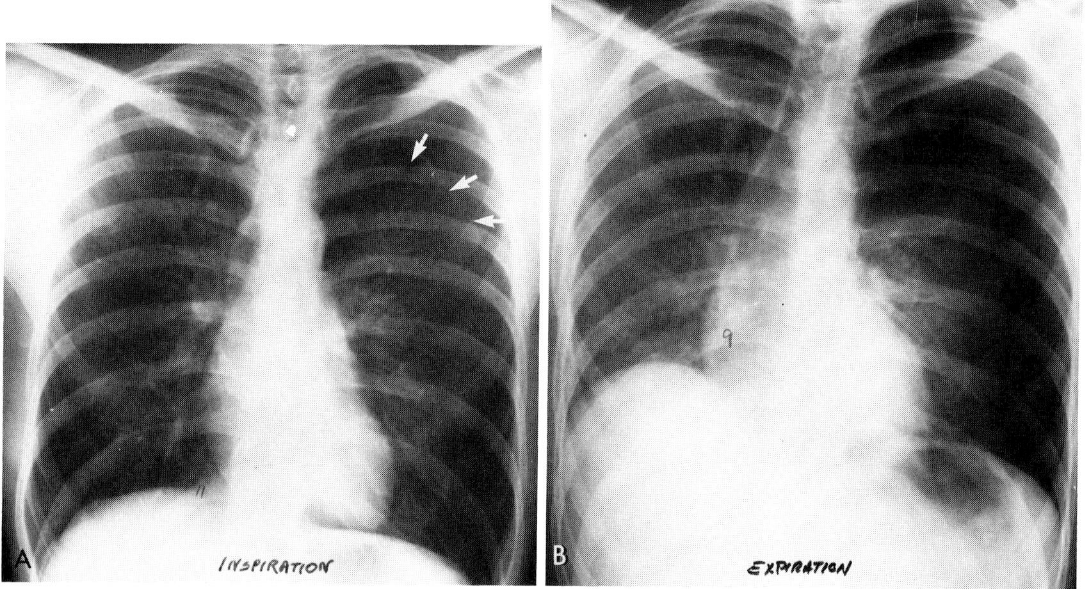

Figure 8–44. Pneumothorax. *A*, A left apical pneumothorax can be seen on the inspiration view (*arrows*). *B*, On the expiration view, note that the pneumothorax becomes more obvious.

There is a suggestion of a pneumothorax at the left apex. What would you do now? Inspiration and expiration views have a number of uses, one of which is to visualize diaphragmatic motion. An expiration view, however, reduces the intrapulmonary pressure, so that a pneumothorax will apparently expand and so become more visible (Fig. 8–44B). Conversely, on a full inspiration view, the pneumothorax will appear smaller.

A small pneumothorax requires no specific treatment, although recurrent small pneumothoraces may require treatment by one of the procedures used to seal the visceral pleura to the parietal pleura (talc, tetracycline, or an inflammatory agent may be used). Larger pneumothoraces should be treated by using a chest tube to empty out the free air (Fig. 8–45). A tension pneumothorax may be life-threatening.

Staphylococcal pneumonia may be extremely necrotizing and may produce enormous cavity-like appearances in the lung fields resembling pneumothoraces or lung abscesses. These cavities, known as *pneumatoceles*, are entirely contained by the visceral pleura. They are relatively common in infants but rare in adults. A history of untreated pneumonia with increasing dyspnea

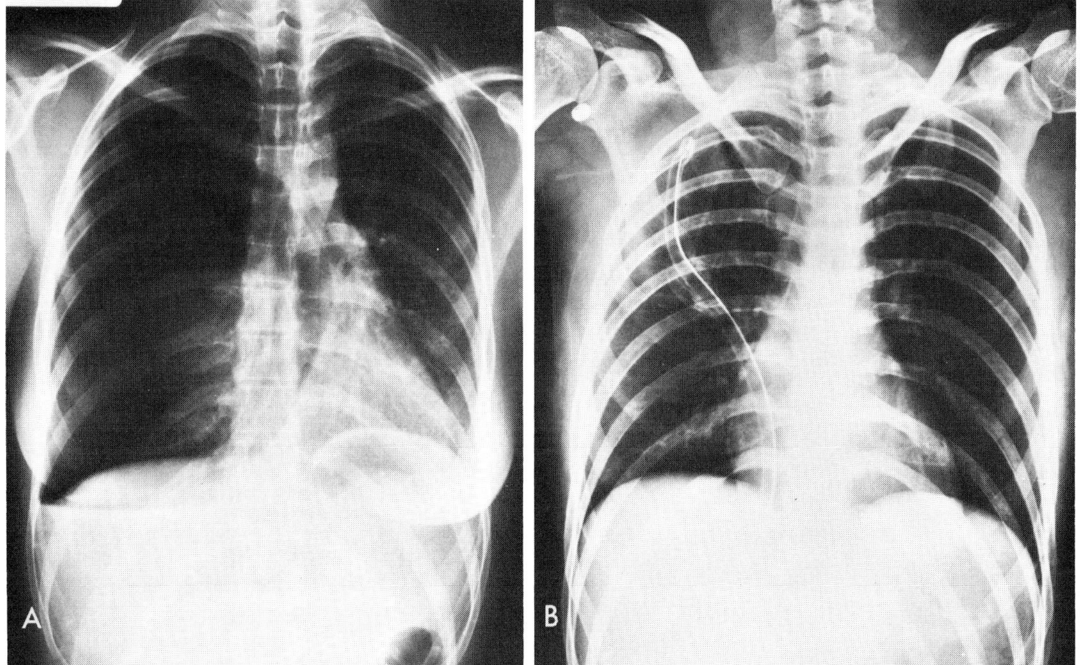

Figure 8–45. Tension pneumothorax with expansion following insertion of chest tube. *A*, On the initial film, note the shift of the heart and mediastinum to the left and the very large tension pneumothorax in this 21-year-old girl who had had a skiing accident and complained of severe pain and increasing dyspnea. *B*, Following insertion of the chest tube, there has been total reexpansion of the lung, and the anatomy has returned to normal.

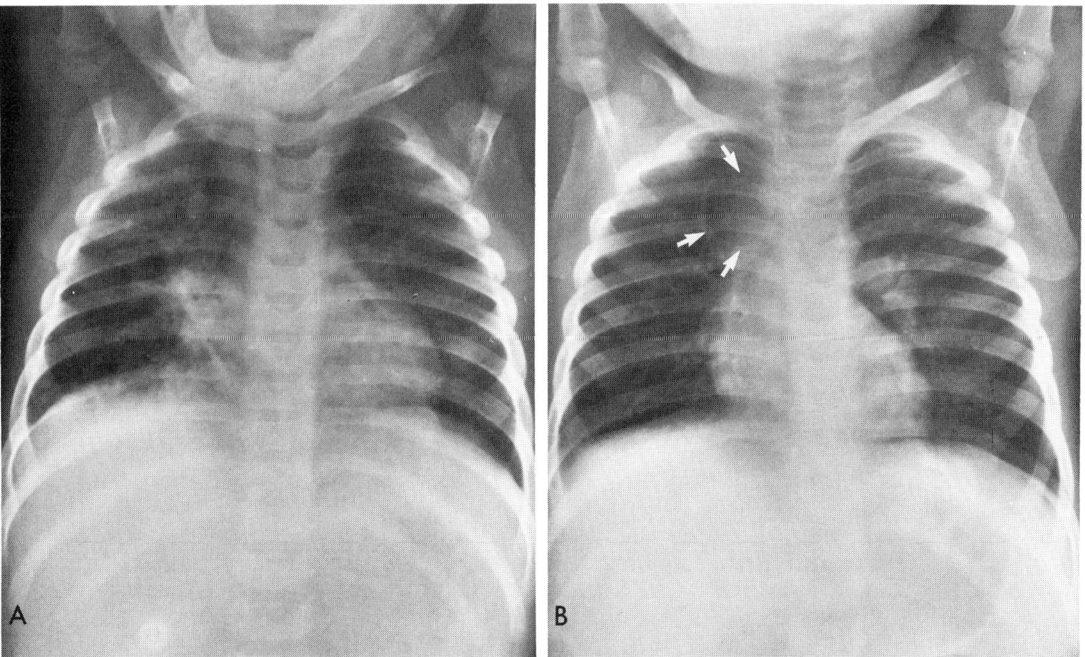

Figure 8–46. Pneumatoceles. *A*, On the initial film there is patchy opacification throughout the lung fields but most marked in the right midzone. *B*, On a film taken ten days later, a well-defined lucency is obvious (*arrows*); it can be detected on the initial film if comparison is made. The lung fields are clearing, although there is now some hyperlucency of the right lung, presumably due to air trapping. A mucous plug was found in the right main stem bronchus. This 2½-year-old child had been admitted five times previously for recurrent staphylococcal pneumonia.

over several days and a characteristic radiographic appearance make diagnosis relatively simple (Fig. 8–46). Pneumonia may be caused by any number of different microorganisms. Most commonly, pneumonia occurs in very young or in elderly, debilitated patients.

Case C21

Shrivel D. Gross, age 29, was a hard-working young medical resident who slept an average of 4 hours a night. He had been holding a retractor for his surgical colleagues in the operating room for ten hours when he noticed he was feeling worse than usual. While rushing through the radiology department, he stopped long enough to have a chest x-ray taken (Fig. 8–47). What does it show?

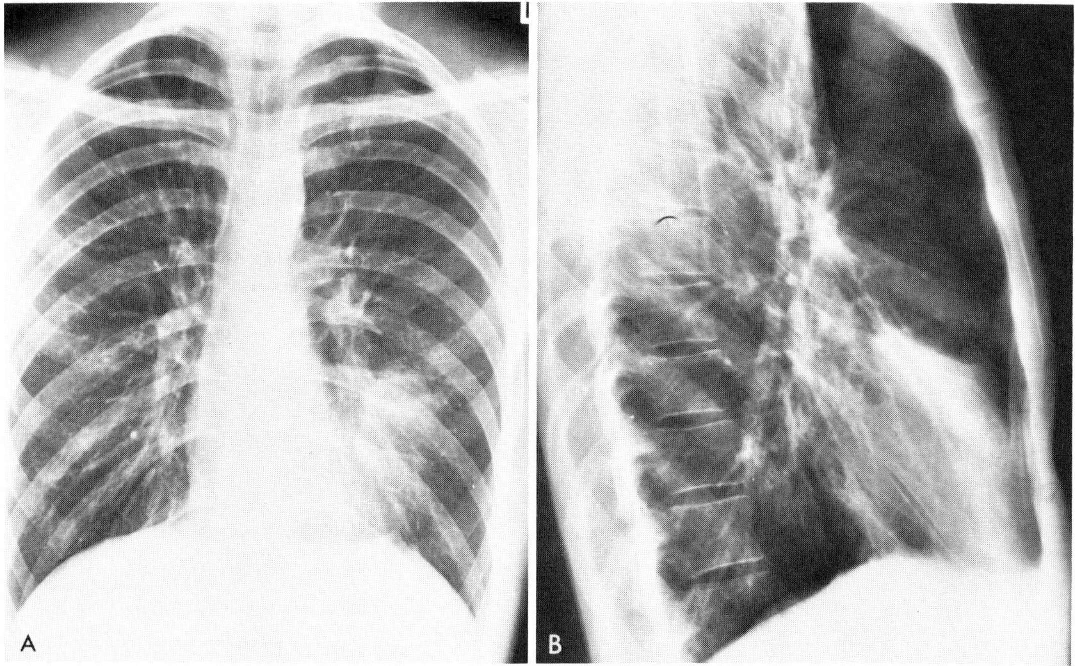

Figure 8–47. Lobar pneumonia (lingular), PA view (*A*) and lateral view (*B*). Opacification in the left lower zone obliterates the left heart border (silhouette sign). On the lateral view this wedge-shaped area of consolidation lies over the heart and represents a lingular pneumonia.

The classic signs of lobar pneumonia are opacification of a segment of the lung with obliteration of the adjacent soft tissue shadows, i.e., the diaphragm or heart borders; this is known as the *silhouette sign.* Pneumonia is usually associated with some loss of volume, and bowing of one of the fissures. It should be possible to identify the lobe or segment involved on the basis of the PA view alone, but a lateral view is often helpful (Figs. 8–48 and 8–49). In a typical pneumococcal pneumonia, opacification takes 10 to 14 days to clear, and it is not necessary to take another chest x-ray until the end of that time unless the patient's condition seems to be worsening. The decision to send the patient home depends on how he feels and whether his temperature has returned to normal rather than on radiographic evidence. In many people involvement of a whole segment or lobe does not occur, because either they are extremely fit or the bacterial agent is less potent than usual. These people develop small patches of pneumonia, or pneumonitis.

The most common cause of true atelecta-

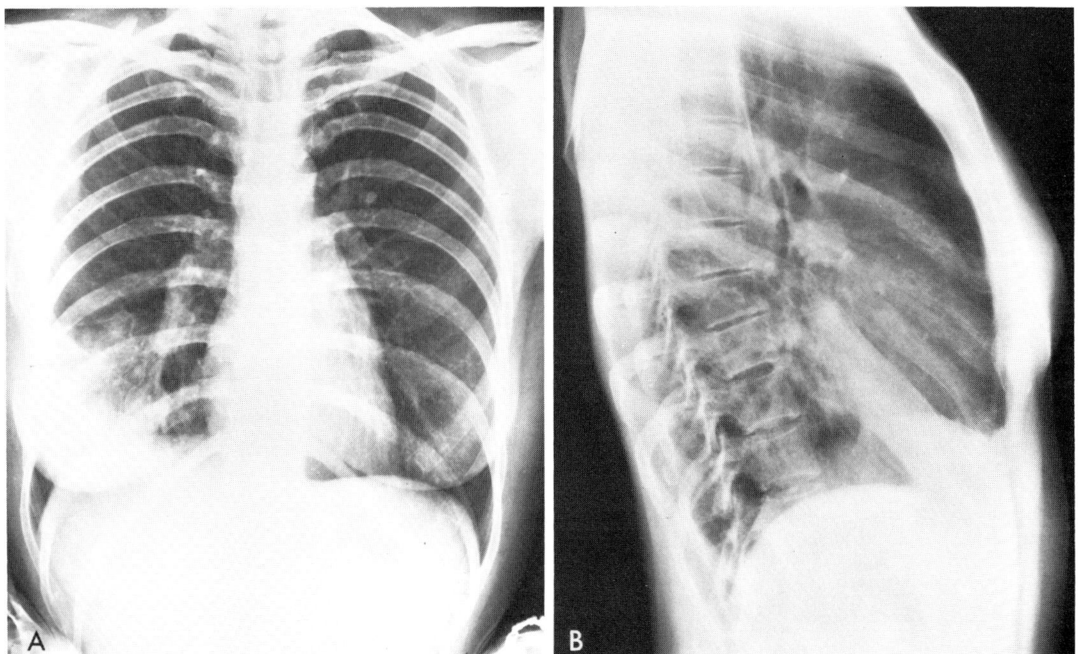

Figure 8–48. Right lower lobe pneumonia, PA view (*A*) and lateral view (*B*). This 45-year-old female patient presented with a nine-day history of muscle pains and a productive cough. On these chest films, the consolidation in the anterior segment of the right lower lobe can be clearly seen.

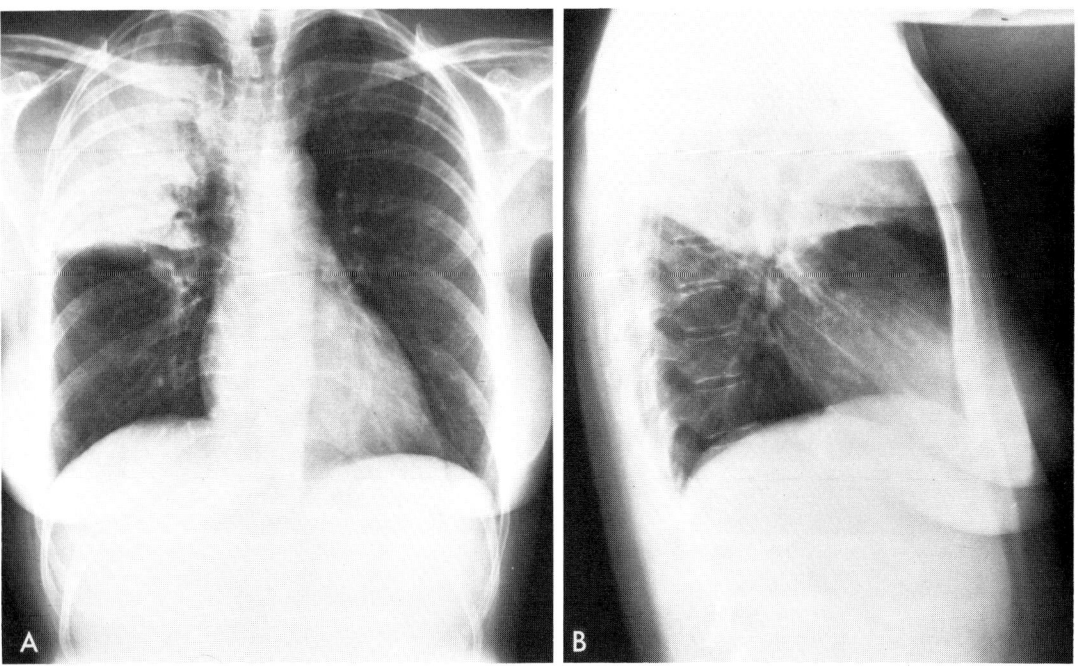

Figure 8–49. Right upper lobe pneumonia, PA view (*A*) and lateral view (*B*). There are clear-cut margins between this right upper lobe consolidation and the horizontal fissure on the PA view and between the consolidation and the oblique and horizontal fissures on the lateral view. This 61-year-old female patient presented with fever, malaise, pleuritic chest pain, and dyspnea.

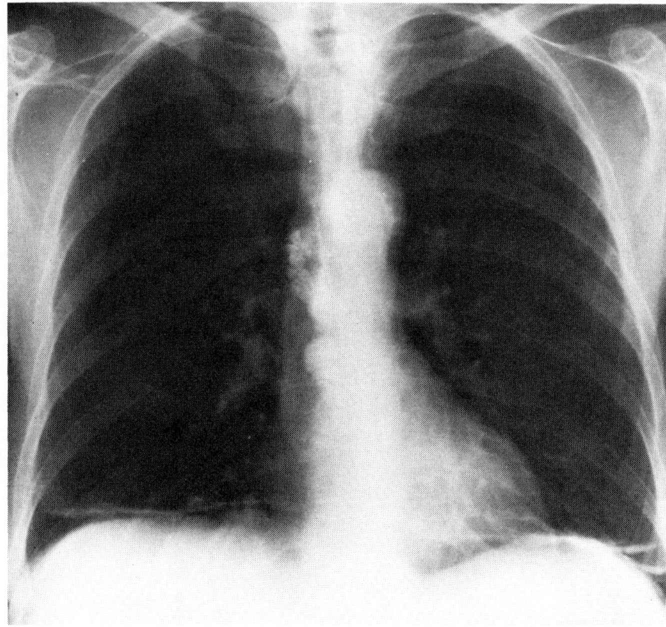

Figure 8–50. Deflation atelectasis. Two days after having an elective gastrectomy, this patient developed linear atelectasis, because his abdomen hurt and he was not breathing properly. Note the calcification of the lymph nodes from previous healed tuberculosis.

sis is probably failure to ventilate properly. After an abdominal operation, deflation atelectasis is extremely common (Fig. 8–50). *Deflation or nonobstructive atelectasis* is caused by lung compression due either to poor breathing or to an adjacent tumor, bulla, or fluid. *Obstructive atelectasis* may be caused by a neoplasm, foreign body, or mucous plug within one of the bronchi. Absorption of air distal to the obstruction occurs, producing the atelectasis.

Viral pneumonia may, however, exhibit no radiographic findings other than a slight increase in interstitial markings, which will require comparison with noninvolved parts of the lung or with a previous film for positive diagnosis of pneumonia. In some cases, however, the diagnosis is relatively easy to make radiographically because of widespread pneumonitis (Fig. 8–51) or an area of consolidation. There may also be concomitant pleurisy with a small pleural effusion. Frequently, diagnosis of viral pneumonia can be made clinically, and without diffi-

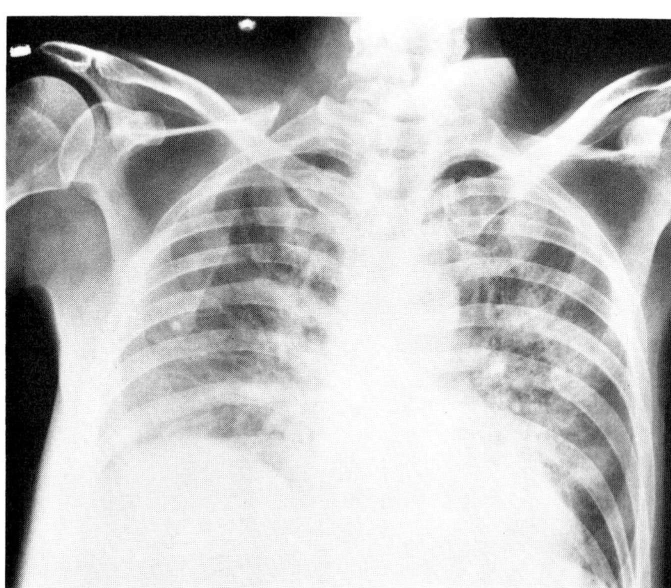

Figure 8–51. Viral pneumonia. This 53-year-old man was admitted with severe dyspnea and chest pain. The single AP film shows a diffuse patchy opacification not unlike that seen in interstitial pulmonary edema. The patient died; autopsy proved these findings were caused by diffuse viral pneumonitis.

culty. The rationale for taking a chest x-ray is to exclude the possibility of other diseases or complications and to differentiate viral pneumonia from upper respiratory tract infection.

Case C22

Sigmoid Frond, age 72, was a retired social worker who presented with increasing dyspnea and some chest pain. She complained of coughing up small amounts of blood-stained mucus. On examination, it was found that she had lost weight. A chest x-ray was taken (Fig. 8–52). What does it show?

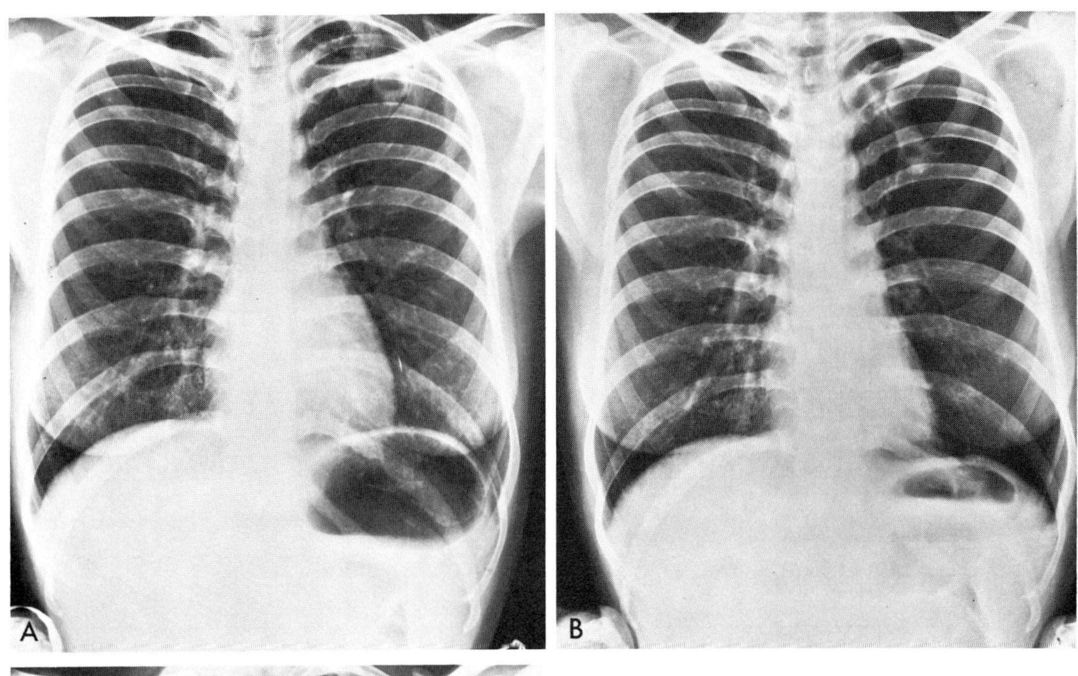

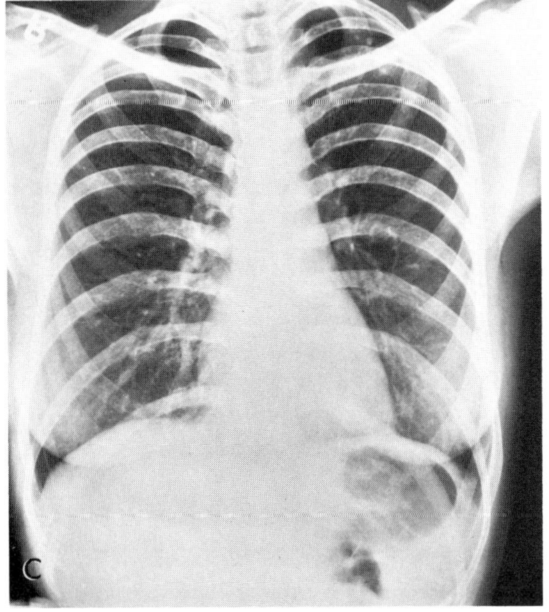

Figure 8–52. Healing of cavitary tuberculosis. *A*, The initial film shows a cavity in the left apex with an air-fluid level. The patient was complaining of fatigue, and many members of her family had had tuberculosis. *B*, Before the advent of antituberculous chemotherapy, the treatment of choice was to collapse the cavity, often by producing a pneumothorax. *C*, Five years later, there are several small calcified foci in the left apex with apparent complete healing.

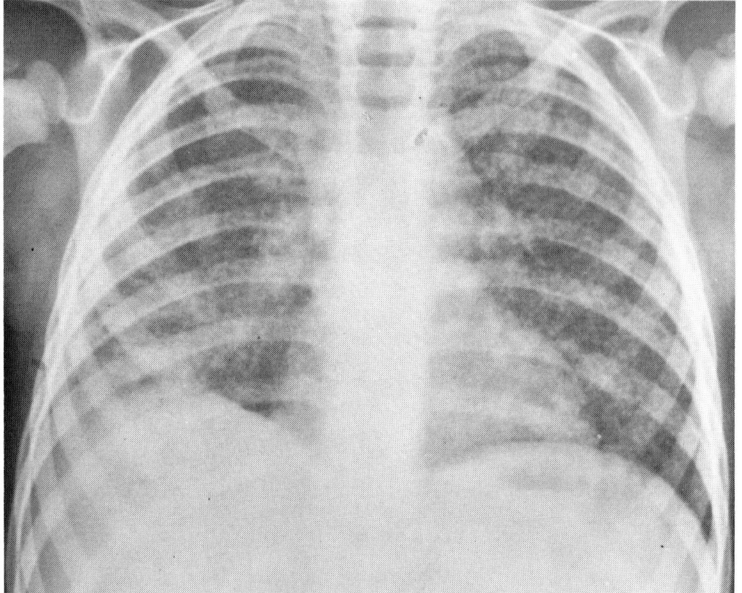

Figure 8–53. Miliary tuberculosis. The diffuse nodular pattern in both lung fields on the AP film of this child, who was severely ill, is characteristic of miliary tuberculosis. He succumbed a few days later, and the diagnosis was confirmed at autopsy.

Patients with pulmonary tuberculosis often present with cavitary upper lobe pneumonia, and if the diagnosis is uncertain, tomography is helpful not only to identify cavities but also to look for underlying calcification. A comparison with previous chest x-rays is most helpful.

Pulmonary tuberculosis may first appear radiographically as a small area of consolidation, usually in the apex of the lung. Con-

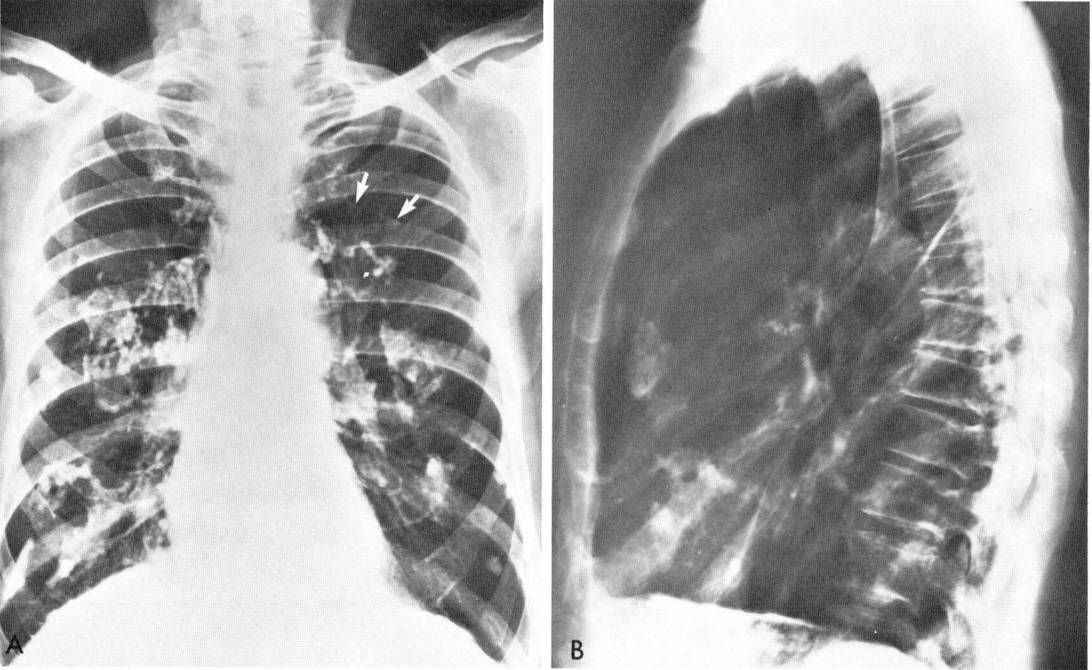

Figure 8–54. Pleural calcification, AP view (*A*) and lateral view (*B*). This 69-year-old patient had had tuberculous pleurisy 40 years previously. Apart from some intrapulmonary calcifications seen at the upper part of the left hilum (*arrows*), the remainder of the sheets of calcification are in the pleura.

solidation may be associated with hilar adenopathy with some interstitial or peribronchial reaction. This combination, characteristic of true primary tuberculosis, is rarely seen on a radiograph in the acute phase of the disease. When a consolidation calcifies, it is easily seen. The combination of a peripheral lung lesion (the Ghon lesion) and a central calcified node is known as a *Ranke complex*.

If reinfection occurs, which happens often in elderly or debilitated patients, it can take many forms: patchy infiltrates, cavitating pneumonia, or tuberculous pneumonitis (which is nearly always rapidly progressive and fatal). The classic presentation is that of miliary tuberculosis, so called because the visualized nodules are the size of millet seeds (Fig. 8–53). The possible diagnoses of a miliary mottled pattern on chest x-ray include miliary tuberculosis and interstitial pulmonary fibrosis. Unfortunately, the diagnosis of miliary tuberculosis is often made only at autopsy. Pleural calcification as a result of old tuberculosis is one of the few causes of vertical longitudinal lines on a chest x-ray (Fig. 8–54). Most anatomical divisions in the lung run centrally, toward the hilar regions. Previous hemothorax is probably the most common cause of massive pleural calcification; other causes include asbestosis and previous empyema.

Case C23

Kit N. Stocking, age 52, was a retired female prize fighter who attempted to console herself for frequent losses in the ring by drinking an extract of grain. She was found in the gutter outside the emergency room one night and was admitted to the hospital in a semicomatose state and singing "My Little Chickadee." She was cleaned up as much as possible and sent to the radiology department. What does her chest x-ray show (Fig. 8–55)?

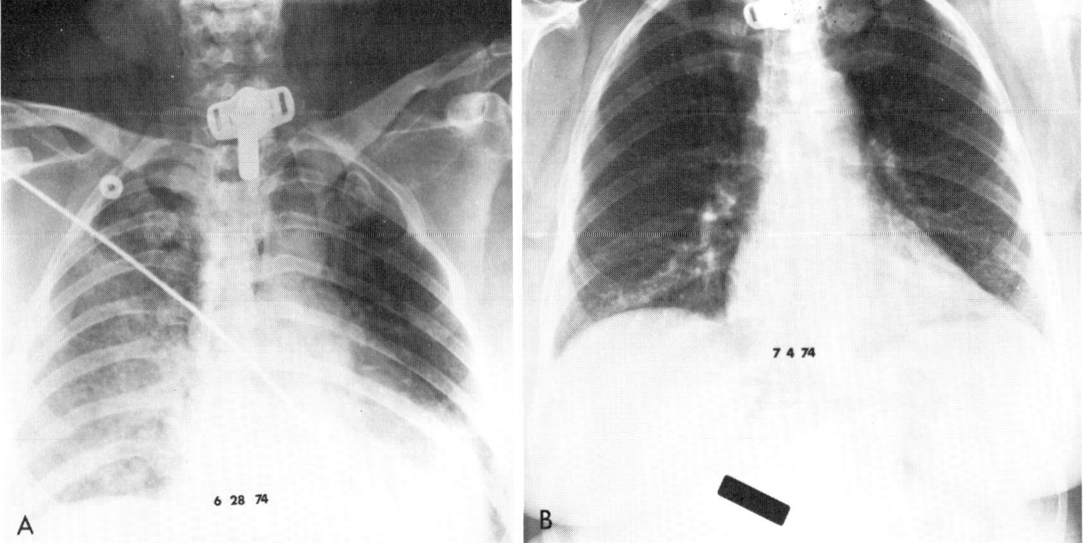

Figure 8–55. Aspiration pneumonia. *A*, The AP initial film shows diffuse opacification throughout the right lung and at the left base. The fact that this process is very patchy suggests an aspiration pneumonia rather than pulmonary edema, although the differential diagnosis is often difficult. A tracheostomy tube has been inserted because of the patient's severe dyspnea. *B*, Follow-up film taken one week later.

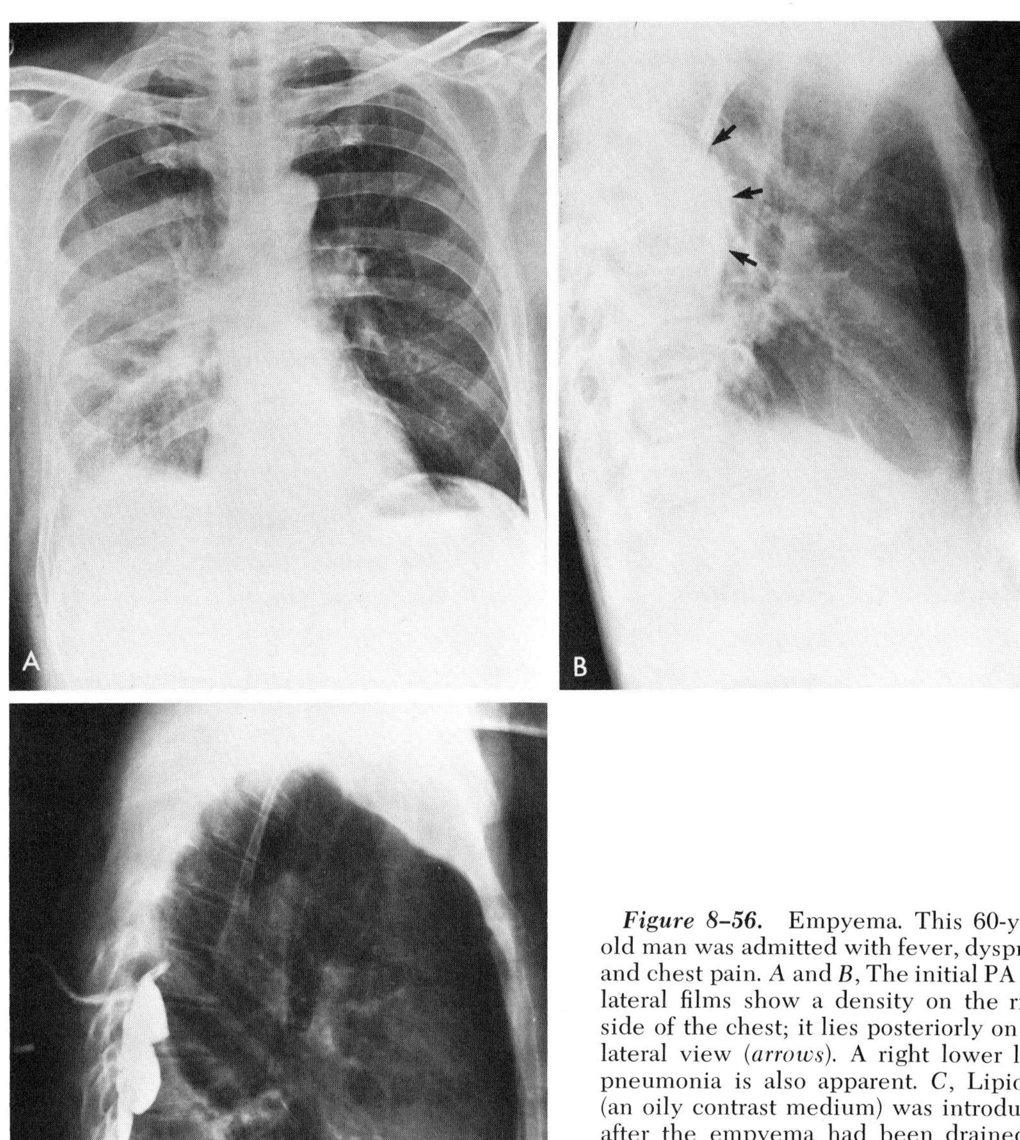

Figure 8–56. Empyema. This 60-year-old man was admitted with fever, dyspnea, and chest pain. *A* and *B*, The initial PA and lateral films show a density on the right side of the chest; it lies posteriorly on the lateral view (*arrows*). A right lower lobe pneumonia is also apparent. *C*, Lipiodol (an oily contrast medium) was introduced after the empyema had been drained to show the extent of the cavity.

Aspiration pneumonia commonly occurs in debilitated patients and alcoholics as well as in children, who may aspirate peanuts or teeth. The aspirated substance will settle in the lowest-lying part of the bronchial tree, depending on the position of the patient. For example, an alcoholic or a severely ill patient who aspirates while supine, characteristically develops pneumonia in the apical segment of the right lower lobe. In patients who have aspirated foreign matter while erect, the medial segment of

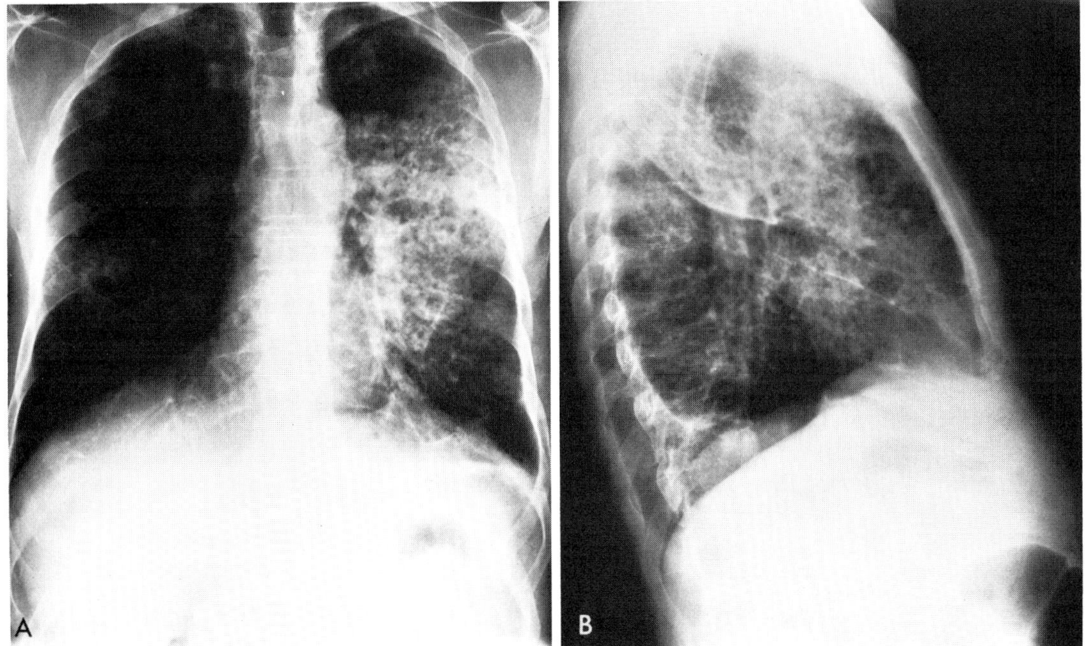

Figure 8–57. *Klebsiella* pneumonia with lobar expansion, PA view (*A*) and lateral view (*B*). There is irregular patchy opacification predominantly in the left upper lobe. On the lateral projection, bowing backwards of the oblique fissure implies an increase in lung volume. The sputum contained *Klebsiella* gram-negative rods.

the right middle lobe is the most frequently involved, because of the topography of the bronchial tree.

Recurrent pneumonia and, in debilitated patients, the presence of unusual organisms may lead to chronic infection or to pleurisy or may cause an intrapleural abscess or *empyema* (Fig. 8–56). Abscesses are often loculated in a costophrenic angle but may occur within a fissure or adjacent to the

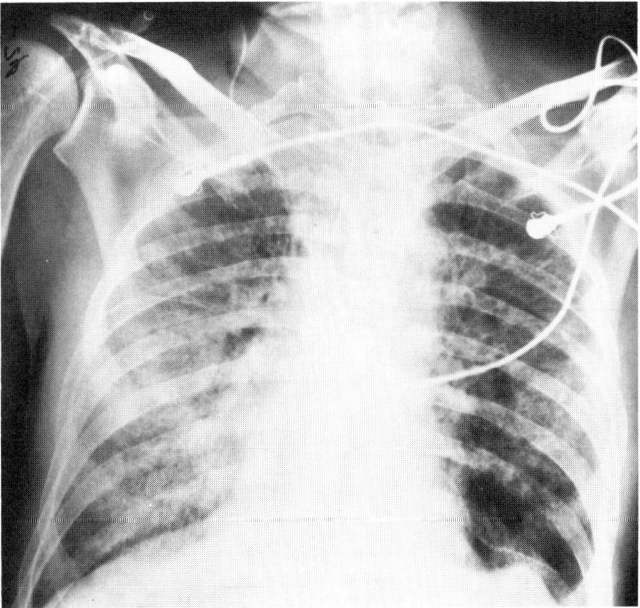

Figure 8–58. *Pneumocystis carinii* and cytomegalovirus pneumonitis. This 47-year-old man had a five-year history of progressive Hodgkin's disease for which he had received six cycles of chemotherapy. During the last cycle he had become severely dyspneic. The AP chest x-ray shows diffuse poorly defined areas of opacification. A lung biopsy revealed pulmonary fibrosis as well as focal pneumonitis due to *Pneumocystis carinii* and cytomegalovirus.

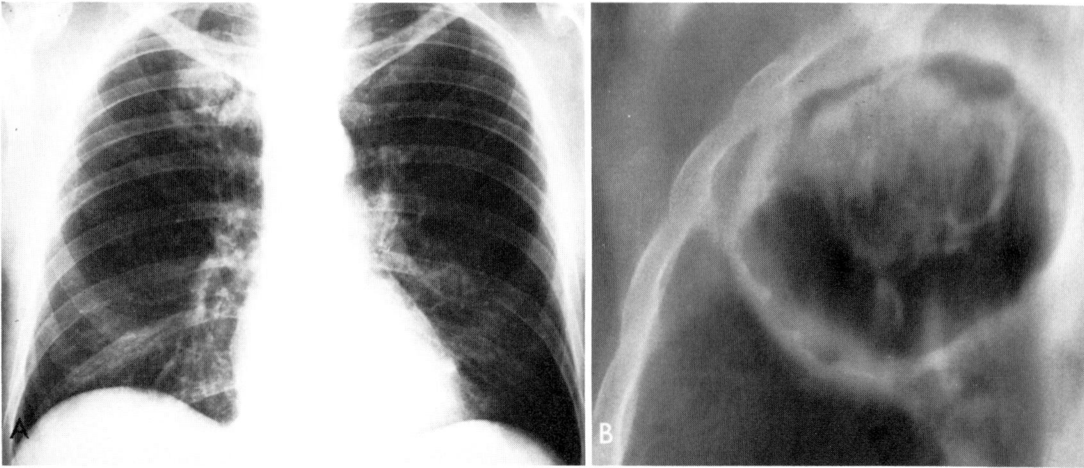

Figure 8–59. Aspergillosis with a fungus ball. *A*, On the PA view, there is a poorly defined opacity at the right apex. *B*, A tomogram shows a large cavity containing a fungus ball. At thoracotomy, this proved to be aspergillosis in a previously healed tuberculous cavity.

pleura. If an empyema communicates with an airway, it may have an air-fluid level on an erect chest x-ray. Empyema may develop secondary to an infected pneumothorax, following a thoracentesis, or in patients with bronchial fistulae. The radiographic appearance of an empyema varies, from that of a pleural effusion or mass to that of a classic loculated air-fluid level. Pleurisy is often associated with small effusions, although it may have no radiological findings. Diagnosis may be easier to make if one considers that pleurisy occurs in some 10 per cent of patients with pneumococcal pneumonia, whereas true empyema is considerably rarer, occurring in less than 2 per cent.

The presence of acute cavitary pneumonia suggests that the organism responsible is staphylococcus or *Klebsiella* (Fig. 8–57). *Klebsiella* is also one of the rare causes of a consolidation with an increase in the volume of the affected lobe that causes the fissure to bow *away* from the pneumonia. Gram-negative organisms such as *Escherichia coli* frequently produce pneumonia in patients in hospitals, and other gram-negative organisms may cause pneumonia in debilitated patients. In patients who are taking cytotoxic drugs, who are receiving steroids for immunosuppressive therapy such as that following renal transplantation, or who are severely burned, rarer infections caused by such organisms as *Pneumocystis carinii* and *Aspergillus* may occur (Figs. 8–58 and 8–59).

Pneumonia may also have other symptoms or other causes. A patient with pneumonia may present with abdominal pain due to pleural irritation. Unusually persistent or recurring pneumonia may be the presenting feature of a neoplasm that is partially blocking off a bronchus and causing stasis, atelectasis, and pneumonia.

Case C24

Suzy Creamcheese, age 34, was admitted to hospital with severe dyspnea and increasing chest pain. The only relevant feature in her clinical history was that following her tenth child she began taking "the Pill." A chest x-ray was taken and was assessed as normal (Fig. 8–60A). What would you do now?

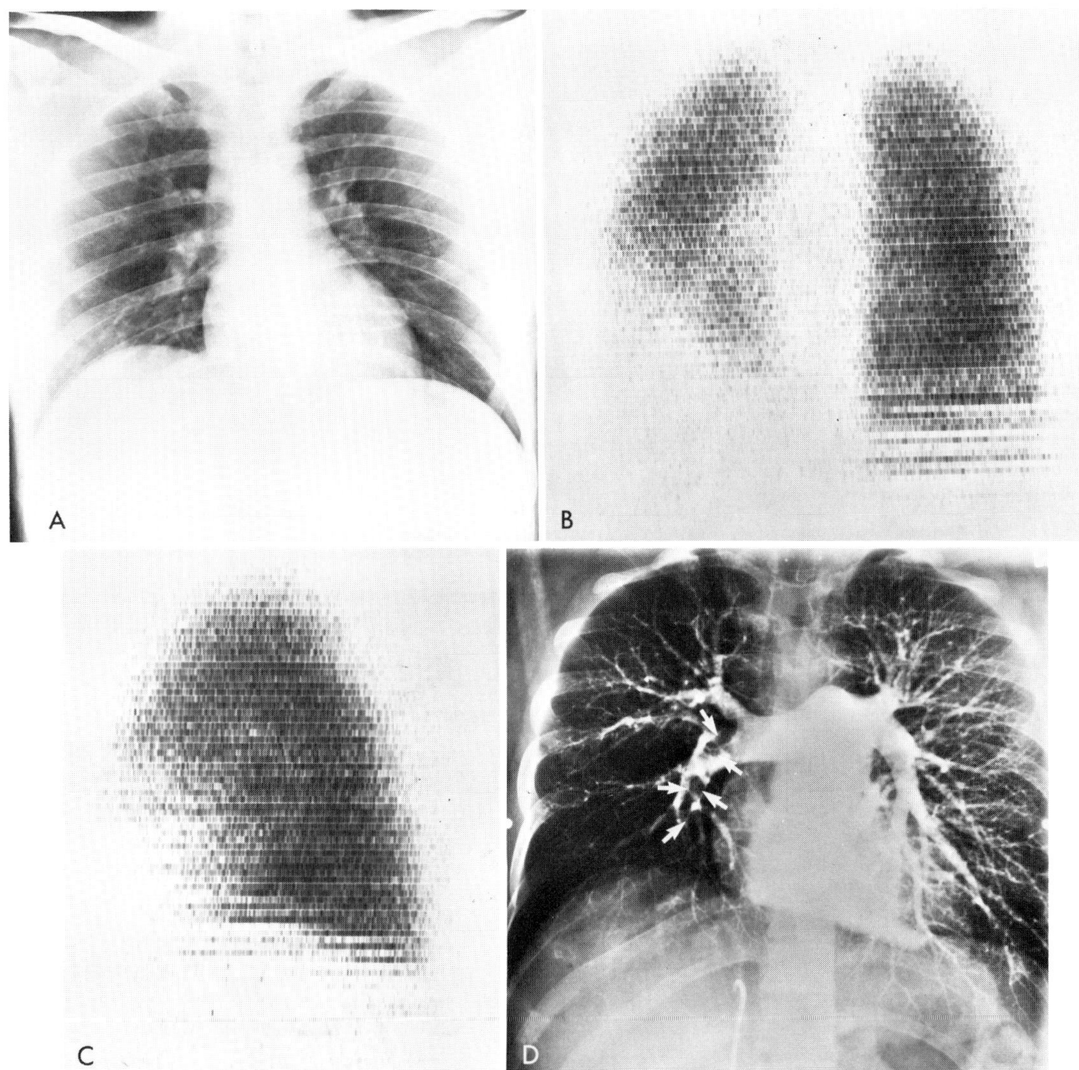

Figure 8–60. Pulmonary emboli. *A*, The PA chest x-ray shows minimal elevation of the right hemidiaphragm but is otherwise normal. *B* and *C*, On the AP and lateral views from a lung scan, a number of defects at the right base can be seen. *D*, An angiogram confirms that the defects are due to pulmonary emboli.

Plain film findings of a pulmonary embolus, if they occur, include an area of oligemia (Westermark's sign), a pleural-based area of consolidation with a characteristic convexity toward the hilum (Hampton's hump), and enlargement of a main pulmonary artery. Moreover, when actual pulmonary infarction occurs, there is often elevation of the hemidiaphragm with a small pleural effusion and a discrete area of opacification.

Radionuclide ventilation-perfusion studies are the investigation of choice and will demonstrate most pulmonary infarcts (Figs 8–60B and 8–60C). It is imperative, however, to perform a radionuclide study in conjunction with a chest radiograph in order to eliminate the possibility of other causes of a filling defect such as pleural effusion, pneumonia, or tumor. If the chest x-ray does show a cause for the filling defect seen on the scan, the radiologist must look for other defects on the scan that have no corresponding radiographic abnormality in order to confirm the diagnosis of pulmonary embolus. If this is not done, an angiogram must be performed; moreover, angiography may be valuable in determining the exact position of the clot or clots if surgical removal of the thrombus is contemplated (Fig. 8–60D). Diagnosis of pulmonary emboli on angiography includes finding filling defects or cut-offs of major arteries and "pruning" of smaller vessels in association with poor arterial filling and late venous return. Venography is useful to demonstrate thrombi in leg veins and extension of the thrombus into the inferior vena cava.

Pulmonary emboli may result from a number of conditions. The most common cause is thrombophlebitis in the legs, which occurs particularly in patients who are confined to bed after surgery. Emboli may also be associated with infection, and staphylococcal emboli may cavitate. They occur in drug addicts who inject major veins with dirty needles and in patients with chronic renal failure who are on dialysis and whose arteriovenous shunts have become infected.

Case C25

Persephone Mansi, age 25, was a tightrope walker in a traveling circus visiting town. She was performing one afternoon when she developed increasing dyspnea and a constricting feeling across her chest. She finally felt so ill that she ended her act early and dropped into the safety net. Examination by the circus doctor revealed rales and rhonchi and pericardial friction rub, and she was coughing up yellowish sputum. A chest x-ray was taken at the local hospital (Fig. 8–61). What does it show?

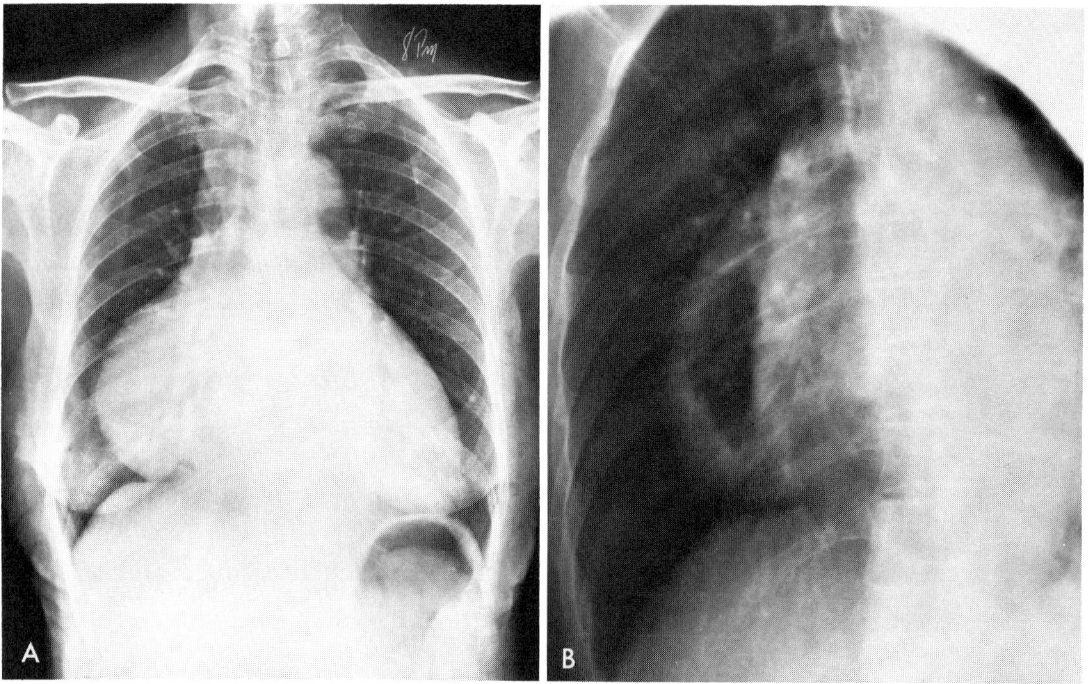

Figure 8–61. Pericardial effusion, PA view (*A*) and lateral decubitus view (*B*). There is massive cardiomegaly without specific chamber enlargement or evidence of pulmonary congestion. Carbon dioxide introduced into the venous system collects along the lateral margin of the right atrium and demonstrates the presence of a pericardial effusion; it can be seen as a vertical air-fluid level in this picture.

The diagnosis of pericardial effusion on the basis of plain film findings alone is difficult, and even fluoroscopy demonstrates only decreased ventricular pulsations. On a lateral view, separation of the anterior epicardial fat line can be seen in about 40 per cent of patients with pericardial effusions larger than 200 ml. One method of detecting an effusion involves instilling carbon dioxide into the venous system as the patient lies on his left side so that the gas is carried into the right atrium; the gas acts as a contrast agent on an x-ray, defining the distance between the endocardium and the outside of the pericardium (Fig. 8–61B). Radionuclide angiography is often used to define an effusion, which appears as a zone of decreased radioactivity around the blood pool within the heart chamber, separating it from the blood pool in the lungs. Ultrasonography has largely replaced these radiographic methods of diagnosing pericardial effusions (Fig. 8–62). Definitive diagnosis, however, can usually be made on the basis of electrocardiography (an effusion causes characteristic changes such as loss of Q waves, elevation of ST waves, and notching or inversion of T waves) and the patient's clinical history.

There are many causes of pericarditis and pericardial effusion. They include: inflammatory causes such as viral and bacterial infections as well as myocardial infarction, trauma, connective tissue disorders, allergic and metabolic disorders, and direct neoplastic involvement by lymphoma, leukemia, or metastatic disease.

Complications of acute pericarditis include chronic pericarditis (adhesive or constrictive) and cardiac tamponade: diminished lung markings and an increase in heart size.

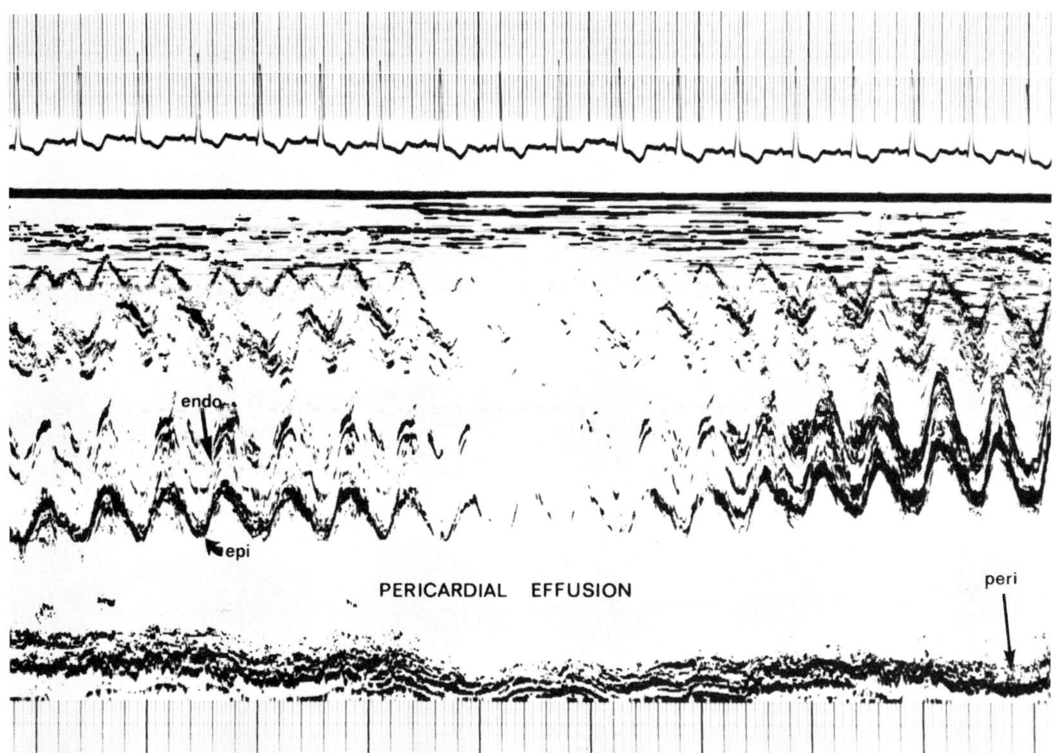

Figure 8–62. Ultrasonogram of a pericardial effusion. This is a time-motion study of the heart demonstrating a large pericardial effusion. The reflecting interfaces of the heart can be seen, including the endocardium (endo), epicardium (epi), and pericardium (peri). The anechoic area represents a pericardial effusion.

Case C26

Virginia Slim, age 68, was a heavy smoker with a chronic cough who was admitted to the hospital with a fever. When questioned, she revealed that she had lost weight recently and was occasionally coughing bloody sputum. On examination, she was noted to be cachectic, and rales were heard at the right apex. A chest x-ray was taken (Fig. 8–63). What does it show?

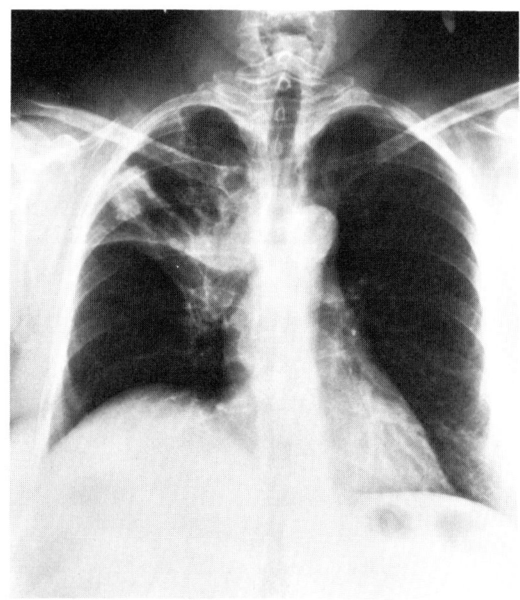

Figure 8–63. Bronchogenic carcinoma. On the PA view, there is a large central mass distorting the upper right hilum with a peripheral opacity that proved to be a pneumonia. Note the loss of volume in the right upper lobe and elevation of the right hemidiaphragm.

A neoplasm of the lung may present as an asymptomatic mass seen on a routine chest x-ray and may be associated with hemoptysis, dyspnea, lethargy, fatigue, loss of weight, or pain, which may be caused by pleural involvement, metastatic spread, or hypertrophic pulmonary osteoarthropathy (which is discussed elsewhere).

The bronchogenic carcinoma seen on Ms. Slim's chest x-ray is a central lesion adjacent to the right hilum. The peripheral opacity represents an area of pneumonic consolidation secondary to partial bronchial obstruction caused by the tumor, not an infrequent occurrence. Tomograms may be used to demonstrate the characteristic radiological findings: narrowing and irregularity of the bronchus (Fig. 8–64). The diagnosis can be confirmed by fiberoptic bronchoscopy.

Bronchogenic carcinoma may be peripheral or central (Fig. 8–65), small or large, and it may be associated with hilar and mediastinal lymphadenopathy. The lesion may often have secondary manifestations such as peripheral pneumonia, atelectasis, lung abscess, unresolving pneumonia, or even obstructive emphysema. Occasionally, necrosis occurs within the tumor itself, producing an irregular thick-walled cavity. The presenting features of bronchogenic carcinoma may sometimes be pain in the arm, Horner's syndrome, and involvement of the apex of the lung; this combination of findings is known as a Pancoast tumor (Fig. 8–66).

Secondary spread of a lung tumor may

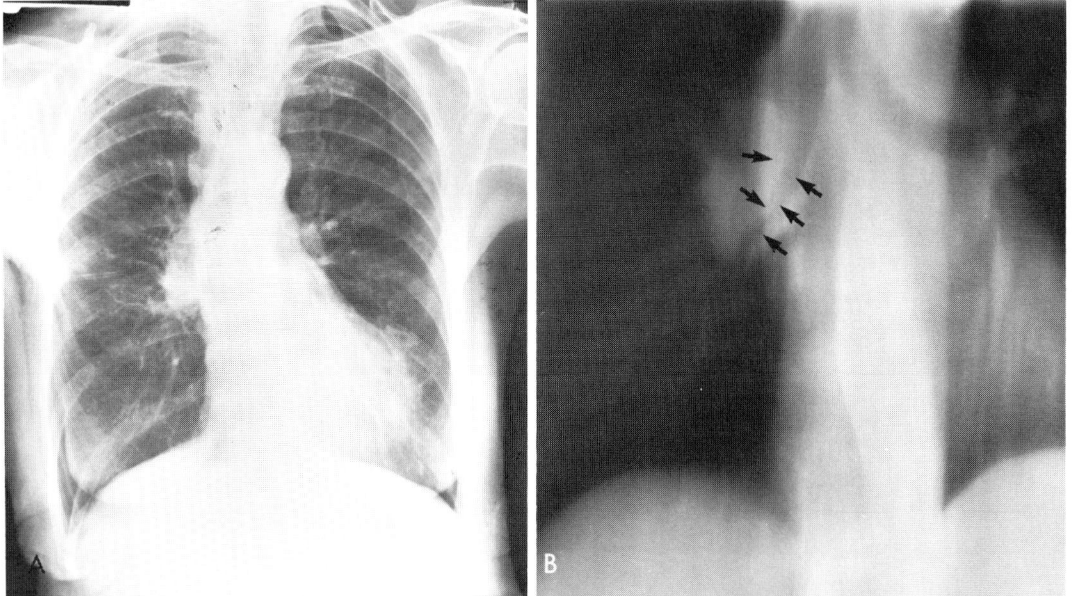

Figure 8–64. Bronchogenic carcinoma. PA view (*A*) and tomogram (*B*). Although the right hilar mass can be seen on the plain film, the narrowing and irregularity of the lower lobe bronchus is well shown on the tomogram (*arrows*).

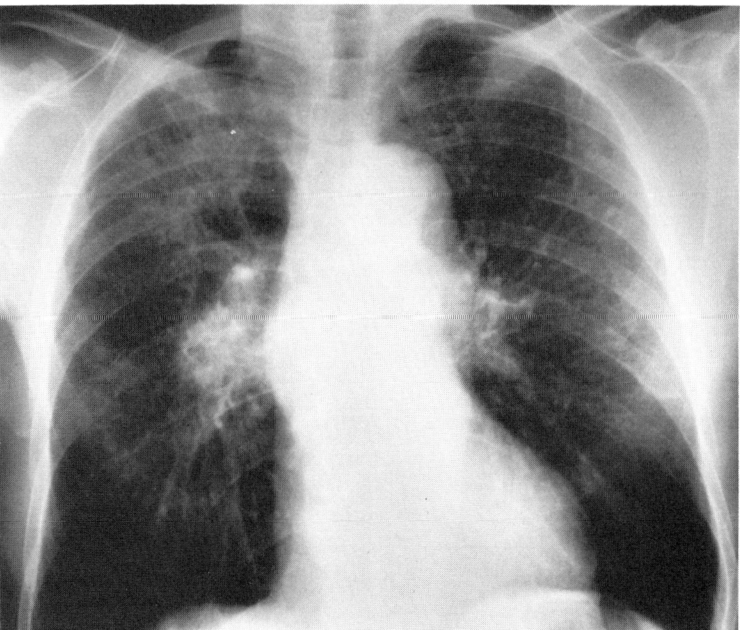

Figure 8–65. Bronchogenic carcinoma. This 72-year-old man had been a heavy smoker and presented with a chronic cough and some recent hemoptysis. There is a mass adjacent to the right hilum that proved on brush biopsy to be a bronchogenic carcinoma. The increase in peripheral lung markings at the right apex represents a pneumonitis secondary to almost total obstruction of the right upper lobe bronchus. There is also evidence of chronic lung disease.

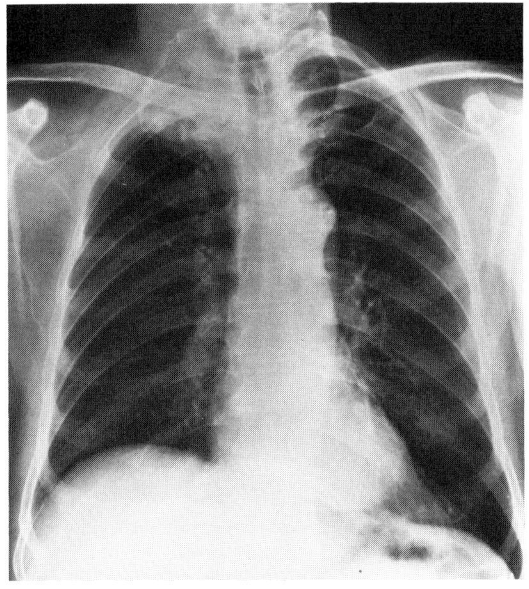

Figure 8–66. Pancoast tumor. This PA film shows a soft-tissue mass at the right apex with destruction of the upper ribs. There is a suggestion of an enlarged node at the right hilum. On percutaneous biopsy, this proved to be an epidermoid carcinoma.

involve the adjacent lung, mediastinum, pericardium, and even the heart, and may directly invade the ribs and sternum. Secondary metastatic spread to the distant skeleton and to the liver is also very common.

The cell type found in malignant lung tumors varies from small round cell carcinoma to squamous cell, adenocarcinoma and non-differentiated tumors. Approximately 5 per cent of primary lung malignancies are alveolar cell carcinomas, which have two characteristic patterns: An ill-defined peripheral opacity with indistinct margins is sometimes seen. A diffuse nodular form with multiple irregular pulmonary infiltrates also occurs (Fig. 8–67); this form is often rapidly progressive with complications such as pleural effusions and lymphangitic spread. The differential diagnosis of this radiographic picture includes sarcoidosis, metastatic lesions, tuberculosis, and chronic granulomatous disease.

Metastases to the lung from distant sources are extremely common (Fig. 8–68). They may spread via the lymphatics or blood stream or directly from an adjacent

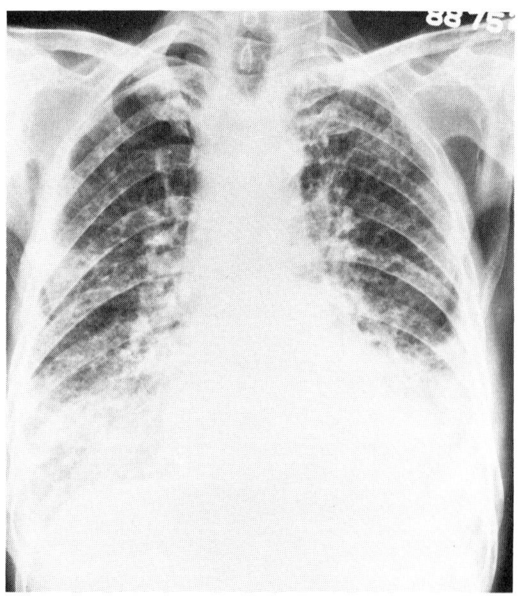

Figure 8–67. Alveolar cell carcinoma. This patchy diffuse increase in lung markings with ill-defined patchy opacities is typical of alveolar cell carcinoma with lymphangitic spread.

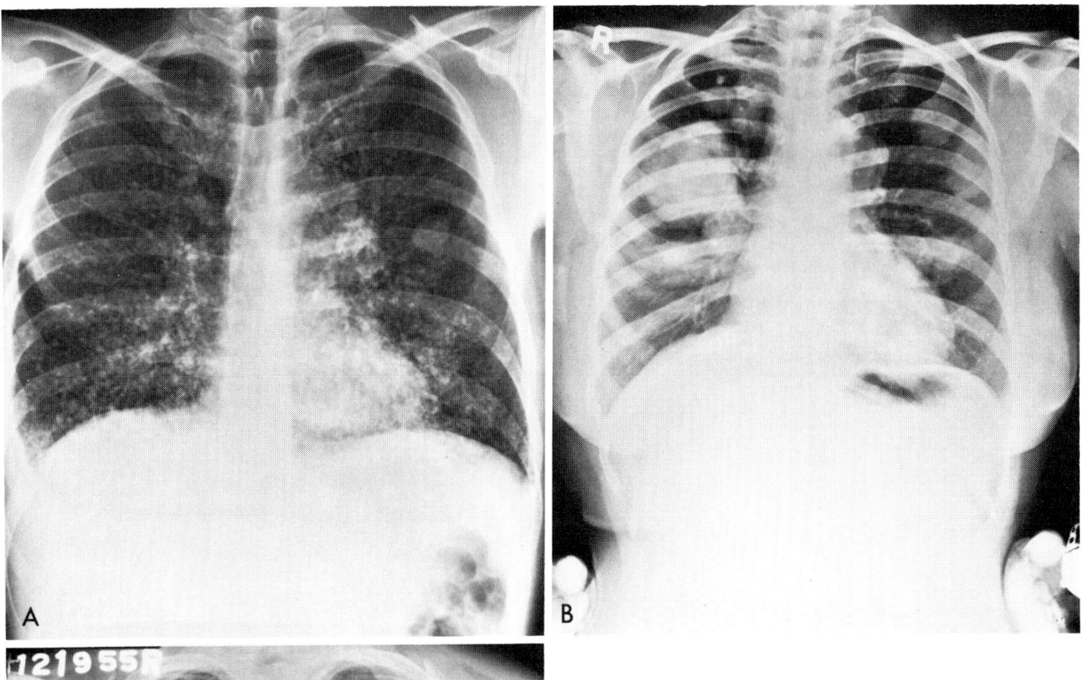

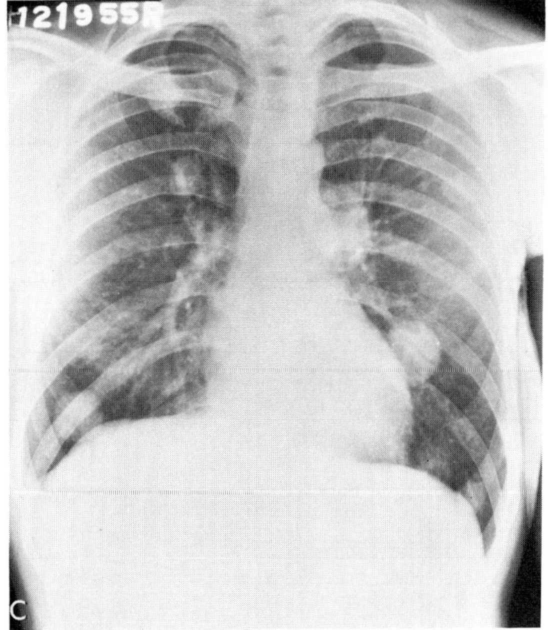

Figure 8–68. Pulmonary metastases from various primary sites. *A*, Malignant melanoma. An overall reticulonodular pattern is visible, although there is one well-circumscribed mass in the left midzone. The patient had had a malignant melanoma removed from his chest wall 18 months previously. *B*, Melanosarcoma from the choroid. There are a number of "cannonball" metastases throughout the lung fields in this 60-year-old female patient. *C*, Fibrosarcoma. This 30-year-old male had had a fibrosarcoma of the left shoulder removed six months previously. The chest x-ray shows multiple pulmonary nodules.

organ (breast, esophagus, stomach). The genitourinary system is characteristically responsible for "cannonball" metastases — multiple, sharply demarginated, rounded densities of appreciable and varying sizes from that of a golfball to a grapefruit. Cannonball metastases are often caused by hypernephroma in middle-aged people, by testicular tumor in young males, and by cervical or uterine tumor in older women. Metastases from osteogenic sarcoma may ossify or cavitate. Miliary metastases from thyroid carcinoma, which usually occurs in adolescents or young adults, may rarely light up on a thyroid scan. Kerley A and B lines and interstitial blurring are radiographic signs of lymphangitic spread, which is usually associated with enlarged hilar lymph nodes and is most frequently seen with tumors of the lung, breast, stomach, and pancreas. Finally, increased incidence of primary pulmonary malignancy is associated with ex-

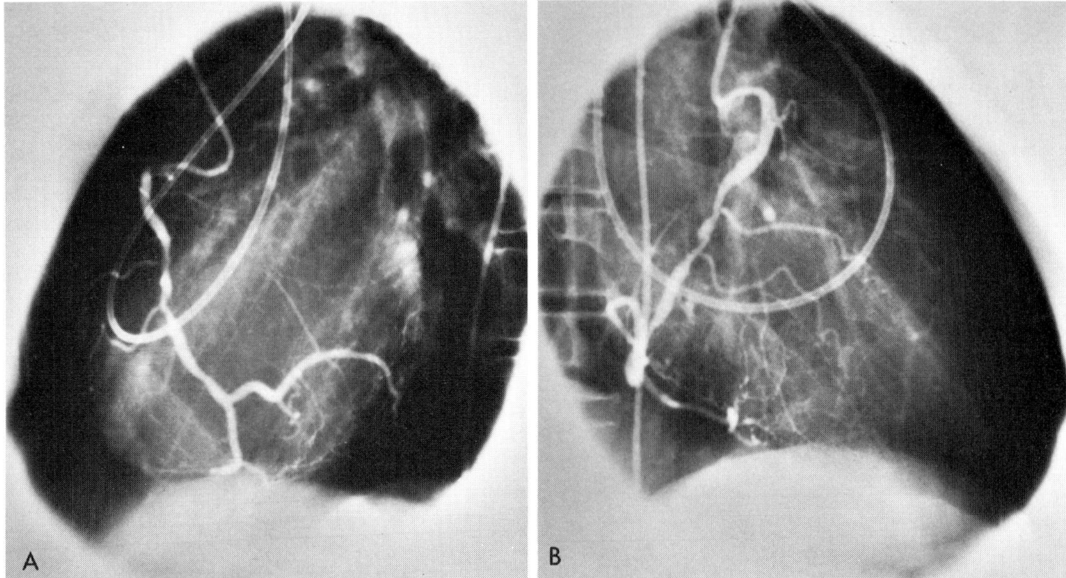

Figure 8–69. Coronary arteriography, LAO view (*A*) and RAO view (*B*). The left coronary artery was almost totally occluded at its origin and cannot be seen here. The right coronary artery shows considerable irregularity and stenosis; it is the dominant vessel supplying the base of the heart.

posure to inorganic dusts, particularly asbestos.

CHEST PAIN

Perhaps one of the most common situations in clinical medicine is that of a middle-aged man complaining of chest pain that becomes particularly noticeable on exertion. *Angina pectoris* is caused by inadequate oxygenation of the heart and is often relieved by rest or sublingual administration of nitroglycerin. Angina produces a pain that is often substernal but may radiate to the mandible or the left arm and shoulder. On examination, the patient usually has elevated blood pressure, tachycardia, and a fourth heart sound. Frequently, the EKG taken with the patient at rest is completely normal, and the only evidence of cardiac ischemia is detected following exercise. The chest x-ray is characteristically normal.

If coronary angiography is performed, however, atherosclerosis of the main coronary arteries and their branches is demonstrated in the majority of the patients with angina (Fig. 8–69). Coronary angiography should be performed with great care in any patient with angina pectoris because of the risk of precipitating acute myocardial infarction or producing arrhythmias and ventricular fibrillation.

Case C27

Horatio Clapworthy, age 38, is a senior executive of a large "publishing" firm famous for its pornography. He began to experience intense precordial chest pain while racing from his office to one of his "specialist" movie theaters. The pain radiated to his chin and down his left arm. Mr. Clapworthy described it as "crushing." When he was admitted to the emergency room, the pain had persisted for 45 minutes and he was sweating, appeared ill and restless, and was severely hypotensive. An EKG showed elevated ST segments (Fig. 8–70). On his way up to the ward, an admission chest x-ray was performed; it was normal.

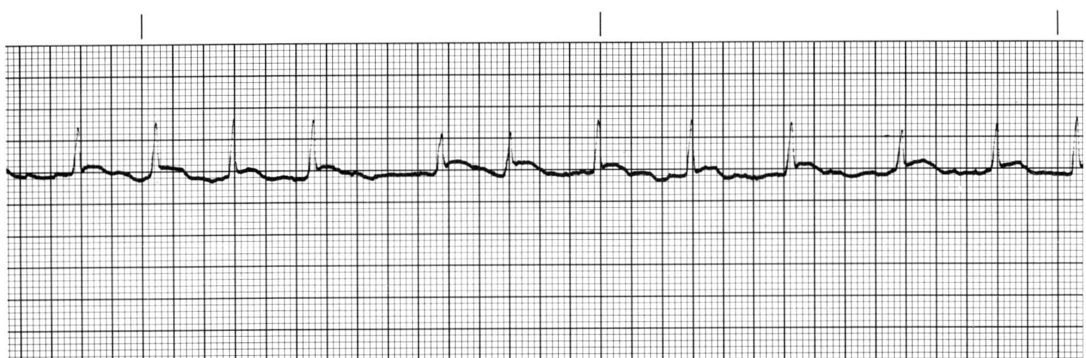

Figure 8–70. Acute myocardial infarction. This EKG shows S-T elevation with T wave inversion and atrial fibrillation. The patient, a 38-year-old man, had an acute myocardial infarct.

The clinical complications of an acute myocardial infarction such as sudden death and various arrhythmias will not be discussed because they have few if any radiological manifestations. A number of complications do concern the radiologist, however. Some two thirds of patients who have acute myocardial infarction develop acute congestive heart failure. This CHF may be the initial manifestation, in which case the patient will present with dyspnea and pain. Radiological diagnosis of congestive heart failure is discussed earlier in this chapter. Since it is such an important subject, however, a further radiographic example is given. A 45-year-old woman with a long history of angina pectoris and coronary artery insufficiency had a myocardial infarction and rapidly developed acute pulmonary edema (Fig. 8–71). The development of pulmonary edema following an infarct can be caused by a number of conditions, in-

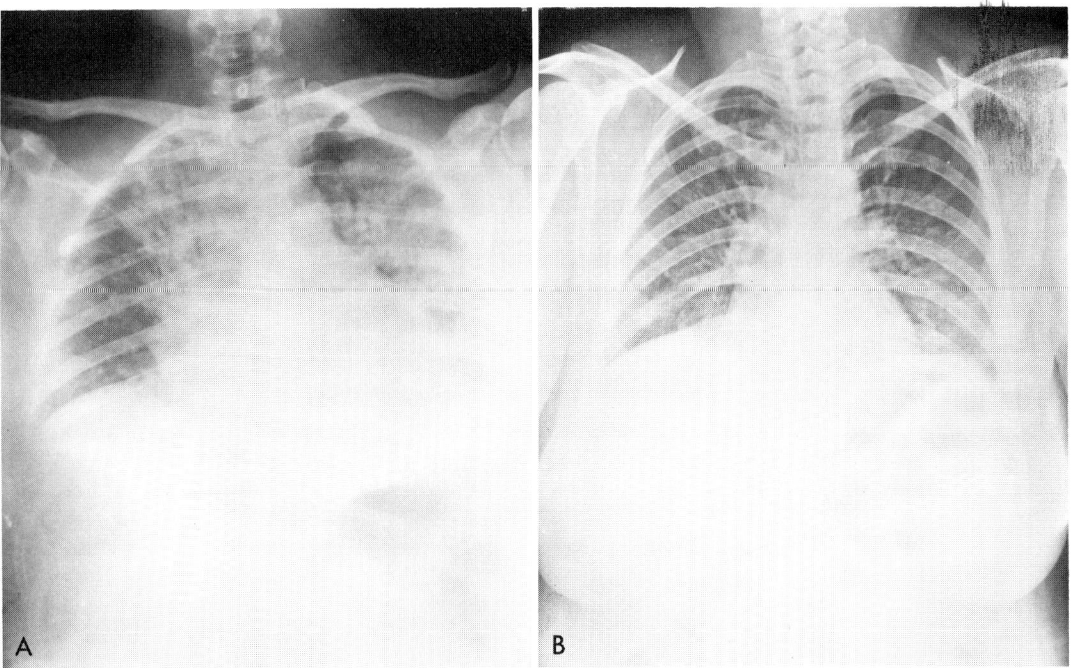

Figure 8–71. Pulmonary edema, caused by an acute myocardial infarct, with clearing. This 45-year-old female patient suffered an acute myocardial infarct and was admitted with severe dyspnea and chest pain. *A*, The initial AP film shows widespread pulmonary edema, which cleared rapidly following digitalization and diuresis. *B*, Film taken one week later.

cluding failure of the ventricular muscle to contract properly, various arrhythmias, and rupture of the papillary muscles, which causes acute mitral insufficiency. Older patients often develop chronic congestive heart failure and then have recurrent episodes of pulmonary edema with the least provocation; this situation is often complicated by chronic pleural effusions.

Case C28

Cornelius Cornpopper, age 78, was a debilitated man well known to the emergency room staff because of malnutrition and frequent bouts of congestive heart failure. The last time he was admitted to the hospital percussion and auscultation of his chest revealed widespread rales and dullness at both bases. A chest x-ray was taken which confirmed the clinical diagnosis of bilateral effusions and pulmonary edema, although comparison with a radiograph of this patient taken one year earlier showed there had been no change (Fig. 8–72A). A new young house officer took a liking to Mr. Cornpopper and decided to treat him rather more enthusiastically than predecessors had. Bilateral thoracenteses were performed that removed 600 ml of fluid from the left chest and 1500 ml from the right. Another chest x-ray was taken to look for a pneumothorax, and the astute intern wondered if the effusion at the right base was obscuring a pathological process (Fig. 8–72B). What would you do now?

A decubitus film was taken, and although some fluid remains at the right base, there appears to be an underlying pathological process in the right lower lobe (Fig. 8–72C). Often, a decubitus view with the patient lying on the opposite side is most helpful, because the fluid will run into the paraspinal gutters, clearing the costophrenic angle on the side where a tumor or lesion is suspected. Another pleural tap was performed on Mr. Cornpopper, and the fluid was sent for cytologic examination. After a few days, the patient was well enough to be taken to the radiology department for tomographic study, which revealed a mass in the right lower lobe that encroached upon and narrowed one of the major bronchi (Fig. 8–72D). On the following day, the diagnosis of bronchogenic carcinoma was confirmed by percutaneous lung biopsy under fluoroscopic guidance.

It is not uncommon for an elderly patient to have more than one lesion at the same time, and effusions often effectively mask underlying pulmonary pathological processes. Judicious use of decubitus views and tomography may reveal other conditions, including metastases, lung abscesses, chronic atelectasis, and collapse of a segment or lobe.

A further but later complication of acute myocardial infarction that is radiologically interesting is the development of a left ventricular aneurysm. Following myocardial infarction, routine chest radiographs are taken for most patients at stated intervals (at discharge from hospital, and then at one, three, six and twelve months later, and then yearly). The first radiographic clue to the presence of a left ventricular aneurysm is bulging and squaring off of the left cardiac border (Fig. 8–73). If this were a radiograph of your patient, what would you do now?

Fluoroscopy is the procedure of choice. If a left ventricular aneurysm has occurred, the area of ventricular wall involved shows either paradoxical contraction or no evidence of contraction, and it will fail to propel a normal cardiac impulse to the apex of the heart. This paradoxical or limited pulsation is best documented using cineradiography. Calcification may also occur, either within the ventricular wall itself or in the underlying thrombus in the ventricular cavity (Fig. 8–74). Should surgical intervention be considered, coronary arteriography in association with angiocardiography is performed to demonstrate the state of the coronary blood supply as well as to delineate the area involved.

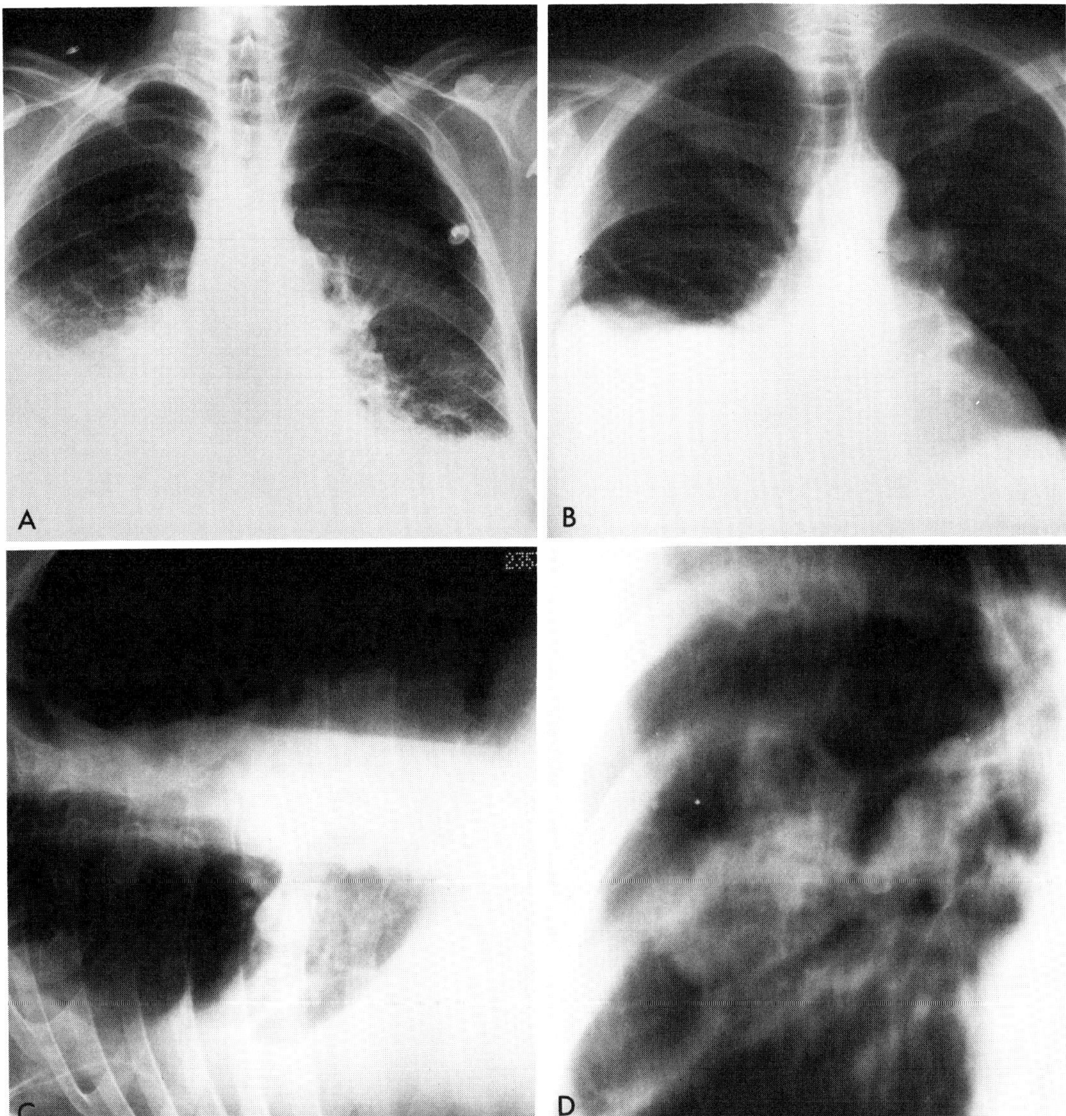

Figure 8–72. Longstanding pulmonary effusions and chronic congestive failure. *A*, The initial AP film shows redistribution, pulmonary edema, and bilateral effusions with the effusion on the right being the larger. *B*, This AP film taken one year later shows progressive cardiac enlargement but clearing of the left pleural effusion. The effusion on the right appears to be subpulmonary and *C*, a right decubitus view, also taken one year later, shows that the fluid layers out. However, a mass has become apparent at the right base. *D*, Tomography at a later date shows an ill-defined mass with narrowing, irregularity, and obstruction of the right main stem bronchus. On biopsy, this was found to be a bronchogenic carcinoma.

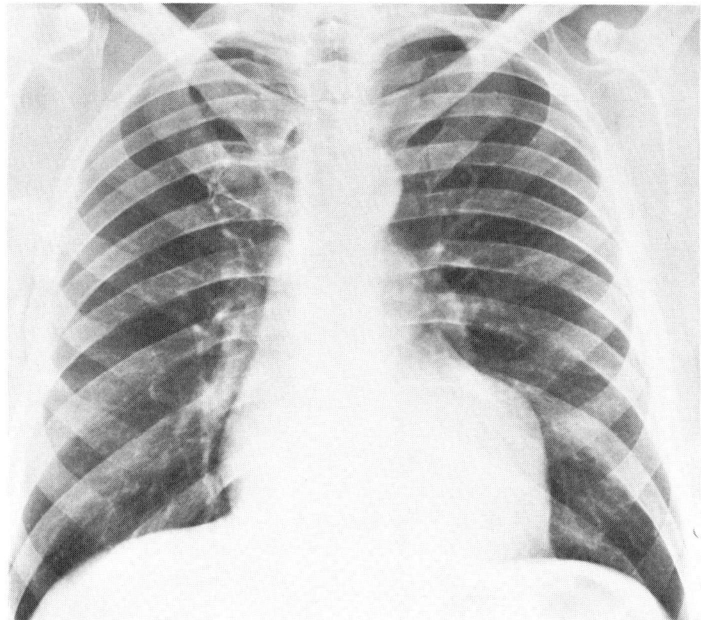

Figure 8–73. Left ventricular aneurysm. This 44-year-old male patient had suffered a myocardial infarction ten months previously. The chest radiograph is normal, apart from squaring of the left heart border, which is characteristic of a left ventricular aneurysm.

For many patients who have had one myocardial infarction, revascularization procedures or coronary artery by-pass operations will be considered. It is necessary to delineate the area of ischemia as well as to ascertain which vessels are either totally or partially occluded. Although coronary arteriography has traditionally been used to delineate the area of infarction, radioisotope studies of the myocardium have been shown to have lower morbidity and mortality rates (Fig. 8–75). A further advantage of radioisotope studies is that they can be performed at any stage of the infarction process, from admission to the hospital through evolution of the infarct, so revascularization can be easily observed. A high correlation has been found between the evidence shown on the scan and the actual size of the infarct at autopsy; it seems likely that radioisotope imaging of the cardiac infarct will be the procedure of choice in the future for following a myocardial infarction.

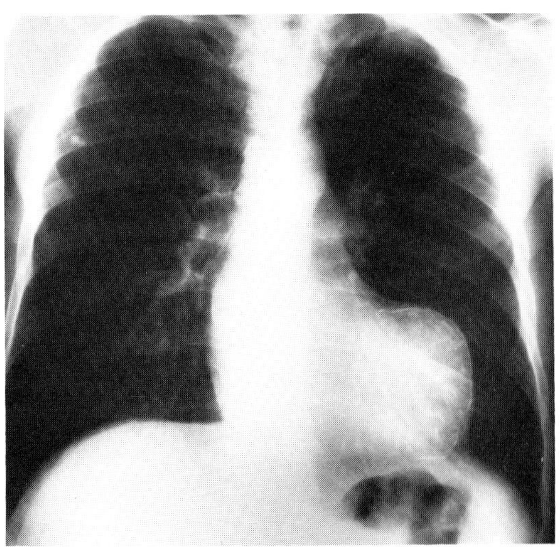

Figure 8–74. Calcification in the left ventricular wall. There is massive left ventricular wall calcification in this 52-year-old patient who had suffered a myocardial infarct three years previously. The calcification was found on a routine follow-up film.

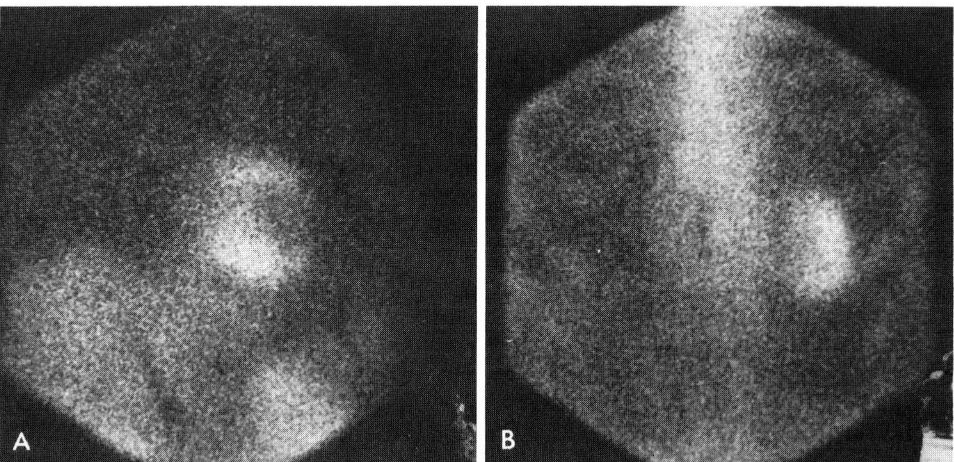

Figure 8–75. Isotope cardiac imaging. This 54-year-old woman had severe chest pain 48 hours before these studies were performed. *A*, A thallium-201 scan shows a defect in the region of the left ventricle of the heart. *B*, On a subsequent ^{99m}Tc-pyrophosphate study, the myocardial infarct shows up readily and fits like a piece of a jigsaw puzzle into the defect seen on the thallium scan. Images of the ribs can be seen, produced by this predominantly bone-seeking radioisotope.

Case C29

S. Meli Grunge, age 68, was a retired income tax inspector with a long history of hypertension. One day while running for the senior citizens' picnic bus, he experienced severe central chest pain and

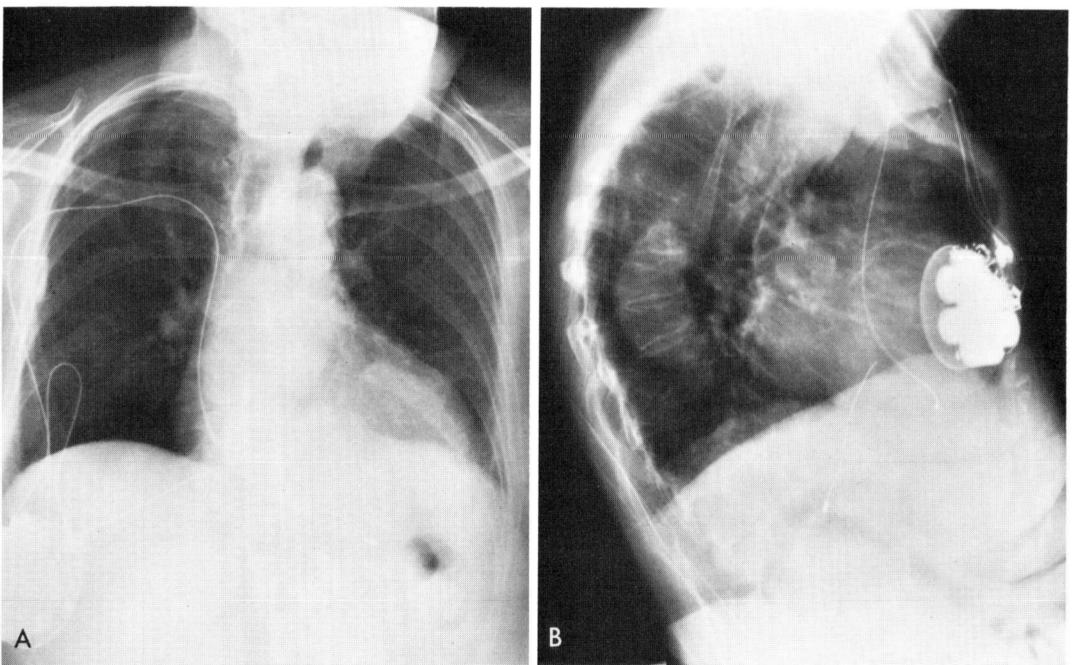

Figure 8–76. Hypertension, PA view (*A*) and lateral view (*B*). The left ventricle is enlarged, with dilatation and unfolding of the aorta. Note the pacemaker. There is a broken wire apparently in the liver. How did it get there?

Case C29 (Continued)

had an acute desire to move his bowels. He was rushed to the local hospital, where his blood pressure was found to be elevated. An EKG was normal. There were no other physical signs. A recent routine chest x-ray was obtained from Mr. Grunge's physician, which showed the classic radiographic signs of hypertension (Fig. 8–76). A supine chest x-ray was taken at the patient's bedside using a portable x-ray machine. Comparison with the previous film demonstrated widening of the aortic arch.

Dissecting aortic aneurysm can produce severe pain without noticeable dyspnea. The dissection occurs when blood bursts through the intima of the aorta and dissects down the media because of some weakness inherent in the vessel wall itself. Medial cystic necrosis may occur in Marfan's syndrome but is more commonly associated with atherosclerosis and hypertension.

Often, there are no previous films available for comparison. Since people with this condition are gravely ill, it is frequently possible to take only a supine film. Definitive diagnosis of dissecting aortic aneurysm is difficult to make on the basis of a single AP film, because this view causes the heart and great vessels to appear magnified. Should the patient survive, progressive enlargement of the aorta is the only radiographic sign of dissection apparent in the first few weeks. The patient, however, frequently develops clinical signs suggestive of dissecting aortic aneurysm, including unequal or absent pulsations in the arms and legs and, if the aortic root is involved, aortic regurgitation. Thus, the progress of the dissection can be followed clinically, although radiographically the diagnosis is difficult to make until better films can be taken in the radiology department (Figs. 8–77A and 8–77B). Ultimately, an aortogram is performed; this may demonstrate the extent of the dissection and is particularly useful to locate the re-entry point of the dissection in relation to major arteries such as the renal vessels (Fig. 8–77C and 8–77D). The prognosis of a patient with a dissecting aortic aneurysm is very grave, and many patients die within the first few days. In those patients who survive the initial insult, it is occasionally possible to reanastomose the false lumen to the true one.

Many aortic aneurysms are asymptomatic and in fact may first be detected on a routine chest radiograph (Fig. 8–78). Fusiform and saccular aneurysms of the aorta are associated with atherosclerosis, and the incidence of this type at autopsy is 2 per cent of the population. Some of these aneurysms are associated with calcification either in the aortic wall itself or in an underlying thrombus. The classic cause of a calcified aortic aneurysm, particularly in the ascending aorta, is syphilis; this type of aneurysm may grow so large as to erode the under surface of the sternum and ribs (Fig. 8–79).

Two other clinical radiological situations are worthy of note: In a number of elderly people, the descending aorta unfolds to such a degree that it kinks upon itself, possibly owing to the remnants of the fibrous ligamentum arteriosum. On the PA view this condition appears as an aortic dilatation. It is known as *pseudocoarctation* and has no significance. A second type of aortic aneurysm, which is rare but important, is the traumatic aneurysm caused by rapid deceleration of the aorta as occurs in a motor vehicle accident. The aorta is torn just beyond the origin of the left subclavian artery, where it is anchored down firmly. The diagnosis is usually obvious both clinically and radiologically. The patient can be saved by immediate surgical intervention.

OTHER CONDITIONS CAUSING CHEST SYMPTOMS

Most of the common causes of chest disease have been discussed in this chapter. There are conditions we have not covered that should at least be mentioned briefly. Not every cause of chest symptomatology lies within the thorax, and some brain tumors will actually cause dyspnea. Also, signs or symptoms appertaining to the respiratory tract are an integral part of many systemic diseases.

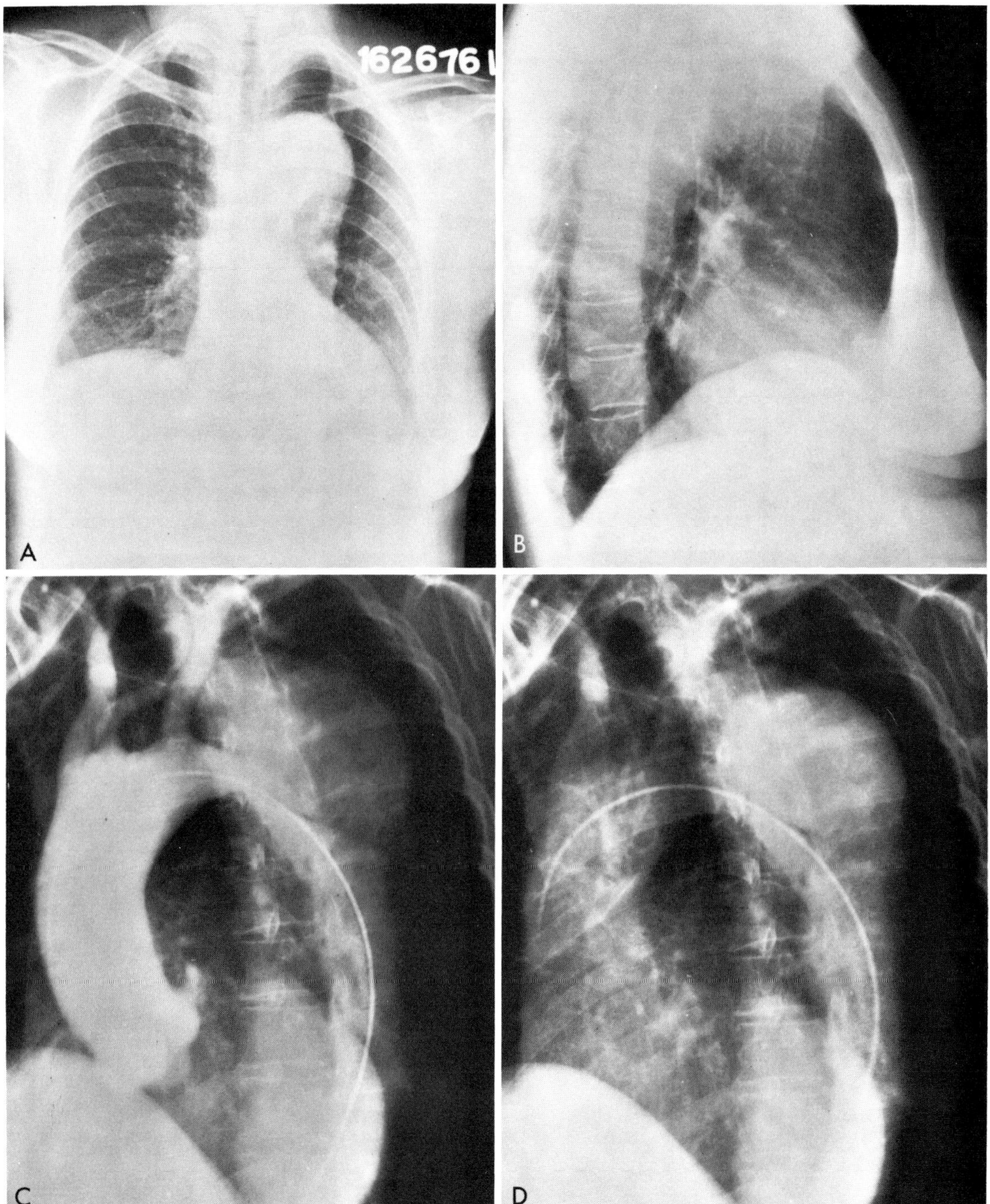

Figure 8–77. Dissecting aneurysm of the aortic arch. *A* and *B*, The PA and lateral chest films show marked widening of the aorta from the aortic arch down into the descending aorta. *C*, An oblique film taken early in aortography reveals a large saccular aneurysm lying distal to the left subclavian artery and compressing the aortic lumen. *D*, A delayed aortogram shows the aneurysm filled with contrast and apparently reentering the thoracic aorta in the region of T10.

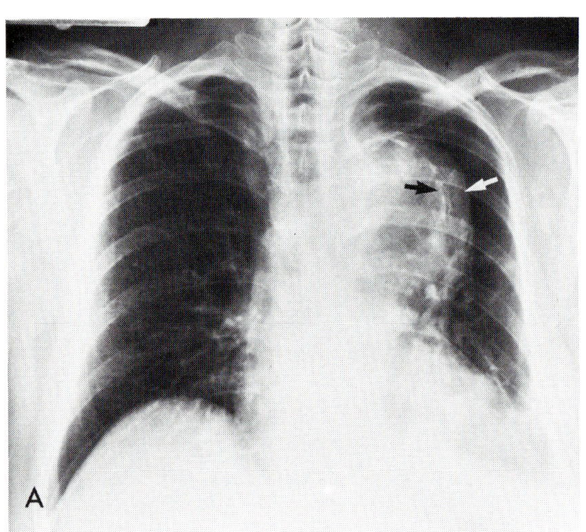

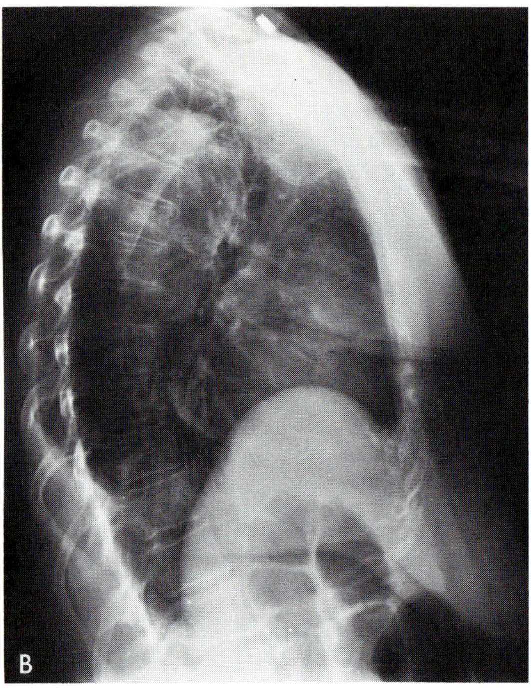

Figure 8–78. Saccular aneurysm of aortic arch, PA view (*A*) and lateral view (*B*). This 65-year-old female patient had had two recent episodes of chest pain and had a long history of hypertension. A large saccular aneurysm of the proximal descending aorta is seen in association with a left pleural effusion. Some atherosclerotic calcification is visible within the aneurysm. The space between this calcification and the outer wall (*arrows*) suggested a dissecting aneurysm, but this was not confirmed at angiography.

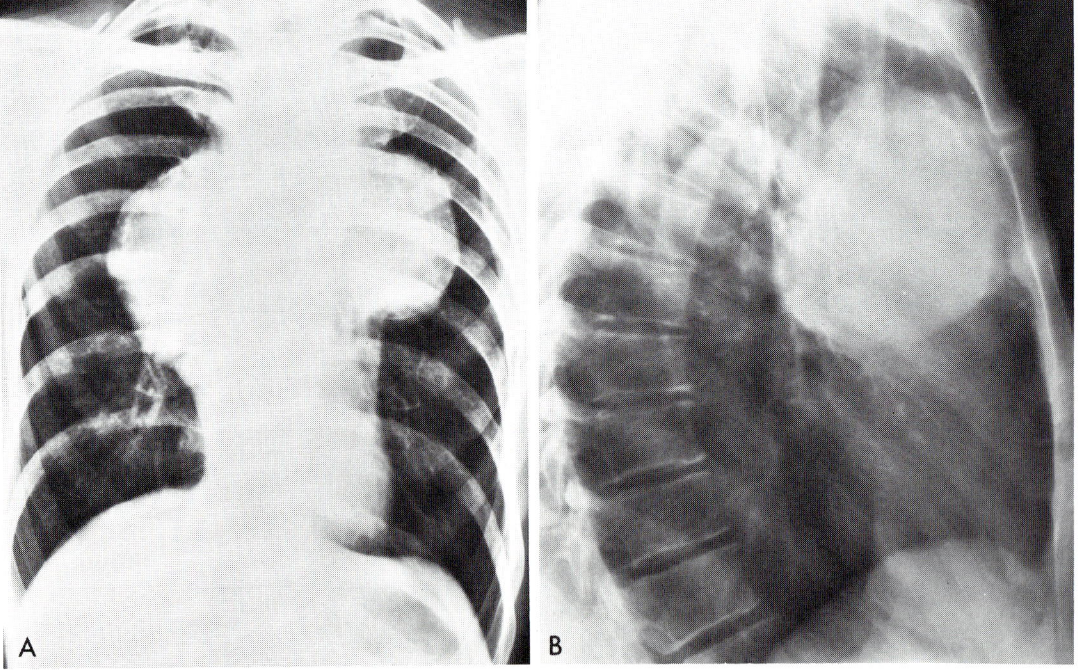

Figure 8–79. Syphilitic aneurysm of ascending aorta. This 40-year-old man had a history of lues, which was treated with arsenicals before the advent of penicillin in 1925. The huge aneurysm grew in size between 1931 and 1938. Note the calcification in its wall, a typical finding in old, burnt-out syphilitic aortitis.

Case C30

Lucretia Mellanzani, age 36, came to the hospital complaining of weight loss, pyrexia, arthralgias, and a butterfly rash on her face. On examination she was found to be dyspneic and anemic. Results of a lupus erythematosus cell test and an antinuclear antibody test were "positive." A chest radiograph was taken (Fig. 8–80A). What does it show?

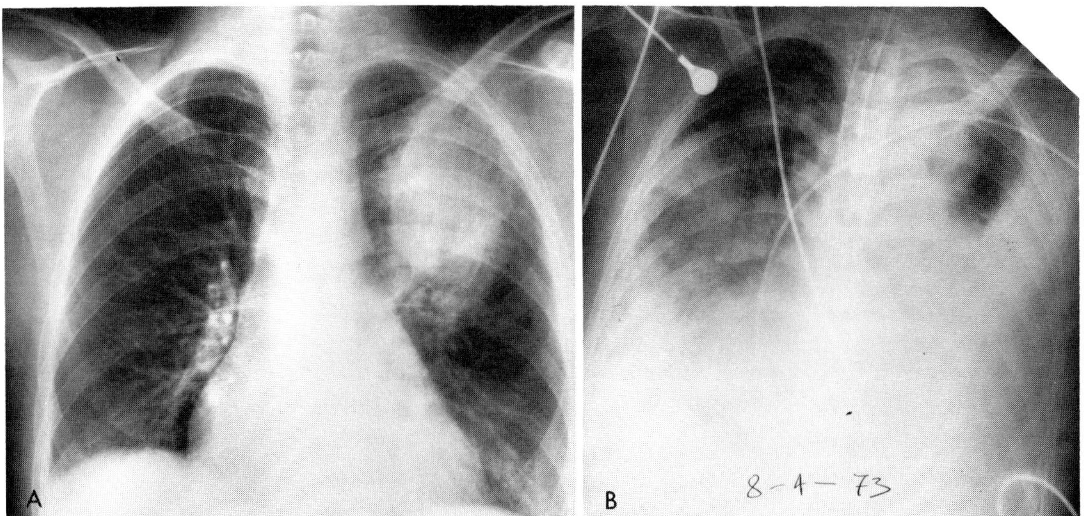

Figure 8–80. Systemic lupus erythematosus. This 36-year-old woman presented with dyspnea. *A*, The initial PA chest radiograph showed a left upper lobe pneumonia with small bilateral effusions. The patient became very ill. *B*, In an AP film taken ten days later, note the bilateral effusions, pulmonary edema, and widespread opacification of both lung fields. The patient succumbed on the twelfth day to an overwhelming infection and pulmonary congestion.

Pleural effusions occur in about half of patients with systemic lupus erythematosus (SLE), which is also frequently associated with atelectasis, hilar adenopathy, pleuritis, or characteristic fluffy infiltrates (Fig. 8–80B). Pericarditis with or without pericardial effusions is also common. Since this is a systemic disorder, patients with systemic lupus erythematosus may develop the nephrotic syndrome and hepatosplenomegaly. About 90 per cent of patients with SLE develop arthralgias, and a few develop rheumatoid arthritis. The majority of these side effects respond to steroids to a variable extent, although the disease is often ultimately fatal.

Many of the connective tissue disorders also give rise to chest symptoms, although pulmonary involvement in pure periarteritis nodosa is rare. Other systemic illnesses may produce dyspnea, such as ankylosing spondylitis (because of the fusion of the costovertebral joints) as well as leukemia and lymphoma (because of disseminated infiltration of the pulmonary parenchyma). One other rare cause of dyspnea is of interest, although it will be discussed more fully in Chapter 9. Occasionally, in a patient with a perforated duodenal ulcer with free intraperitoneal gas and stomach contents, the diaphragms become irritated, and the patient may actually present with "difficulty in breathing." This is an interesting counterpart to a patient with lower lobe pneumonia who presents with abdominal pain. Patients with renal failure may present with many of the conditions we have outlined above; in fact, they usually have a combination of symptoms, such as pericardial and pleural effusions or pneumonia and congestive heart failure. Some viral illnesses are also associated with pneumonitis if not frank pneumonia, and with pleurisy, pericarditis, and even cardiomyopathy.

CHAPTER 9

THE ABDOMEN

It is as difficult to subdivide diseases of the abdomen into related groups as it was diseases of the chest. Any subdivision is complicated by the fact that there are two separate anatomical systems, the gastrointestinal tract and the genitourinary tract, in the abdomen as well as the retroperitoneal structures. The disorders discussed here are therefore artificially divided according to symptom groups: pain, change of bowel habit, gastrointestinal bleeding, hematuria, and various combinations of symptoms.

ABDOMINAL PAIN

Many causes of abdominal pain have no other signs or symptoms. In this section we will deal principally with conditions that can be diagnosed from a plain film of the abdomen or from simple contrast studies, although there are some exceptions. There are also a number of "silent" abdominal conditions that may occasionally cause pain.

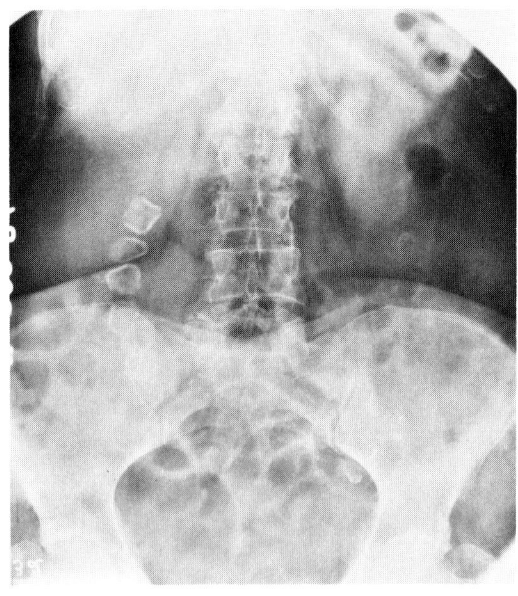

Figure 9–1. Gallstones. On the KUB film, there are a number of facetted gallstones to the right of the midline.

Case A1

Deciduous Klutz, age 40, was fair and fat, having spent her life working on a dairy farm eating the products of her labors. She presented with pain in the right upper quadrant, which on examination was tender. A KUB was taken and revealed multiple gallstones (Fig. 9–1). What would you do now?

The answer to this question is somewhat controversial. Most surgeons would say there is enough evidence on this film to indicate a cholecystectomy without further radiological procedures. Occasionally, however, an oral cholecystogram may be performed to observe gallbladder function, particularly by using a fatty meal. Only about 15 per cent of gallstones are radiopaque. In the patient with right upper quadrant pain and a normal KUB, an oral cholecystogram must be performed to exclude the possibility of radiolucent gallstones, which account for the remaining 85 per cent.

Case A2

Hermione Longcure, aged 97, was diabetic and had had recurrent attacks of acute cholecystitis in the past. On this occasion she developed severe abdominal pain associated with nausea, vomiting, and increasing abdominal distension. A KUB was taken (Fig. 9–2). What does it show?

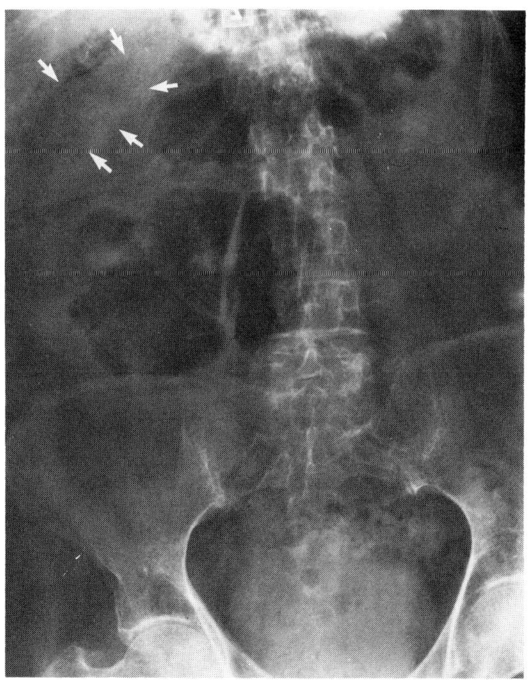

Figure 9–2. Emphysematous cholecystitis. On the KUB, a collection of gas in the right upper quadrant appears to surround a rounded structure (*arrows*). At laparotomy, a gangrenous gallbladder was found.

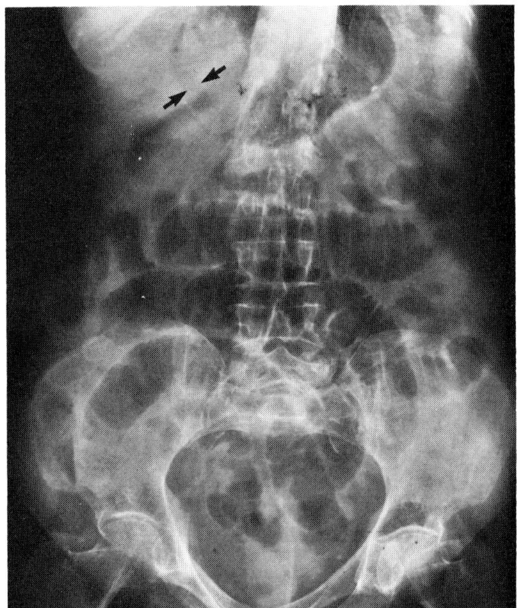

Figure 9–3. Gallstone ileus. Gas is present in the common bile duct (*arrows*) and biliary radicals on the KUB. Many loops of small intestine are distended, with the appearance of an ileus.

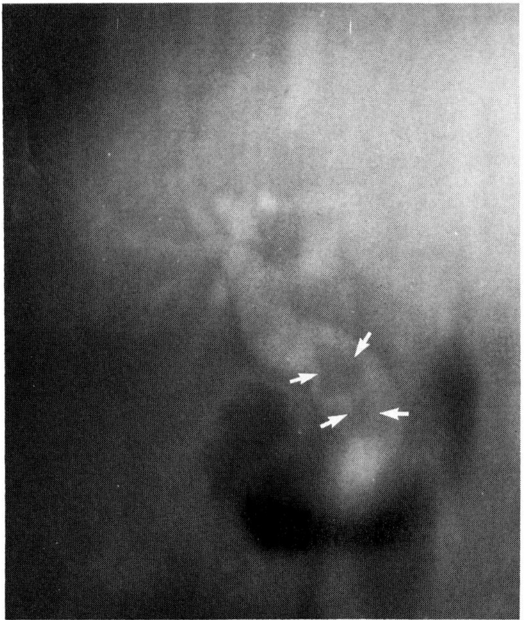

Figure 9–4. Radiolucent stones in the common bile duct. On this 45-minute IVC tomogram of the right upper quadrant, contrast agent can be seen outlining the hepatic biliary radicals and a dilated common bile duct. At least two large facetted stones can be seen in the lower part of the duct (*arrows*).

This radiograph demonstrates the appearance of emphysematous cholecystitis, a rare presentation of acute cholecystitis that has been caused by obstruction of the common bile duct by a stone that has led to infection, usually with a gas-forming organism such as *E. coli* or *C. welchii*. Emphysematous cholecystitis is more common in diabetics, and one of the sequelae may be rupture of the gallbladder into the lesser sac.

The patient with acute cholecystitis usually presents with a localized right upper quadrant ileus known as a *sentinel loop*, which can also occur in association with any abdominal inflammation such as appendicitis and pancreatitis. Chronic cholecystitis causes gallstones, which may be opaque or non-opaque, as well as a poorly functioning gallbladder. Occasionally in a patient who has had recurrent attacks of cholecystitis, a gallstone ruptures through the inflamed gallbladder wall. If there are adhesions in the right upper quadrant, the gallstone ruptures into the duodenal bulb, where it may cause a high obstruction, or more frequently moves down the intestine until it obstructs the terminal ileum; this is known as *gallstone ileus* (Fig. 9–3).

Case A3

Polly Whistle, age 72, had her gallbladder removed some years previously for multiple gallstones, but she was experiencing recurrent attacks of right upper quadrant pain. More recently, she became jaundiced (although she thought the brown coloration of her skin was the result of her annual sojourn in Miami). How would you investigate this patient?

An oral cholecystogram in this case is inappropriate because the gallbladder has been removed. An intravenous cholangiogram may not be productive until the serum bilirubin has dropped to about 3 mg per dl. Opacification of the biliary tree, however, may be obtained with a transhepatic cholangiogram, which may demonstrate the offending lesion. After surgical extirpation of the stone and relief of the obstruction, the surgeon usually inserts a T tube in the common bile duct. Before the tube is removed, contrast material is injected into it in order to check for other retained stones, in either the common bile duct or the biliary radicles. If a stone is found on subsequent study, it is possible to remove the offending calculus percutaneously through the T-tube tract. Such a system of postoperative T-tube cholangiography is performed routinely after cholecystectomy with T-tube insertion. In the absence of a T tube, however, only two routes are available for biliary tract opacification: transhepatic cholangiography and intravenous cholangiography. In this case, an intravenous cholangiogram was performed that showed a common bile duct stone (Fig. 9–4).

Case A4

Uffizi Klintwallop, age 45, was admitted complaining of sudden acute left flank pain and hematuria that occurred after he climbed to the top of the Leaning Tower of Pisa. A KUB revealed a possible ureteric stone (Fig. 9–5A), and IVP demonstrated the exact level of the stone (Fig. 9–5B).

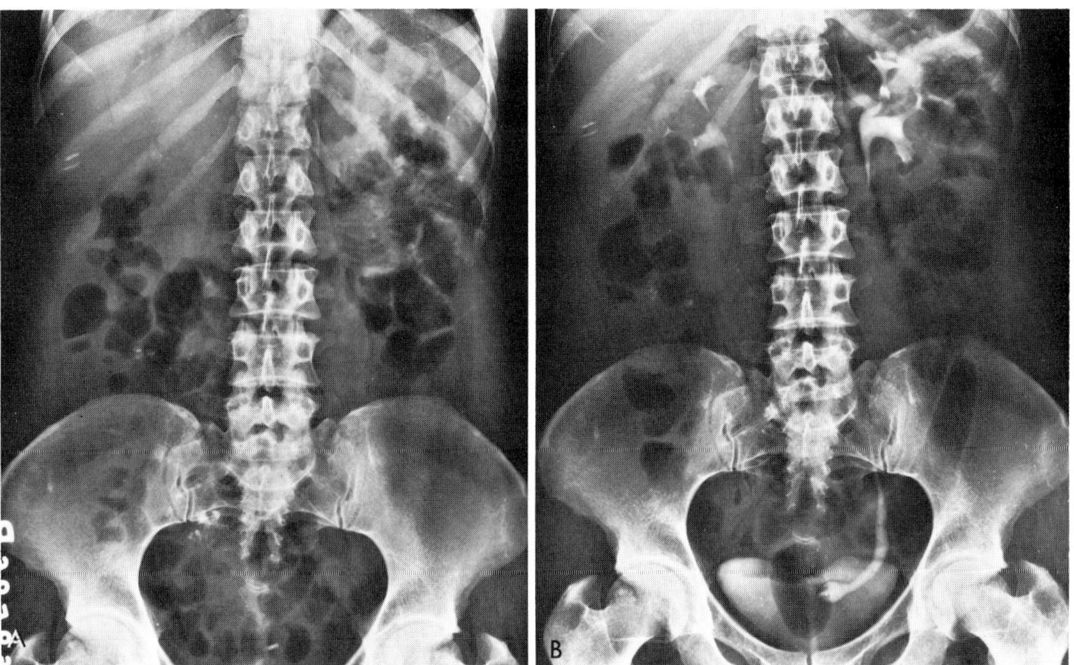

Figure 9–5. Ureteric calculus. *A*, The KUB shows an opaque oblong shadow in the region of the left vesicoureteric angle. The renal shadows are obscured by gas. *B*, The 60-minute IVP film shows the delayed excretion on the left as well as the dilatation of the lower ureter surrounding this opaque shadow. The dilated "cobra head" appearance of the distal ureter represents a ureterocele, which is a congenital anomaly.

Over 90 per cent of symptomatic renal calculi contain calcium phosphate or calcium oxalate and can be seen on plain films. There are a number of underlying causes of renal calculi, including renal tubular disorders, gout and hyperuricemia, hyperparathyroidism and papillary necrosis. In chronic long-standing stasis and recurrent infections, both of which are common predisposing causes of renal calculi, "staghorn" calculi often form and may totally fill the renal pelvis and collecting system (Fig. 9–6). *Nephrolithiasis*, stones within the collecting system, pelvis, ureter and bladder,

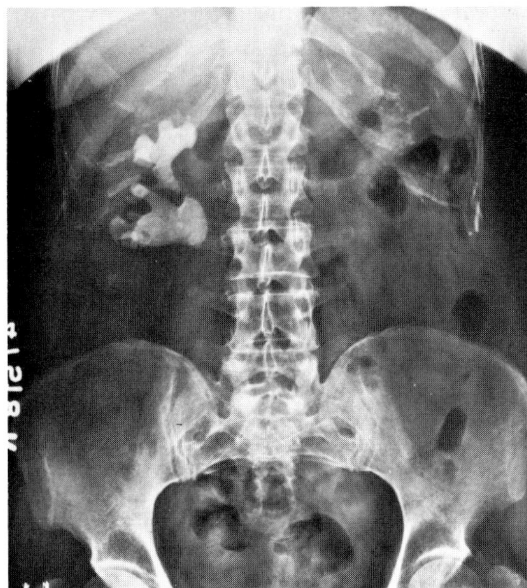

Figure 9–6. Staghorn calculus. On first glance this calculus gives the appearance of the pelvicalyceal system filled with contrast. However, this is a plain film (KUB), and a large staghorn calculus outlines the renal pelvis, infundibulae, and calyces on the right. The 50-year-old male patient with multiple sclerosis was bedridden.

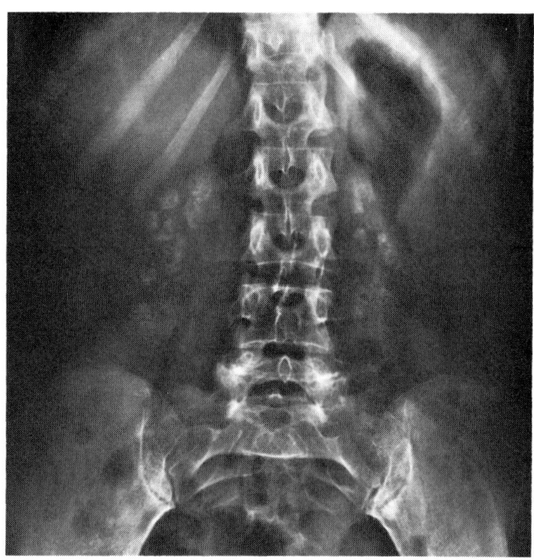

Figure 9–7. Nephrocalcinosis secondary to vitamin D intoxication. Widespread renal parenchymal calcification can be seen on the KUB. The patient, a 58-year-old woman, has taken large quantities of vitamin D over the past five years.

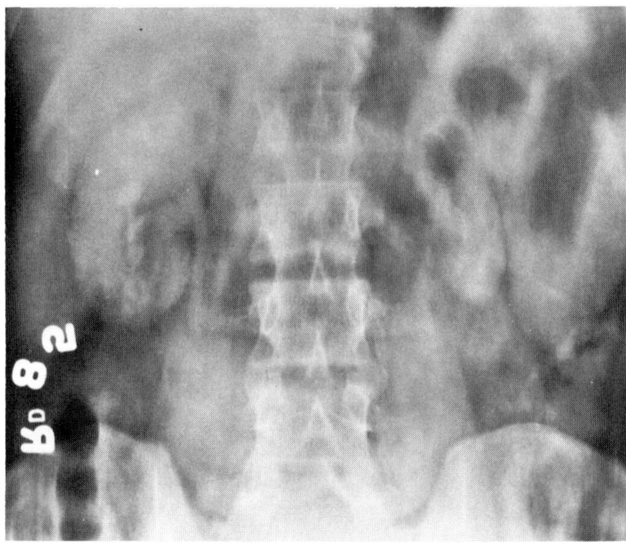

Figure 9–8. Chronic pyelonephritis. On a 5-minute tomogram, both kidneys are seen to function poorly. The left kidney is small and scarred. The calyces in the right kidney are poorly seen and appear dilated and scarred.

should be separated from *nephrocalcinosis*, in which the calcium deposits are scattered throughout the renal parenchyma. The chief causes of nephrocalcinosis are various metabolic disorders, including hyperparathyroidism, renal tubular acidosis, sarcoidosis, and milk-alkali syndrome (Fig. 9–7).

Case A5

Hildegard Boonpickle, age 25, had an acute onset of right-sided flank pain that was colicky in nature and was associated with a stinging sensation on urination. On examination, she was tender over the right kidney, and the urine contained white and red blood cells. A KUB and IVP were normal.

Usually there are no radiographic findings in acute pyelonephritis, although in severe cases the renal parenchyma may be swollen or excretion may be diminished. As the attacks become more pronounced or more frequent, however, chronic pyelonephritis ensues with scarring and distortion of the renal parenchyma. The calyces become blunted, and the renal outline becomes irregular, with subsequent loss of renal size (Fig. 9–8). Ultimately, chronic pyelonephritis leads to failure of renal function; it is the most common cause of chronic renal failure.

Case A6

Casper Longbranch, age 29, had a long history of recurrent urinary infections. He was making his usual milk deliveries one day when his horse kicked him in the left side. He took little notice of this at first, but over the next few days he developed fevers, cramps, and left-sided colic. He went to his doctor and a KUB was taken (Fig. 9–9). What does it show?

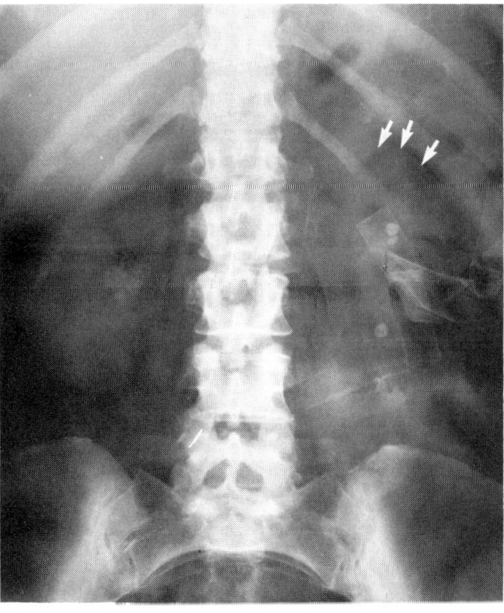

Figure 9–9. Perinephric abscess. The left renal outline is somewhat ill-defined, and there are a number of poorly defined lucencies in the region of the renal bed. Gas outlines the upper pole of the kidney (*arrows*). Note that the patient has multiple calcified renal calculi.

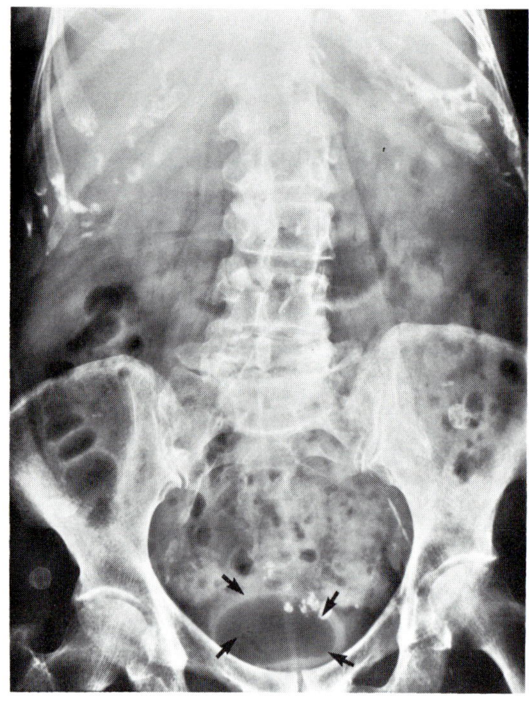

Figure 9–10. Emphysematous cystitis. This 67-year-old woman complained of dysuria and smelly urine. The KUB shows gas in the bladder (*arrows*). (Culture of the urine specimen yielded *Escherichia coli.*) The patient has some calcified fibroids.

The enlarged renal contour outlined by poorly defined bubbles of gas is definitive evidence of a perinephric abscess. An IVP would confirm the blurring of the renal outline but would probably show no changes other than those produced by underlying chronic pyelonephritis. A perinephric abscess is often precipitated by mild injury to an already inflamed kidney or develops as an extension from a renal carbuncle or abscess.

One other urinary tract infection should be mentioned here. Although cystitis usually has no characteristic radiographic features, in some cases caused by gas-forming organisms, gas may actually be seen in the bladder wall or the bladder itself (Fig. 9–10).

Abdominal abscesses do not of course occur only in relation to the kidney, and infection may occur in association with any abdominal organs. There are two other intra-abdominal abscesses of great medical importance.

Case A7

Nanny Bloomers, age 84, had a partial colectomy for a small "apple-core" carcinoma in the descending colon. Two weeks later, it was apparent that things had not gone well. Apart from recurrent bouts of congestive heart failure, there was evidence of sepsis: fever, sweats, abdominal pain, elevated erythrocyte sedimentation rate (ESR), and elevated white blood count (WBC). A subphrenic abscess was suspected. How would you diagnose this patient's condition?

A chest x-ray may show elevation of a hemidiaphragm, and there may be a pleural reaction with free fluid. Limited diaphragmatic motion may be demonstrated by fluoroscopy. With these signs, it is not possible to differentiate between pul-

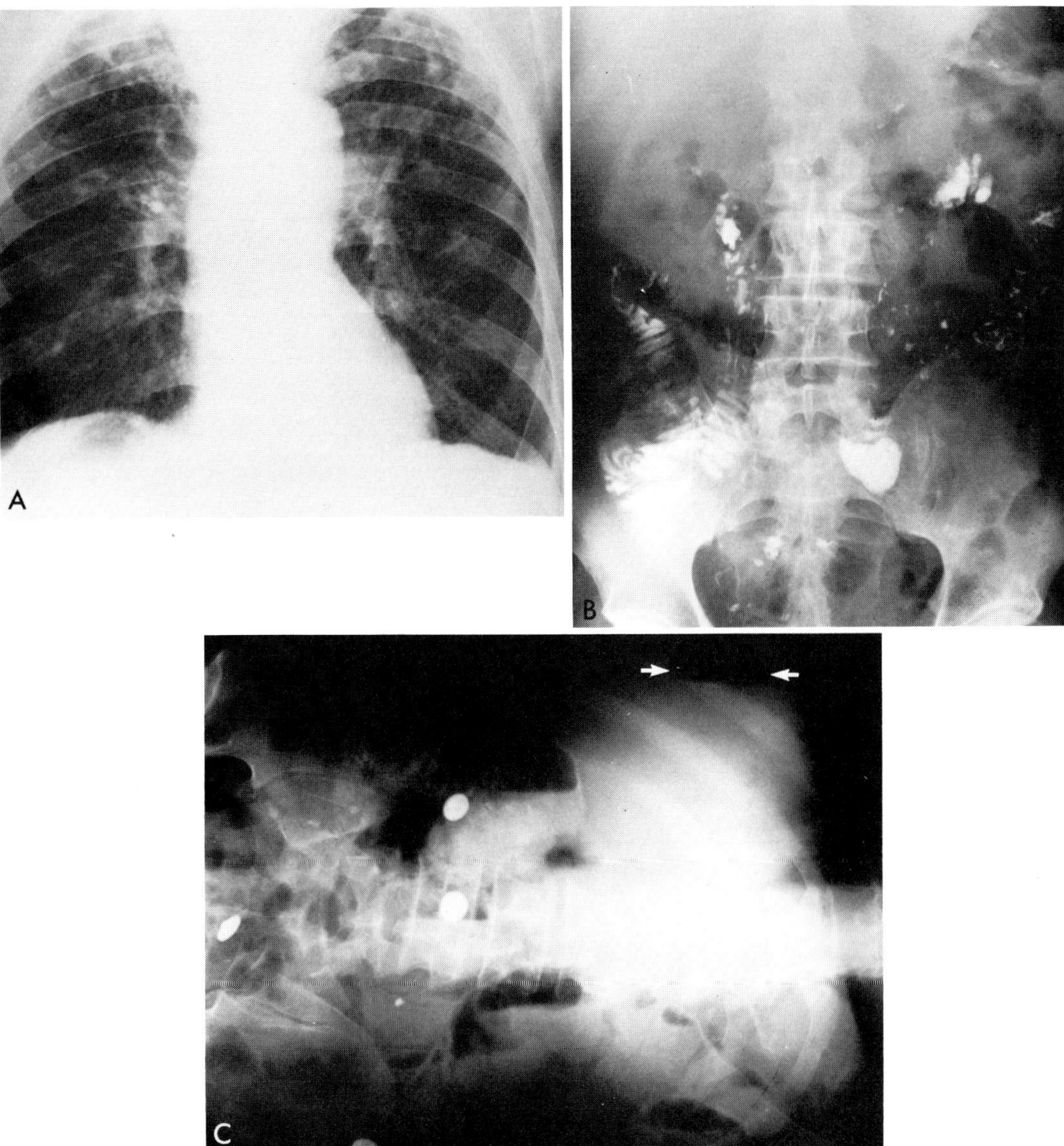

Figure 9–11. Subphrenic abscess. This 63-year-old man developed a spiking fever ten days after gastrectomy for a malignant gastric ulcer. *A* and *B*, The PA chest film shows some air under the right hemidiaphragm, and the KUB shows a featureless right upper quadrant. *C*, A lateral decubitus film taken 48 hours later shows a large air-fluid level (*arrows*) under the right hemidiaphragm that was caused by a subphrenic abscess.

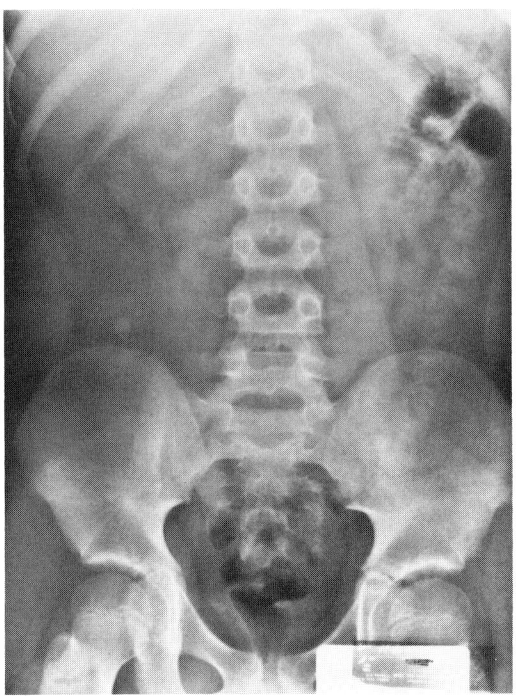

Figure 9–12. Acute appendicitis with an appendicolith. There is a calcified density in the right lower quadrant and a lack of bowel gas shadows in this 11-year-old child with proven acute appendicitis.

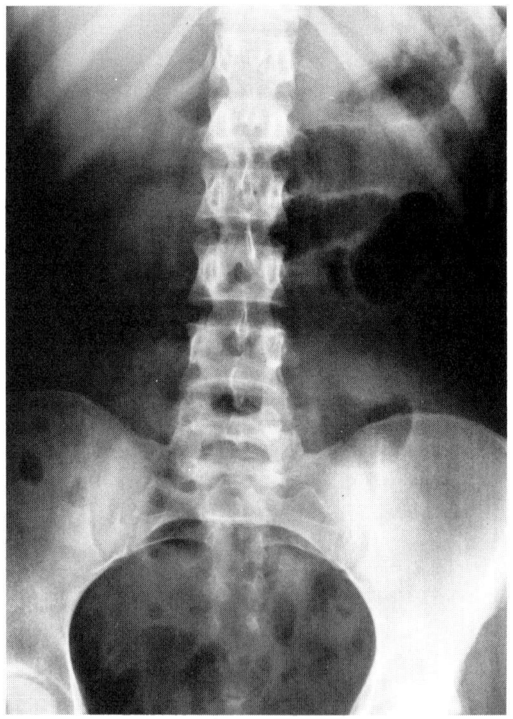

Figure 9–13. Appendix abscess. This 24-year-old man had pain in the right lower quadrant. Three months later, he presented with increasing pain and tenderness, and a plain film of the abdomen was taken. There is an area containing ill-defined gas bubbles to the right of the lower lumbar spine; at operation this was found to be an appendix abscess. Note the distended loops of small bowel in the left upper quadrant (sentinel loops).

monary infarction, postoperative atelectasis or pneumonia, postoperative diaphragmatic changes, and subphrenic abscess. A KUB often shows no irregularity, although it may demonstrate an abscess or air-fluid level, which can also be seen on an upright chest x-ray, particularly if the abscess is on the left side (Fig. 9–11). Usually, however, the diagnosis of subphrenic or subdiaphragmatic abscess is not easy, and more sophisticated techniques are required. Diagnostic pneumoperitoneography has dropped out of fashion and has been replaced by nuclear medicine and ultrasound techniques.

Acute appendicitis is a clinical diagnosis, but occasionally an appendicolith may be seen on a KUB (Fig. 9–12). It is associated with a sentinel loop of small bowel, which is caused by localized ileus due to the inflammation. When the appendix perforates, it can cause either a generalized peritonitis with a paralytic ileus or a localized periappendiceal abscess, which may appear as a right lower quadrant soft-tissue density. It may rarely appear as an abscess with a number of small gas bubbles speckled in it (Fig. 9 –13).

Other causes of intestinal ileus do not involve infection. These include: postoperative adynamic ileus, the ileus that accompanies various biochemical disorders such as hypokalaemia, the toxic ileus seen in association with pneumonia (particularly pneumococcal) and typhoid fever, and the ileus that accompanies localized intraperitoneal disease (appendicitis and pancreatitis).

Case A8

Virginia Plain, age 99, was admitted comatose and desperately ill. She had been diabetic for at least 50 years and had survived bilateral leg amputations, multiple bouts of congestive heart failure, and recurrent pneumonia. A chest x-ray and KUB were taken (Fig. 9–14). What does the KUB show?

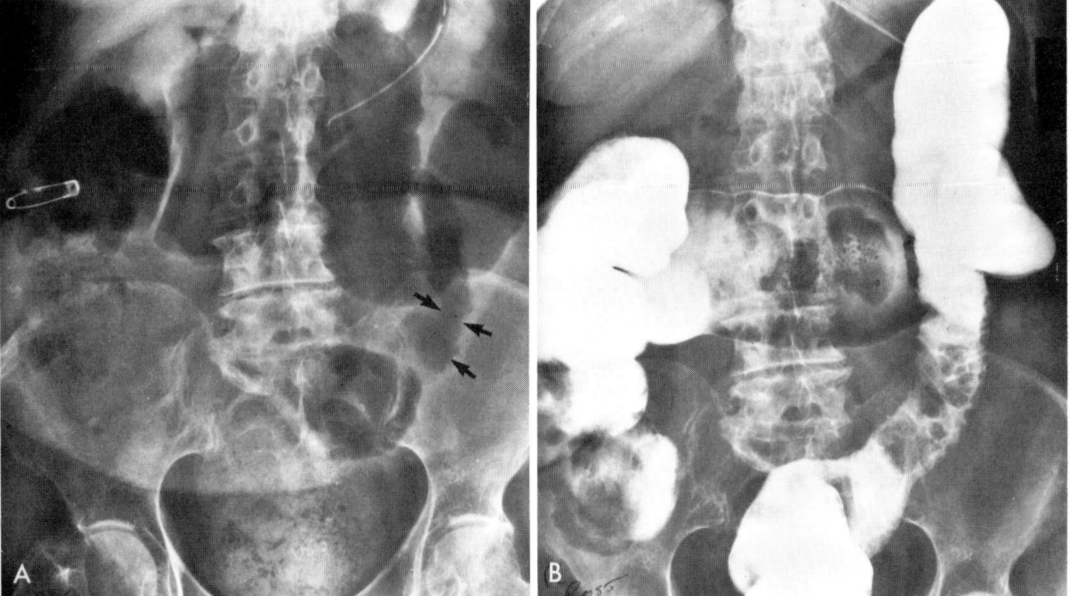

Figure 9–14. Intestinal ischemia and "thumbprinting," plain film (*A*) and barium enema (*B*). Thickened mucosal folds with some "thumbprinting" in the descending colon (*arrows*) can be seen on both the plain film and the contrast study.

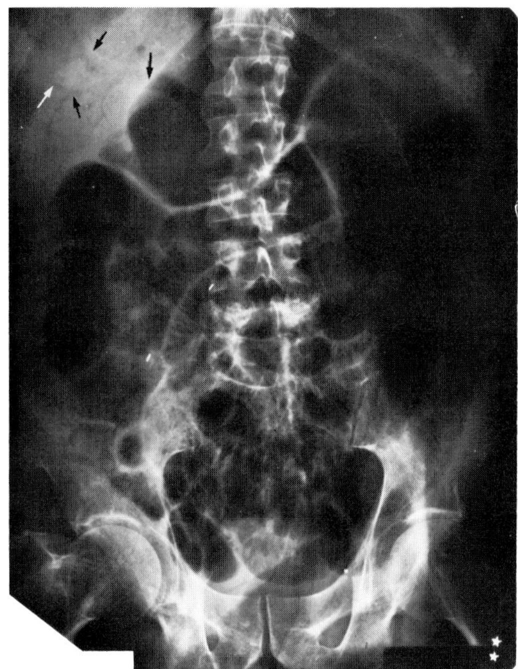

Figure 9–15. Mesenteric artery thrombosis with gas in the portal veins. Numerous air-filled small bowel loops are seen, and there is some air in the colon. In the right upper quadrant, gas can be seen in the portal veins (*arrows*). At autopsy, thrombosis of the mesenteric artery and infarction of the bowel were found.

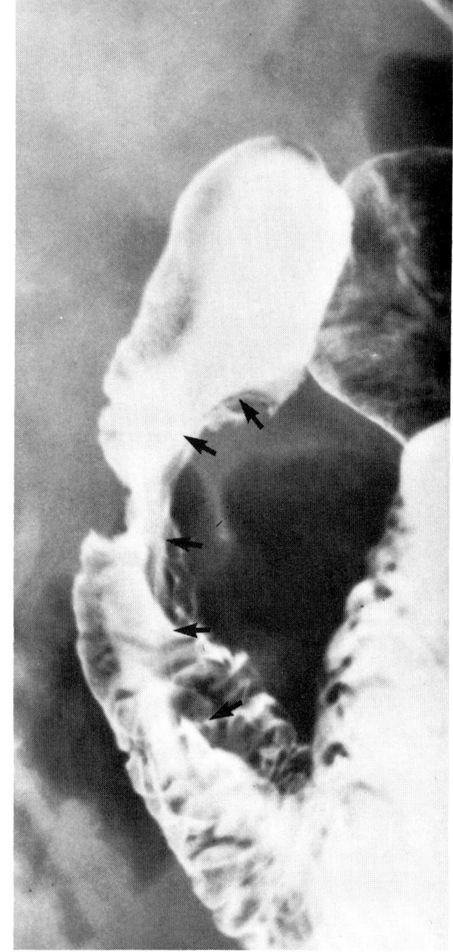

Figure 9–16. Pancreatic mass. On this hypotonic duodenogram, a mass lesion can be seen encroaching on the duodenal sweep and narrowing the duodenum. A double contour can also be seen (*arrows*). Both of the findings are signs of a mass in the head of the pancreas.

Intestinal ischemia is another cause of adynamic bowel; it may be an acute manifestation of sickle cell anemia or mesenteric embolic disease, but it may also occur chronically as a result of vascular compromise in patients with severe arteriosclerosis. As intestinal ischemia progresses, "thumb printing" occurs and a KUB taken at a later date shows no appreciable change in the position of the bowel gas. Closer inspection may show the presence of gas actually within the bowel wall (gangrene), a bad prognostic sign. There is one other interesting if rare complication: the presence of gas within the portal venous system, also signifying intestinal gangrene (Fig. 9–15). The usual cause of ischemic bowel disease is occlusion of the mesenteric artery; in more chronic cases, mesenteric vein thrombosis may be the cause.

Case A9

J. N. B. Loophole, age 63, a well-known local lawyer with a long history of drinking, presented with abdominal and back pain. He complained of increasing weight loss. On examination, he appeared to be cachectic and in some distress. A physical examination, chest x-ray, and KUB were all normal. How would you investigate this patient? An IVP, a barium enema, and an oral cholecystogram were also normal. An upper gastrointestinal series was also performed (Fig. 9–16). What does it show?

The pancreas is one of the most difficult organs to evaluate clinically and radiologically, because it is a hidden organ and disorders of the pancreas may have "silent" manifestations. Widening of the duodenal sweep is highly suggestive of a lesion lying within the head of the pancreas, whereas lesions in the tail of the pancreas may be totally silent and lesions in the body may displace the stomach anteriorly. With the possibility of a lesion in the head of the pancreas of this patient, what would you do next? Until recently, an angiogram would have been performed, often with equivocal results. Now, however, ultrasonography or CT scanning is the procedure of choice (Fig. 9–17). CT scanning has been hailed as the ideal method of diagnosing pancreatic lesions, but in actual practice it has proven to be rather less useful than first hoped be-

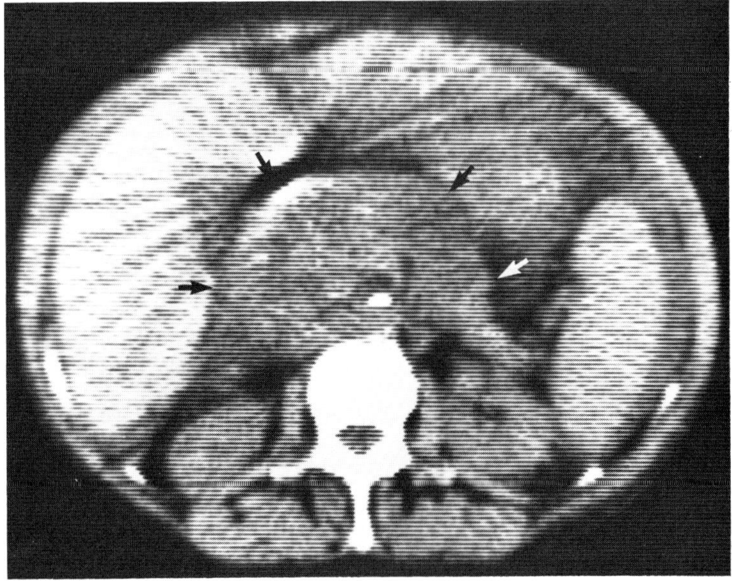

Figure 9–17. Pancreatic carcinoma. This CT scan shows a huge mass replacing the pancreatic outline (*arrows*).

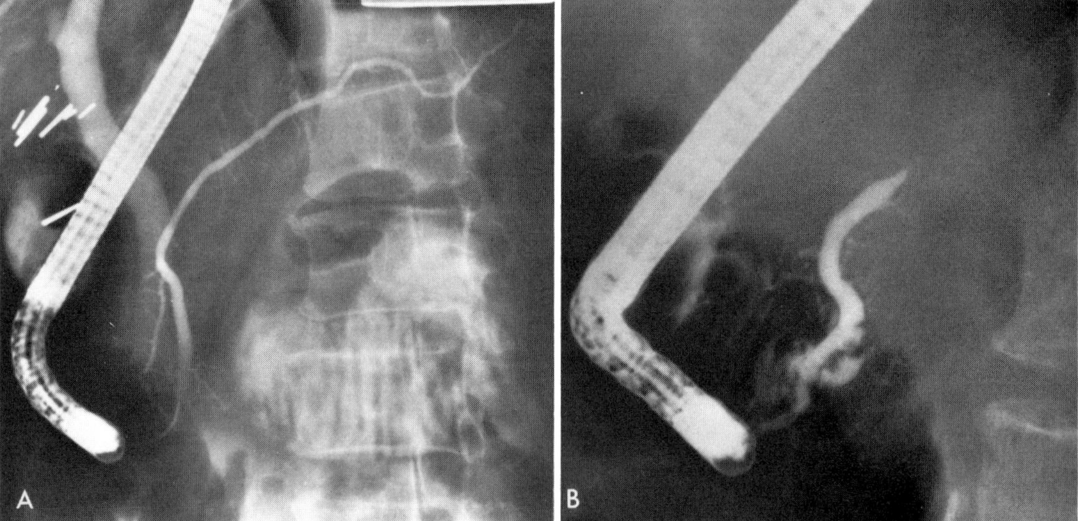

Figure 9–18. Pancreatic duct cannulation. *A*, Normal film. A flexible fibro-optic endoscope is introduced into the duodenal sweep from the mouth and the pancreatic duct is cannulated under fluoroscopic guidance. Following an injection of water soluble contrast agent, the duct and its ramifications are clearly seen, as is the filling of the common bile duct and the gallbladder. *B*, In this 60-year-old male with a pancreatic mass, the irregularity and distortion of the duct is characteristic of a carcinoma of the head of the pancreas.

cause of the inability of the CT scanner to differentiate between the pancreas and overlying bowel shadows in many patients. In this patient, there is a suggestion of a mass in the head of the pancreas; a "skinny needle" biopsy performed under ultrasonic guidance revealed pancreatic carcinoma.

In spite of all our relatively sophisticated techniques, the pancreas is still the most difficult organ in the body in which to diagnose pathological changes. To the usual armamentarium of plain films, barium studies, and angiography, we can now add CT scanning and pancreatic duct cannulation, both of which may be helpful. Endoscopic retrograde pancreatic duct cannulation is particularly useful in the diagnosis of inflammatory diseases of the pancreas (Fig. 9–18).

There is one plain film finding of use in chronic pancreatitis: the presence of multiple calcifications within the pancreas itself. Figure 9–19 illustrates the radiographic appearance of this condition.

Another complication of pancreatitis that is worthy of mention is the rare occurrence of a pseudocyst, in which a loculated collection of fluid may originate from any part of the pancreas and may cause pressure de-

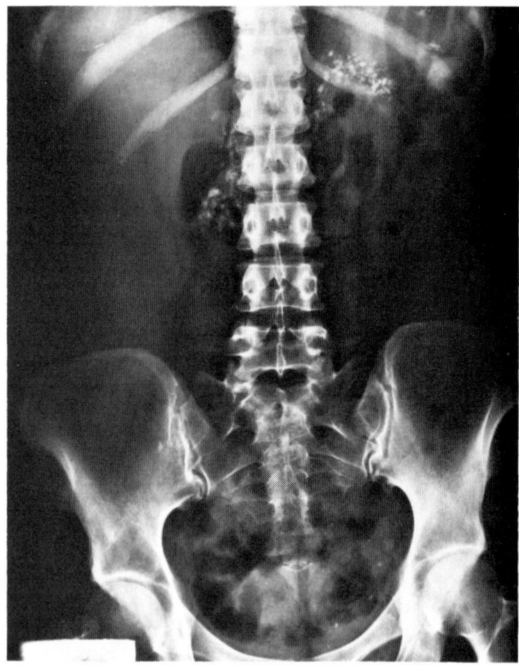

Figure 9–19. Pancreatic calcification. This 41-year-old female alcoholic had a long history of chronic pancreatitis. The KUB shows numerous tiny flocculant calcifications in the region of the pancreas. Note the enlarged liver.

fects in the stomach, duodenal sweep, or proximal small intestine. The diagnosis of pancreatic pseudocyst is facilitated by the use of ultrasonography and CT scanning (Fig. 9–20).

Acute pancreatitis is difficult to diagnose radiographically; an elevated serum amylase level is a much more dependable indication. Sometimes pancreatitis causes radiological symptoms such as localized ileus (sentinel loop), a colon cutoff sign (no air in the descending colon), reactive pleurisy and effusion at the lung bases, or even a retroperitoneal abscess. Secondary inflammatory changes may be seen in the mucosal pattern of the lesser curve of the stomach, the inside of the duodenal sweep, and the superior surface of the transverse colon. A distant secondary finding is medullary infarction in the metaphyseal and diaphyseal regions of the long bones, which leads to avascular necrosis.

There are a number of other causes of abdominal pain, some of which are obvious (for example, trauma) and some more subtle. Trauma to the abdomen may involve both soft tissues and bones. Direct injury to a flank may cause rupture of a kidney, and direct injury to the lower ribs can produce abdominal pain.

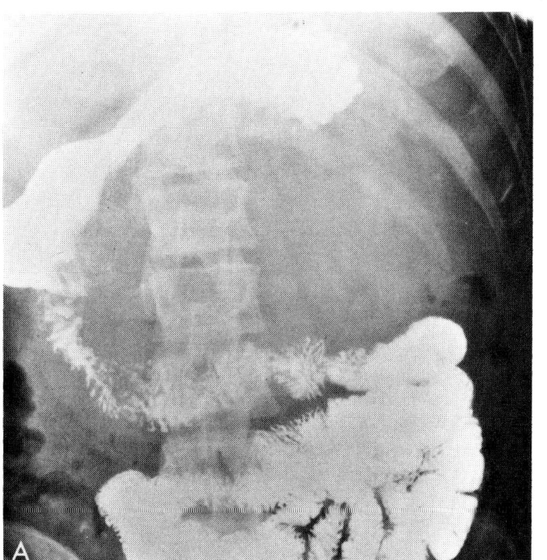

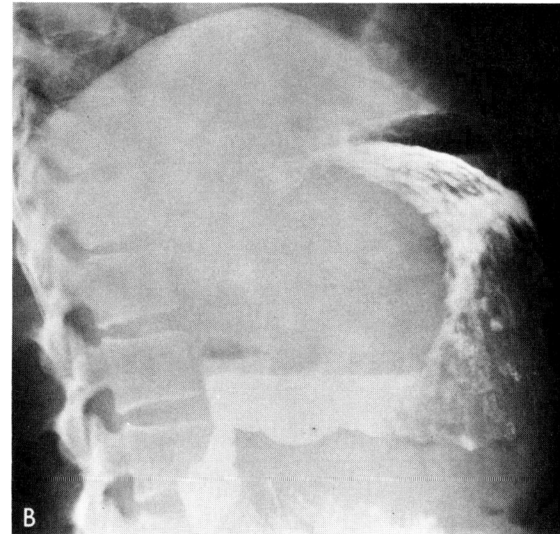

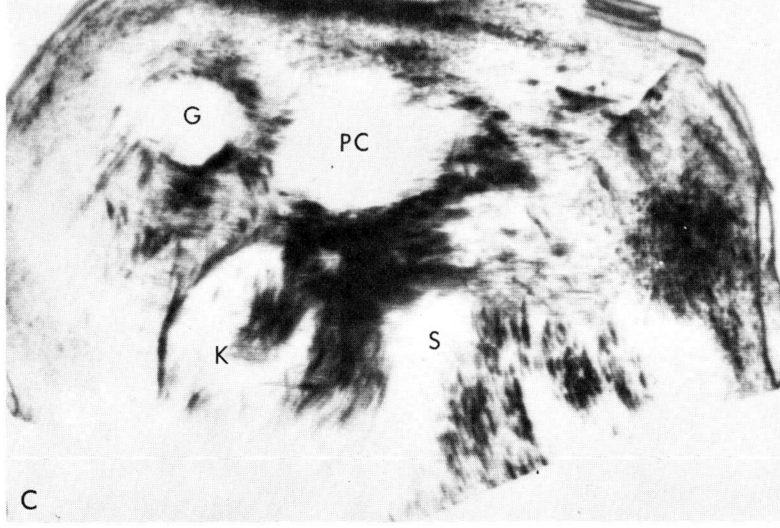

Figure 9–20. Pancreatic pseudocyst. *A* and *B*, In films from the UGI, the barium-filled stomach is displaced anteriorly and upwards with indentation of the duodenal sweep. *C*, The sonogram shows a large sonolucent mass in the region of the pancreatic head, representing a pseudocyst (PC). Note the gallbladder (G), right kidney (K), and spine (S) on this transverse image.

Case A10

Iggi Poppins, age 25, a distant cousin of Mary, was admitted to the hospital after having had her nether regions run over by a steamroller. It was obvious that her pelvis was badly shattered (Fig. 9–21). What complications could one anticipate?

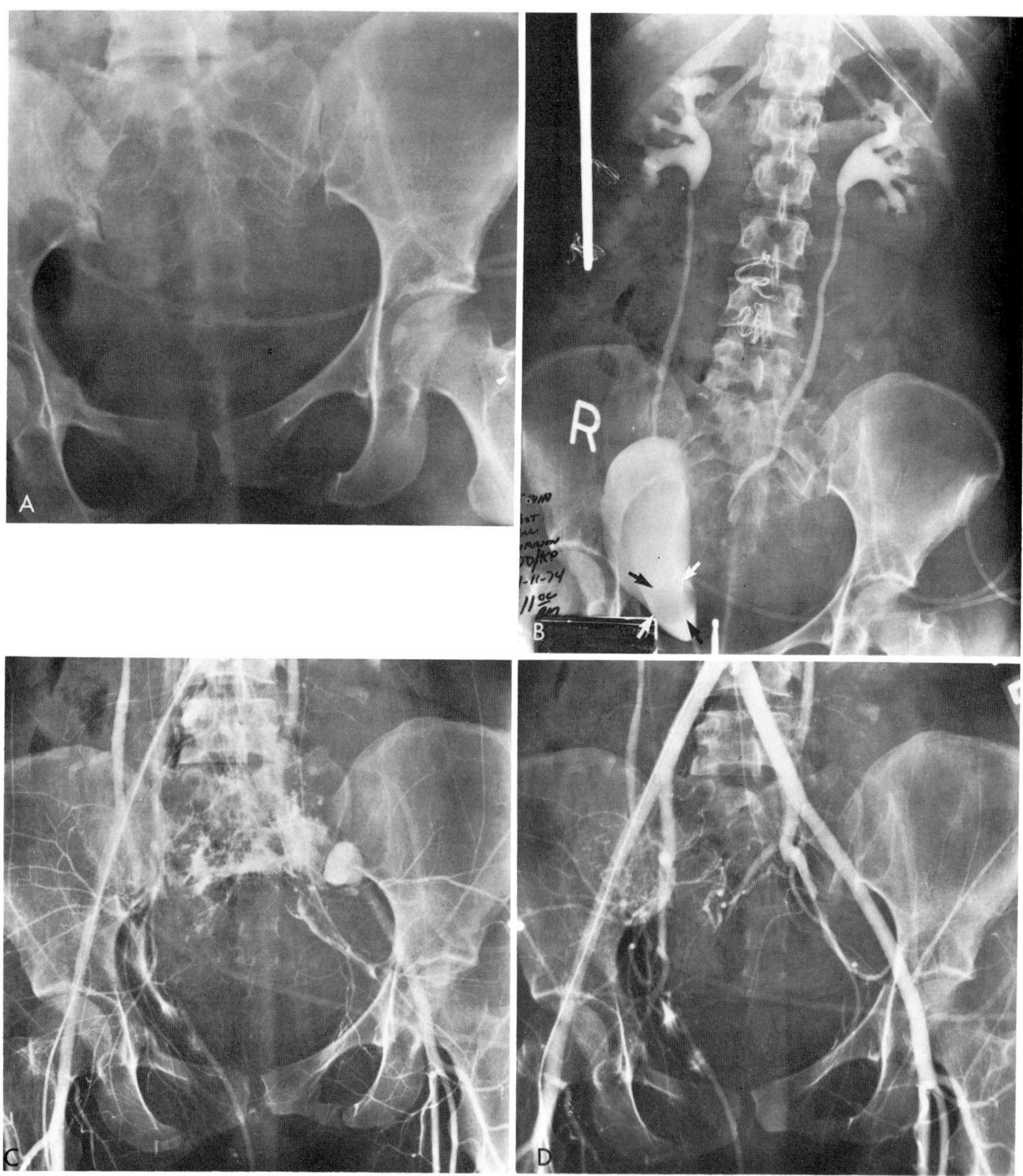

Figure 9–21. Fractured pelvis with rupture of the urethra and a large retroperitoneal bleed from a traumatic aneurysm of the superior gluteal artery. *A*, The plain film shows multiple fractures of the pelvis and diastasis of the left sacroiliac joint. *B*, During IVP, pronounced displacement of the bladder and rupture of the urethra, were found, and cystoscopy and catheterization were performed. On this 15-minute film, the Foley catheter balloon can be seen in the bladder (*arrows*). *C*, Angiography demonstrated continued bleeding and extravasation from a torn vessel just proximal to a false aneurysm, which were controlled by injection of autologous clotted blood. *D*, An aortogram performed two weeks later shows almost total recovery.

This case illustrates some points of particular importance to the clinician and the radiologist as well as the patient. First, the radiologist should be involved in decisions concerning a severely injured patient from the outset of the investigation. Second, it is important to ascertain the extent of damage to the urological system from above and not from below, for fear of introducing infection. Third, the radiologist is able to stop major arterial bleeding by using drugs or emboli introduced directly via an angiocatheter.

Case A11 Fontilroy Belcher, age 9, came in complaining of abdominal pain and fever. His pediatrician diagnosed a ruptured appendix. The KUB was read as normal, and a chest x-ray was taken (Fig. 9–22). What does it show?

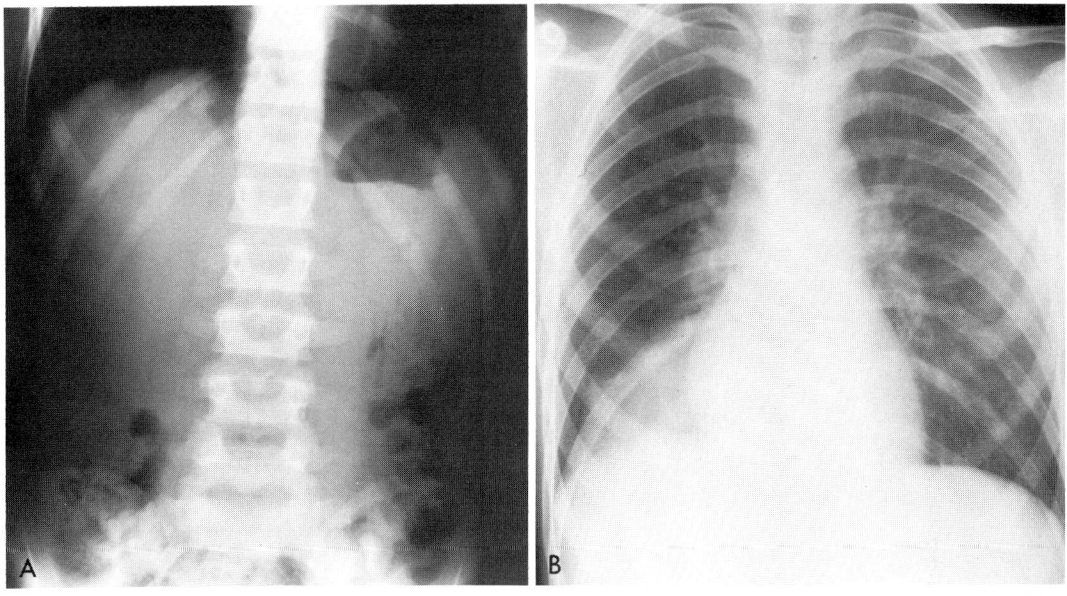

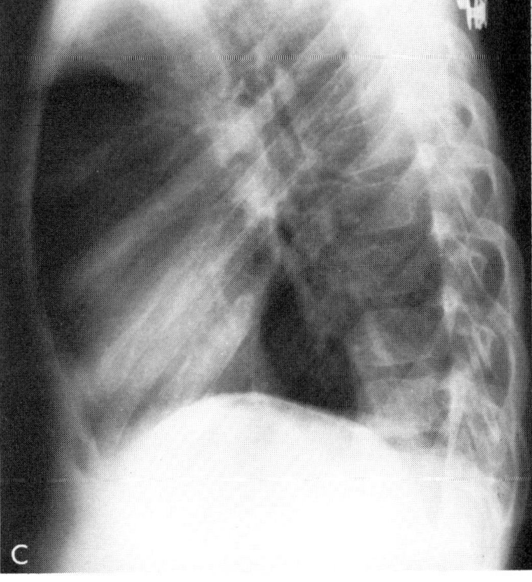

Figure 9–22. Right lower lobe pneumonia. *A*, On a plain film of the abdomen, the bowel gas pattern is within normal limits. There is a suggestion of density in the right upper quadrant, just under the hemidiaphragms. *B*, The PA view of the chest demonstrates obliteration of the right diaphragm and opacification of the right lower zone. *C*, A lateral view of the chest confirms the presence of a right lower lobe pneumonia.

There is obliteration of the right hemidiaphragm, confirming the presence of a right lower lobe pneumonia. Lower lobe pneumonia is not an uncommon cause of abdominal pain, particularly in children and adolescents.

Case A12

Ureta Twatts, age 23, was what used to be known as a courtesan and "no better than could be expected." She was admitted complaining of abdominal pain, but on clinical examination, no abnormality could be found. A KUB revealed all (Fig. 9–23).

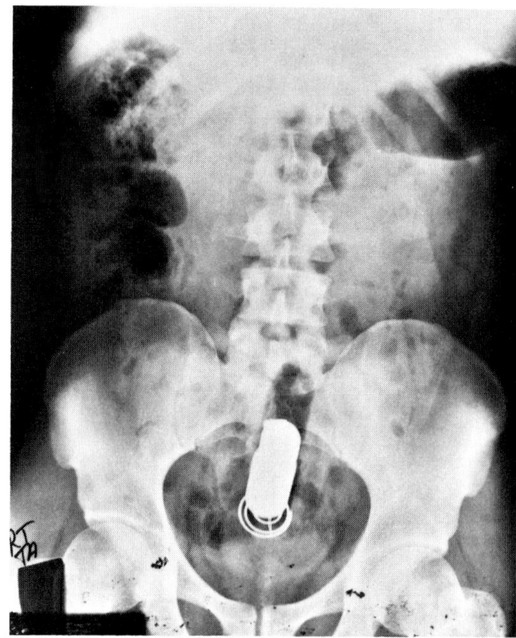

Figure 9–23. Foreign body in rectum. The KUB shows a vibrator at the rectosigmoid junction; it was removed successfully.

Case A13

Posy Parsnip, age 37, was married to an incompetent parson who practiced more than he preached. After her first 15 children, the gynecologist insisted that Mrs. Parsnip use an intrauterine device for birth control. Some years later she came to her physician complaining of intermittent abdominal pain. On physical examination, no abnormality could be found. What does the KUB show (Fig. 9–24)?

A radiologist is often asked to identify the position of an IUD from a single KUB. Because the normal uterus may be anteverted or retroverted, large or small, and laterally or centrally placed, it is frequently impossible even with a lateral view to determine whether the IUD is in place. The best way to document the intrauterine location of an IUD is with ultrasonography, because the IUD is densely echogenic and easily identified within the uterus.

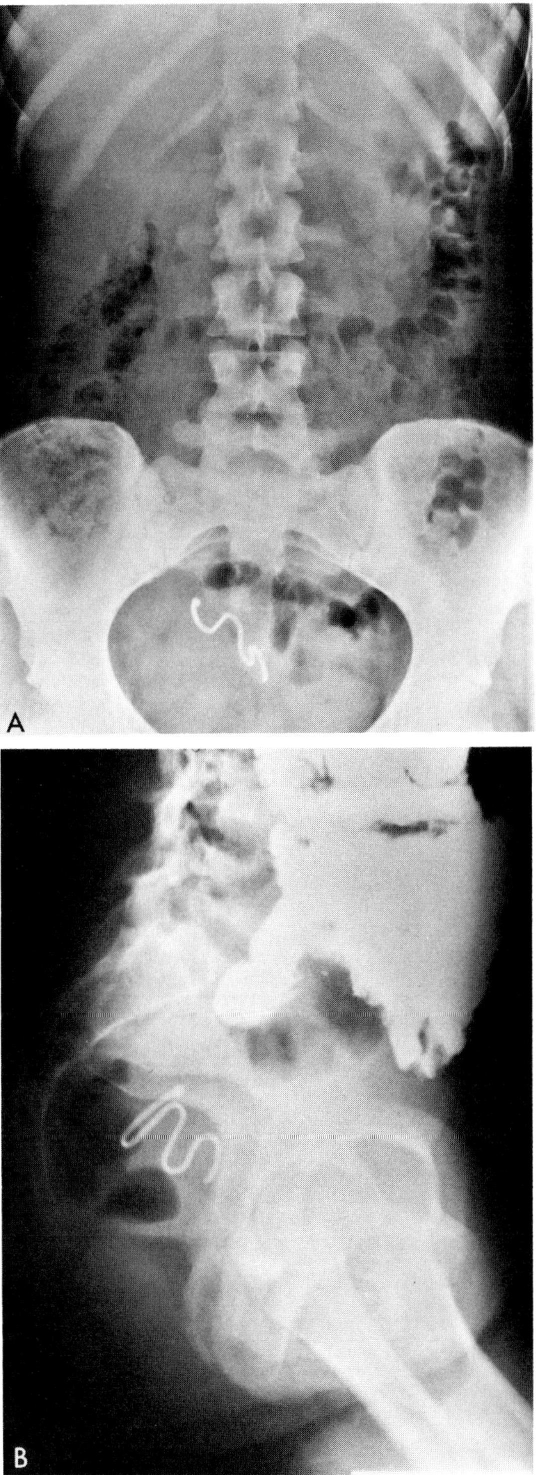

Figure 9–24. IUD out of the uterus, AP view (*A*) and lateral view (*B*). This radiopaque IUD was seen on the AP view to lie somewhat too high and to the left and on the lateral view to lie too central. It was actually between the uterus and rectum. Note the spreading of the coils of the loop, which cannot occur inside the uterus.

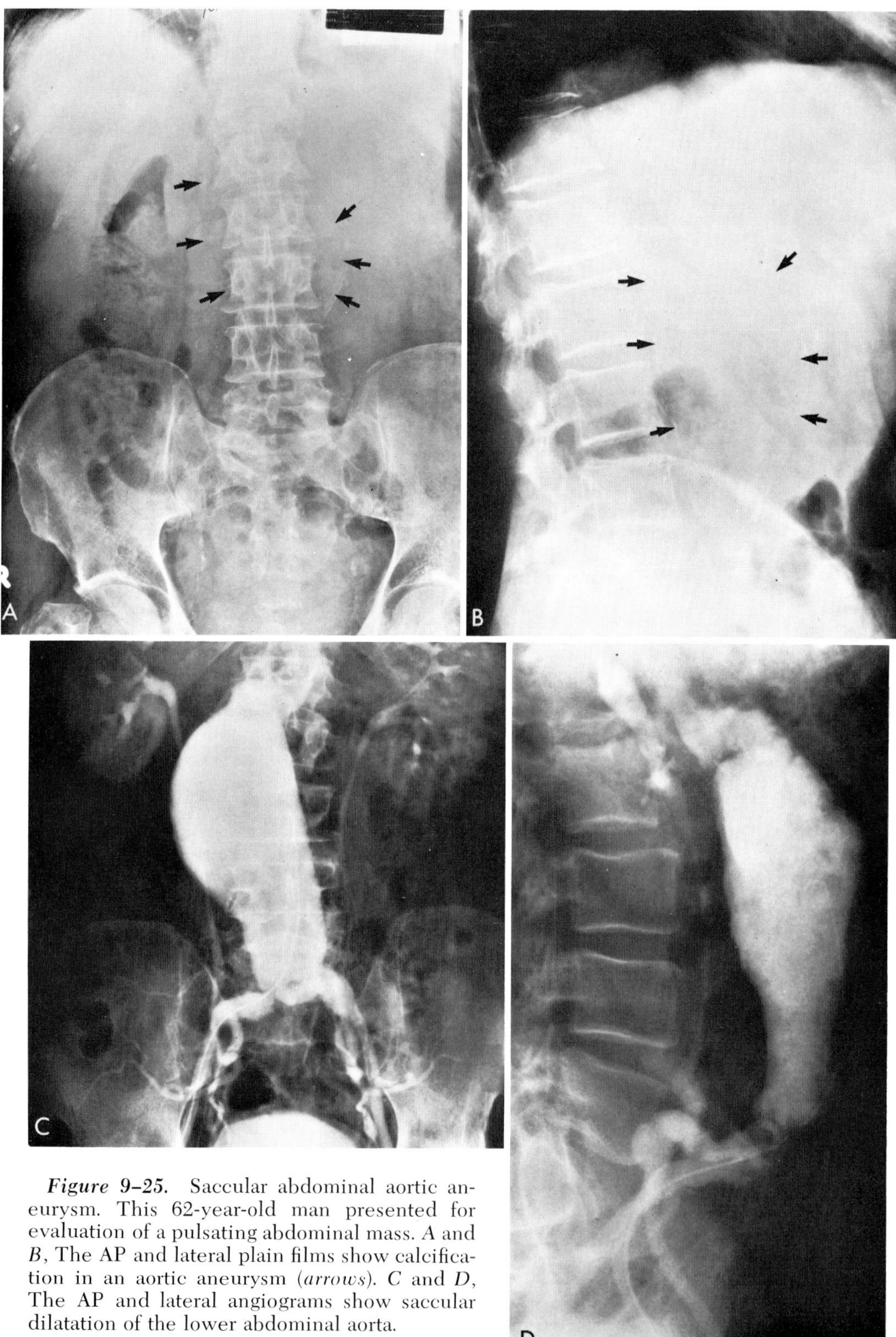

Figure 9–25. Saccular abdominal aortic aneurysm. This 62-year-old man presented for evaluation of a pulsating abdominal mass. *A* and *B*, The AP and lateral plain films show calcification in an aortic aneurysm (*arrows*). *C* and *D*, The AP and lateral angiograms show saccular dilatation of the lower abdominal aorta.

Case A14

Jeremiah Bleeder, age 62, came in complaining of abdominal discomfort. On examination, there was an obvious pulsatile mass in the lower abdomen. A KUB and a lateral view revealed an 8-inch saccular abdominal aortic aneurysm (Fig. 9–25).

To operate or not to operate? Basically, the age and state of health of the patient has to be taken into account, as well as the size and rate of growth of the aneurysm. The basic measurement above which abdominal aortic aneurysms are considered to be clinically significant is 6 cm, and one may have to use angiography and ultrasonography to confirm the exact dimensions.

Case A15

Silenzio Trash, age 38, was admitted with abdominal discomfort, increasing girth, and loss of weight. The KUB was equivocal, but it did show a suggestion of a retroperitoneal mass.

How would you further investigate a retroperitoneal tumor? The classic approach is to perform an IVP to look for renal or ureteric deviation, then to do a lymphogram and possibly an angiogram before an exploratory laparotomy. With the advent of CT scanning we have at last acquired a reasonable technique for looking at the retroperitoneal area. In this patient a large retroperitoneal mass was shown (Fig. 9–26).

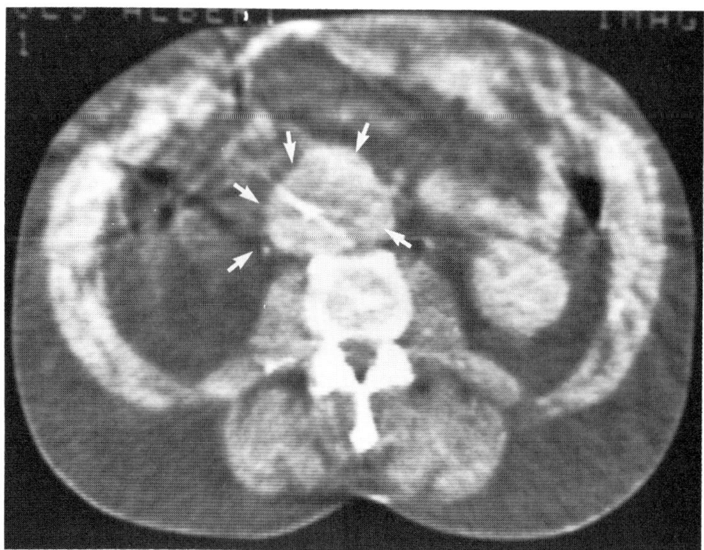

Figure 9–26. Retroperitoneal tumor. The CT scan shows a large retroperitoneal mass (*arrows*) obliterating the normal contours of the abdominal aorta. At biopsy, the mass proved to be a fibrosarcoma. The artefact from a surgical clip within the mass can be seen.

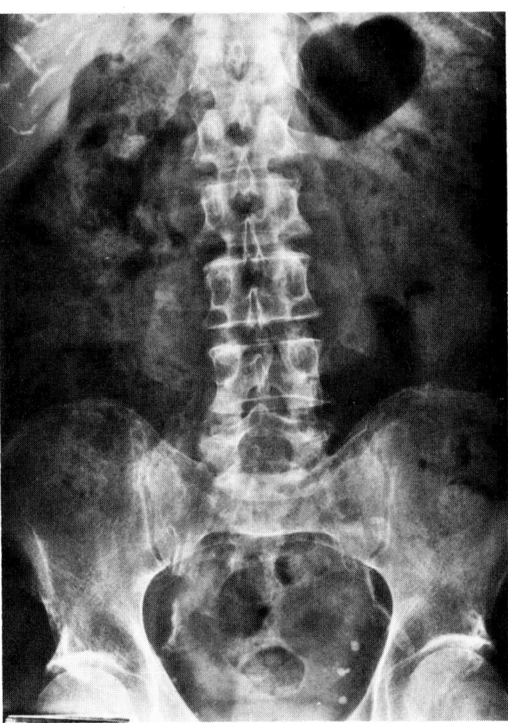

Figure 9–27. Fecal impaction. Solid feces are visible throughout the colon from the cecum to the rectum in this 79-year-old man.

Although we have by no means covered all the plain film findings possible in the abdomen, we have attempted to provide an introduction to the investigation of intra-abdominal pathology. Calculi and calcifications, infections and abscesses, lesions of the pancreas and retroperitoneum, tumors and aneurysms, ruptures, perforations, and fractures have all been mentioned. The basic approach to abdominal symptoms is obvious: (1) plain films, (2) special views or techniques, (3) contrast studies with barium and water-soluble agents, (4) special procedures such as angiography, pancreatic duct cannulation, and lymphography, and (5) such techniques as biopsy under ultrasonographic guidance and CT scanning.

ABDOMINAL PAIN AND CHANGE OF BOWEL HABIT

Undoubtedly the most common cause of abdominal pain associated with a change in bowel habit is constipation. The diagnosis is usually a clinical one, but it is surprising how frequently a radiologist is able to evaluate a bowel as "FOF" (full of feces) on a KUB (Fig. 9–27). It is essential to exclude all the other possible causes before diagnosing the cause of abdominal pain as constipation. One should look for calculi, tumors or masses, intestinal obstruction, and ileus and should exclude the possibility of vascular or bony lesions. It is difficult to specify what is a "normal" amount of fecal material visible on a plain film of the abdomen. Looking at some of the other examples of abdominal radiographs in this book may help, but it is difficult. Many radiologists maintain that solid feces should not be present in the cecum, and its presence or absence may be a useful parameter in evaluating constipation.

In older patients, constipation is often a symptom of an underlying disorder such as diverticulitis or carcinoma. Once the majority of feces have been cleared from the colon, a barium enema should be done. In patients with true chronic constipation, dilatation of the bowel (acquired megacolon) is common, and often the sigmoid becomes redundant and tortuous.

Case A16

Anemone Gurkin, age 28, a waitress in the local speakeasy, presented with severe abdominal pains and cramps. She had had no bowel action for two days. Examination revealed increased bowel sounds and a somewhat tympanic abdomen on percussion. What does the plain film of the abdomen show (Fig. 9–28)?

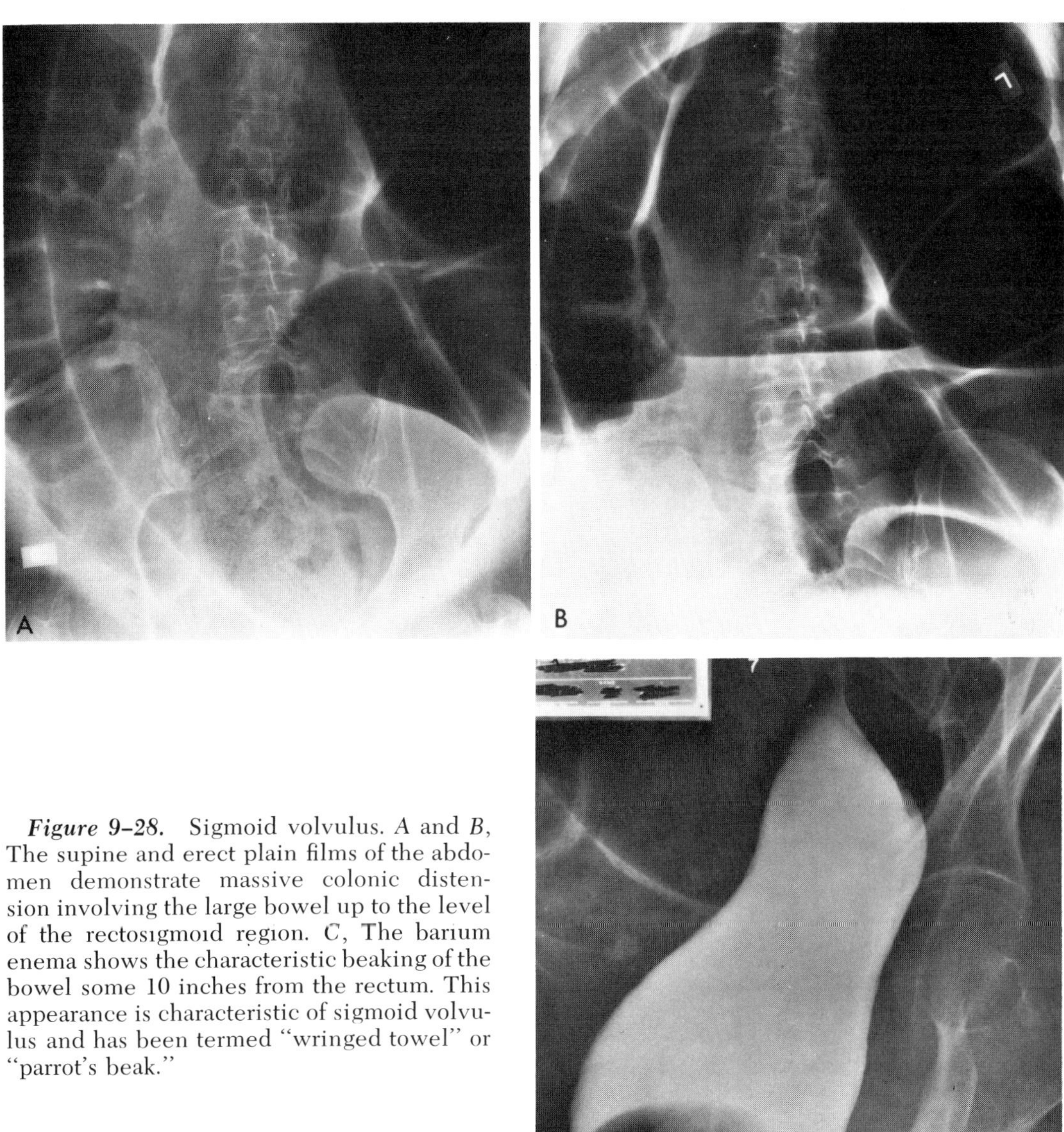

Figure 9–28. Sigmoid volvulus. *A* and *B*, The supine and erect plain films of the abdomen demonstrate massive colonic distension involving the large bowel up to the level of the rectosigmoid region. *C*, The barium enema shows the characteristic beaking of the bowel some 10 inches from the rectum. This appearance is characteristic of sigmoid volvulus and has been termed "wringed towel" or "parrot's beak."

Although theoretically much of the small bowel and some of the colon may undergo volvulus, the two major segments of the bowel that twist upon themselves in the adult are the sigmoid colon on its mesentery, and the cecum. For the cecum to do this requires it to have a separate mesentery rather than lying in its normal retroperitoneal fixed location. Any cause of mechanical large bowel obstruction will produce gaseous distension of the colon proximal to the level of obstruction, so that volvulus of the cecum is associated only with small bowel distension. The dilated cecum lies characteristically in the left upper quadrant or the central abdomen and may measure up to 30 cm in diameter.

The sigmoid characteristically twists and then folds back on itself, usually ending up either lying centrally or going up into the right upper quadrant (Fig. 9–28). Volvulus is usually associated with large bowel ob-

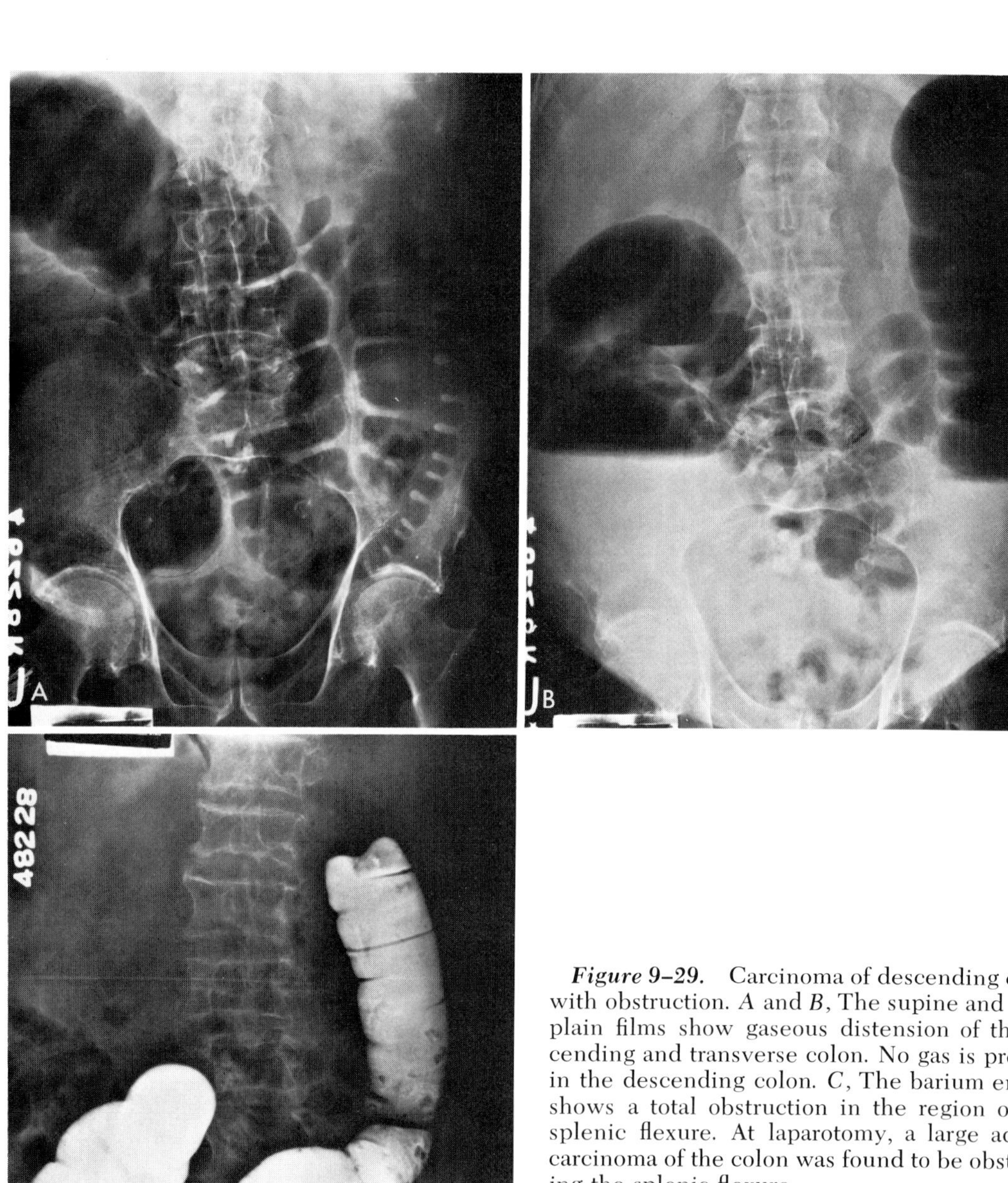

Figure 9–29. Carcinoma of descending colon with obstruction. *A* and *B*, The supine and erect plain films show gaseous distension of the ascending and transverse colon. No gas is present in the descending colon. *C*, The barium enema shows a total obstruction in the region of the splenic flexure. At laparotomy, a large adenocarcinoma of the colon was found to be obstructing the splenic flexure.

struction and gaseous distension of the ascending, transverse, and descending colons. Volvulus of the small bowel is rare but does occur in infants and produces a radiographic picture similar to that of small bowel obstruction, except that occasionally the twisted loop fills with fluid and appears as a pseudotumor.

Case A17

Sabin Beauchamp, age 68, a poetry reader well known to the Mothers Union, presented with abdominal pain and increasing constipation. On examination, no abnormality was found apart from increased bowel sounds. A plain film of the abdomen was taken (Fig. 9–29A). What does it show?

The gaseous distension of the transverse colon suggests obstruction, but this appearance may also be seen in ileus. The bowel wall appears to be of normal thickness (i.e., there is no edema), and no gas can be seen in the descending colon. This suggests a constricting lesion in the region of the splenic flexure. A barium enema confirmed the presence of carcinoma of the descending colon at this site (Fig. 9–29B).

Mechanical obstruction of the small bowel also leads to differential air-fluid levels as well as to gaseous distension. One way to differentiate small-bowel from large-bowel obstruction is to look for the linear shadows of the valvulae conniventes, which traverse the distended loops of small bowel and are not present in the colon (Fig. 9–30). Also, if one remembers normal intestinal anatomy, it is often relatively easy to distinguish the distended bowel and to make an educated guess about the level of obstruction.

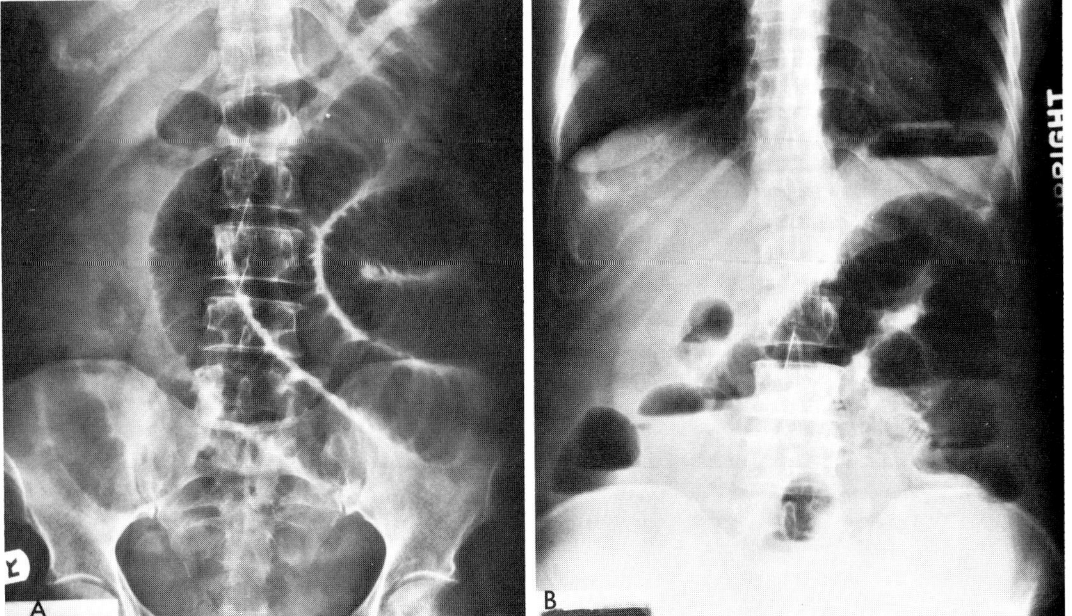

Figure 9–30. Small bowel obstruction, *(A)* supine, *(B)* erect films. In this 53-year-old woman with adhesions due to previous surgical procedures obstructing the terminal ileum, the characteristic appearances of small bowel obstruction can be seen. On the supine film the transverse valvulae conniventes are well seen running transversely across the distended loops of bowel. On the erect film multiple differential fluid levels can be seen.

Case A18

Ursula Tarrystone, age 86, had her appendix removed as a precaution before setting out as the cook on an expedition up Mount Everest. Five days following the operation, however, she was complaining of abdominal distension, some pain, and a total lack of bowel motion. On examination, there were no bowel sounds. A plain film of the abdomen was taken (Fig. 9–31). What does it show?

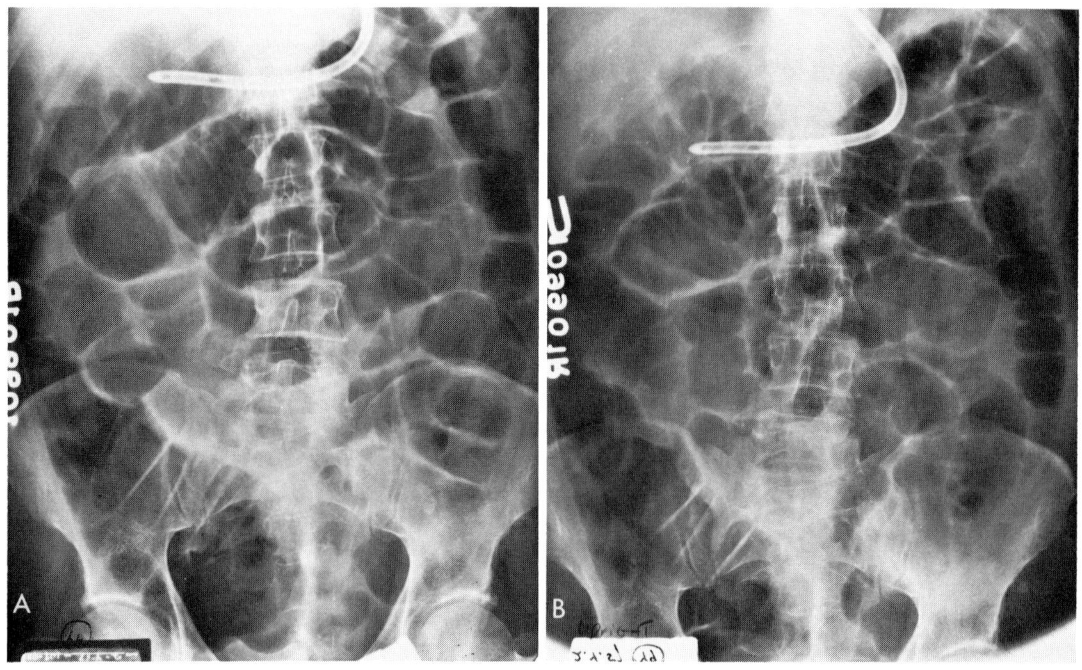

Figure 9–31. Intestinal ileus, supine KUB (*A*) and erect KUB (*B*). Note the widespread dilatation of bowel loops with gas apparently in the intestine from the stomach to the rectum, a typical finding in ileus.

The diagnosis of intestinal ileus is usually easy to make. Bowel sounds are absent, and gas is present from the stomach to the rectum and is visible in both small and large bowel. If present, air-fluid levels are usually at an equal level in a single loop of bowel.

There are many causes of generalized adynamic ileus, but ileus occurs in most patients after intra-abdominal surgery and may last as long as 10 days postoperatively. Ileus also occurs as a result of biochemical calamities such as severe hypokalemia, in association with various drug therapies and infections—particularly peritonitis—and in pneumonia, myocardial infarction, and spinal cord injury. Earlier in this chapter, ileus in the form of a "sentinel loop" was illustrated in association with cholecystitis, pancreatitis, and appendicitis. Most forms of ileus respond to treatment of the underlying disorder. If ileus is more than minimal and temporary, an intestinal decompression tube (Miller–Abbott, Kantor, or Harris) is used.

One other cause of pain and change of bowel habit reminds us that in certain parts of the world diarrhea is not uncommonly caused by parasitic infestations (Fig. 9–32). One in every four people in the world is infested with *Ascaris lumbricoides*, and if the worm settles in the intestine, the patient experiences colicky abdominal pain, distension, and diarrhea. Occasionally, so many worms are present that a mechanical obstruction may occur.

The three most common causes of diarrhea in North America and Europe are probably ulcerative colitis, gastroenteritis, and

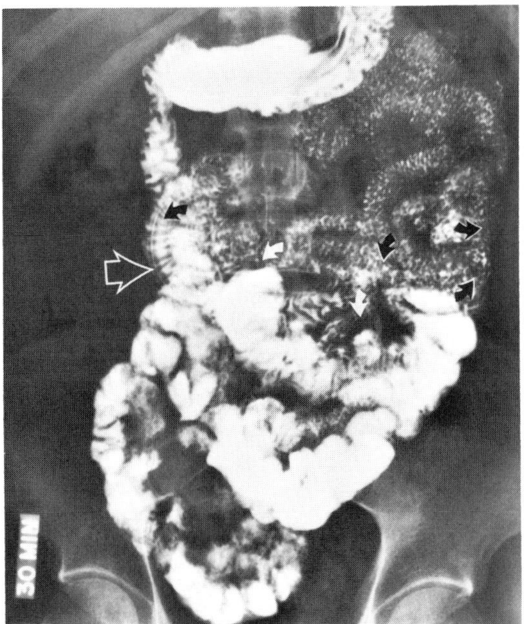

Figure 9–32. Ascariasis. On the small bowel follow-through film, the proximal jejunum shows tubular filling defects (*arrows*) with a streak of barium running down within one of these shadows (*hollow arrow*). These defects represent ascaris worms, one of which has swallowed barium outlining its alimentary tract! This young man had recently visited Mexico.

diverticulitis; these are dealt with later in the chapter.

CHANGE OF BOWEL HABIT

For a patient to present with a change of bowel habit alone is fairly unusual, because most forms of obstruction are accompanied by pain. Ileus is usually associated with abdominal discomfort. Ulcerative colitis is nearly always associated with some bleeding and may or may not be accompanied by pain. Many cancers of the bowel are associated with weight loss, blood in the stools, and pain. Diverticulitis is usually very painful. Thus, although the subdivisions used in this chapter may seem artificial, there is probably only one true cause of chronic diarrhea without other symptoms: a malabsorption syndrome.

The term *malabsorption syndrome* describes a large group of conditions of extremely varied etiology, including sprue, celiac disease, blind loop syndrome, pancreatic insufficiency, parasitic infections, collagen diseases, some inflammatory diseases of the bowel, and several infiltrative disorders such as lymphosarcoma and Whipple's disease.

The radiographic picture bears little relationship to the severity of the disorder, and in fact a small bowel follow-through may seem normal even in a patient with severe non-tropical sprue. Attempts have been made to challenge the bowel by adding sucrose, lactose, gluten, and other antagonists, but the results have not been constant.

Case A19

Crustacea Wigwam, age 44, was a missionary in Malaysia, where it was difficult for her to adhere to the strict gluten-free diet that her doctor had prescribed for long-standing non-tropical sprue. A routine examination showed that she had lost a considerable amount of weight, and she reported having liquid and semisolid stools 10 to 12 times a day. A small bowel follow-through was performed (Fig. 9–33). What does it show?

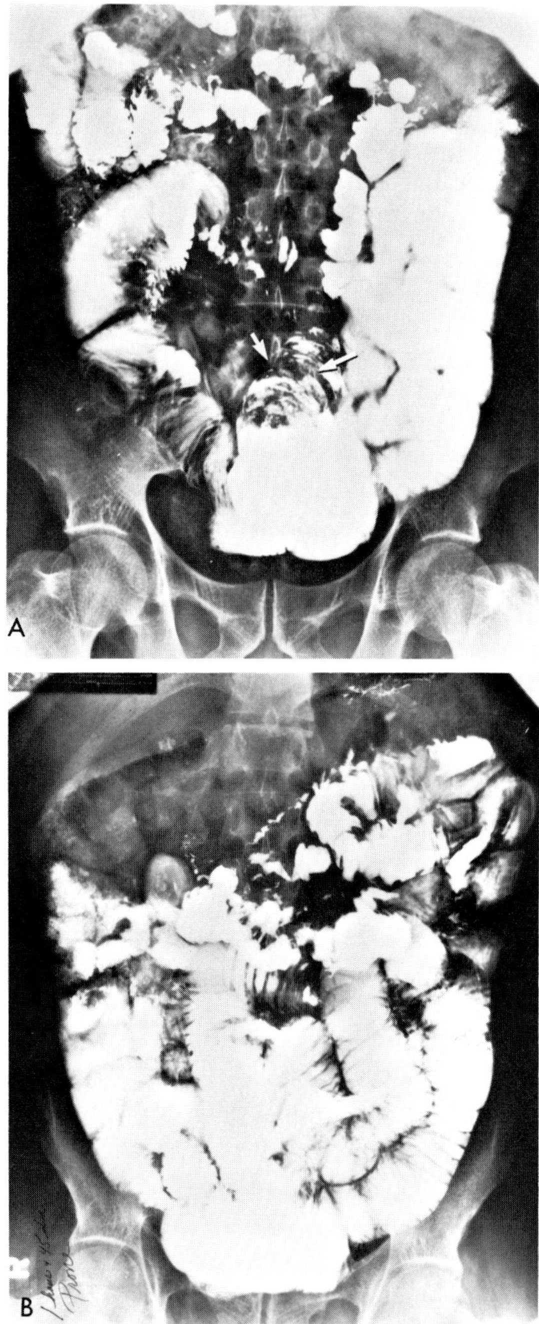

Figure 9–33. Malabsorption syndrome. *A* and *B*, Small bowel follow-through films. Curious appearance of the barium with flocculation, separation, and poor mixing as well as the featureless appearance of the dilated small intestinal loops are characteristic of malabsorption syndrome, in this case typical nontropical sprue. Note the "coiled spring" appearance of the barium-filled bowel loops (*arrows*) in *A*.

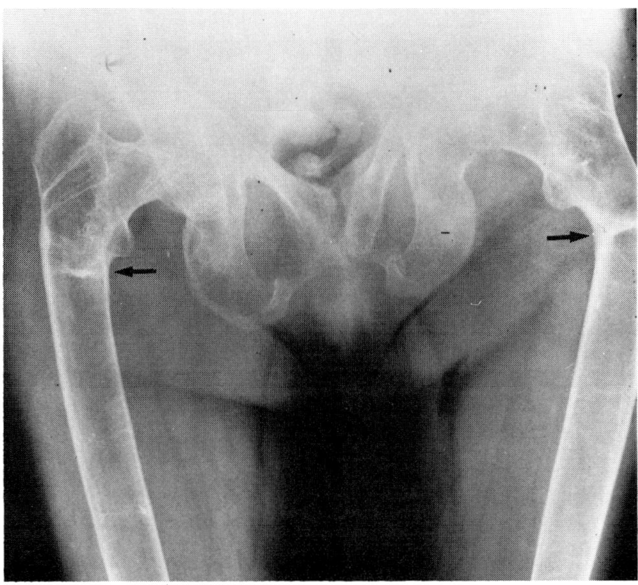

Figure 9–34. Osteomalacia. This 45-year-old female patient had longstanding osteomalacia secondary to biliary cirrhosis. In the film of the upper femurs, extreme demineralization and loss of trabeculae of the whole skeleton with pseudofractures, Looser zones (*arrows*), and bending can be seen.

The classic radiographic features of malabsorption include flocculation and segmentation of barium (although to some extent this will depend on the type of barium used), effacement of the mucosal pattern, dilated loops of bowel with thickened folds, decreased motility, apparent discontinuity of bowel loops, and evidence of hypersecretion. Different barium mixtures may give different appearances, and a colloidal barium small bowel follow-through may look relatively normal in a patient with a malabsorption syndrome. The problem for the patient, however, is not the intestine's radiographic appearance, but the underlying metabolic sequelae of malabsorption. Obviously, severe loss of weight occurs, and it may be associated with protein-losing enteropathy, steatorrhea, anemia (particularly megaloblastic), and deficiency of various minerals and vitamins. Figure 9–34 is a film of a patient with a malabsorption disease. What does it show?

"SILENT" GASTROINTESTINAL BLEEDING

"Silent" gastrointestinal bleeding is very common in patients complaining of either frank blood in the feces or tarry stools. The level of bleeding as well as the volume of blood lost determines the color of the stools, which may range from black to bright red. The most common cause of bright red blood in the stools is hemorrhoids, but they are usually associated with some anal discomfort and are easily diagnosed clinically. Most patients with severe gastrointestinal bleeding have associated symptoms, such as pain with a bleeding gastric or duodenal ulcer or loss of weight and discomfort with most intestinal malignancies. Two sources of relatively silent gastrointestinal bleeding, the first in the upper alimentary tract and the second in the colon, are discussed.

A routine procedure for investigating silent gastrointestinal bleeding should be established. After a carefully obtained clinical history and examination, the patient should first have a barium enema and then an upper gastrointestinal series. If the symptoms are initially suggestive of a lesion in the upper intestine, the UGI should be done first. Because the barium may remain in the colon for 24 to 48 hours or even longer following a UGI, however, an adequate barium enema must be postponed until the barium has been passed.

Case A20

Mr. Lionel Fegato, age 62, was a well-known society figure who had been seen propping up most of the bars in town. He was admitted with anemia and complaining of weakness and black tarry feces. On examination, he was found to be slightly jaundiced, and his liver was not palpable. A chest x-ray and plain film of his abdomen were normal. A barium enema was performed, and apart from showing a few colonic diverticula it was normal. A barium swallow and an upper gastrointestinal series were then performed (Fig. 9–35). What do they show?

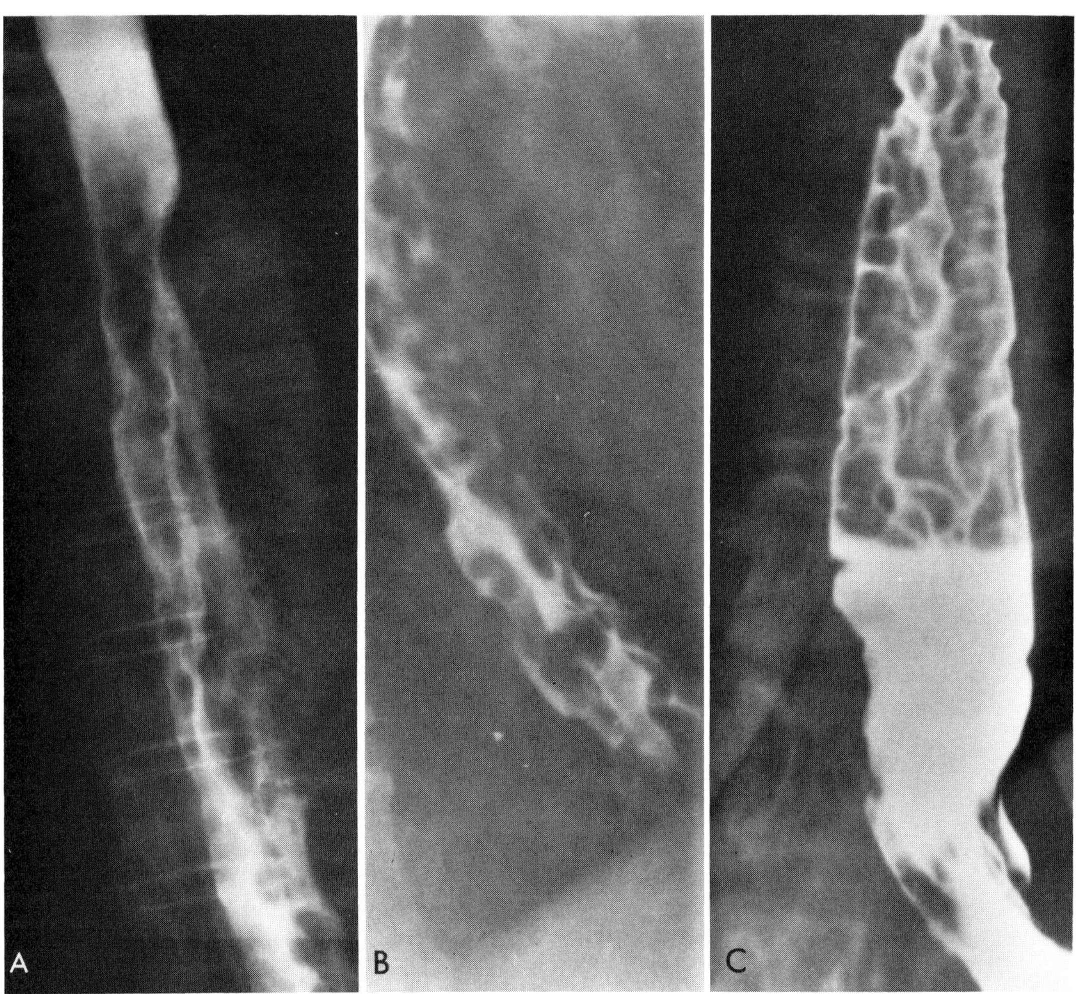

Figure 9–35. Esophageal varices. *A* and *B*, Films from the barium swallow show multiple rounded filling defects as well as the longer linear irregularities throughout the distal esophagus. *C*, When the patient performs the Valsalva maneuver, these defects become more obvious. These appearances are typical of esophageal varices.

The diagnosis of esophageal varices often depends entirely on the radiologist, although the clinical history may be suggestive. In portal hypertension (an increased pressure gradient in the blood vessels of the liver, which can result from several conditions), collateral veins that allow drainage from the portal to the systemic venous system may open up at the sites of anastomosis between portal and systemic veins. Collateral veins (*varices*) usually develop in the fundus of the stomach and in the lower esophagus. The radiologist attempts to visualize the varices by having the patient perform a Valsalva maneuver, which raises the pressure within the varices, thus distending them. It is usually possible to differentiate between varices and reflux esophagitis, another cause of upper gastrointestinal bleeding.

Case A21

Mrs. Charlton F. Bluebottle, age 72, the wife of a well-known entomologist, was admitted for investigation following persistent spotting of blood in the feces. Hemorrhoids had been excluded by clinical examination and proctoscopy. After adequate preparation, a barium enema was performed (Fig. 9–36). What does it show?

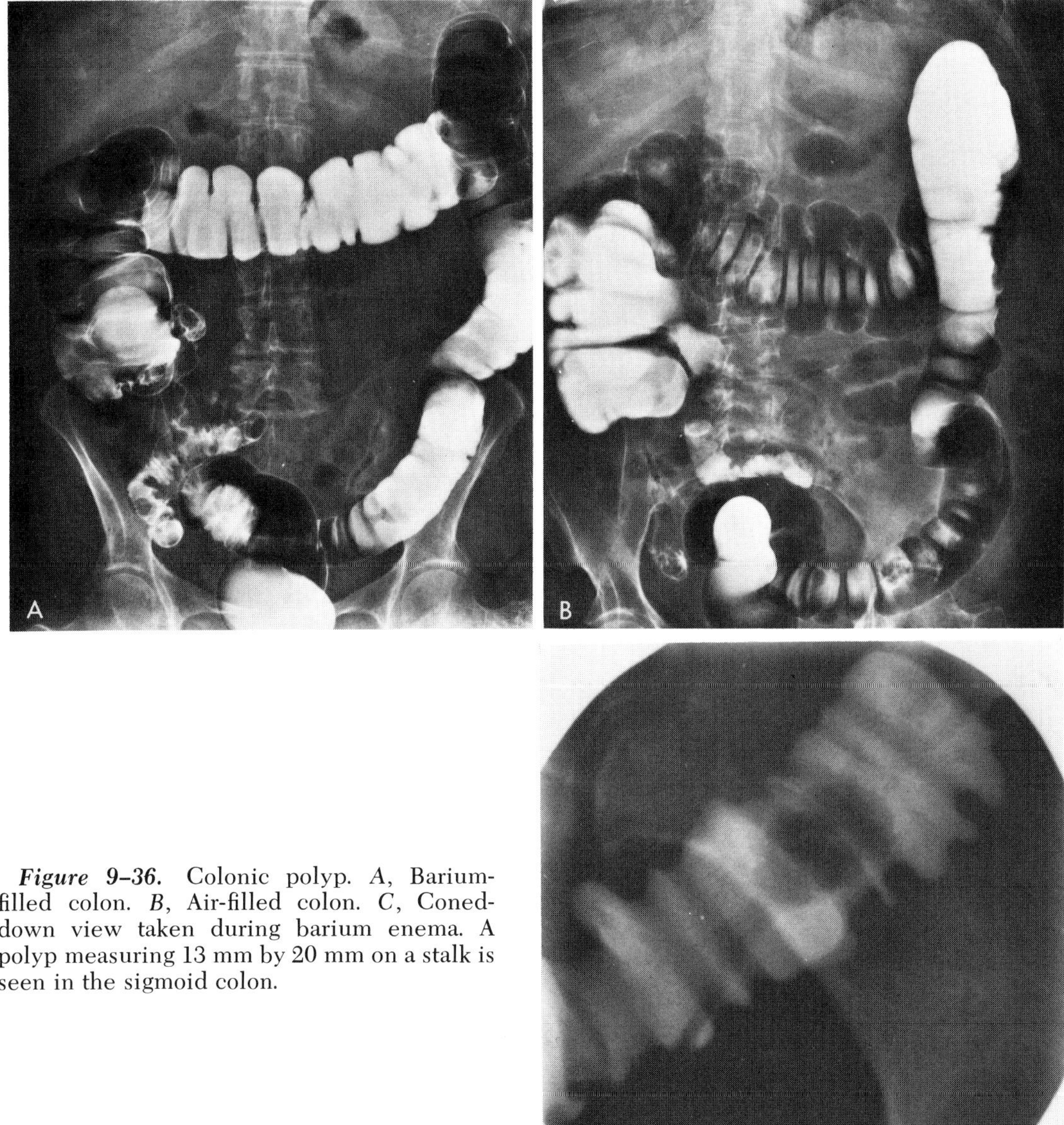

Figure 9–36. Colonic polyp. *A*, Barium-filled colon. *B*, Air-filled colon. *C*, Coned-down view taken during barium enema. A polyp measuring 13 mm by 20 mm on a stalk is seen in the sigmoid colon.

Most causes of upper gastrointestinal bleeding are accompanied by pain, and most causes of lower gastrointestinal bleeding are associated with both pain and a change of bowel habit. But there is one cause of "silent" lower gastrointestinal bleeding of importance; Mrs. Bluebottle's x-ray shows a large solitary polyp on a stalk in the colon. Treatment of this is controversial, because according to pathologists, all polyps greater than 10 mm are actually or potentially malignant. If this patient were your mother, what would you recommend?

If the polyp is less than 10 mm in size and has a long stalk, it can be followed by periodic barium enema studies. If it is greater than 10 mm, it can be removed, a procedure that has been facilitated by the use of the fibro-optic endoscope. If the radiologist finds one polyp, he should always look for more because they are often multifocal. Finally, one must remember that there are various syndromes associated with both small and large bowel polyps, including Peutz-Jeghers syndrome (multiple gastrointestinal polyps and perioral pigmentation).

Perhaps a more important radiological factor in the diagnosis of polyps is whether the filling defect seen on the barium enema film is actually a polyp or some retained fecal material. As has been mentioned previously, it is important to adequately cleanse the colon prior to performing a barium enema. Surprisingly, this procedure is often neglected. It is frequently necessary to perform a second barium enema to confirm the presence of a polyp before subjecting the patient to colonoscopy.

GASTROINTESTINAL BLEEDING AND PAIN

Now we can turn our attention to a group of important gastrointestinal disorders that present primarily with pain and bleeding.

Case A22

Ponsonby Guzzler, age 27, had had recurrent abdominal pain for 5 years that came on about 2 hours after meals. He was a junior executive with a large x-ray machine manufacturing company, and often the strain of talking to radiologists every day became too much for him. He ate irregularly and frequently supplemented his food with martinis. He was admitted to hospital complaining of black tarry stools and vomiting blood. An upper gastrointestinal series was performed (Fig. 9–37). What does it show?

There is an obvious "trefoil" deformity of the duodenal cap, with distortion of the first part of the duodenal sweep. The diagnosis of duodenal ulceration is easy to make, but can it be identified as an acute or chronic ulcer on the basis of radiographs alone? Not unless there are previous films for comparison. Often with a clinical history of acute ulceration, one can see marked mucosal edema in the duodenum on the UGI films. Should a second study be performed four to six weeks later, the edema is seen to have subsided, although the crater is usually still present. Thus, in patients with a long history of ulceration, differentiating between an acute ulcer and a scarred crater is often impossible. Over 80 per cent of duodenal ulcers occur in the bulb, but they will sometimes occur in the post-bulbar part of the duodenum, where they are often easier to diagnose because of the localized spasm they produce. Also, multiple and recurrent peptic ulceration both in the duodenal bulb and in the stomach may be a manifestation of the Zollinger-Ellison syndrome, which is caused by a non-beta cell islet tumor of the pancreas.

Another complication of duodenal ulceration is perforation. Since perforation often occurs after an alcoholic debauch, the diagnosis may be facilitated by the presence of a large air-fluid level in the abdomen or of air under the diaphragm on an erect chest radiograph (Fig. 9–38).

A single duodenal ulcer is usually managed by medical therapy, and in many hospitals a second upper gastrointestinal series is performed six to eight weeks after the

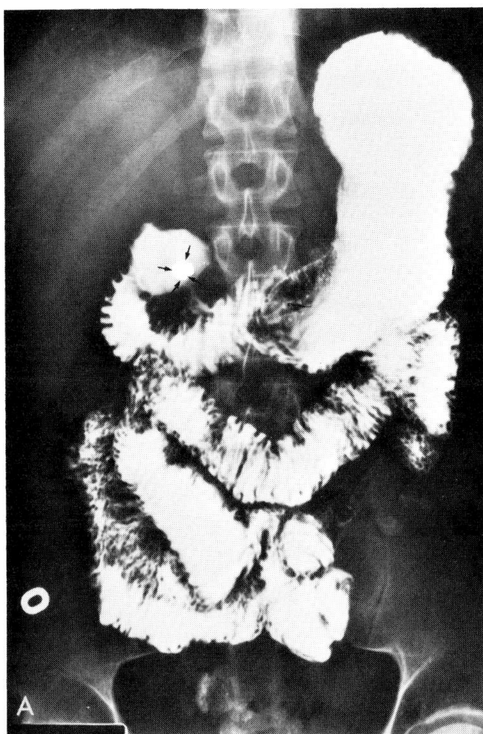

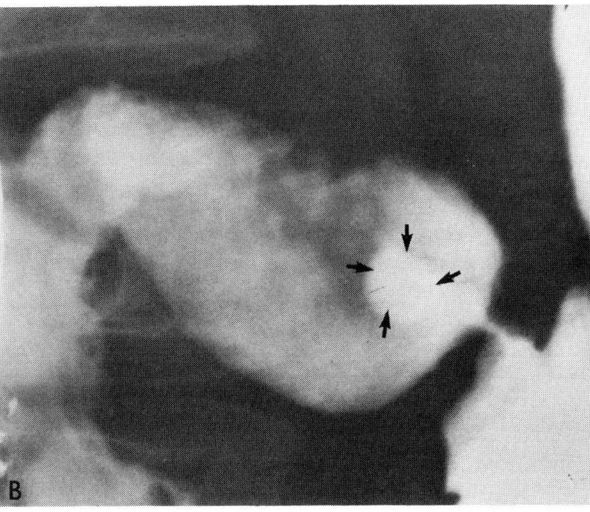

Figure 9–37. Duodenal ulcer. *A*, Film from upper gastrointestinal series. *B*, Coned-down view. A duodenal ulcer measuring 1 cm in diameter and 0.5 cm in depth is demonstrated on the posterior aspect of the bulb (*arrows*). No other abnormality can be seen. Note the normal small bowel mucosal pattern.

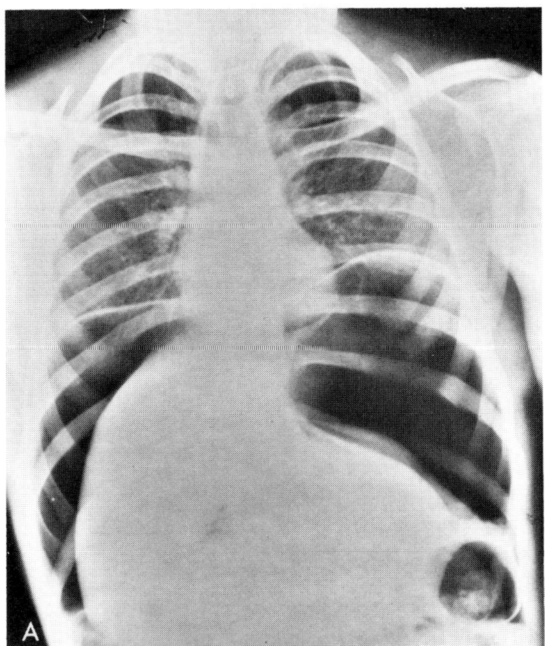

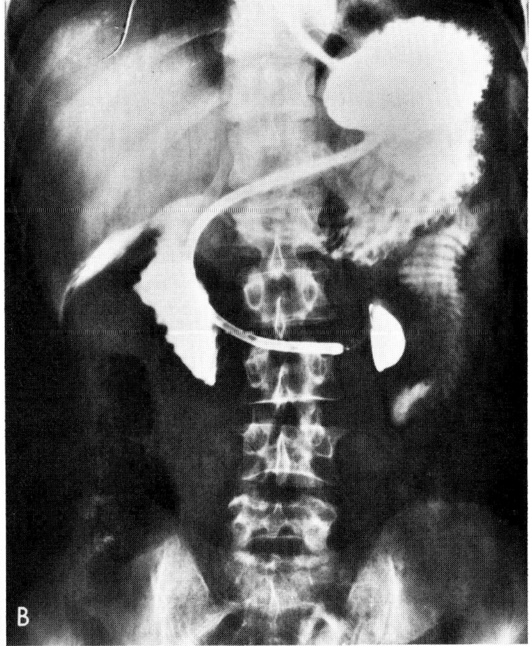

Figure 9–38. Duodenal ulcer and perforation in a patient with Zollinger-Ellison syndrome. This 37-year-old man had a long history of repeated gastric and duodenal ulceration. On this occasion he presented with intense abdominal pain. *A*, A PA chest x-ray reveals a large amount of free intraperitoneal air. *B*, Some Gastrografin given by mouth shows edematous gastric mucosal folds, obstruction of the third part of the duodenum, and a perforation just beyond the duodenal bulb. The patient had voluminous gastric secretion with a high acid content. At laparotomy, multiple pancreatic adenomata of the benign islet cell type were found.

initial study. This second study is often relatively useless because of the scarring that frequently occurs as a result of the initial insult to the mucosa. In the opinion of many authorities, a second UGI series is unnecessary unless complications occur. In any case, an upper gastrointestinal series should not be performed too soon after the initiation of therapy, and radiographic studies performed at frequent intervals should not be expected to show dramatic changes.

Recurrent hemorrhage or severe scarring may lead to a surgical bypass operation, and a partial gastrectomy with a jejunogastric anastomosis (Billroth II) operation is commonly used both for chronic duodenal ulceration and for other lesions of the gastric antrum. One complication of this operation is that ulcers may develop in the stomal area if there is still an increased level of secretion of gastric acid (Fig. 9–39). These ulcers may be difficult to diagnose because of surgically produced mucosal irregularities, although mucosal edema and spasm frequently accompany stomal ulcers.

Another complication of upper gastrointestinal ulceration is hemorrhage, which may be either catastrophic bleeding or just gentle oozing over a long period of time. If bleeding is severe, a selective angiogram to determine the site is important. Formerly, approaches to control bleeding included oral medication and diet or surgical resection, depending on the severity of the bleeding. The radiologist now has a highly valued role to play in the management of bleeding. He can embolize the bleeding vessel by injecting prepared coagulant or Gelfoam, or he can slow and stop the bleeding by administering vasoconstrictors to the site via a precisely placed intravascular catheter.

Subphrenic abscess is also a complication of perforated ulcer or of surgery for ulceration; the diagnosis and radiographic appearance of this lesion are discussed earlier in this chapter.

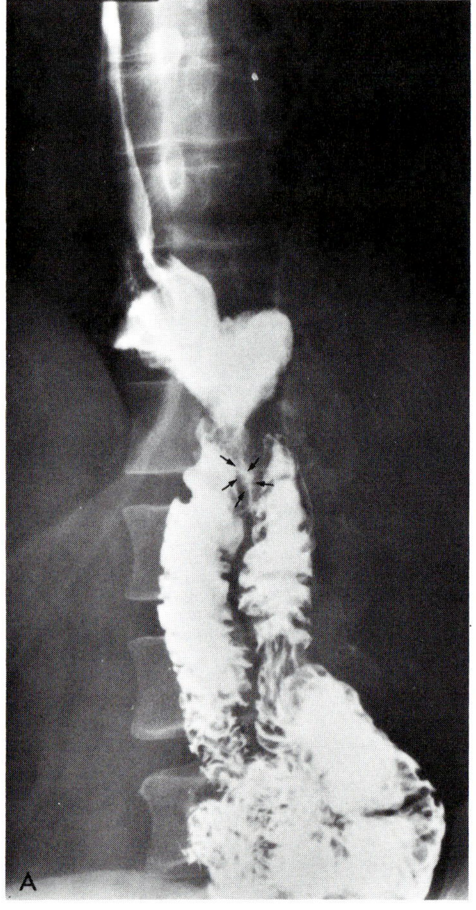

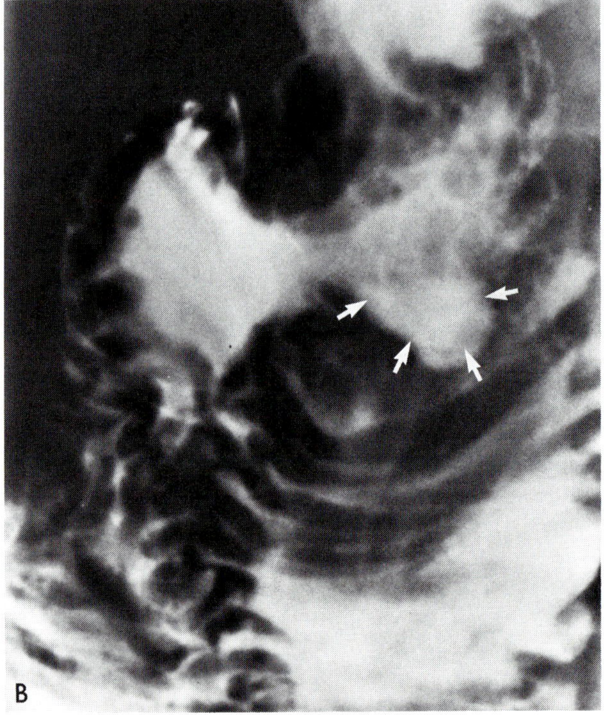

Figure 9–39. Marginal ulcer. *A*, Film from upper gastrointestinal series. *B*, Coned-down view. Ten years before these films were taken, the 45-year-old male patient had a subtotal gastrectomy, vagotomy, and gastrojejunostomy for ulcer disease. The barium outlines a small gastric remnant with free flow into both the efferent and the afferent loops. The small bowel appears normal except for a 1-cm ulcer in the jejunum just distal to the anastomosis (*arrows*).

Case A23

Wilfreda Swaine, age 68, widow for 28 years of a well-known multimillionaire, came to her family doctor complaining of abdominal pain and black stools. The laboratory reported that her stools were guaiac-positive, but the clinical examination found that she was normal except for mild tenderness in the left upper quadrant. A chest x-ray and plain film of the abdomen were taken, and an upper gastrointestinal series was performed (Fig. 9–40). What does it show?

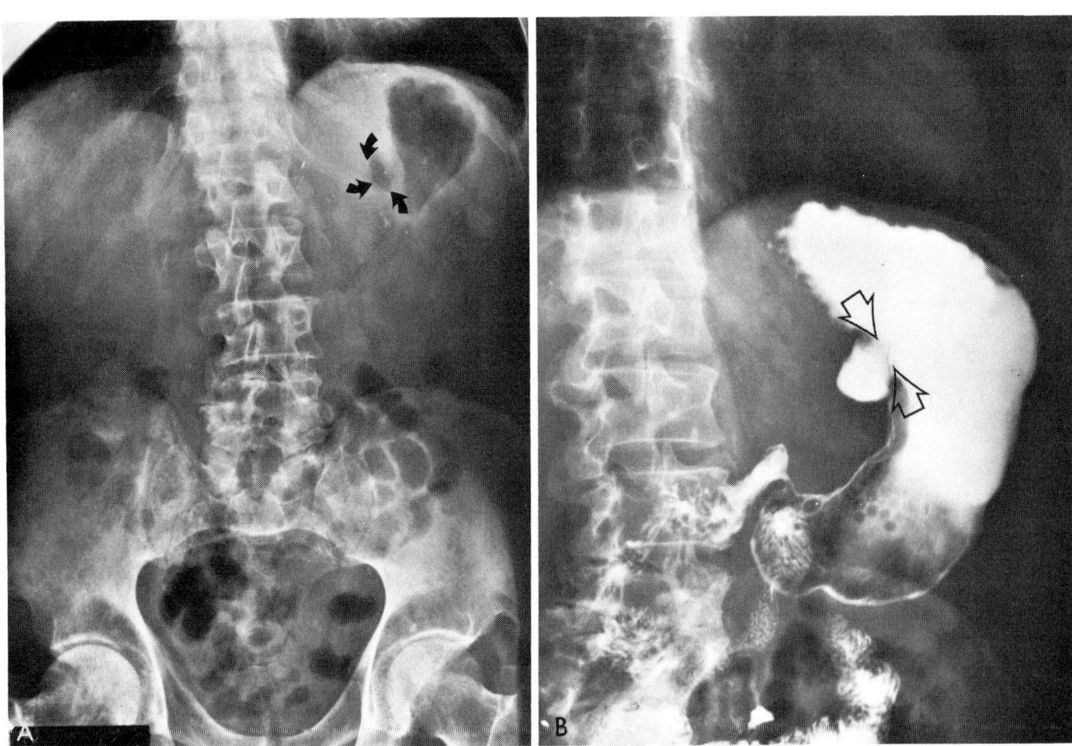

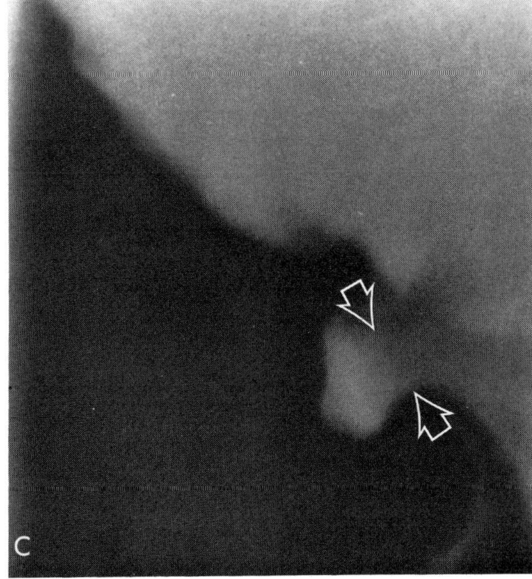

Figure 9–40. Benign gastric ulcer. *A*, The ulcer crater is outlined by gas (*arrows*). *B*, A film from an upper gastrointestinal series confirms the diagnosis. *C*, On a coned-down view from a UGI in a different patient, the appearances are similar. Note that the ulcers in both patients project outside the normal contour of the lesser curvature. The mucosal collar can be clearly seen (*hollow arrows*). Both ulcers proved on endoscopy to be benign.

Gastric ulcers behave differently from duodenal ulcers. On Mrs. Swaine's x-ray, there is a large crater lying on the lesser curvature of the stomach. The mucosal edema separating the ulcer from the stomach can also be seen as well as thick mucosal folds radiating in toward the crater. The ulcer appears to project beyond the stomach wall. These are all signs that the ulcer is probably benign, and radiographically one should be able to differentiate benign and malignant gastric ulcers in a high percentage of patients. In a malignant ulcer, the crater occurs in the mass that projects into the stomach, the mucosa both inside the crater and surrounding it are irregular, and there is often rigidity and the absence of peristalsis.

The correct procedure to follow radiographic diagnosis of a benign gastric ulcer is antacid therapy. About six to eight weeks later, a second upper gastrointestinal series should be done, at which time the crater should have decreased in size or should have healed completely. In some elderly patients, the radiographic appearance may remain virtually unchanged in spite of adequate medical therapy. If the patient is still clinically considered to have a benign gastric ulcer, another upper gastrointestinal series may be performed in a month or so. If there is any doubt at all about the diagnosis, however, endoscopy with biopsy is easy to perform, and the correct diagnosis can be easily made.

ABDOMINAL PAIN, CHANGE OF BOWEL HABIT, AND GASTROINTESTINAL BLEEDING

Four of the most important conditions of the gastrointestinal tract cause abdominal pain, a change of bowel habit, and some gastrointestinal bleeding. The most common condition is diverticulosis of the colon, which may be asymptomatic until the diverticula become inflamed (diverticulitis). The most serious condition is cancer of the stomach or colon; the initial sign of cancer may, however, be unexplained loss of weight. Two other conditions, ulcerative colitis and Crohn's disease, produce similar signs but have different consequences.

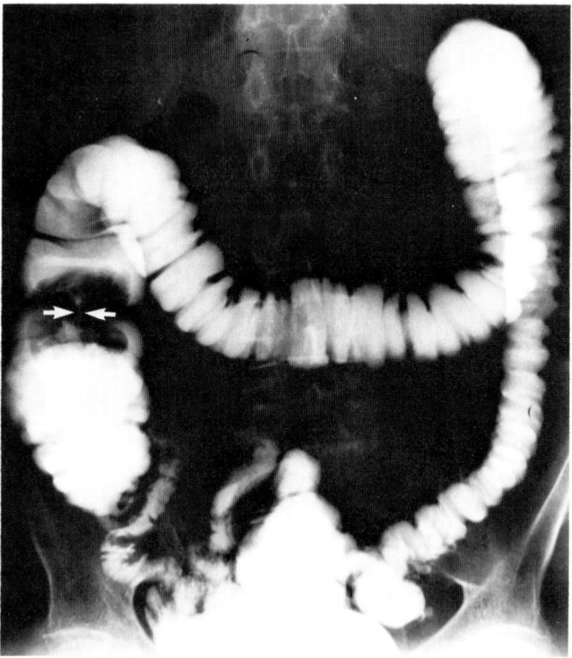

Figure 9–41. Carcinoma of the colon. On a film from a barium enema, there is a classic "apple-core" carcinoma of the ascending colon that shows the typical shoulders and narrow lumen (*arrows*), which has not yet become obstructed.

Case A24

Virgil Prunus, age 44, headmaster of an old established private boarding school who had a history of duodenal ulcer, went to his doctor complaining of vague upper abdominal pains, some loss of weight, and blood in the stools. On examination the doctor found no abnormality and sent him to the hospital for a barium enema study. The clever radiologist thought an upper gastrointestinal series was more appropriate. It demonstrated a duodenal ulcer, but the internist perservered and a barium enema study was performed at a later date (Fig. 9–41). What does it show?

There is a small apple-core constriction of the ascending colon that has not yet produced obstruction. The appearances are typical of a carcinoma of the colon. In this case it was found serendipitously, perhaps supporting the suggestion that all men over 40 should be given a yearly barium enema to detect such lesions, because the patient has a better chance of survival if colonic carcinoma is caught early.

Case A25

Felonious Fundworthy, age 64, was a nice man who resided in jail only because his occupation involved robbing banks. He complained of decreasing appetite and loss of weight associated with a fullness in his stomach. On examination the patient looked cachectic, and there was a large mass in the upper abdomen. An upper gastrointestinal series was performed (Fig. 9–42A). What does it show?

The clue to radiographic diagnosis is lack of peristalsis in the stomach (Figs. 9–42B and 9–42C). If this finding is associated with displacement of loops of jejunum, so that the stomach appears to be lying all by itself, the diagnosis of a large mass surrounding a small rigid infiltrated stomach becomes obvious. This appearance is typical of linitis plastica. Infiltration of the wall can be inferred from the fixed irregularity of the mucosal lining.

Linitis plastica is a relatively rare form of gastric carcinoma. Most carcinomas of the stomach are more localized and can cause gross deformities: they may be fungating or polypoid, they are usually associated with a large mass, and they occur most usually in the antrum or body of the stomach. Earlier in this chapter, benign ulcers of the stomach and the criteria for differentiating between benign and malignant lesions were discussed. It is possible to successfully differentiate between benign and malignant ulcers on the basis of a radiograph in a high percentage of cases. Figure 9–43 is a good example. Unlike a benign gastric ulcer, this lesion lies within the confines of the stomach, a large mass is associated with it, the mucosa is irregular, and there are no radiating folds running toward it. All these radiographic criteria suggest that this ulcer is malignant rather than benign.

Cancer may occur elsewhere in the gastrointestinal tract, and we have briefly dealt with carcinoma of the esophagus earlier in this chapter. Carcinoma of the small bowel is rare; it usually appears as a mass with mucosal infiltration and the presenting symptom may be small bowel obstruction. Large fungating carcinomas of the colon can be found in elderly patients presenting with constipation, and carcinoma of the pancreas is often silent, causing some secondary manifestations.

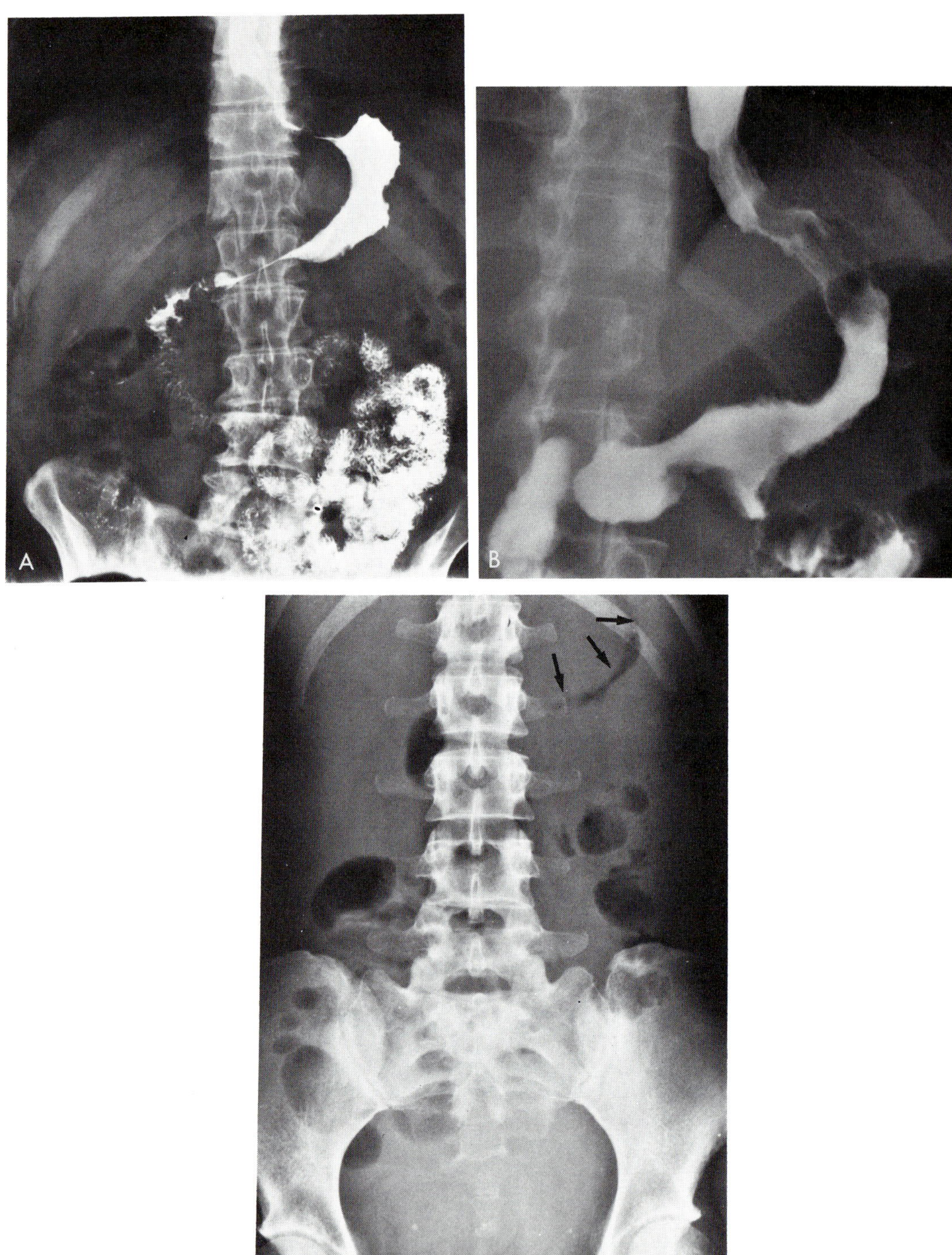

Figure 9–42. Linitis plastica or scirrhous carcinoma of the stomach. *A*, Upper gastrointestinal series. *B*, Upper gastrointestinal series from a second patient. *C*, Plain film of the second patient. The rigid appearance of the stomach, the mucosal irregularity, and the luminal narrowing are all characteristic of a scirrhous carcinoma of the stomach. The total lack of peristalsis is demonstrated by the fact that the rigid stomach contains gas even on the plain film (*arrows*). Note that the small bowel is displaced away from the stomach.

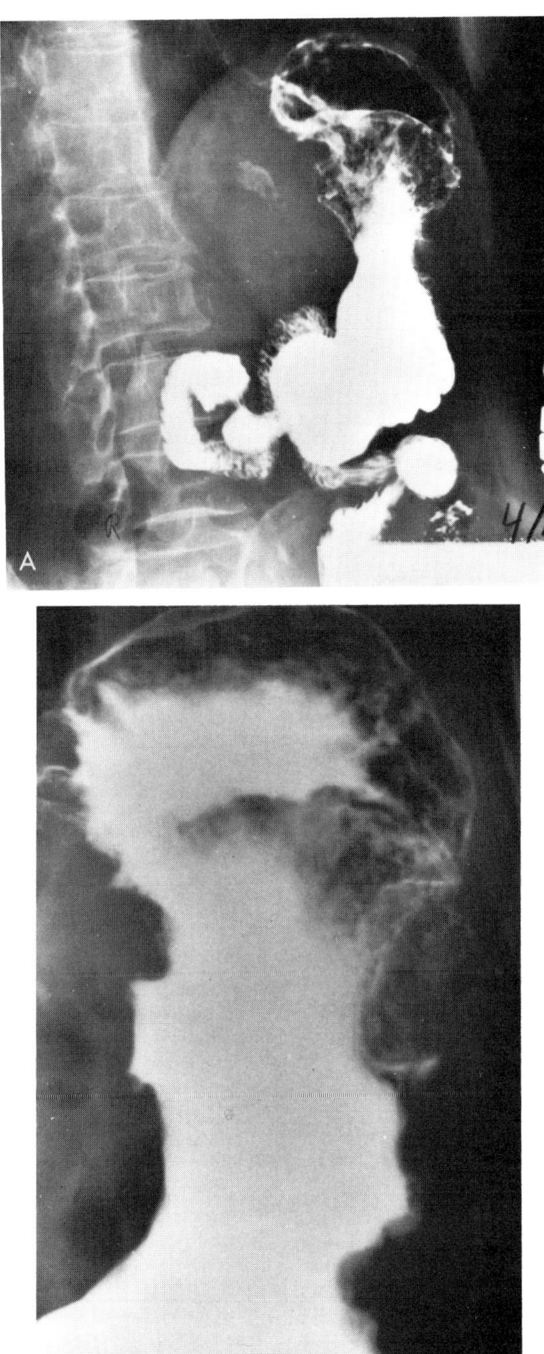

Figure 9–43. Malignant gastric ulcer. RAO view (*A*) and spot film from a UGI series (*B*). There is a large mass with marked distortion of the mucosal pattern involving both the greater and lesser curvatures of the stomach. The patient, a 60-year-old woman, had complained of weight loss and increasing fatigue.

Case A26

Mrs. Windi Van Passluft, age 72, was the proprietor of a small restaurant. She presented to her G.P. complaining of lower abdominal crampy pain, diarrhea, and some blood in the feces. On examination, she was found to have a tender mass in the left lower quadrant, and the doctor diagnosed a probable carcinoma. A barium enema shows otherwise (Fig. 9–44).

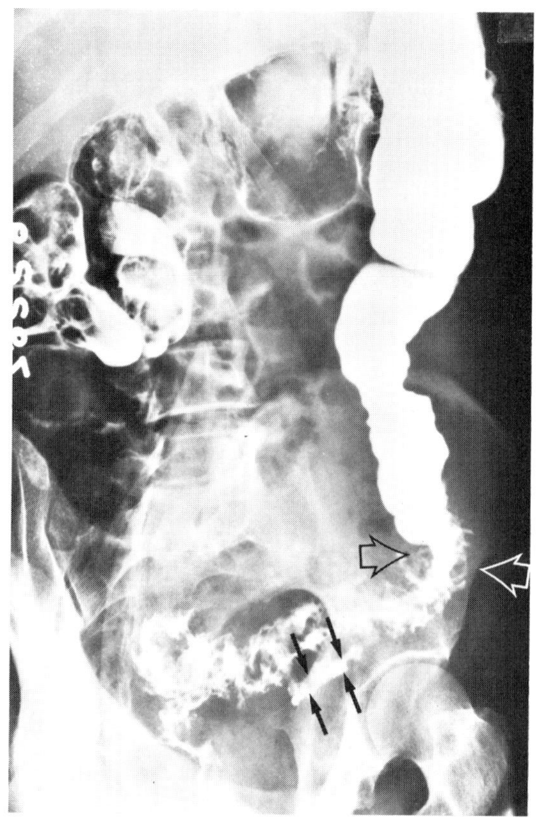

Figure 9–44. Diverticulitis with perforation. On a film of a barium enema, there is an area of narrowing with irregular mucosa in the sigmoid colon, and a collection of barium can be seen to lie outside the normal lumen (*arrows*). This represents a perforation with abscess formation. The spiky appearance of the mucosa is highly suggestive of diverticulitis (*hollow arrows*).

Diverticulitis accounts for more days off work or in hospital for elderly patients than all carcinomas of the gastrointestinal tract. With age, most people develop a chronic diverticulum or two, and although diverticulosis is rare under 40, most elderly patients will have some degree of involvement — usually of the sigmoid colon, although diverticula can occur in any segment of the colon.

Differentiating between diverticulitis and a colonic carcinoma may be difficult without endoscopy. The clinical picture of a tender lower-quadrant abdominal mass with bloody diarrhea, however, is more typical of diverticulitis. The radiographic appearances may also be misleading, but usually the irritability and colonic spasm seen in diverticulitis do not occur in cancer. Radiological differentiation between diverticulitis and diverticulosis is usually simple; a clinical history of pain and tenderness and the radiological picture of spasm, irritability, and a "spiked" appearance to the colon are diagnostic of diverticulitis. Several complications of diverticulitis can develop. Hemorrhage may occur, and selective angiography can be useful to pinpoint the bleeding site. Abscess formation is not uncommon, and occasionally fistulae will occur.

Diverticulosis is more common in North America and in Europe than in many of the developing countries, and the reason is said to be that people in this area of the world fail to eat enough "roughage." If cineradiography is employed, incoordination in the peristaltic waves of the affected segments of bowel may be documented. This localized increase in intraluminal pressure may force small outpouches of mucosa through the muscularis layer of the colon at the point of penetration of the blood vessels from the serosa to the submucosa. Figure 9–45 shows some examples of diverticulosis in older patients.

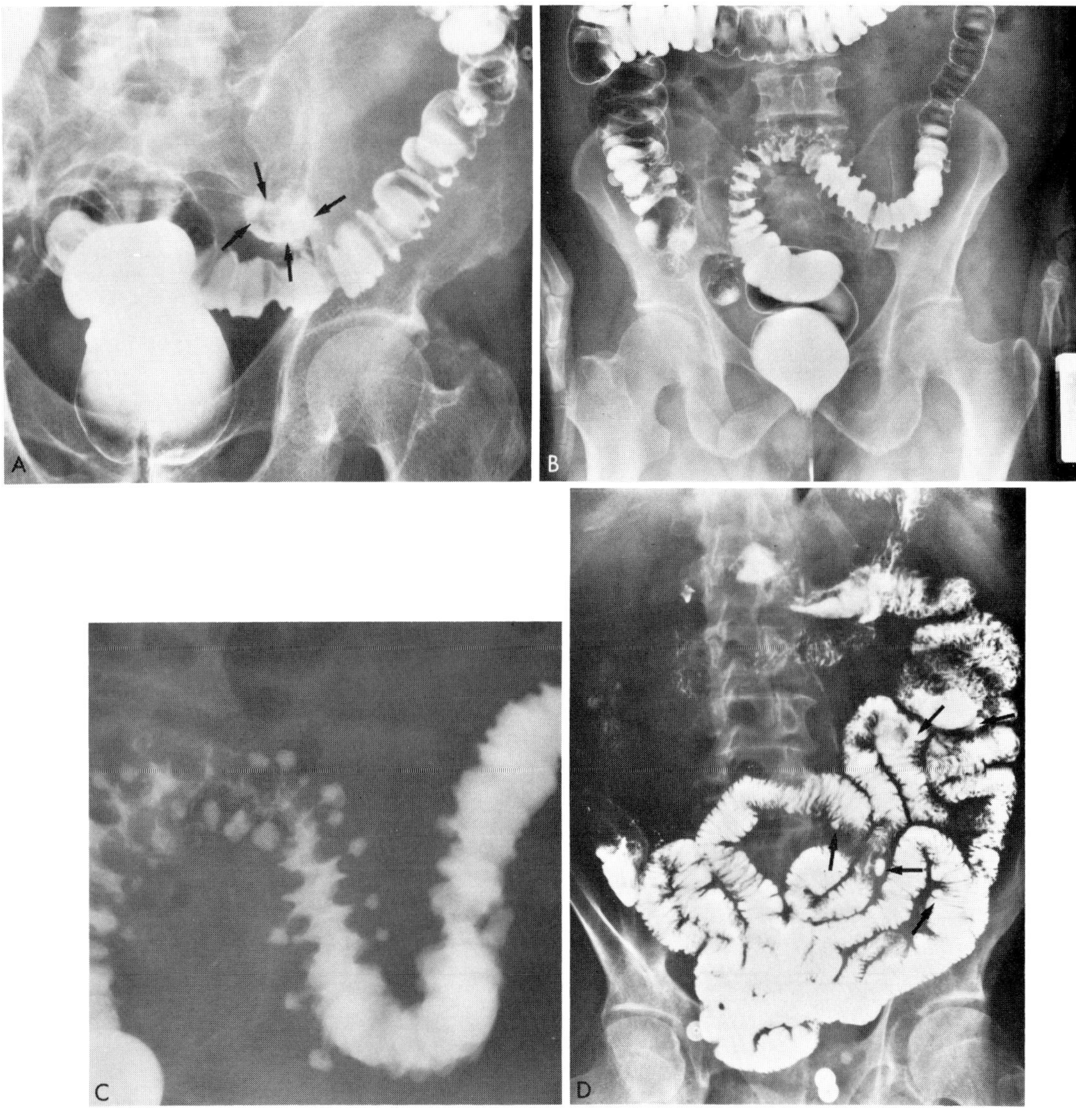

Figure 9–45. Diverticulosis. *A*, Barium enema showing some diverticula with a perforation and abscess (*arrows*). The 64-year-old man presented with rectal bleeding. *B* and *C*, Barium enema in a 60-year-old man with multiple colonic diverticula. The coned-down view (*C*) shows the characteristic appearance of sigmoid diverticulosis. *D*, Upper gastrointestinal series and small bowel follow-through showing multiple small bowel diverticula (*arrows*). This was considered to be an incidental finding in the 61-year-old man.

Case A27

Jeremiah Bookbasher, age 24, was a serious-minded, hard-working medical student who presented with loss of weight, decreasing appetite, and some diarrhea. Examination revealed no abnormality. A barium enema was normal. What would you do now? When the colon had been cleared of barium, a small bowel follow-through was performed which showed the classical changes of regional enteritis, or Crohn's disease (Fig. 9–46).

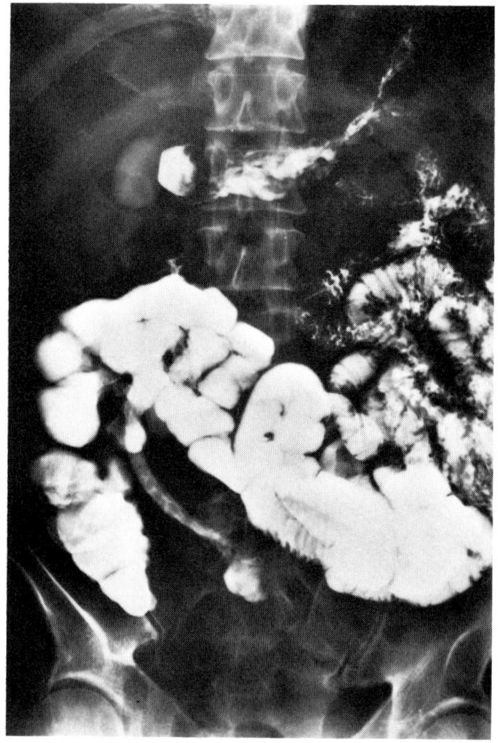

Figure 9–46. Regional enteritis involving terminal ileum. On a film taken during the small bowel follow-through, the distal part of the ileum shows loss of normal mucosal pattern, with marked narrowing of the last 12 inches of the terminal ileum (string sign). There are also some pressure defects on the cecum.

These films demonstrate the classic changes of regional enteritis: "skip" areas, mucosal irregularity, thickened folds, and evidence of fibrosis surrounding the area of the terminal ileum (*string sign*). In more severe cases, fistulae may develop, a large inflammatory mass may surround the involved segments, and small-bowel obstruction may occur. Rarer complications include perforation, subphrenic abscesses, sacroiliac arthritis, and liver disease.

Regional enteritis was originally described as involving the small intestine, predominantly the terminal ileum. It has been recently shown to involve any part of the gastrointestinal tract, including the esophagus and duodenum, and in approximately 40 per cent of cases the colon is also involved (Fig. 9–47). In fact, in many patients examined before this discovery, the originally described localized areas of ulcerative colitis in the large bowel probably represented solitary areas of granulomatous colitis. The radiographic appearance can be very similar to that of ulcerative colitis or even diverticulitis, although granulomatous

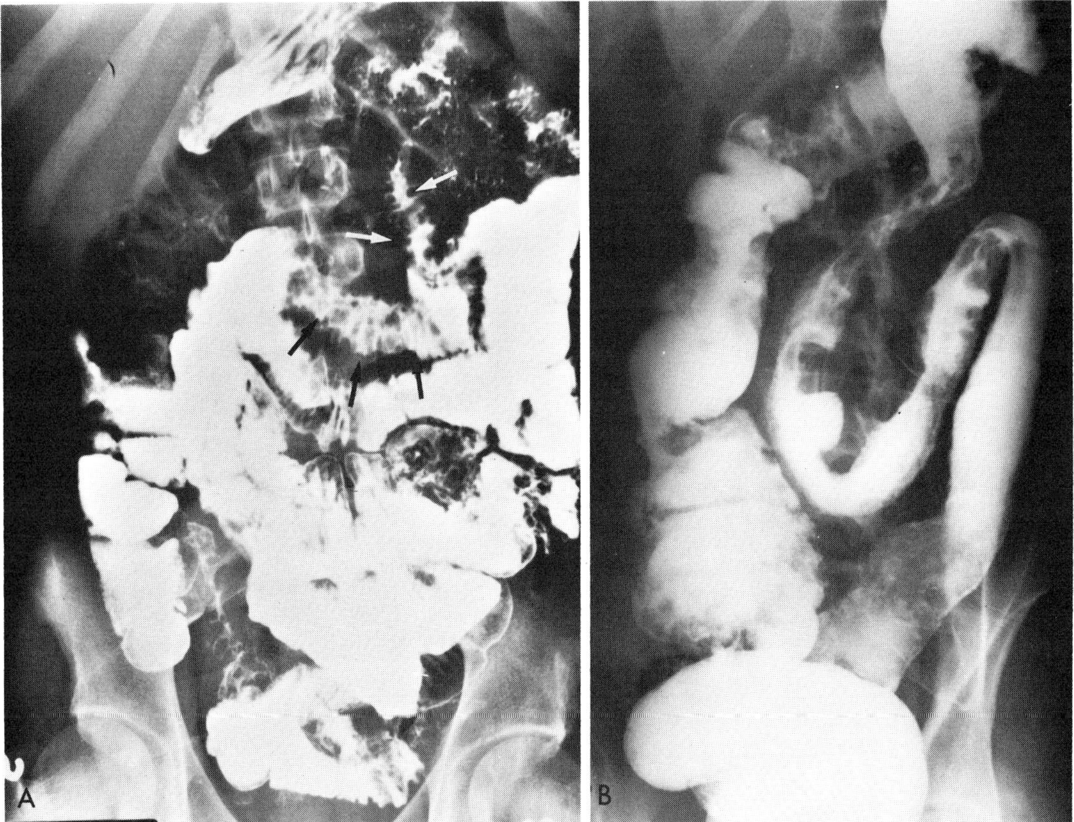

Figure 9–47. Regional enteritis. *A*, Jejunal involvement. This 17-year-old male patient had a five-year history of ileal involvement; note the similarity to the ileal involvement shown in Figure 9–46. The jejunum shows straightening, lack of coiling, and obvious mucosal abnormalities. *B*, Colonic involvement. Thickened mucosa is present throughout the colon but is most noticeable in the descending colon. Longitudinal ulceration with "skip areas" is present. These appearances are typical of granulomatous colitis.

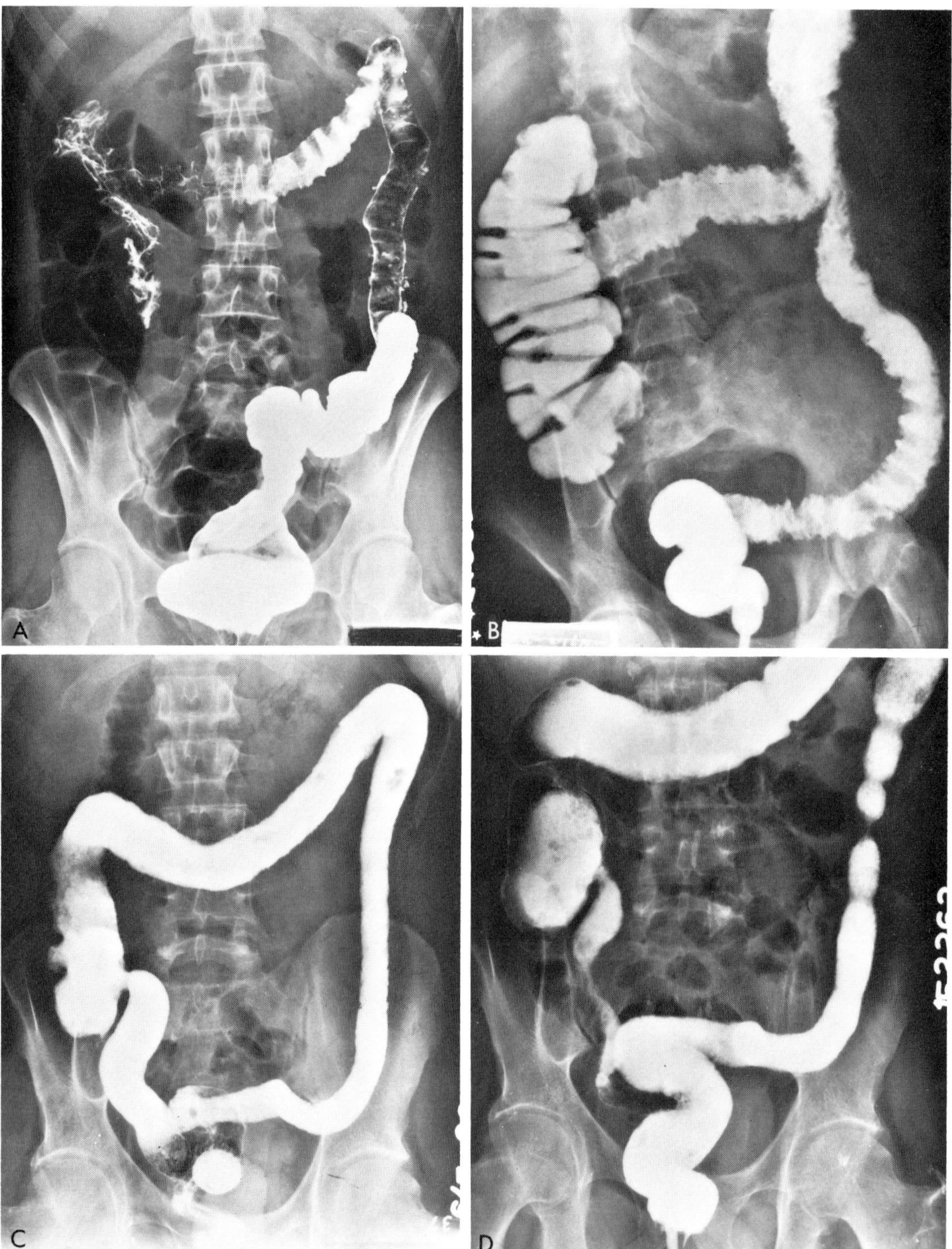

Figure 9–48. Ulcerative colitis. *A*, A barium enema shows the serration and ulceration of the mucosa of the left transverse and descending colon in this 40-year-old woman with early ulcerative colitis. *B*, In a young man with a more advanced case of ulcerative colitis, the loss of haustral pattern and marked mucosal irregularity and ulceration are seen in the transverse and descending colon. *C*, A film of the same patient taken five years later shows that the colon has become shrunken, scarred, and rather featureless. Note that similar changes involve the cecum and terminal ileum (backwash iliitis). *D*, This film of a 28-year-old man shows "lead piping" of the colon, with loss of haustra and narrowing, shortening, and rigidity of the colon. Multiple small filling defects, which can be seen particularly in the cecal area, represent remaining islands of normal mucosa and are known as "pseudopolyps." Note that backwash iliitis is also present.

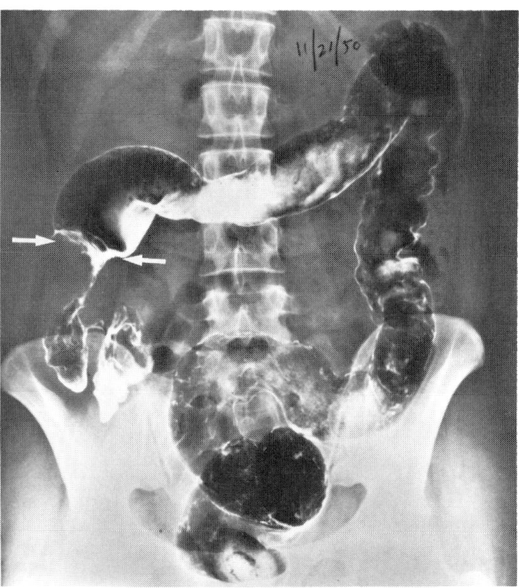

Figure 9–49. Carcinoma of the colon in association with ulcerative colitis. This 32-year-old woman had had severe colitis since age 8. On a film from the barium enema, the featureless character of the colon can be seen with some shortening and rigidity. There is a stricture of the ascending colon with shoulders (*arrows*); this is characteristic of a carcinoma.

colitis predominantly involves the right side of the colon. The appearance of thickened mucosal folds in association with colonic wall thickening, fistula formation, longitudinal ulcerations, and skip areas should suggest granulomatous colitis rather than ulcerative colitis (Fig. 9–47B).

The early diagnosis of ulcerative colitis is rarely made radiologically, however, because the barium enema often initially appears normal except possibly for some irritability of the colon. On closer scrutiny, very fine serrations representing minute ulcers can be seen to lie outside the normal contour of the bowel; they usually occur in the sigmoid region. As ulcerative colitis progresses, the submucosal ulcerations become larger, and the normal mucosal pattern is totally effaced, with loss of the normal haustral markings and decreased peristalsis. These changes mainly involve the left colon, and the presacral soft-tissue space is often widened (Fig. 9–48).

As ulcerative colitis evolves, a characteristic appearance of pseudopolyps and large mucosal ulcerations occurs producing a "cobblestone" appearance. The individual ulcerations are described as "collar-button" ulcers. In long-standing ulcerative colitis there is rigidity and shortening of the bowel, and reflux will occur into the terminal ileum *(reflux ileitis)*, causing dilatation and mucosal irregularity. There is an increased incidence of colonic carcinoma associated with ulcerative colitis, which characteristically occurs in younger patients who have had the disease for a long period of time. Detection of this malignant change is frequently difficult (Fig. 9–49).

Case A28

Cynthia Megabeli, age 24, specialized in a certain kind of nightclub dancing. She had had ulcerative colitis for ten years, with remissions and exacerbations. One night, after gyrating for several hours, she presented to the local hospital with a fever and a painful distended abdomen, and she appeared very ill. A plain film of the abdomen was diagnostic (Fig. 9–50).

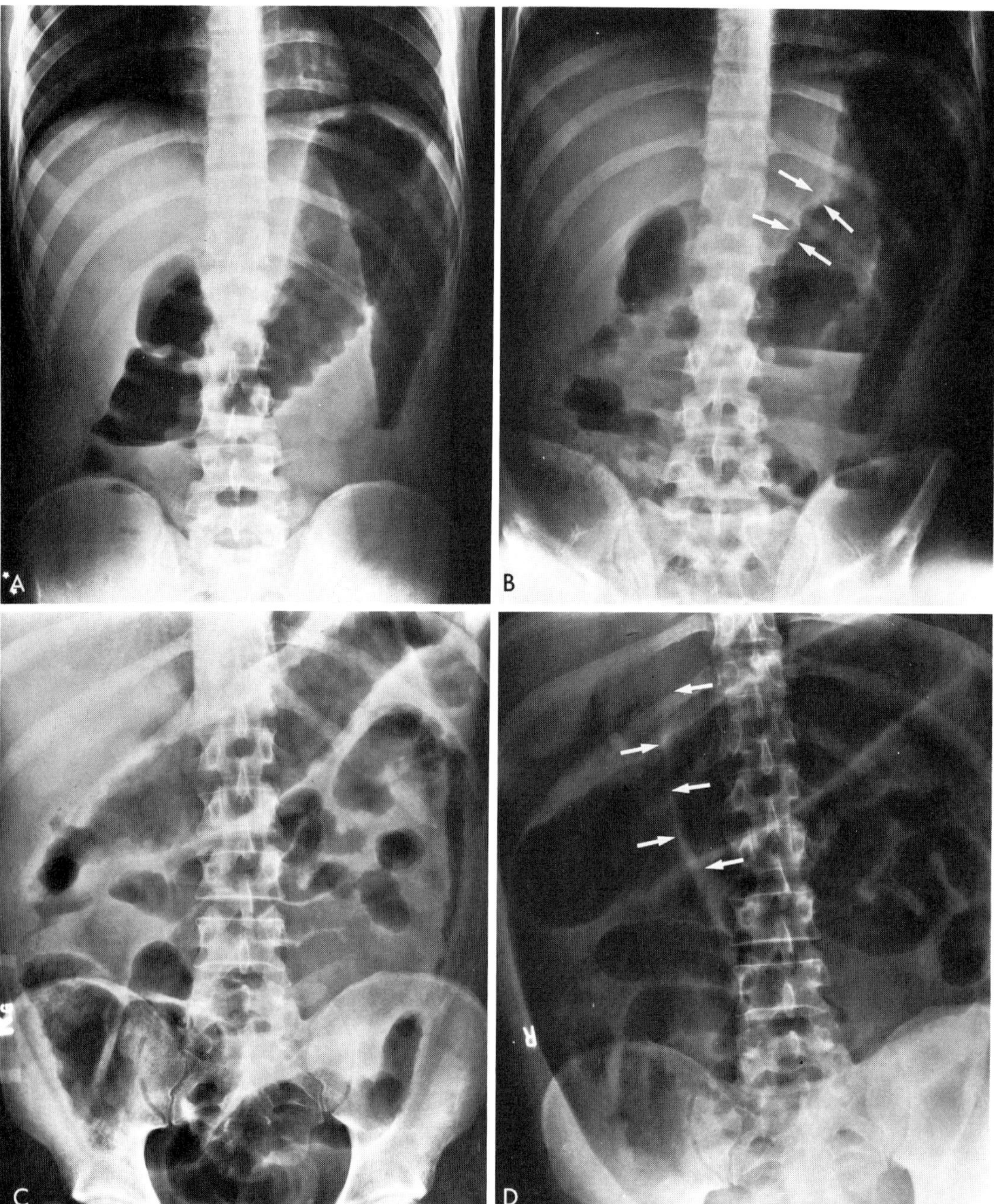

Figure 9–50. Toxic megacolon. *A* and *B*, Supine and erect plain films of the abdomen show distension of the large bowel with a number of air-fluid levels. The mucosal edema is well seen (*arrows*). *C* and *D*, Supine plain films taken six days apart of a different patient. The initial film shows air in both small and large bowel, and mucosal edema is present. This 48-year-old man presented with fever, bloody diarrhea, and abdominal cramps. The second film shows a large pneumoperitoneum outlining the falciform ligament (*arrows*). On emergency proctocolectomy, multiple perforations were found, and the entire colonic mucosa was found to be edematous, with multiple microabscesses typical of ulcerative colitis.

There is obvious distension of much of the colon, and the mucosal irregularity with pseudopolyps can be seen outlined by gas. Few radiologists would risk a barium enema at this stage because of the danger of colonic perforation. Once the condition has defervesced through correction of the fluid and electrolyte imbalance and treatment with steroids and antibiotics, a barium enema can be performed. If toxic megacolon fails to respond to this therapy, there is an increasing danger of perforation and peritonitis, and emergency subtotal colectomy is the treatment of choice.

HEMATURIA

The most common causes of hematuria in young patients are renal stones and pyelonephritis, which have already been illustrated earlier in this chapter. There are, however, other causes that should be discussed.

Case A29 Sanguine Nephropolis, age 45, was on his way to Paris for an annual mortician's meeting when he suddenly developed hematuria. He was otherwise well and had no pain or other symptoms. On examination no abnormality could be found. An intravenous pyelogram was performed (Fig. 9–51). What does it show?

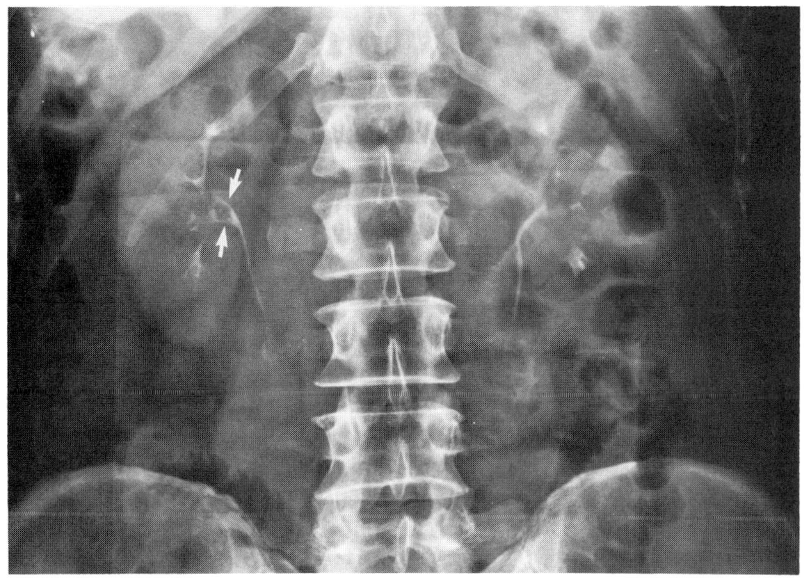

Figure 9–51. Transitional cell carcinoma of the right renal pelvis. A 5-minute IVP film shows a filling defect in the right renal pelvis (*arrows*) that has a somewhat lobulated appearance. It was constant on subsequent films. At laparotomy, the defect was found to be a papillary transitional carcinoma.

The differential diagnosis of a filling defect in the renal pelvis includes blood clot, stone, and tumor. Which would be more likely? In this patient's case, the filling defect was caused by a transitional cell carcinoma. This tumor is of interest because it occurs in chemical workers in the rubber industry, apparently because of a toxin excreted into the urine. It may arise de novo and become multifocal, involving a renal pelvis, a ureter, or the bladder. The treatment of choice is to remove the kidney and ureter on the involved side and to examine the patient with intravenous pyelography every six to twelve months.

Case A30

Sisto Nephropolis, age 50, who was the sister of the previous patient, came in complaining of cramping abdominal pains mainly in the left flank. On examination, a painless mass was found. A chest x-ray and a plain film of the abdomen were normal. Some red blood cells were found in her urine, and an intravenous pyelogram showed a mass in the left kidney (Fig. 9–52). What would you do now?

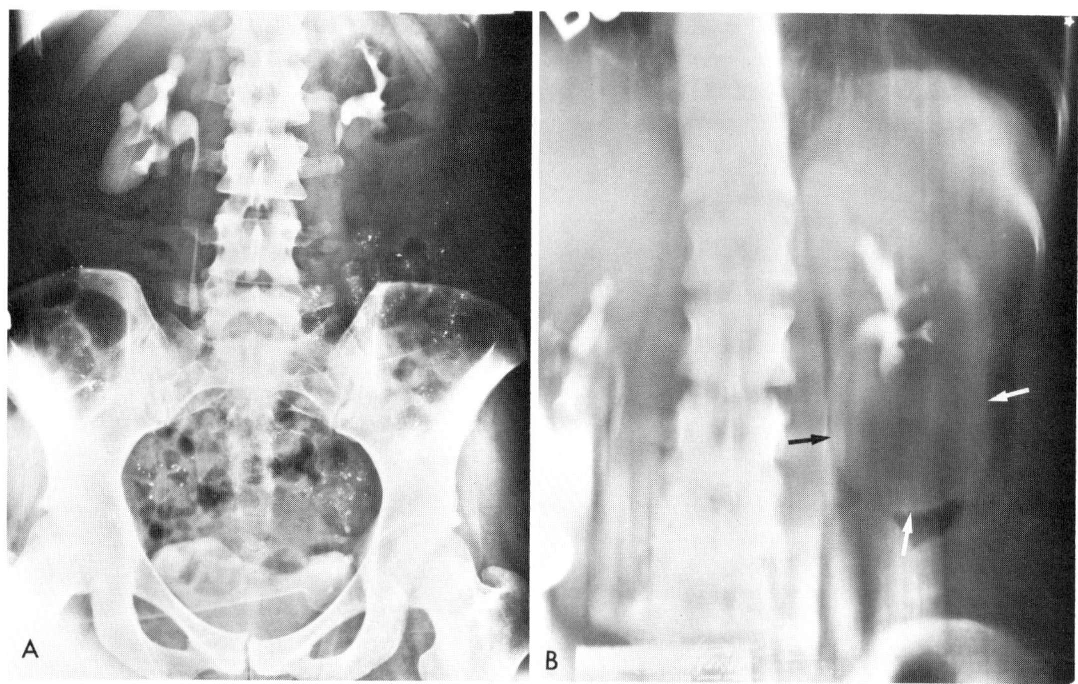

Figure 9–52. Solitary benign renal cyst. The preliminary film of the abdomen showed that the left kidney was increased in size. *A*, A 15-minute IVP film showed that the lower pole calyces were blunted. *B*, On a nephrotomogram, a large lucent defect with a rim (*arrows*) was present in the left lower pole. At laparotomy, a benign cyst was excised. (The gallbladder is opacified because oral cholecystography and intravenous pyelography were performed on the same day.)

This patient represents a classic radiographic situation. The correct approach is to make sure that the intravenous pyelogram is of reasonable quality and that tomography is employed to obtain a good nephrogram. The next non-invasive procedure is an ultrasonographic scan to determine whether the lesion is cystic or solid (Fig. 9–53); in this patient it was found to be cystic. The possibility of a cystic hypernephroma is not excluded at this point, and there is some disagreement about the correct sequence of radiographic investigations indicated by these preliminary findings. If the nephrotomograms show the lesion to have a very clear margin (the "*rim*" *sign*), if the patient is young and without other symptoms or frank hematuria, and if the ultrasonographic scan shows that the lesion has a smooth wall, the diagnosis is almost certainly a benign renal cyst. The patient should then be checked by intravenous pyelography at intervals of six months to one year. If there is any doubt at all, however, angiography is the correct diagnostic procedure to use (Fig. 9–54). A direct cyst puncture can be performed, usually with ultransonographic guidance, and contrast material may be instilled into the cyst itself (Fig. 9–55). Multiple lateral, oblique, and decubitus views are taken in order to ascertain that the cyst wall is smooth and does not contain a small

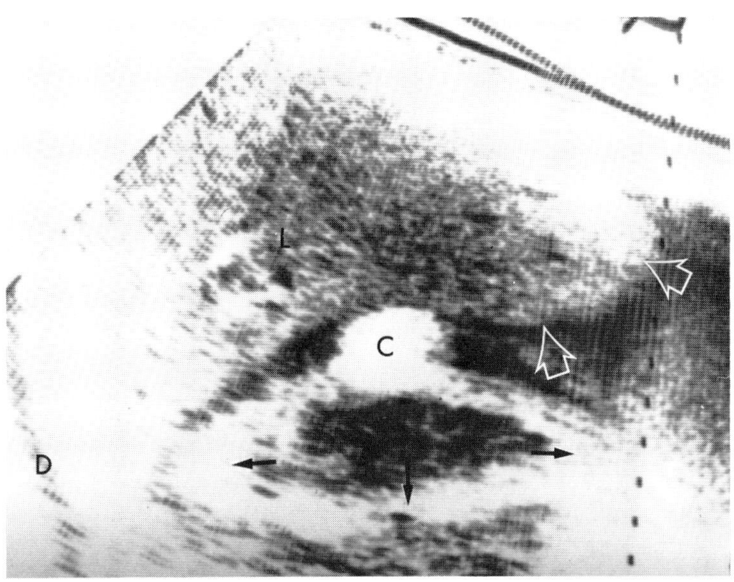

Figure 9–53. Renal cyst. On this ultrasonogram, the sonolucent renal parenchyma is well seen (*arrows*), with the centrally placed collecting system appearing darker. Note the large anterior renal cyst (C). The diaphragm (D), liver (L), and liver edge (*hollow arrows*) are well shown. (The patient's head is to the left.)

mural malignancy (which is found in about 2 per cent of so-called "benign" cysts at autopsy).

Renal cysts are usually solitary but may be multiple in either one or both kidneys. Adult polycystic disease is progressive, often familial, and more common in men. It is associated with cysts in the liver in one third of patients. Death is caused by progressive renal failure, because the cysts become so large that they compress the normal renal parenchyma and compromise renal

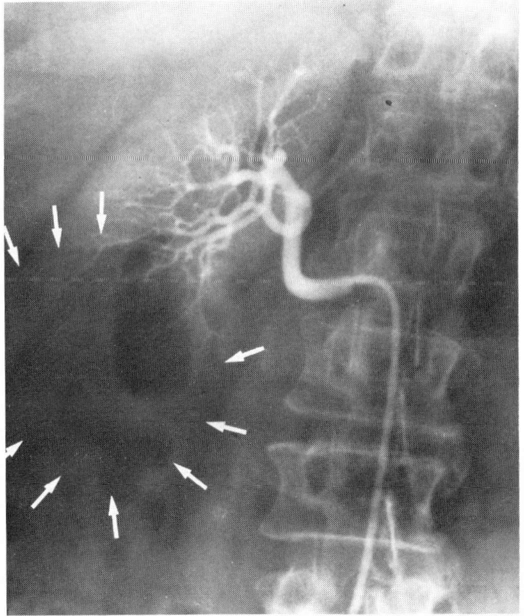

Figure 9–54. Selective angiogram showing a simple renal cyst. There is a well-circumscribed avascular filling defect in the lower pole of the right kidney (*arrows*), and the vasculature around it is stretched. These appearances are characteristic of a simple renal cyst.

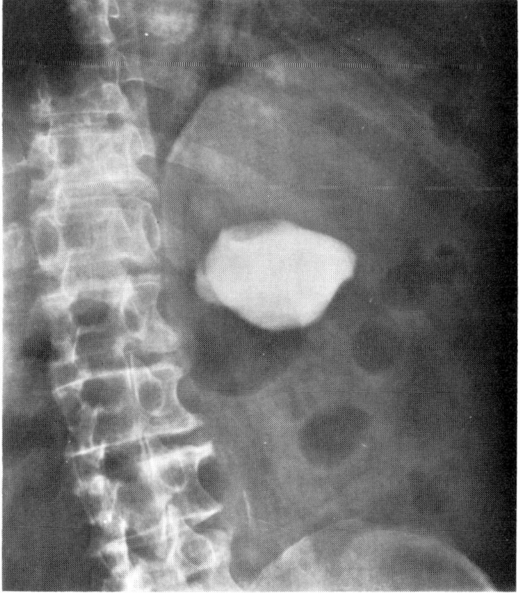

Figure 9–55. Renal cyst. A single film following cyst puncture shows contrast medium in a left upper pole renal cyst.

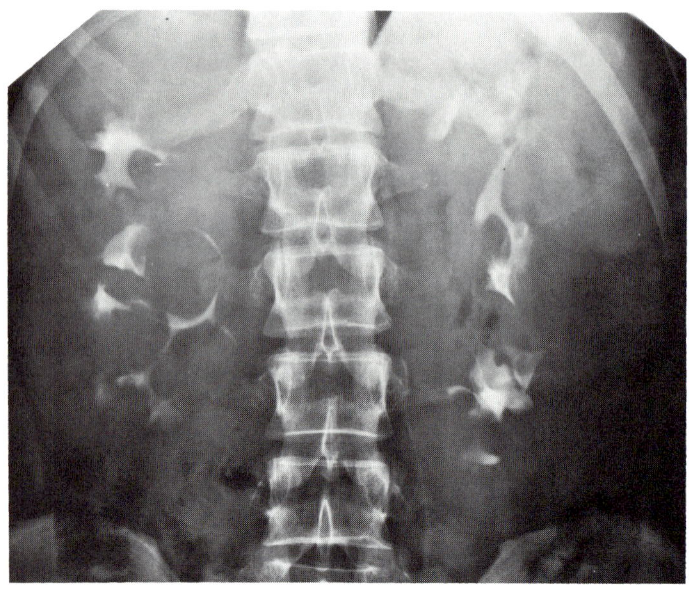

Figure 9–56. Polycystic kidneys. On the 15-minute IVP film, there is marked enlargement of both kidneys with distortion of the calyces, infundibula, and renal pelvis. Many of the calyces appear to stretch around smooth circular masses that represent multiple bilateral cysts.

function. The radiographic findings are characteristic, with enlargement of the renal outlines and bilateral but asymmetrical compression and elongation of the calyceal systems (Fig. 9–56). Ultrasonography or arteriography can be performed but is usually unnecessary, because the diagnosis should be obvious on the basis of the plain films and the intravenous pyelogram. In patients with terminal renal failure from polycystic renal disease, retrograde pyelography is sometimes useful to demonstrate calyceal distortion.

Medullary cystic disease is a rare form of familial salt-losing nephritis in which the radiographic appearance is similar to that of polycystic disease. Congenital multicystic kidney (or unilateral renal dysplasia) is probably a developmental defect in which one kidney has been replaced by multiple cysts and is usually non-functioning.

Case A31

Fanny Flapper, age 48, who was still dancing with the Rockettes, went to her general practitioner's clinic complaining of pain in the left flank and hematuria. She was otherwise well. A chest x-ray and a plain film of the abdomen were normal. An intravenous pyelogram demonstrated a space-occupying lesion in the left kidney (Fig. 9–57A). Ultrasonography showed that the mass was solid, and an angiogram was performed (Fig. 9–57B).

By far the most common malignant renal tumor in the adult is hypernephroma. Although it is usual for the primary neoplasm to cause symptoms first, various secondary manifestations such as "cannonball" metastases in the lungs or a solitary skeletal metastasis in a long bone may cause the presenting symptoms. About 20 per cent of hypernephromas calcify, and some undergo either necrosis or cystic degeneration. The angiographic findings are characteristic: multiple tortuous new blood vessels going into the tumor (neovasculature) as well as arteriovenous shunts and early venous filling. Injection of epinephrine makes the neovasculature more easily visible, because

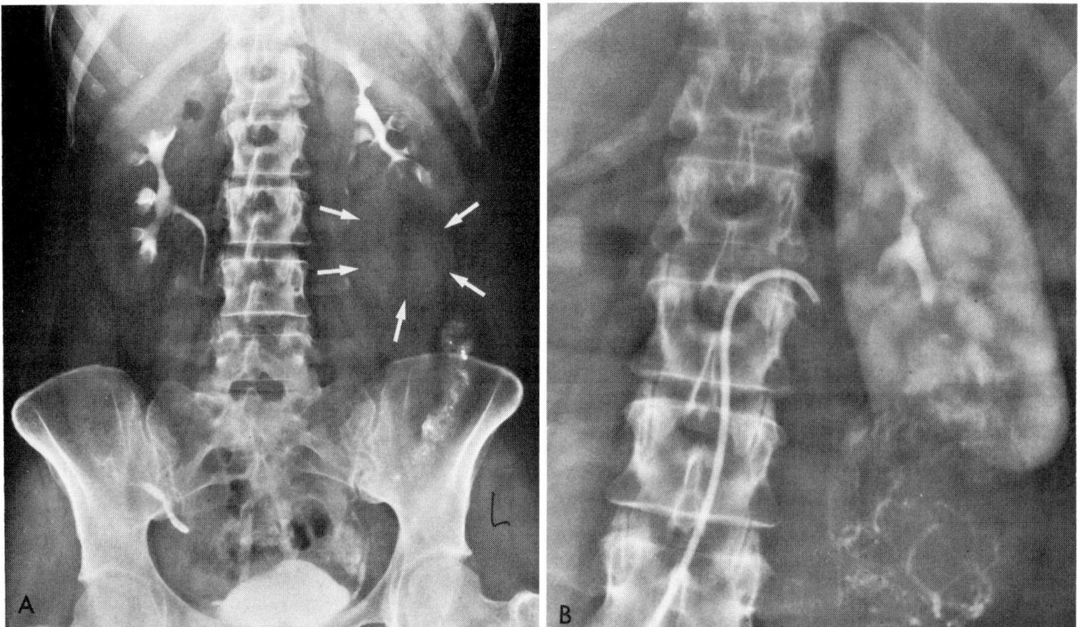

Figure 9–57. Hypernephroma. The plain film of the abdomen revealed a large mass adjacent to the left kidney. *A*, On the 15-minute IVP film, the mass can be seen in the lower pole of the left kidney (*arrows*) displacing the calyces upwards. *B*, Renal arteriography revealed the vascular nature of the tumor, with some cork-screw vessels ("neovasculature").

normal vessels are constricted by the epinephrine whereas the malignant vessels do not respond.

Differentiating between a simple cyst and hypernephroma depends to some extent on the findings on IVP films (the cyst remains lucent but the tumor, although initially lucent, will appear of equal or greater density than the normal renal parenchyma in later films), on ultrasonography (the cyst is sonolucent but the tumor is solid), and on angiography (the cyst is avascular but the tumor has neovasculature).

Another malignant tumor of the kidney is Wilm's tumor, the second most common cause of an abdominal mass in a child (the most common cause is hydronephrosis). The mass is usually discovered by accident in an asymptomatic child. A plain film of the abdomen reveals the mass, and an intravenous pyelogram shows an intrarenal space-occupying lesion distorting the collecting system on that side (Fig. 9–58). Other malignant tumors of the kidney include infiltration by lymphoma and leukemia as well as the occurrence of metastases from distant primary sites.

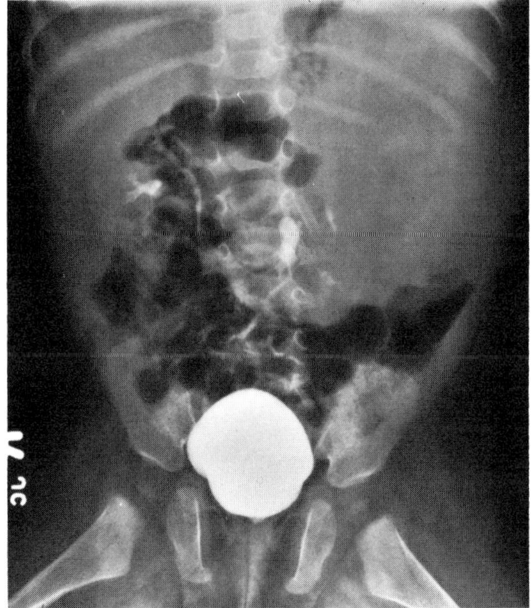

Figure 9–58. Wilm's tumor. This 1-year-old baby had a large abdominal mass displacing the small bowel medially and anteriorly. The 20-minute IVP film showed the marked displacement of the left kidney with stretching and thinning of the calyces. A nephrectomy revealed this to be a Wilm's tumor and the patient was treated with Actinomycin D. He was still alive five years later.

Case A32

Pythagoras Pillpopper, age 64, had a long history of back problems for which he took vast amounts of phenacetin. He was also a diabetic and had had many urinary infections. He came in complaining of hematuria. Considering that the patient has three predisposing causes of hematuria, what could he be suffering from, and what should an intravenous pyelogram show (Fig. 9–59)?

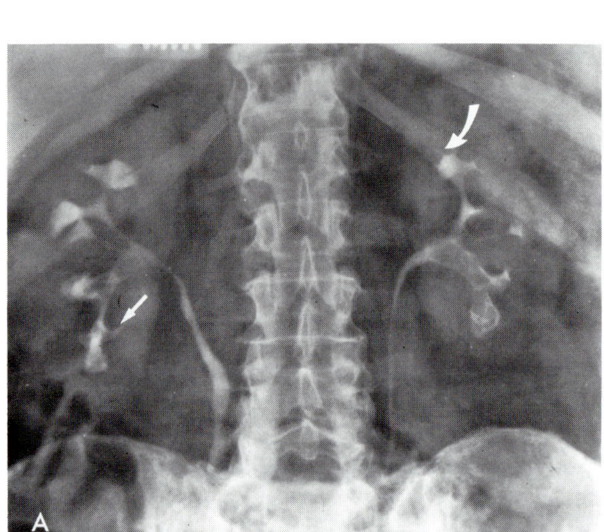

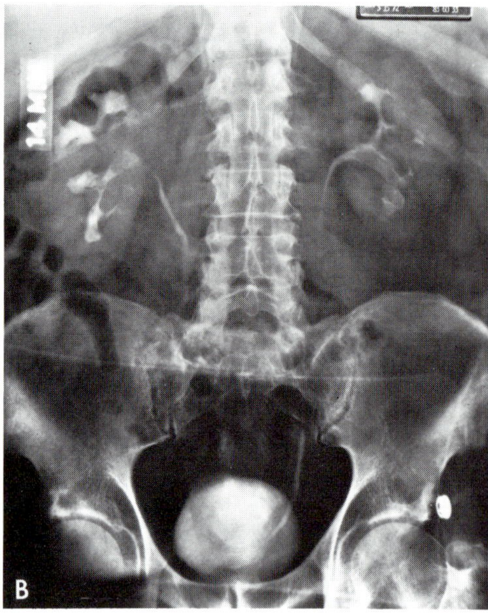

Figure 9–59. Papillary necrosis, 6-minute coned-down view, and 14-minute IVP film taken during IVP. Both films show the distortion of the calyces, with blunting, cupping, and dilatation as well as multiple filling defects, many of which were seen on the plain film to be calcified. Note that there are a few scars, but on the whole the renal parenchyma is of normal width. There is a "lobster claw" deformity in the lower pole on the right (*small arrow*) and a central abscess (*curved arrow*) in the upper pole on the left.

There are many predisposing causes of renal papillary necrosis, but the most common is undoubtedly recurrent pyelonephritis. Now that large volumes of contrast agent are being used routinely for intravenous pyelography and compression techniques are better, papillary necrosis is being found more frequently than previously. Several stages of papillary necrosis are described (Fig. 9–60). At one time a distinction was made between *papillary* necrosis and *medullary* necrosis, but it was largely artificial and is no longer used. The predisposing causes of papillary necrosis include recurrent infections (both bacterial and tuberculous), diabetes, sickle cell anemia, chronic

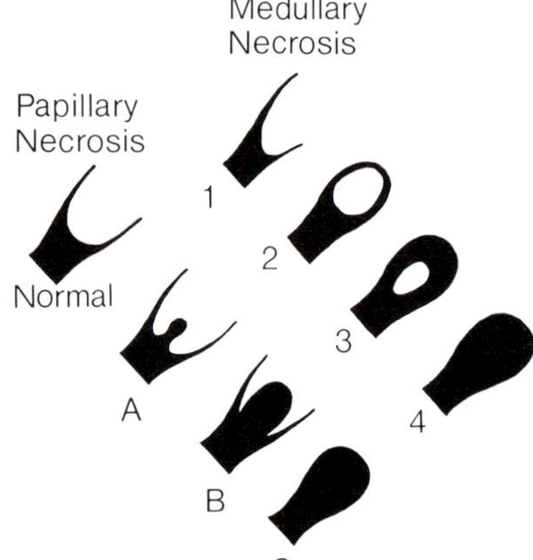

Figure 9–60. The stages of papillary necrosis. In the condition known as papillary necrosis, a small pool of contrast medium can be seen lying centrally within the renal pyramid. This usually communicates with the calix (A). If this destruction enlarges, clubbing will ensue (B and C). Medullary necrosis begins as elongation of the arms of the calix, producing the so-called lobster claw deformity (1). This will continue until the papilla falls off and lies free-floating in the calix itself (2 and 3). Here it may either calcify or be passed as a small stone and then only clubbing remains (C/4).

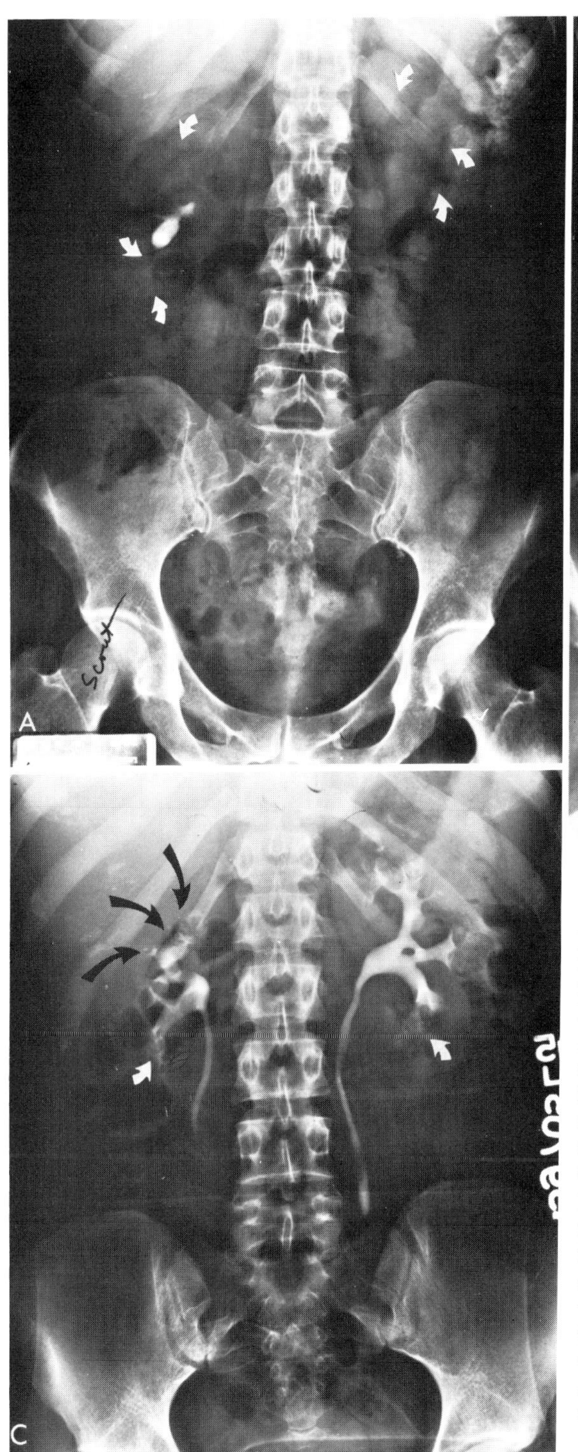

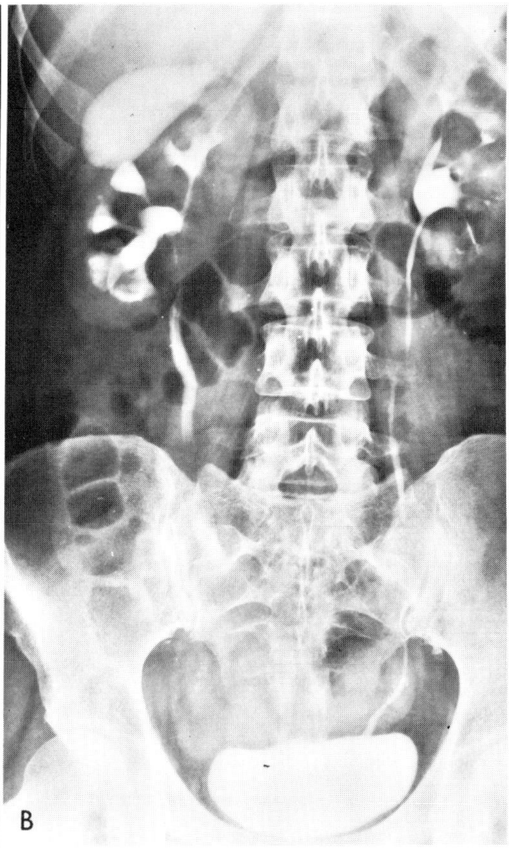

Figure 9–61. Papillary necrosis. *A* and *B*, plain film and 15-minute IVP film. The plain film reveals one large calcified stone and multiple small poorly defined calcifications overlying both kidneys (*arrows*). On the IVP film, most of these appear to lie within the dilated blunted calyces. This middle-aged female patient had a history of multiple urinary tract infections and hypertension, and these appearances were considered to be typical of papillary necrosis. (*C*), A 15-minute IVP film of a different patient. The plain film showed multiple minute pinpoint calcifications. The IVP film reveals the central abscesses of papillary necrosis (*black arrows*) as well as the linear opacification typical of tubular ectasis (or dilated collecting tubules), which is best seen in the lower poles (*white arrows*). This 20-year-old patient had a history of recurrent urinary tract infections.

ingestion of phenacetin and aspirin, and recurrent urinary obstruction. The sloughed-off papillae may be passed as "stones" or may remain in the collecting system, where they calcify (Fig. 9–61). Renal function is only rarely affected, and with proper treatment of the underlying process, no renal impairment occurs in most patients.

One other condition that is of radiographic interest and has a similar appear-

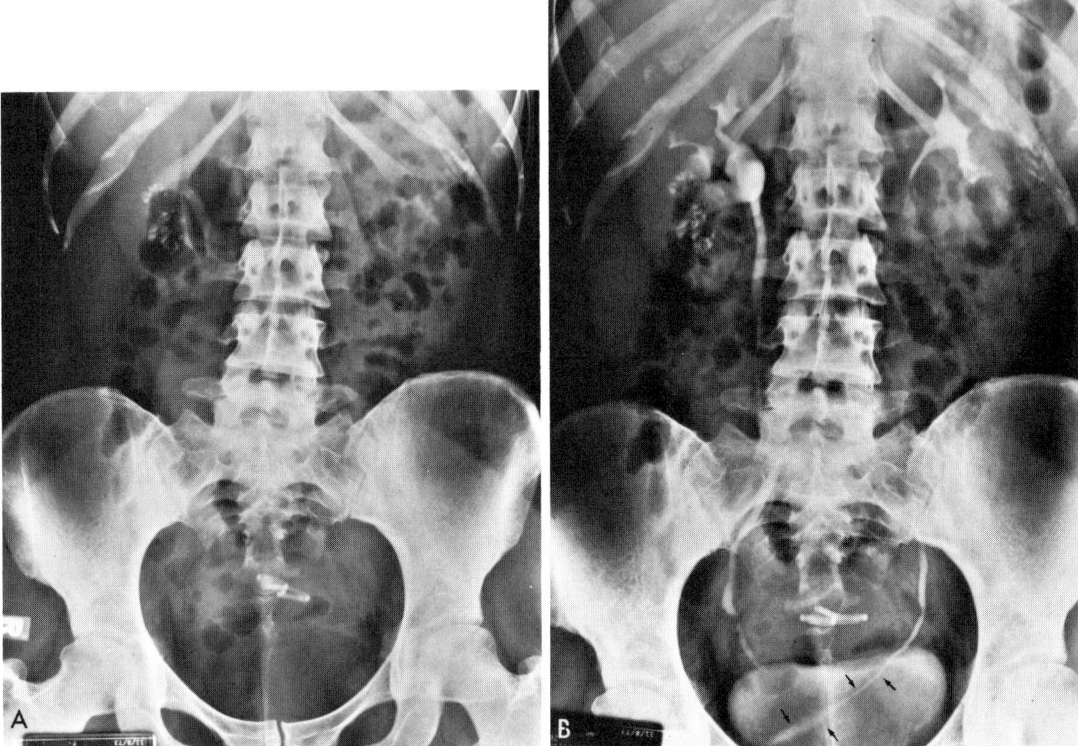

Figure 9–62. Medullary sponge kidney. *A*, The plain film demonstrates an IUD in normal position as well as multiple calcifications in the lower pole of the right kidney. *B*, The 20-minute IVP film shows that these calcifications are within the lower pole pyramids, a typical finding in medullary sponge kidney. Note the ureteral "jet" phenomenon *(arrows)*, which is normal and represents opacified urine from the ureter spurting into the less opacified urine in the bladder.

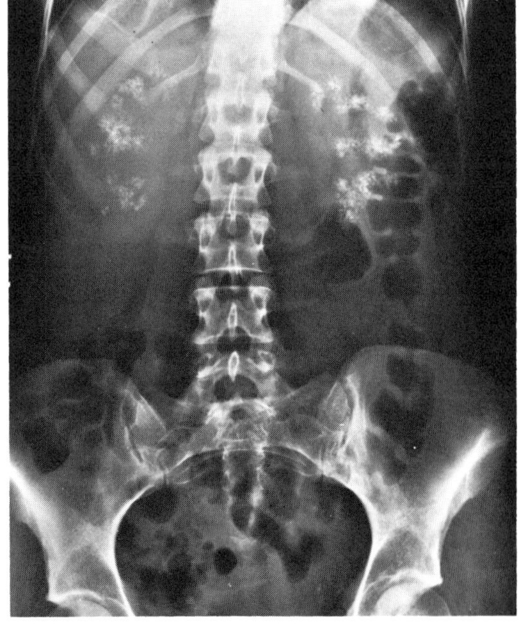

Figure 9–63. Nephrocalcinosis. This 45-year-old woman has renal tubular acidosis. Note the calcifications in the region of the tubules, typical of this condition. On biopsy, there was no evidence of medullary sponge kidney.

ance is medullary sponge kidney, in which multiple congenital cysts arise from the distal collecting tubules. The cysts lead to retention of urine, with recurrent infections and stone formation (Fig. 9–62). On biopsy or section, the kidney looks like a "sponge"; hence, the name of this condition. Medullary sponge kidney is usually asymptomatic and like papillary necrosis rarely leads to impairment of renal function. It is of some importance to differentiate the radiographic appearances of renal calculi, calcified renal papillae, and medullary sponge kidney from that of nephrocalcinosis (Fig. 9–63), which is usually caused by an underlying metabolic disorder and should be investigated further.

Case A33

Aneuryn Piddle, age 82, had been experiencing difficulty in micturition for the past 20 years, although recently it had been gradually getting worse. He complained of hesitancy, a poor stream, and having to urinate a second time immediately after the first; more recently, he had developed hematuria. The story is characteristic, and the rectal examination confirmed the suspicion of a huge prostate gland. An intravenous pyelogram was performed to exclude the possibility of renal damage as well as to assess the degree of obstruction (Fig. 9–64).

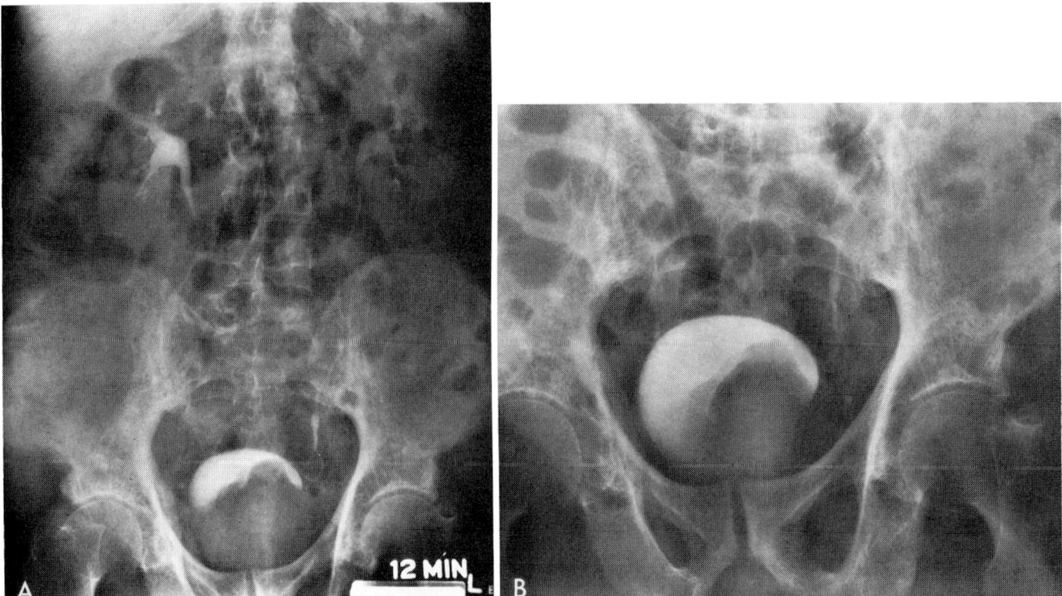

Figure 9–64. Benign prostatic hypertrophy, 12-minute IVP film (*A*) and coned-down view of the bladder (*B*). This vast mass arising from the floor of the bladder and indenting the bladder outline proved to be prostatic hypertrophy, not a bladder tumor as had been first thought. The patient has evidence of Paget's disease in the pelvis (thickened cortices and irregular trabecular pattern), a finding not uncommon in elderly patients.

Hematuria is often the presenting symptom of bladder and prostatic conditions, and many elderly male patients with benign prostatic hypertrophy will have accepted their difficulties with urination but will present to their physician at the first sign of bleeding.

Choice of surgical procedure depends on

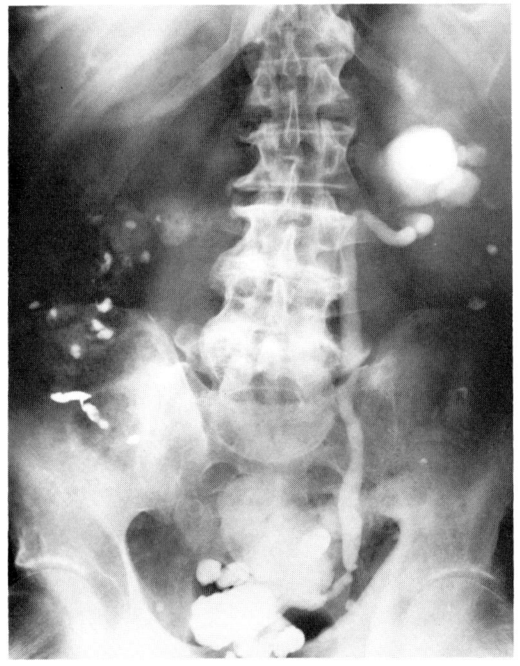

Figure 9–65. Benign prostatic hypertrophy and hydronephrosis. This 72-year-old man had a long history of prostatic problems, and this film shows delayed emptying, hydronephrosis, and a dilated ureter on the left. The bladder is severely distorted and shrunken, although it is difficult to assess because retained barium in the rectum overlies the bladder region.

the degree of urinary obstruction rather than on the associated radiographic findings, and either transurethral prostatectomy or suprapubic removal of the whole gland is performed. In some patients, chronic benign prostatic hypertrophy will lead to obstructive nephropathy, with dilatation of the collecting systems, tortuosity and dilatation of the ureters, a hypertrophy of the bladder wall, formation of diverticula, pseudodiverticula, and mucosal irregularities (Fig. 9–65). Most men develop some degree of benign prostatic hypertrophy, which reaches maximum obstructive potential after age 60, and about one man in four requires some form of surgical treament.

Case A34

Clyde Derringer, age 16, was in a "house of correction" for armed robbery. He was admitted to the hospital complaining of hematuria, and a plain film revealed the problem (Fig. 9–66).

Pushing objects into the urethra, either for sexual stimulation or to gain sympathy, is not an uncommon practice that perhaps curiously appears to be more common in males than females. This young man underwent cystoscopy, and the foreign body was successfully removed. The next morning, he was found to have pushed a thermometer into his urethra and deliberately to have broken it. He was referred for psychiatric help.

Case A35

Hector Flopper, age 71, presented with frank hematuria of recent onset. On cystoscopy, a large fungating carcinoma was found, and an intravenous pyelogram as well as a retrograde cystogram were performed.

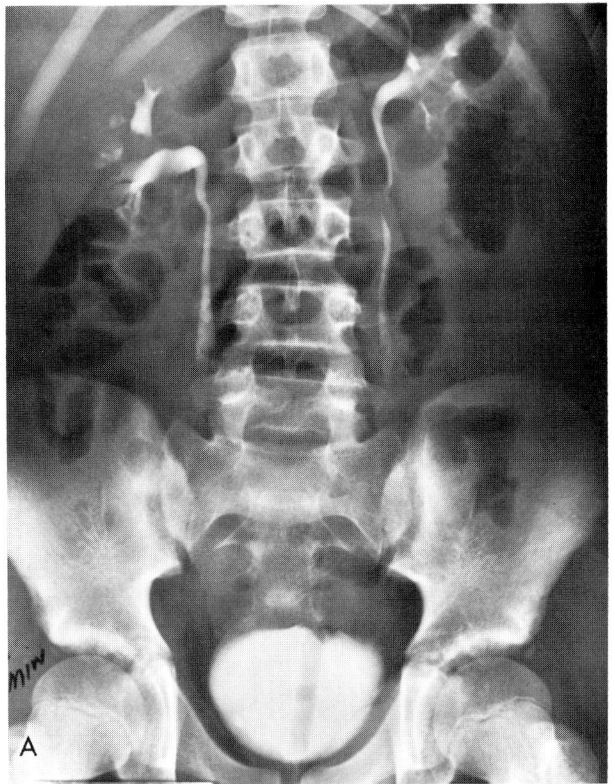

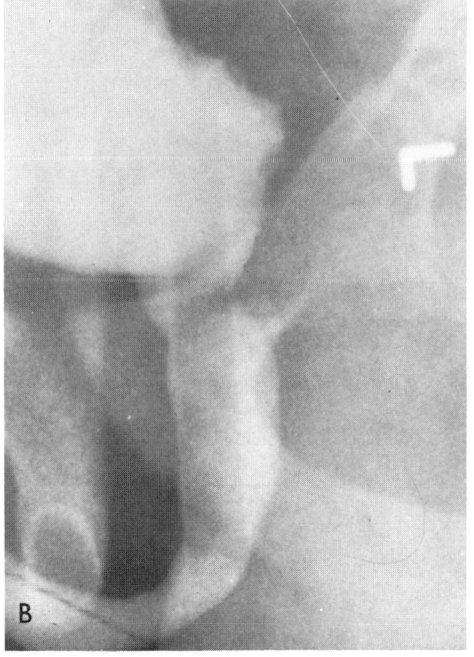

Figure 9–66. Foreign body in the urethra, 25 minute IVP film (*A*) and VCUG (*B*). There is a cylindrical filling defect in the bladder and prostatic urethra; it was a pencil.

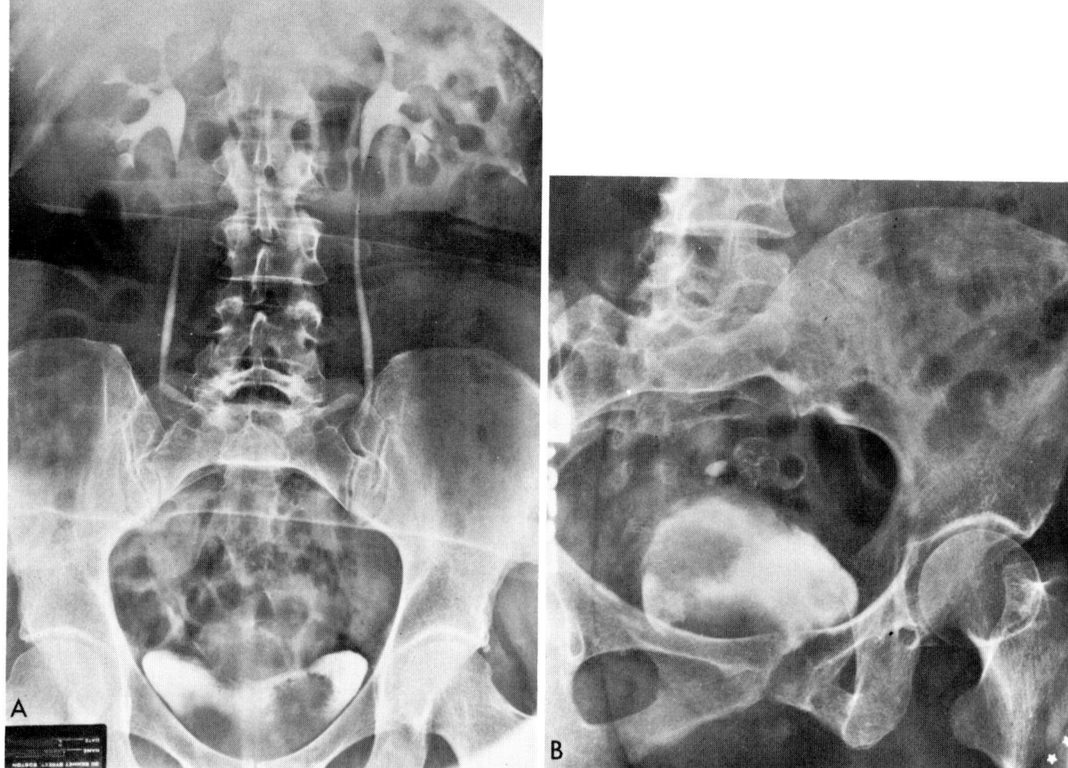

Figure 9–67. Bladder carcinoma, an IVP film (*A*) and a cystogram (*B*) of a different patient. In both patients note the irregular filling defects in the bladder, mainly rising from the bladder floor. In the first patient, the upper urinary tracts are normal. The appearance of multilobular ragged filling defects with loss of part of the circumference of the bladder wall is typical of carcinoma of the bladder. At biopsy both tumors were found to be transitional cell carcinomas.

Hematuria can also be the presenting symptom of a bladder tumor. Like benign prostatic hypertrophy, bladder carcinomas are inclined to occur in elderly patients. An intravenous pyelogram is used to demonstrate the degree of obstruction and involvement of the lower ureters (Fig. 9–67A). A retrograde cystogram is used to demonstrate the extent of bladder wall involvement (Fig. 9–67B). Incidentally, taking plain films of the abdomen and the chest is a useful, simple, and economical method of surveying the skeleton for metastases; the metastases from bladder tumors are usually lytic, but if the carcinoma has spread to the prostatic bed, they often become blastic.

Transitional cell carcinoma of the bladder looks similar to squamous cell carcinoma. Like transitional cell carcinoma of the renal pelvis, it occurs in younger patients and is often multifocal. Finally, prostatic carcinoma presents with blastic skeletal metastases, an elevated serum acid phosphatase level, and a hard craggy prostate gland.

There are, of course, other causes of hematuria such as trauma, benign focal nephritis, tuberculosis, and other infections, and infestations such as schistosomiasis. In some people, ingestion of beet root and some drugs or chemicals produces a red-colored urine. True hematuria, however, necessitates an intravenous pyelogram in every patient who presents with this symptom.

CHAPTER 10

THE NECK

This chapter deals briefly with a heterogeneous group of conditions in which there is disease in the neck. Patients with many of these conditions present with pain or discomfort. Dysphagia, hoarseness, and mass in the neck are also discussed.

Case N1

Antonia Aubergine, age 78, champion tennis player for Golden Arches retirement home, complained of pain that radiated down her arm and into her fingers, particularly when she served. Sometimes when she turned her head rapidly, the pain would be so intense as to make her drop her tennis racket. She went to her family practitioner, who sent her for x-rays of her neck (Fig. 10–1).

These four films demonstrate the classic changes of cervical spondylosis, or osteoarthritis of the neck. Narrowing of the intervertebral foramina caused the patient's symptoms, because osteophytes compressed the cervical nerves. On sudden movement, they produce pain and paresthesia as well as actual muscle weakness. These signs and symptoms become gradually worse with age and may actually be continuous before the patient presents to a physician. Unfortunately, cervical spondylosis is not readily treatable, although the judicious use of a high foam collar, traction ("hanging yourself"), and, occasionally, removal of the offending osteophytes may be successful.

Case N2

Father Aurelius Durst-doisy, age 54, had had severe rheumatoid arthritis for years. The disease predominantly involved his hands, wrists, and feet but had more recently begun to affect larger joints. One Sunday, while preaching about the wrath of God, he experienced a drop attack that, appropriately, brought him to his knees. His doctor, who was attending the church service, called for an ambulance to take the priest to the hospital.

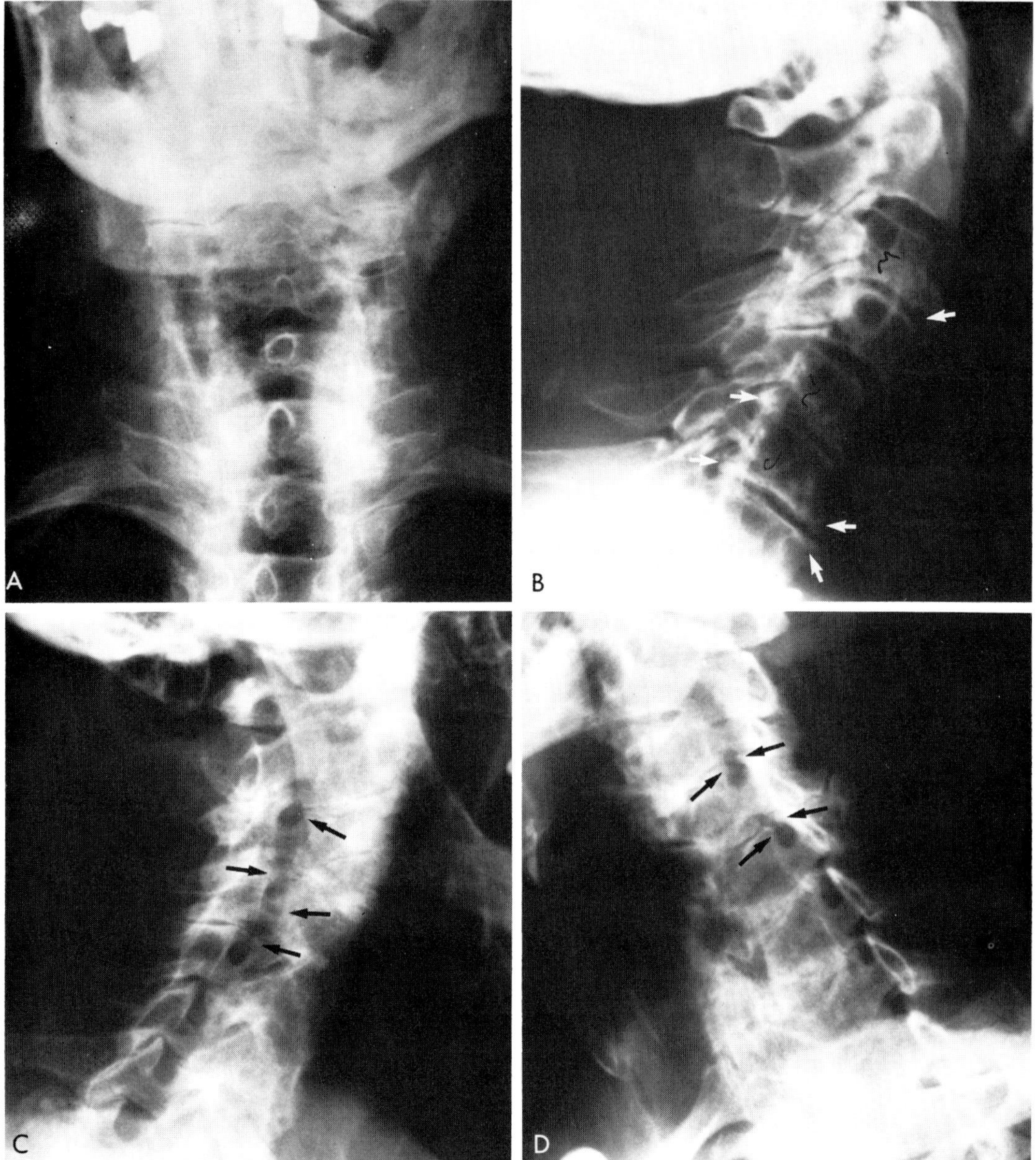

Figure 10–1. Cervical spondylosis, AP view (*A*), lateral view (*B*), and oblique views (*C* and *D*). Note the narrowing of the cervical disc spaces and the sclerosis surrounding them. The vertebral bodies are distorted, and anterior and posterior osteophytes (*arrows*) are encroaching on the intervertebral foramina.

What complication of rheumatoid arthritis would one expect to find in the cervical spine? How would you investigate it?

Flexion and extension views of the atlantoaxial joint are usually performed with the greatest care in patients who have long-standing rheumatoid arthritis (Fig. 10–2). Often, a neurologist is present to assist with the filming, because there is a danger of cord damage. Tomography is frequently needed to demonstrate free movement of the odontoid (Fig. 10–2C), which occurs in rheumatoid arthritis because synovial overgrowth causes disintegration of the transverse ligament holding the two upper cervical vertebrae together (Fig. 10–3). Atlantoaxial dissociation is usually treated by posterior fusion to prevent the patient from pithing himself.

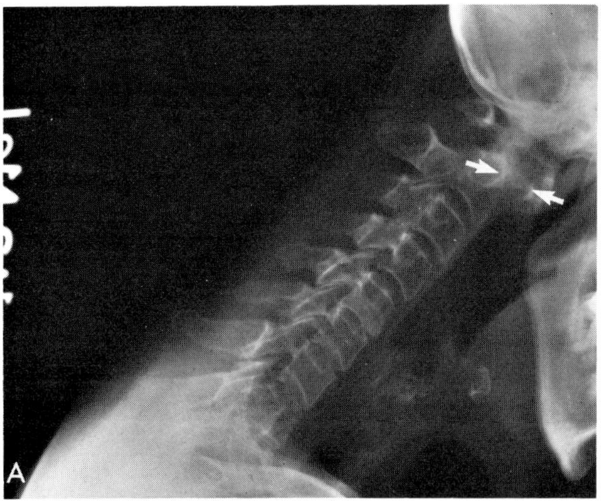

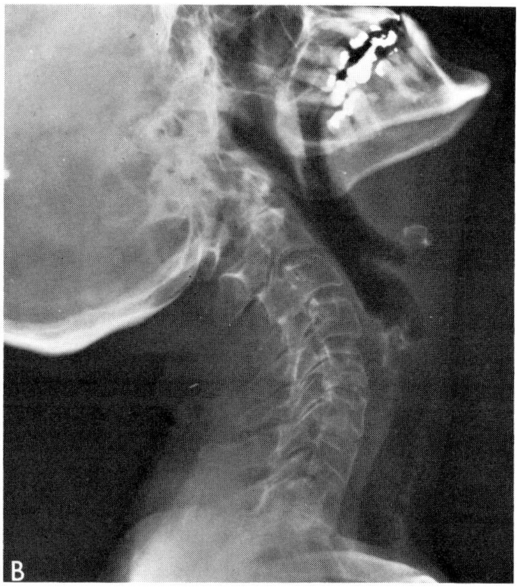

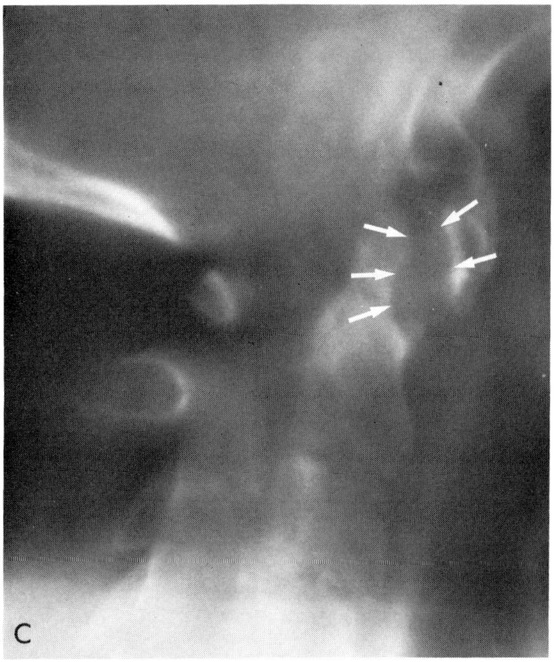

Figure 10–2. Rheumatoid arthritis involving the atlantoaxial joint, flexion view (*A*), extension view (*B*), and tomogram (*C*). On lateral views of the cervical spine in flexion and extension, the free movement of the odontoid in relation to the arch of the atlas can be seen. The space between the back of the arch of the atlas and the front of the odontoid (*arrows*) should measure no more than 2 to 3 mm in normal people.

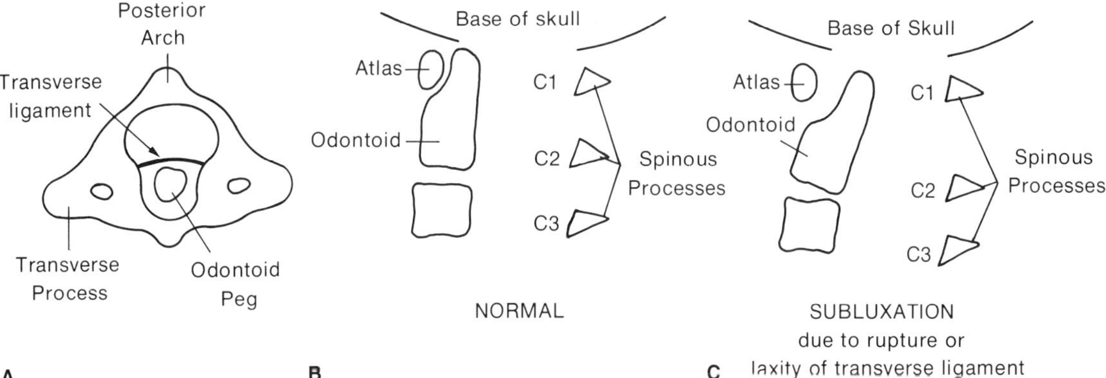

Figure 10–3. The atlantoaxial articulation. These anatomical sketches demonstrate the relationship of the arch of the atlas (C1) to the axis (C2). Note the separation of the spinous processes of C1 and C2 in patients with subluxation.

Case N3

Percival Clod, age 56, a heavy smoker, presented with pain in his shoulder that radiated down his arm and was made worse by movement. His family practitioner thought the symptoms were caused by bursitis, but the soft-tissue x-rays of the shoulder were normal. Neck films revealed a normal cervical spine, but an abnormality in the apex of the right lung was noted. A CXR was diagnostic (Fig. 10–4).

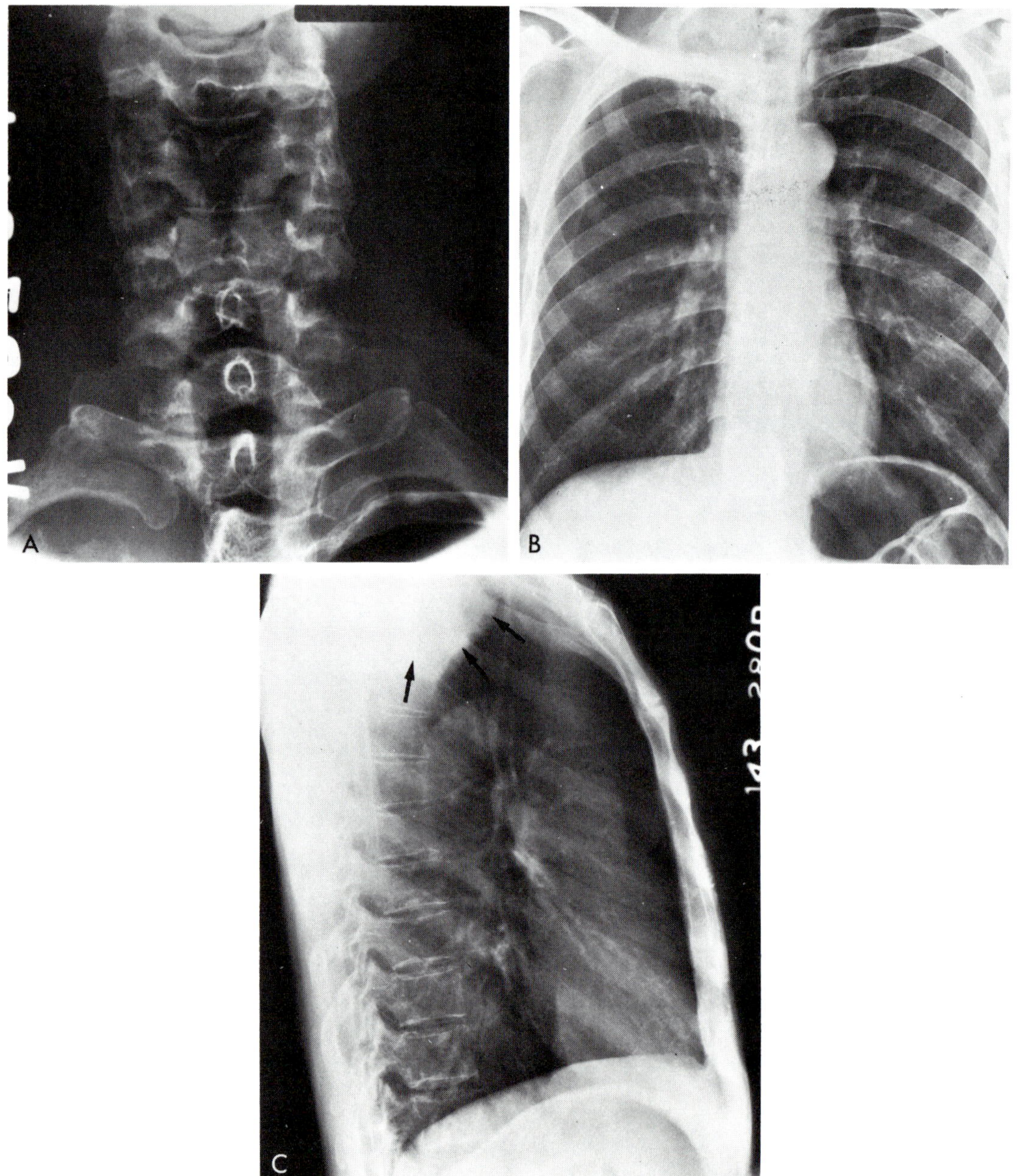

Figure 10–4. Pancoast tumor. *A*, AP view of cervical spine. *B*, PA view of the chest. *C*, Lateral view of chest. The views of the cervical spine and chest show the typical appearances of a Pancoast tumor: destruction of ribs and thoracic vertebrae associated with an apical density in the lung field that can be seen lying apico-posteriorly on the lateral chest x-rays (*arrows*).

A superior sulcus or Pancoast tumor involving the apex of the lung may present with neck or shoulder pain.

Undoubtedly, however, the most common cause of shoulder pain is bursitis or tendinitis (Fig. 10–5). Internal and external rotation views of the soft tissues in the shoulder should be taken. They may be coned down or may be enhanced by the use of xeroradiography. Shoulder arthrography can be useful for looking at the internal anatomy of the joint and in particular for locating rotator cuff tears and for diagnosing "frozen shoulder" (in which the joint capsule becomes fibrotic, with subsequent loss of volume of the shoulder joint).

Incidentally, one of the classic presentations of globus hystericus is a complaint of either pain in the neck or dysphagia, and all the radiological findings will, of course, be normal.

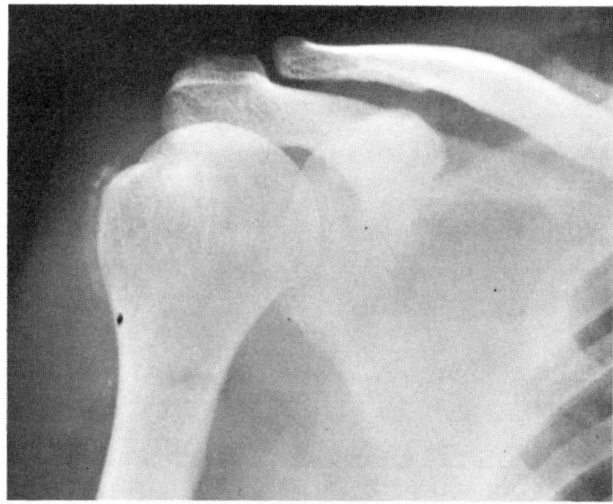

Figure 10–5. Calcific bursitis. Note the calcification overlying the greater tuberosity of the humerus; it lies within the subacromial (subdeltoid) bursa. Calcific bursitis is often best demonstrated using internal rotation views of the shoulder.

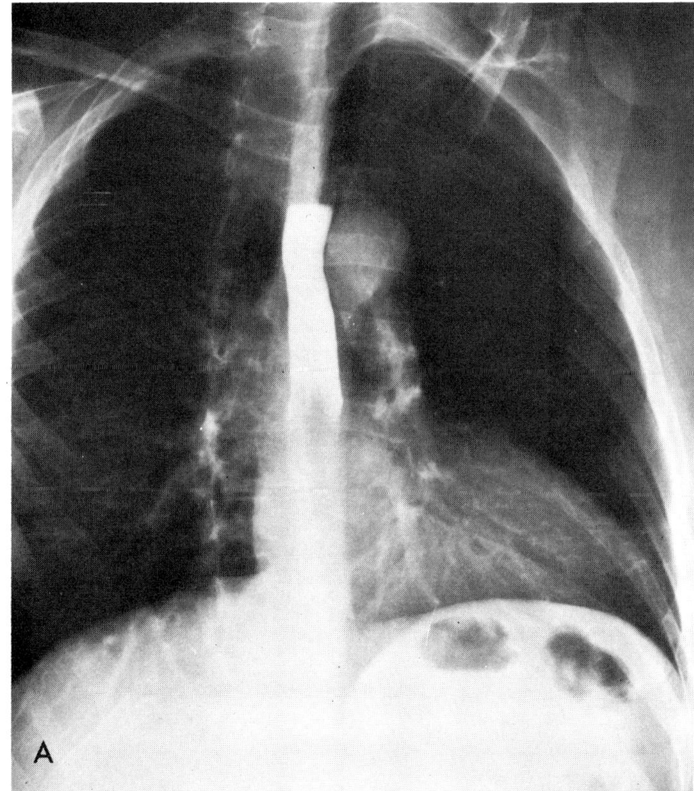

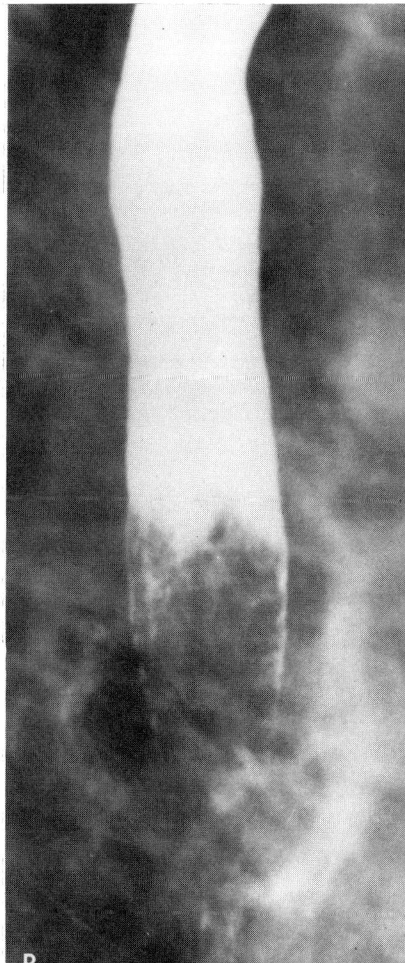

Figure 10–6. Foreign body in esophagus, AP view (*A*) and coned-down view (*B*). A barium swallow revealed a large filling defect in the midesophagus that was causing almost total obstruction. This large piece of turkey was successfully removed through an esophagoscope.

Case N4

Digby Grossgobble, age 52, came to the hospital after having sudden difficulty in swallowing during a banquet. Plain films were negative, and a barium swallow revealed a large foreign body in the esophagus (Fig. 10–6).

Dysphagia is a serious problem and should be investigated carefully, although plain films only rarely show abnormality. The investigation of choice is a barium swallow, which should be combined with cineradiography if problems with motility are suspected. Endoscopy of the esophagus is almost always performed in conjunction with barium studies.

Case N5

Ambrosia Burp, age 62, had a 19-year history of difficulty in swallowing associated with recurrent regurgitation. More recently, she had been able to take only liquid meals (consisting mainly of a byproduct of grain). The CXR was diagnostic, and a barium swallow confirmed the diagnosis (Fig. 10–7).

The density seen on the right side of the thoracic spine from the upper mediastinum to the diaphragm is characteristic of achalasia and represents a dilated fluid-filled esophagus. The gastric air bubble is characteristically absent, and sometimes an air-fluid level may be seen on erect films. Barium studies are best performed after the esophagus has been emptied with a catheter, because the narrowed gastroesophageal junction will then be easier to delineate. This narrowing is caused by a congenital or acquired failure of motility due to a localized absence of Auerbach's plexus in this region. Subcutaneous injection of Mecholyl, which causes a wave of peristalsis to move through the area, is a diagnostic test for achalasia. Esophagomanometric pressure studies are also diagnostic. One complication of long-standing achalasia is common: recurrent aspiration pneumonia may occur and may lead to pulmonary fibrosis and a characteristic pattern in the mid or lower lung fields not unlike that of lipoid pneumonia (Fig. 10–8).

Other causes of megaesophagus are scleroderma (in which there is also a failure in motility) and Chagas' disease, both of which have other clinical features. Presbyesophagus and tertiary contractions of the esophagus are extremely common in people over 65. There are other causes of narrowing of the esophagus, however, and differentiation of carcinoma from achalasia may be difficult on the basis of radiographic findings alone. Endoscopy is essential for correct diagnosis.

Case N6

Ermitrude Hungershall, age 68, had a long history of regurgitation, but she recently developed increasing dysphagia. Plain films showed no abnormality, and a barium study showed an irregular stricture at the lower end of the esophagus (Fig. 10–9). A hiatus hernia and free gastroesophageal reflux had been demonstrated some years previously but were not seen on this occasion.

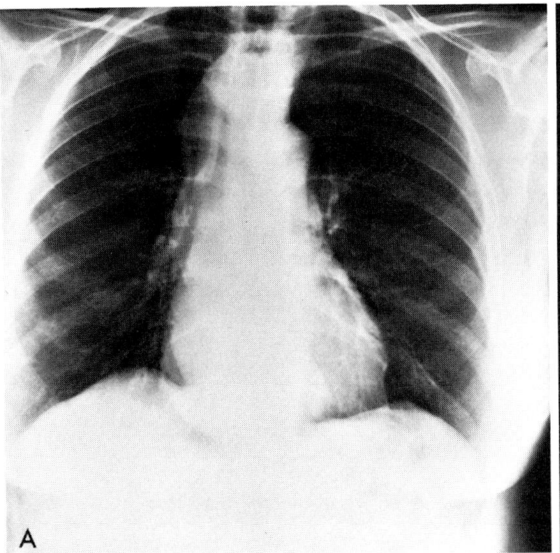

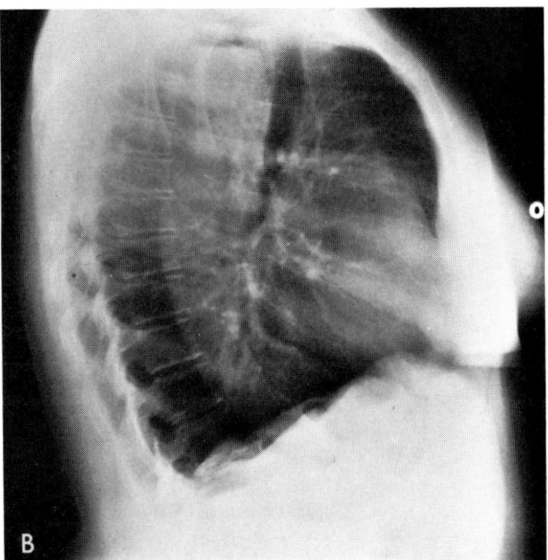

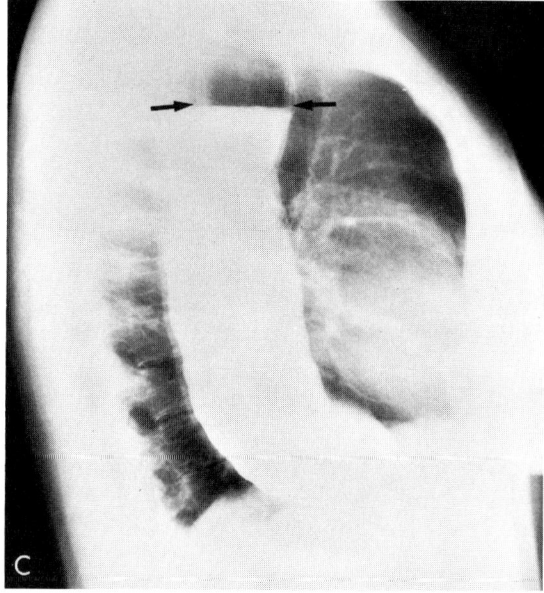

Figure 10–7. Achalasia AP view (*A*), lateral view (*B*), and barium swallow (*C*). The PA chest x-ray shows a large paraspinal density to the right of the spine that on the lateral view seems to lie within the central part of the mediastinum. An air-fluid level may be seen in its upper portion. This represents a fluid-filled esophagus (*arrows*). The barium swallow shows the characteristic dilated patulous esophagus with distal narrowing.

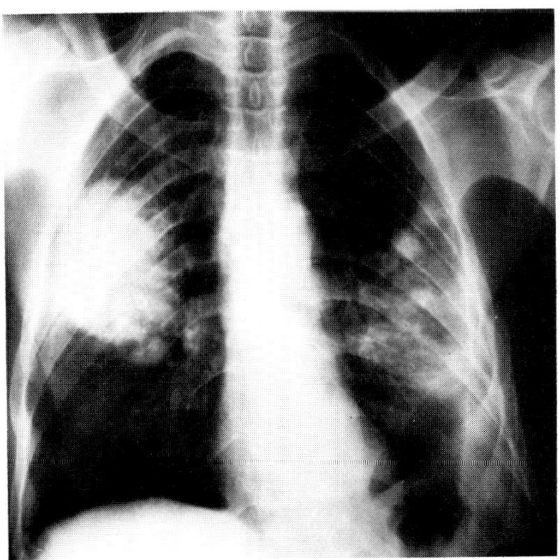

Figure 10–8. Lipoid pneumonia. Recurrent aspiration pneumonia produces areas of chronic consolidation with fibrosis and fatty degeneration (hence the term *lipoid*). In this young male patient with a swallowing disorder, recurrent aspiration had led to these bilateral midzone well-circumscribed areas of consolidation. Note also the left-sided pleural fibrosis, which is due to a chronic inflammatory reaction and pleurisy.

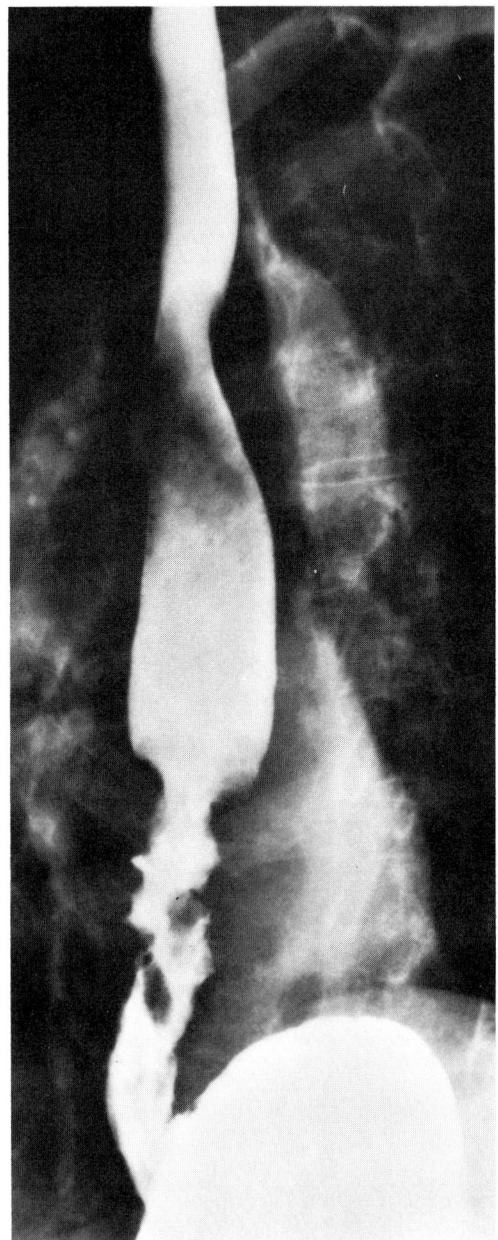

Figure 10–9. Carcinoma of the esophagus. There is an irregular stricture in the lower esophagus. The encroachment on the esophageal lumen is characteristic of a carcinoma, and the appearance of "shoulders" where the normal esophagus meets the tumor is typical of a malignancy anywhere in the gastrointestinal tract.

Reflux esophagitis is almost always associated with symptoms. If there is longstanding irritation anywhere in the body, the risk of malignant change is increased. In the middle and upper thirds of the esophagus, an irregular narrowing is almost always caused by a carcinoma, but narrowing in the lower third makes the differential diagnosis difficult. This patient has carcinoma of the esophagus.

Reflux esophagitis is usually also associated with a hiatus hernia, which may be sliding or rolling (Fig. 10–10). Hiatus hernias may be asymptomatic or may be associated

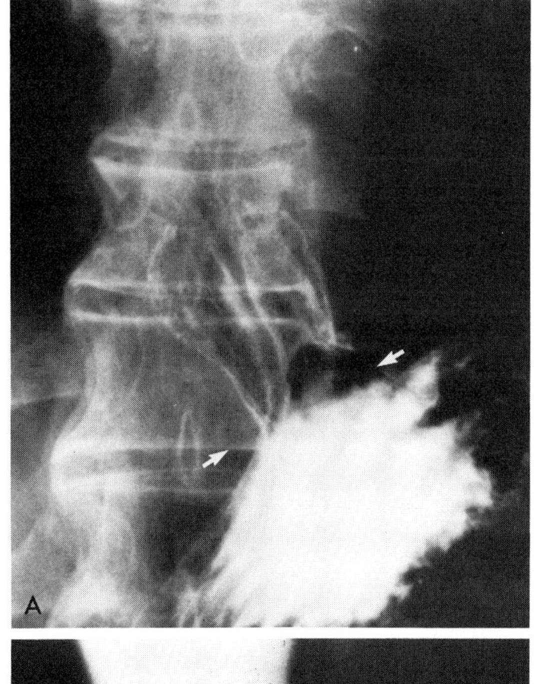

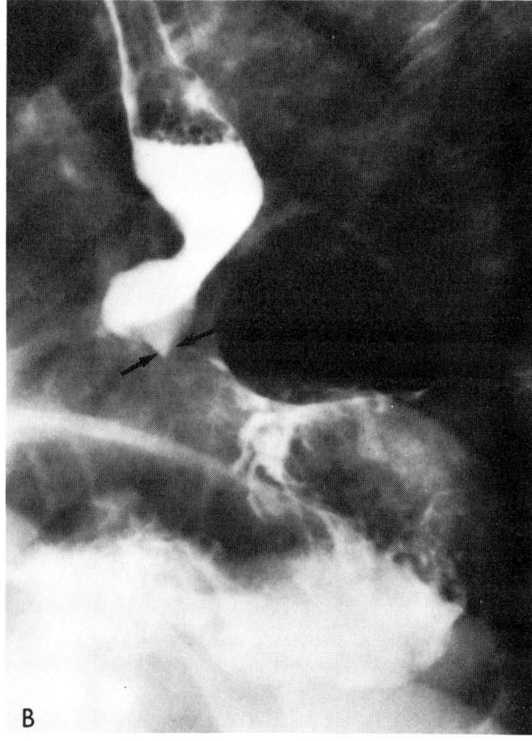

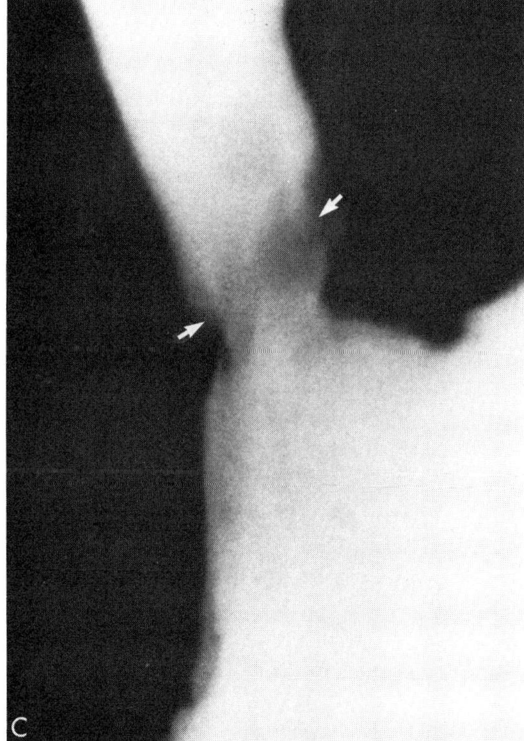

Figure 10–10. Hiatus hernia. *A*, In this man of 58, gastric mucosa is seen above the diaphragm (*arrows*), representing a hiatus hernia sliding through a widened esophageal hiatus into the thorax. *B*, In this elderly obese female patient, the gastric fundus and much of the body of the stomach can be seen above the diaphragm, whereas the gastroesophageal junction (*arrows*) is relatively lower than the top of the fundus. This represents a large rolling hiatus hernia. *C*, In this close-up view of a distended esophagus in a normal young male patient, a distinct ring can be identified (*arrows*). This is a Schatzki ring at the junction of the esophageal and gastric mucosa.

with regurgitation and a feeling of fullness behind the sternum. If the lumen of the lower esophagus is distended sufficiently, a Schatzki ring may be demonstrated (Fig. 10–10C). This occurs at the junction of the squamous esophageal epithelium and the columnar gastric epithelium. It is present in patients with hiatus hernia.

Case N7

Myrtle Peeless, age 28, had chronic renal failure. After renal transplant, she was given high doses of steroids and cytotoxic drugs to avert a rejection. The kidney did not function well however, and the doses of prednisone she was receiving became astronomical. She began complaining of dysphagia, and a barium swallow was performed (Fig. 10–11). What does it show?

Monilial esophagitis primarily involves the upper two thirds of the esophagus and has a characteristic appearance. It occurs in patients receiving high doses of immunosuppressive drugs such as those used in the treatment of lymphoma or leukemia or the control of renal transplant rejection. Monilial esophagitis may be treated with amphotericin.

Case N8

When Edwin Clutternut was 16, he was helping the lady of the manor in her greenhouse on a very hot day. Although he had been told not to touch anything, he became thirsty and, spying a bottle of "lemonade" in the corner, drank it all down in one gulp. He immediately felt a burning sensation and vomited copiously. He was rushed to the hospital and treated accordingly. Twenty years later, he presented with recurrent dysphagia, and a barium swallow was performed (Fig. 10–12). What does it show, and what did he swallow?

The severity of esophageal narrowing depends on the amount and the concentration of the lye or acid swallowed. The stricture usually involves the lower third of the esophagus and is associated initially with spasm, irritability, mucosal edema, and ulceration. During the healing phase, fibrosis and stricture occur in many patients.

In most of the clinical situations discussed above, the investigation of choice has been the barium swallow; but there are, of course, many signs and symptoms involving the cervical region that are not related to the upper gastrointestinal tract. For example, hoarseness is investigated by larynogography, or a patient may present with a mass in the neck, which the clinician is able to diagnose on the basis of other clinical signs and symptoms. This group of conditions includes lymphomas, thyroid and parathyroid adenomas, bronchial cysts, and duplications of the pharynx or larynx. Although plain films may not be helpful in diagnosing these conditions, radionuclide scans are of particular use in one group of diseases.

Case N9

Viola Estherhazy, age 45, presented with a lump in her neck and somewhat staring eyes. The chest x-ray and barium swallow study were normal. What is the investigation of choice?

For 30 years, radioisotope scans have been used for the investigation of thyroid disease. It is now possible to image the thyroid gland with ease and to differentiate between functioning ("hot") nodules from non-functioning ("cold") nodules (Fig. 10–13) as well as to distinguish a single nodule from a multinodular gland (which may not

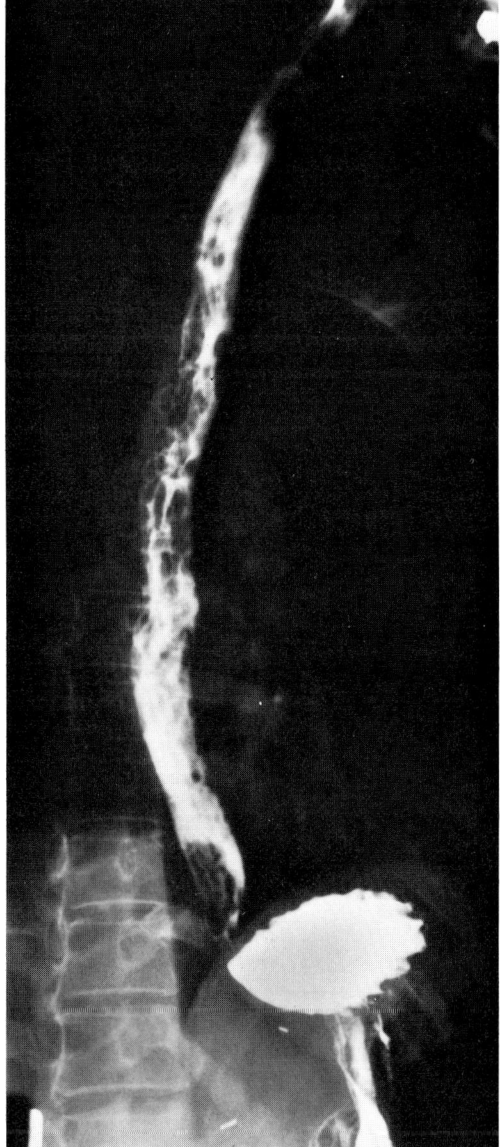

Figure 10–11. Monilial esophagitis. The characteristic irregularity of the esophageal wall can be seen, with nodular defects and deep ulcerations involving both the mucosa and the submucosa.

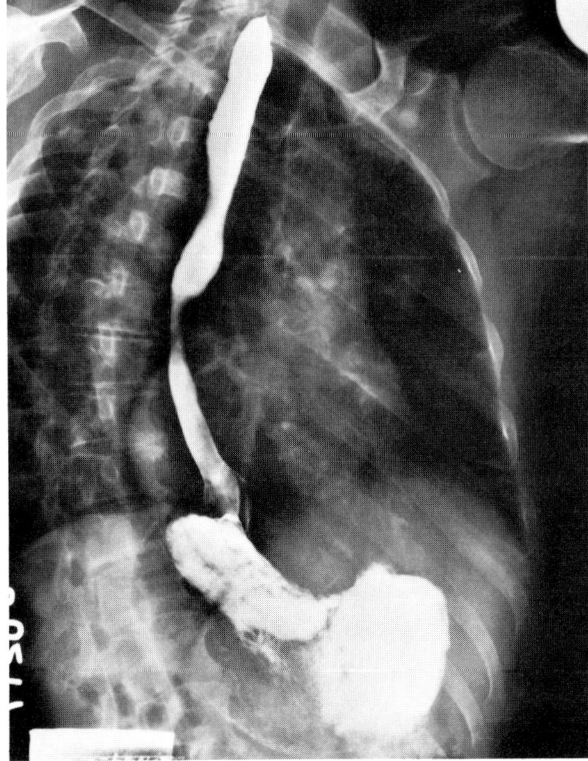

Figure 10–12. Old esophageal stricture from lye ingestion. The smooth narrowing of the midesophagus can be seen 5 cm below the tracheal bifurcation. Fluids passed through freely but solids (e.g., a barium tablet) were held up.

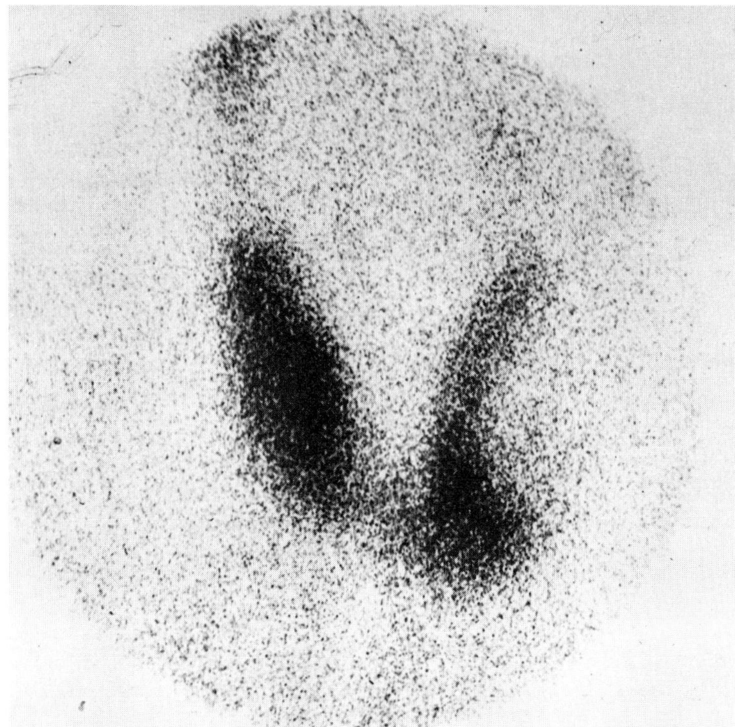

Figure 10–13. Nonfunctioning thyroid nodule. This technetium-99m (pertechnetate sodium) image demonstrates a large (3 by 4 cm) nonfunctioning nodule in the lateral margin of the left lobe of the gland, a finding that correlated exactly with the clinical findings. Such scans should always be interpreted with knowledge of the results of palpation of the neck.

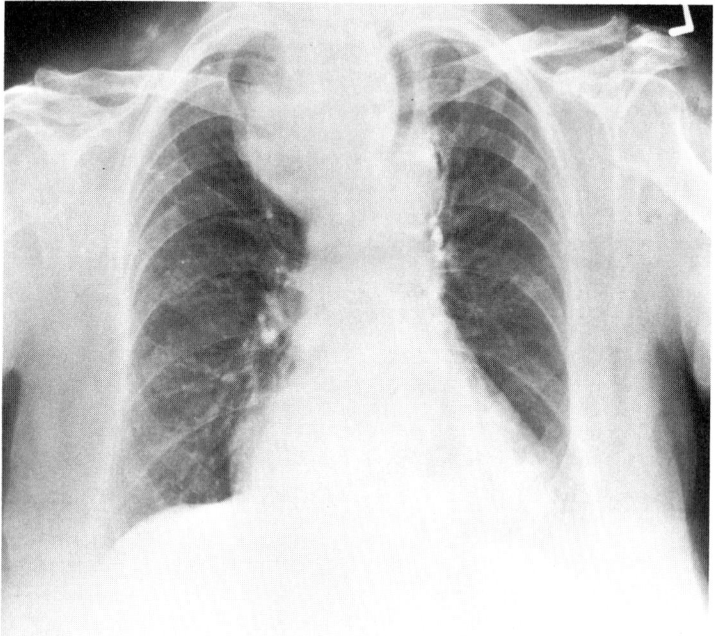

Figure 10–14. Substernal goiter. This chest x-ray shows a large superior mediastinal mass deviating the trachea to the left.

be possible with palpation). Making these distinctions is important, because the potential of malignancy is fairly high in nonfunctioning nodules but extremely low in functioning single nodules or in a multinodular thyroid gland. At times, the combination of a radionuclide scan and ultrasonographic examination of the thyroid is of great help in differentiating the internal structure of large nodules, thus preventing unnecessary operations on such conditions as simple cysts with or without hemorrhage or with areas of thyroiditis.

Finally, a brief mention should be made of substernal goiter, which can present as a superior mediastinal mass on a chest x-ray (Fig. 10–14). It is a common cause of a superior mediastinal density in young and middle-aged patients and can be differentiated from other mediastinal masses or unfolded great vessels by means of a radionuclide scan.

CHAPTER 11

THE BACK

Pain in the back is even more common than pain in the neck, and there are many different causes. Two extremely common disorders, slipped intervertebral disc and osteoporosis, cause low back pain, although they usually affect different age groups. Metastases, various forms of arthritis (particularly those involving the sacroiliac joints), and a number of rarer conditions also cause back pain.

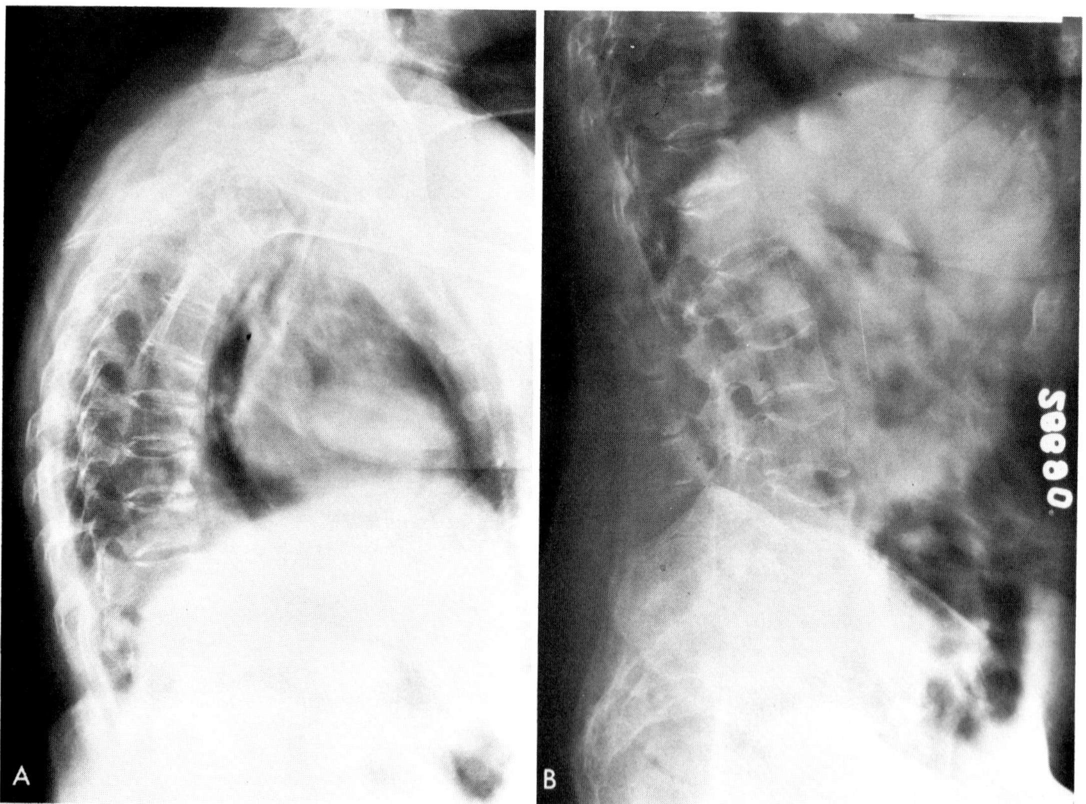

Figure 11–1. Osteoporosis. *A*, Lateral view of the thoracic spine. *B*, Lateral view of the lumbar spine. Note the lack of bone trabeculae in the vertebral bodies as well as the apparent accentuation of the end-plates. Many of the bodies have a biconcave ("codfish") shape, particularly those in the lower lumbar region.

Case S1

Winnie DePooh, age 98, came in complaining of recurrent back pain and the fact that she was definitely getting shorter. She had noticed her loss of height after an annual trip to Florence to be fitted for new clothes. The pain in her back was accentuated each time she collected the honey from the 300 beehives on her husband's farm. On examination she was found to be remarkably fit for her age. Her x-rays were characteristic (Fig. 11–1).

Osteopenia, or loss of bone mineral, is probably a more correct term than *osteoporosis*, unless the etiology of the loss of bone is definitely known. This elderly female patient almost certainly has osteoporosis, an inevitable accompaniment of aging. In females, bone mineral content is at a peak around age 35, and in men the bone mineral remains relatively constant until it begins to decline around age 55. The etiology of "senile" or postmenopausal loss of bone mineral is not well understood, but it appears to be an imbalance between bone formation and bone resorption. Osteoporosis is probably caused by increased resorption rather than decreased formation.

There are many causes of osteopenia (Table 11–1); radiographically it is often difficult to distinguish among them, although the clinical findings can be of great assistance. The classic radiographic features of osteopenia include a loss of bone mineral; this is best seen radiographically in the spine, where initially loss of the trabeculae and accentuation of the endplates occurs. As the disorder progresses, the vertebral bodies become weaker than the intervertebral discs and begin to assume a characteristic biconcave shape ("codfish" or "fishmouth" vertebrae). The patient loses height as a result. Osteopenia involves the whole skeleton, so that loss of bone mineral can be seen in the long bones as well as in the central skeleton. Loss of cortex and thinning of the secondary (non–weight-bearing) trabeculae in the cancellous regions, visible early in the course of the condition, leads to an increase in the number of fractures of the wrist and femoral neck, particularly in older female patients.

Some causes of osteopenia other than the osteoporosis of ageing should be mentioned: Many elderly patients have some degree of osteomalacia as well as osteoporosis, although pure osteomalacia due to malnutrition or malabsorption (such as occurs in sprue) is relatively rare. The radiographic hallmark of osteomalacia is the presence of pseudofractures, or Looser's zones, which occur bilaterally and often symmetrically at right angles to the cortex of the ischial and pubic rami, and at the inner side of the femoral and humeral necks, scapulae, and upper ribs. Radiologists disagree about some earlier radiographic signs of osteomalacia, but intracortical tunnelling may be seen on magnification views of the hands, and there is often a distinct fuzziness of the trabecular margins throughout the skeleton.

TABLE 11–1. Causes of Bone Loss

OSTEOPOROSIS
- Idiopathic or physiological
- Involutional
- Transient
- Heparin-induced or alcohol-induced

ENDOCRINE DISEASE
- Hyperparathyroidism
- Hyperthyroidism
- Hypercortisonism (from Cushing's syndrome or misuse of corticosteroids)
- Turner's syndrome
- Diabetes mellitus

OSTEOMALACIA (WITH OR WITHOUT SECONDARY HYPERPARATHYROIDISM) DUE TO
- Vitamin D deficiency (from malnutrition or malabsorption)
- Renal tubular disorders
- Chronic renal failure
- Alcoholism
- Use of anticonvulsant drugs

OSTEOGENESIS IMPERFECTA

IMMOBILIZATION OR DISUSE FOLLOWING STROKE, PARALYSIS, OR FRACTURE

DIFFUSE MYELOMATOSIS OR CARCINOMATOSIS

CHRONIC DISEASE SUCH AS RHEUMATOID ARTHRITIS

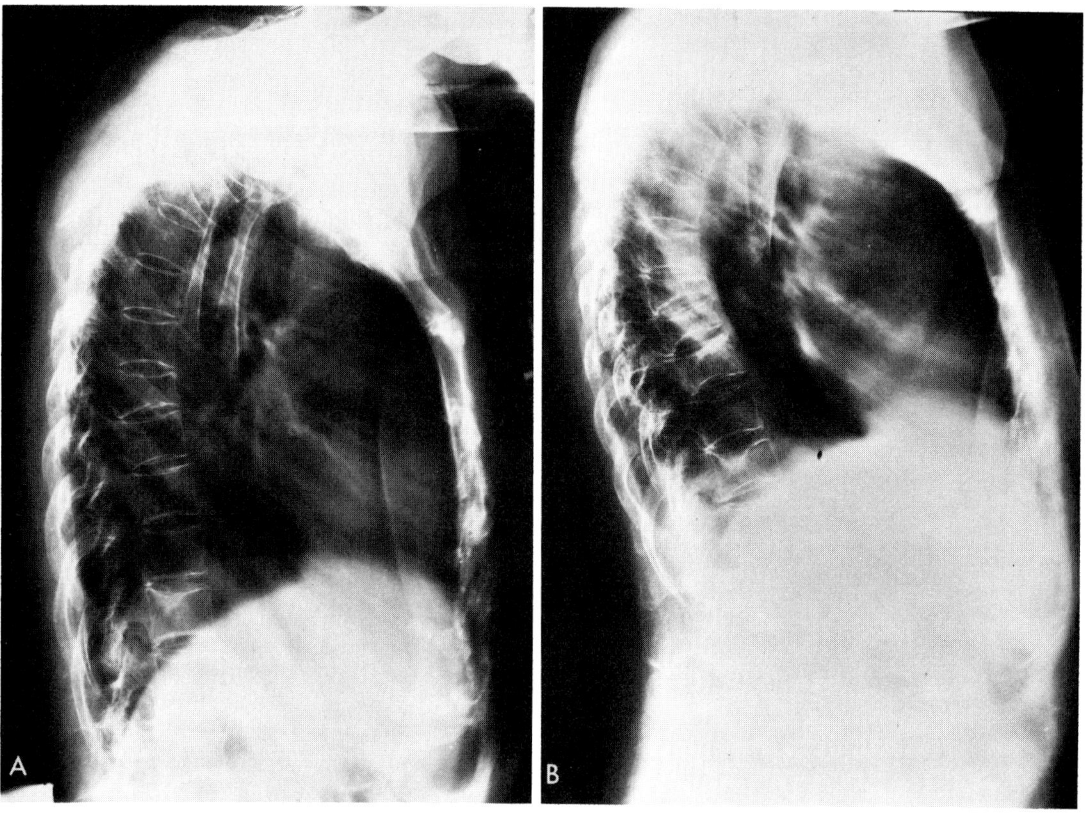

Figure 11-2. Advancing osteoporosis. *A*, Lateral view of the thoracic spine. Severe osteopenia with some early wedging of one of the midthoracic vertebral bodies can be seen. *B*, Lateral view taken two years later. There has been obvious increased anterior wedging of many of the vertebral bodies with apparent widening of the disc spaces.

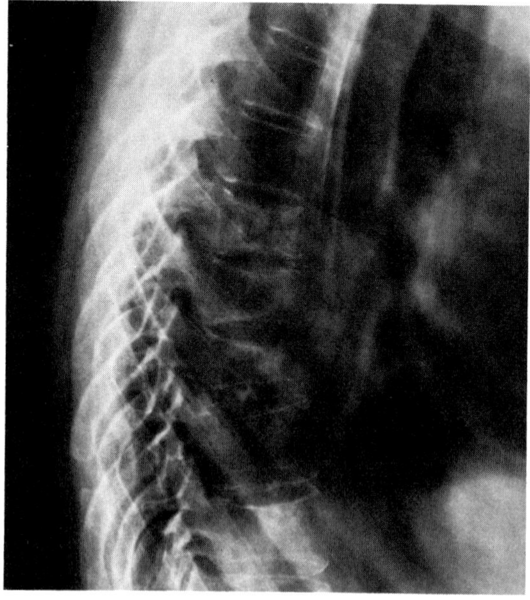

Figure 11–3. Multiple myeloma. In this lateral view of the thoracic spine, note the generalized osteoporosis with wedging of T7, T8, and T9. The mottled lucency and associated density might suggest metastatic disease, but the generalized osteoporosis excludes that possibility. A sternal marrow aspiration revealed the correct diagnosis.

Case S2

Knox Horsefeet, age 51, had a life history of allergies and asthma. Recently he began visiting two different physicians, so that he was able to take massive doses of corticosteroids. He claimed that he required large doses of prednisone to control his asthma, and when he was warned of the consequences, he went off to a third physician to get still more of the drug. He began to compain of low back pain. What will his x-rays probably show (Fig. 11–2)?

Steroid-induced osteoporosis is unfortunately common, even though it has been observed that Cushing's syndrome, which results from hyperadrenocortisonism, causes severe, often irreversible osteoporosis. Doctors try to modify the dosage of steroids for control of such conditions as asthma, systemic lupus erythematosus, and rheumatoid arthritis, so that a balance can be achieved between the clinically useful effects and the untoward side effects of the drug.

Case S3

Ricketty Cushing, age 49, was brushing his teeth one morning when he "felt something snap" in his back and then experienced excruciating back pain. His physician examined him and ordered x-rays of the lumbar spine (Fig. 11–3).

In this young patient with no known disease, there is some evidence of generalized osteoporosis with a number of wedged vertebral bodies that have a mottled appearance. It is all too easy to write this off as a case of early senile osteoporosis. Osteomalacia does not cause these presenting symptoms. Cushing's disease and thyrotoxicosis cause other signs and symptoms. Primary osseous tumors or bone metastases from elsewhere in the body usually involve one vertebral body and only rarely produce generalized osteoporosis. But there is one common neoplasm that may cause generalized osteopenia, particularly in younger male patients. It is imperative to check the blood and urine of every patient under 50 with unexplained osteopenia for the presence of M-type proteins in the blood and of Bence Jones protein, which is present in the urine of 60 per cent of patients with multiple myeloma. This patient had multiple myeloma.

Case S4

Claudius Strain, age 24, was a removal man. While carrying a grand piano across a swimming pool by himself one day, he experienced excruciating pain that radiated down the back of his leg to his calf. Examination revealed guarding and slight scoliosis. Lumbar spine x-rays were normal. A myelogram confirmed the diagnosis of slipped intervertebral disc (Fig. 11–4).

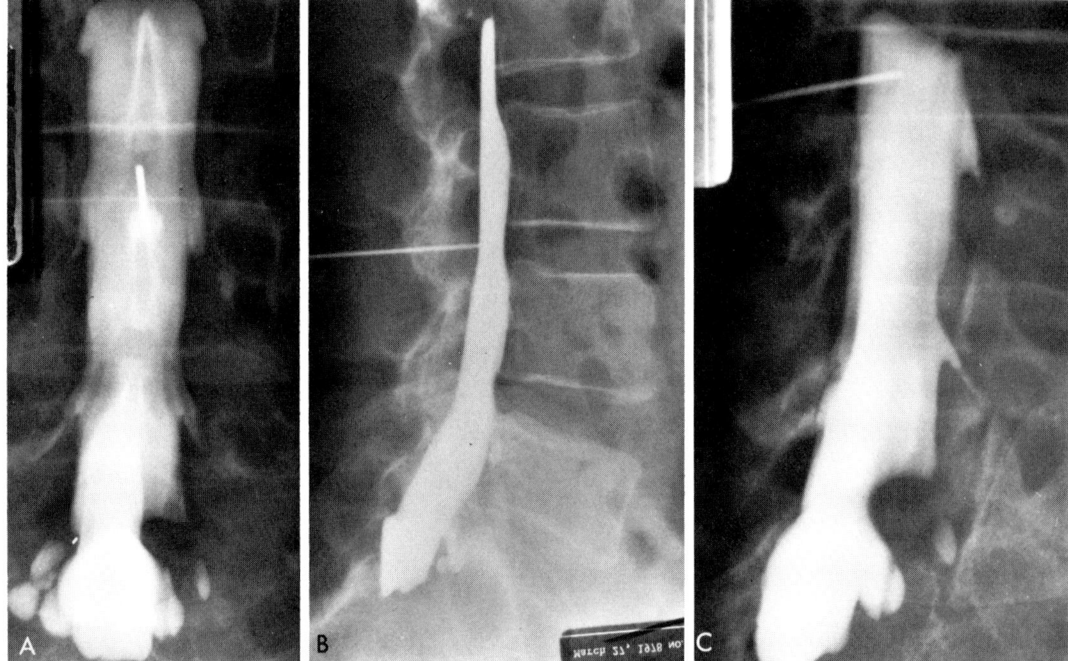

Figure 11–4. Slipped intervertebral disc, AP view (*A*), lateral view (*B*), and oblique view (*C*). Although the lateral view shows indentation at L3 to L4, L4 to L5, and L5 to S1, the AP and oblique views demonstrate a characteristic pressure defect on the left at L5 to S1. At operation, this was found to be a prolapsed intervertebral disc.

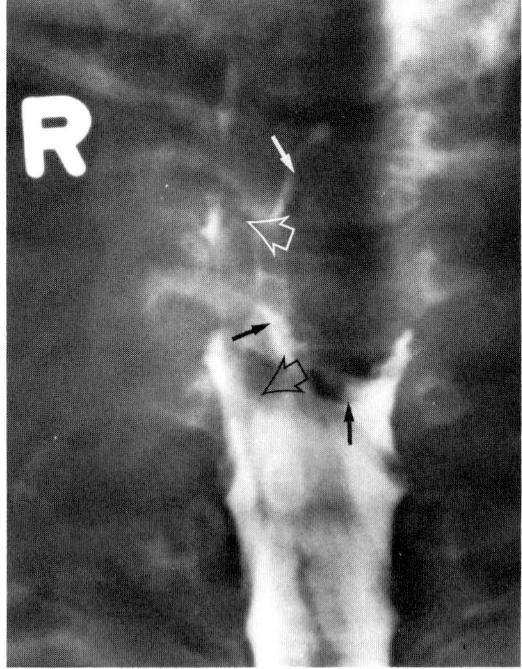

Figure 11–5. Extradural mass. This myelogram shows a large extradural mass (*small arrows*) almost blocking the spinal canal in the upper cervical region. Note the deviation of the cord to the right (*hollow arrows*). At operation, this was found to be a neurofibroma.

Low back pain may be caused by a slipped disc, a condition that usually affects patients younger than those who have osteoporosis. Because of the nature of the pain, the patient usually presents to an orthopedist. Many patients with slipped discs have no abnormal plain film findings, and a myelogram is essential for either confirmation or diagnosis of the disorder. In most cases of low back pain, myelography using an oily contrast medium provides adequate information. Discography may also be performed, but it has largely dropped out of fashion because the results are so frequently equivocal.

Case S5

Quentin Rattenburg, age 64, presented with a 3 1/2-year history of progressive left hemiparesis. Plain films revealed no abnormality, but a myelogram was performed (Fig. 11–5).

Differentiating between intradural and extradural lesions is usually easy with myelography. In this case, an extradural lesion was found in the cervical region. Causes of extradural lesions include hemangioma (in which the coarse vertical trabeculation of the vertebral body is seen), lymphoma, neurofibromatosis (usually associated with osseous defects and widening of the intervertebral foraminae), metastasis, myeloma, hematoma, infection, and abscess.

Intradural lesions (Fig. 11–6), can arise

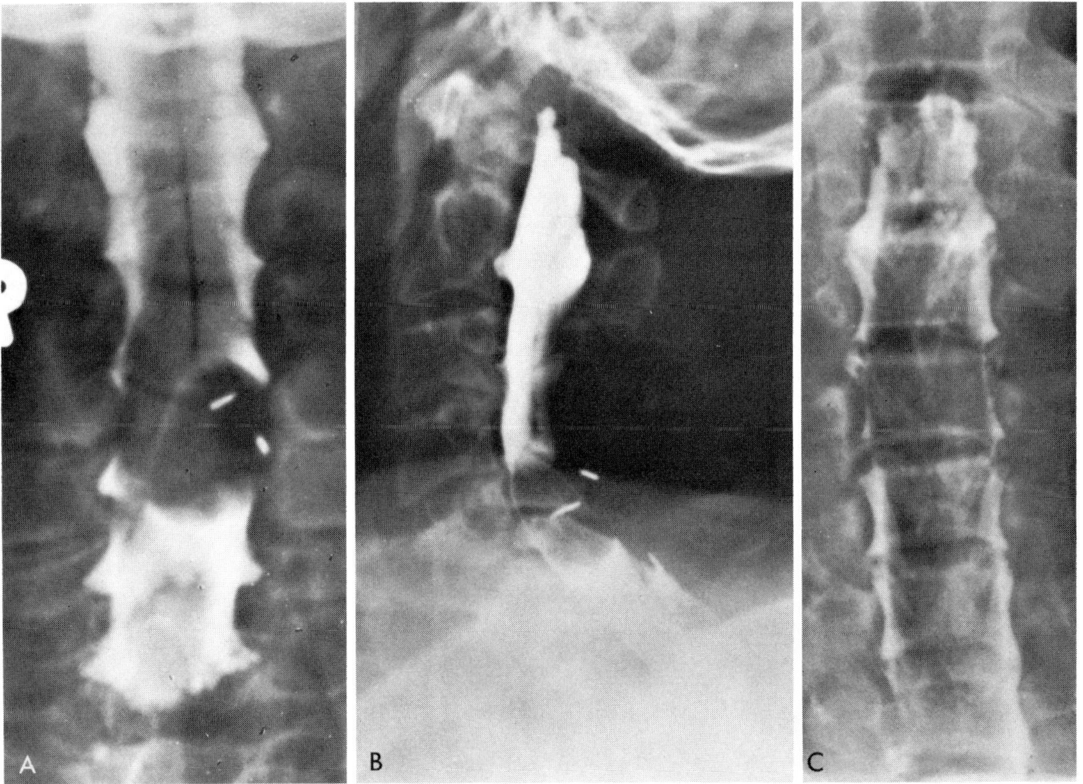

Figure 11–6. Intradural extramedullary mass. *A* and *B*, On the AP and lateral views taken at myelography, there is a large defect indenting the column of contrast from the left and posteriorly at C6. The extramedullary mass was a recurrent meningioma. The original tumor had been removed 20 years previously. *C*, Intradural intramedullary mass. The fusiform enlargement of the cervical cord without deformity of nerve root sheaths is characteristic of syringomyelia.

either within the dural space (extramedullary intradural) or in the cord itself (intramedullary). Myelography is required to differentiate these lesions from each other, but large intramedullary lesions occasionally cause widening of the interpedicular space of the vertebral bodies that is visible on plain films. Intramedullary lesions include ependymoma, glioma, astrocytoma, dermoid, syringomyelia, and vascular tumor. Most extramedullary intradural tumors are benign, and causes include neuroma, meningioma, and neurofibroma (which can be dumbbell-shaped and can be both extradural and extramedullary intradural).

Case S6

Emelia Whipsnade, age 62, entered her doctor's office in great pain. A lion tamer in the local zoo, she was unable to continue her duties because of the pain in her back. On examination, she appeared well but had marked tenderness over the lower lumbar spine. No biochemical abnormality could be found. X-rays of the lumbar spine were taken (Fig. 11–7). What would you do next?

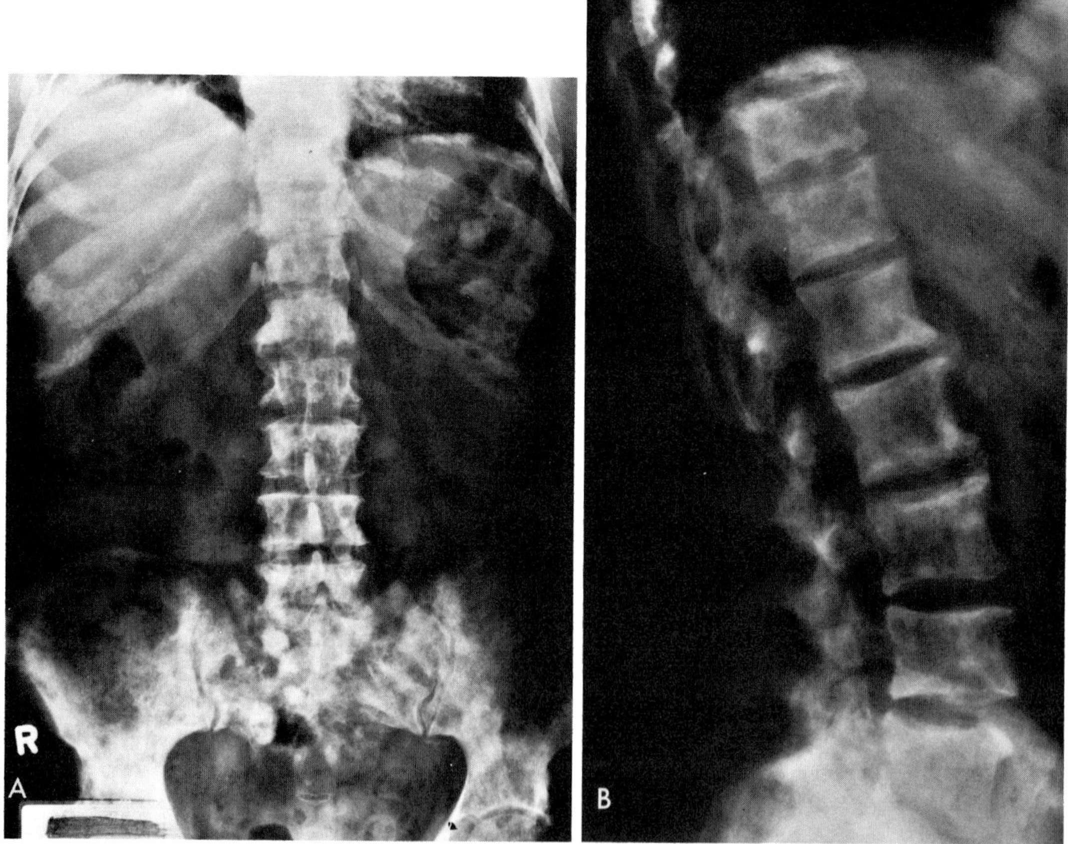

Figure 11–7. Lumbar spine. The AP view (*A*) and the lateral view (*B*) of the lumbar spine and pelvis reveal extensive osteolytic and osteoblastic defects typical of metastatic disease.

We have a lady in her middle years with obvious metastatic disease in all visualized bones. Low back pain may be the presenting feature of a malignancy later in the course of the disease. A bone scan reveals how widespread the condition is, can be referred to in planning therapy, and can be used to locate a metastasis that is accessible to biopsy (although biopsy of the spine can often be successful). The next step is to search for the primary site. What investigations would you choose, and in what order should they be performed?

In a female patient, the radiographic ap-

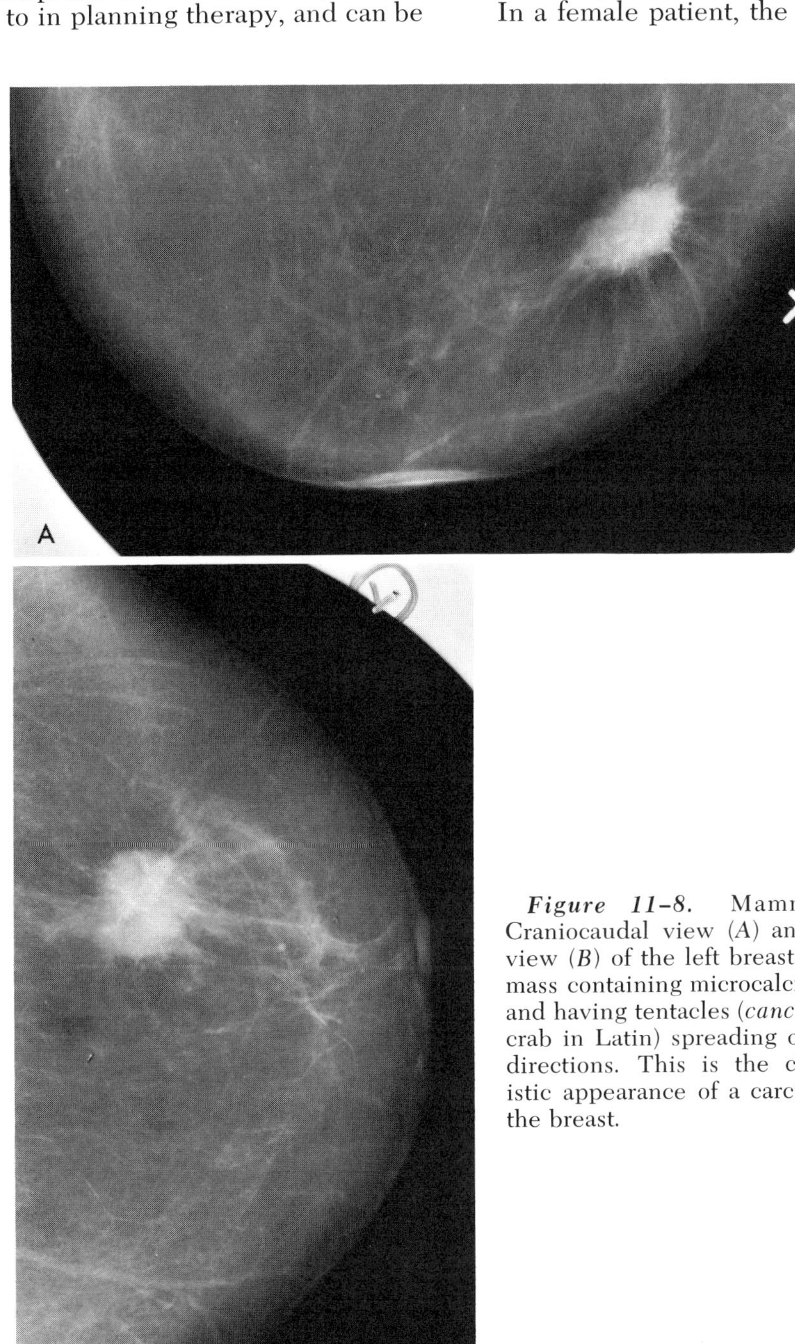

Figure 11–8. Mammogram. Craniocaudal view (*A*) and lateral view (*B*) of the left breast reveal a mass containing microcalcifications and having tentacles (*cancer* means crab in Latin) spreading out in all directions. This is the characteristic appearance of a carcinoma of the breast.

proach should include mammography, a CXR, and studies of the gastrointestinal and genitourinary tracts. Clinical examination of the cervix and uterus should also be made. A mammogram of this patient revealed the primary site (Fig. 11–8). In a male patient, the likely "silent" primary sites for lytic metastases are the lung, genitourinary tract, and gastrointestinal tract (including the pancreas). Metastases from cancer of the prostate are nearly always blastic (sclerotic) and will be discussed elsewhere.

Case S7

Giovanni de Bologna, age 28, was a truck driver who for many years had suffered from migraine, for which he had been treated with large doses of Methysergide. He now complained of a vague low back pain, loss of weight, and a low-grade fever. X-rays of his chest and lumbar spine were normal. What procedure should be performed next?

An intravenous pyelogram was diagnostic of a retroperitoneal process with deviation of the ureters toward the midline (Fig. 11–9). In view of the patient's long history of Methysergide ingestion, a presumed diagnosis of retroperitoneal fibrosis can be made, and the medication should be stopped. If necessary, surgical intervention using blunt dissection to free the ureters is usually successful. Differentiating between retroperitoneal fibrosis and retroperitoneal tumor may be difficult, although many tumors tend to affect only one side and to involve only one ureter.

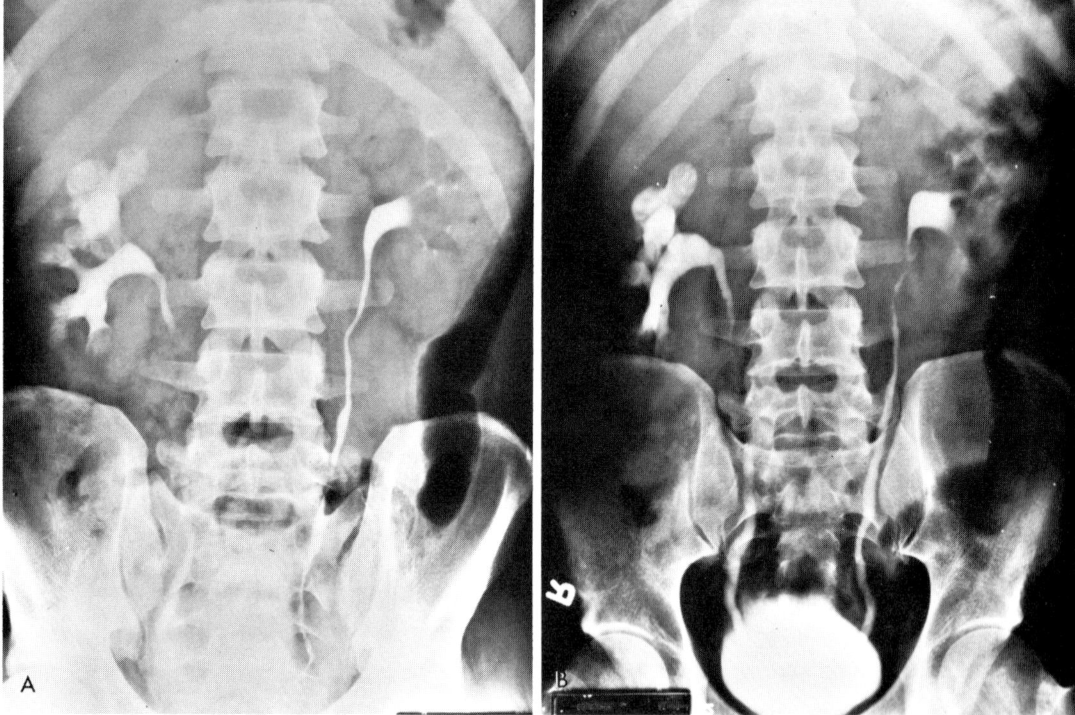

Figure 11–9. Retroperitoneal fibrosis. *A*, 10-minute IVP film. *B*, Prone 15-minute IVP film. Both ureters appear somewhat irregular, rigid, and fixed as well as medially deviated and scalloped, particularly in their distal portions. The bladder also has a somewhat peculiar configuration. At laparotomy, the diagnosis of retroperitoneal fibrosis was confirmed. (Note that the patient also has evidence of tubular ectasia and medullary sponge kidney, both of which are rare benign conditions not usually associated with retroperitoneal fibrosis.)

Case S8

Reuben Machalopolos, age 22, came in complaining of recurrent low back pain over the past few years. Previous visits to various physicians had failed to reveal any abnormality, and the patient had been regarded as a hypochondriac. On examination, he was stiff and had tenderness over the sacroiliac joints. What simple clinical test should be performed now? An x-ray of the pelvis and lumbar spine was diagnostic.

Ankylosing spondylitis often causes low back pain in male teenagers but has no diagnostic radiographic features. If the chest expansion is measured, it will be found to be decreased to 1 or 2 cm (normal is 1 or 2 in) in most patients. The patients are nearly always male, test results for rheumatoid factor are negative, but those for HLA-B27 are almost invariably positive. Ankylosing spondylitis usually begins in the sacroiliac joints, causing blurring of the margins, poorly defined erosions, sclerosis, and bony proliferation, which leads to fusion (Fig. 11–10). The disease progresses inexorably up the spine, with squaring of the vertebral bodies, osteopenia, ossification of the paraspinous ligaments, and involvement of the apophyseal and costovertebral joints (which accounts for the decrease in chest expansion). Ultimately, calcification of the interverte-

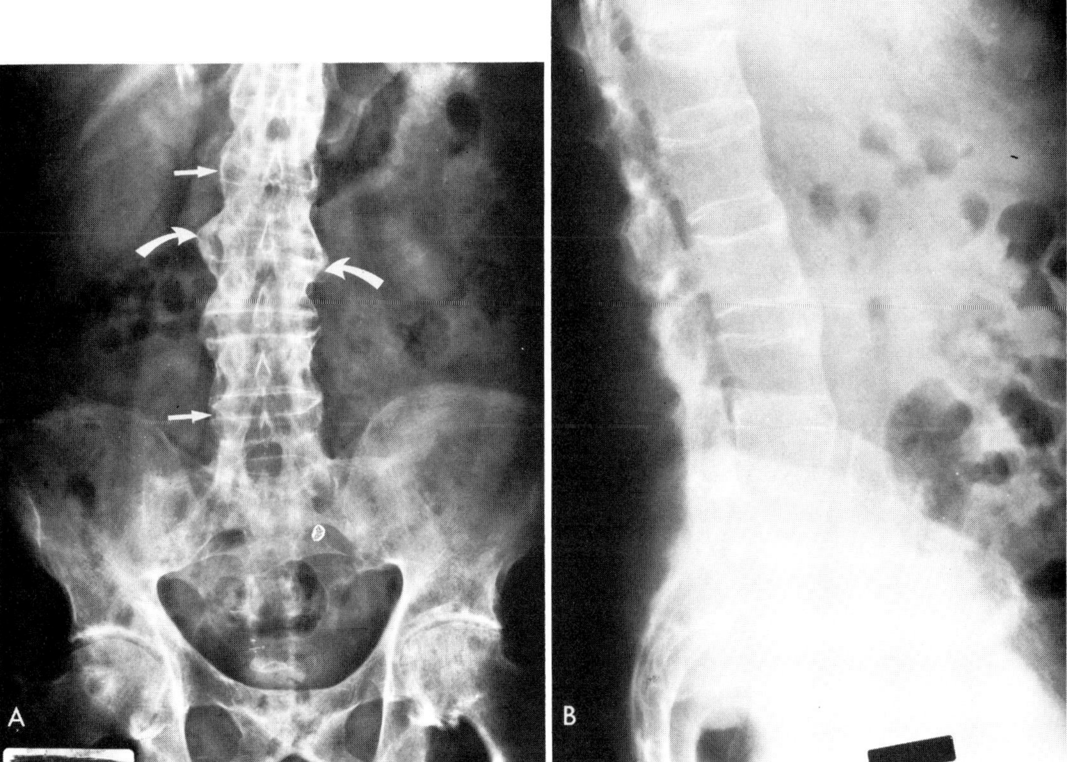

Figure 11–10. Ankylosing spondylitis, AP view (*A*) and lateral view (*B*). Fusion of the sacroiliac joints and the symphysis pubis is seen, with ossification of the anterior spinal ligament and vertebral osteopenia ("bamboo spine"). Degenerative changes in the hip joints and ossification in the paraspinal ligaments (*small arrows*) are also visible. Syndesmophytes (*large arrows*) occur in a number of rheumatoid variants, including ankylosing spondylitis, psoriatic arthritis, and Reiter's syndrome.

bral discs occurs, and fusion of the spine soon follows, producing the "poker" or "bamboo" spine. In about one third of cases there is involvement of the hips and shoulders, and some 5 per cent of patients develop aortitis, which may lead to aortic insufficiency. Death usually results from recurrent pneumonia or congestive heart failure.

Low back pain due to sacroiliitis also occurs in a number of other conditions that appear to be variants of rheumatoid arthritis in that they resemble rheumatoid arthritis but do not cause any change in the peripheral joints. A number of patients with these diseases develop frank rheumatoid arthritis. The constellation of clinical signs and symptoms accompanying sacroiliitis often leads to the correct diagnosis. It is of more than passing interest that test results of patients with these conditions are positive for HLA-B27 but negative for rheumatoid factor (Table 11–2).

TABLE 11–2. Causes of Sacroiliitis

Involvement	Possible Diagnoses
Bilateral	Ankylosing spondylitis Reiter's syndrome Hyperparathyroidism
Unilateral	Pyogenic infection Tuberculosis Infarcts seen in sickle-cell anemia
Bilateral or Unilateral	Enteropathic arthritis Psoriatic arthritis Rheumatoid arthritis Juvenile rheumatoid arthritis Gout

Case S9

Lucillus Cockleberry, age 22, developed nonspecific urethritis, low back pain, and uveitis after having been ill. What disorder could have caused these symptoms? A test for HLA-B27 was positive, and x-rays of the pelvis and oblique views of the sacroiliac joints showed the classic early changes of sacroiliitis (Fig. 11–11).

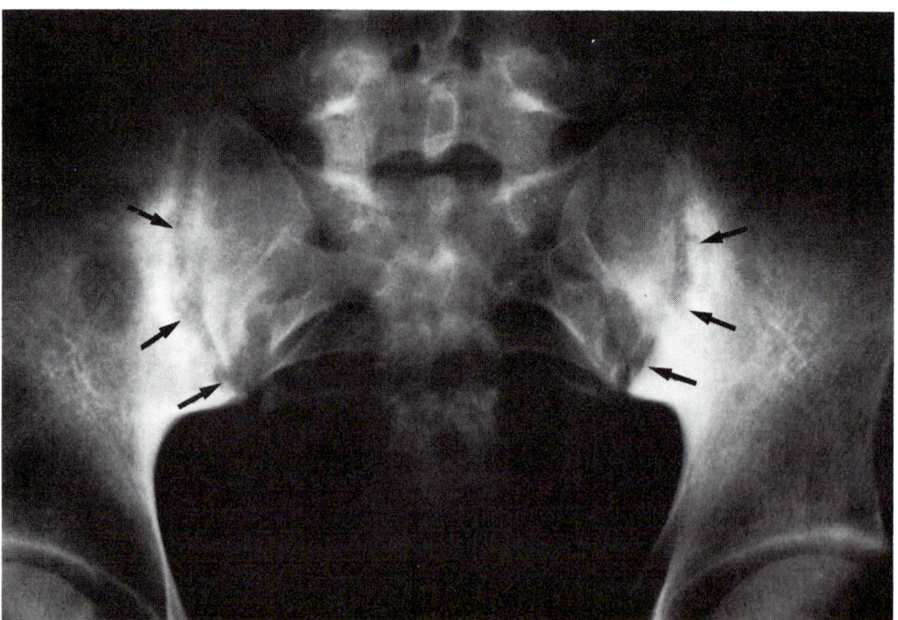

Figure 11–11. Reiter's syndrome. In this AP view of the pelvis, sclerosis surrounds both sacroiliac joints, which have multiple erosions (*arrows*).

This patient has Reiter's syndrome, which is usually preceded by either a venereal disease or bacillary dysentery (as it was in this patient and in Reiter's original case). Most of the patients are male and will experience remissions in a few weeks or months, although occasionally fusion of the sacroiliac joints occurs. A few patients develop either classic ankylosing spondylitis or frank rheumatoid arthritis.

The differential diagnosis of sacroiliitis in a young patient includes ankylosing spondylitis, Reiter's syndrome, and psoriatic arthritis. One should also consider the possibility of enteropathic arthritis, which is the development of joint disease in patients with ulcerative colitis or regional enteritis (Table 11–2).

CHAPTER 12

THE EXTREMITIES

There are many causes of pain in the extremities just as there are many different types of pain, ranging from the acute pain experienced following a fracture or dislocation to the vague pain associated with tumors or the throbbing sensation associated with some forms of Paget's disease. Conditions causing pain in the extremities are discussed in their order of frequency as seen by the radiologist or the clinician.

Case E1 Jessekiah DePooh, age 78, tripped and fell in her apiary and was brought in complaining of pain in her hip. An x-ray of the pelvis was taken (Fig. 12–1). What does it show?

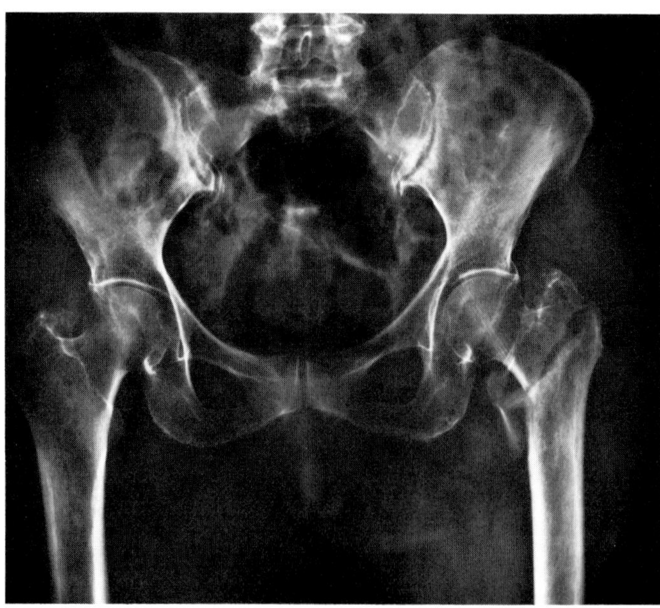

Figure 12–1. Fracture of the femoral neck (AP view). There is a comminuted intertrochanteric fracture of the left femoral neck. Slight impaction of the fracture is present. Note the generalized osteoporosis, which is in keeping with the patient's age.

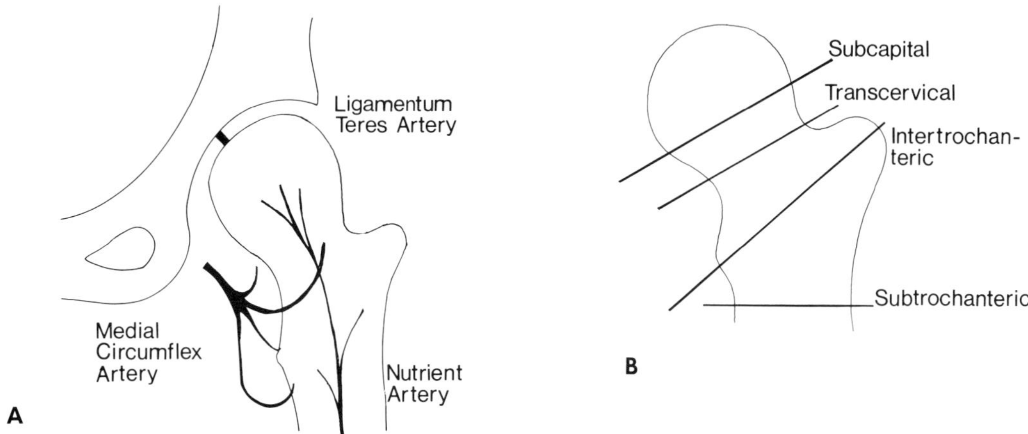

Figure 12–2. *A*, Diagram of the blood supply to the femoral head. *B*, Drawing showing the principal types of fracture of the femoral neck.

Fractures of the femoral neck are usually easy to diagnose from x-rays. Sometimes, however, a fracture impacts and either lateral or oblique views are necessary to confirm the diagnosis. Fractures of the femoral neck are usually categorized according to the anatomical level of the break; this classification is important because of the possible effect on the blood supply to the femoral head. In the fetus and the neonate most of the blood is supplied through the ligamentum teres, but this source usually dries up with age, and in the adult most of the blood is supplied from the femoral nutrient arteries (Fig. 12–2). Thus, subcapital fractures of the femoral neck have a higher incidence (33 per cent) of avascular necrosis of the femoral head than intertrochanteric fractures (10 per cent), for which the body can compensate by opening a collateral supply via the capsular vessels (see Table 12–1).

There are many ways of treating a femoral neck fracture. If it is impacted and not displaced, the fracture is left alone to heal. If the neck is very displaced, resulting in shortening of the leg, internal fixation with a metal pin or screw is required (Fig. 12–3). If the fracture is hopelessly comminuted, the femoral head must be replaced with a prosthesis.

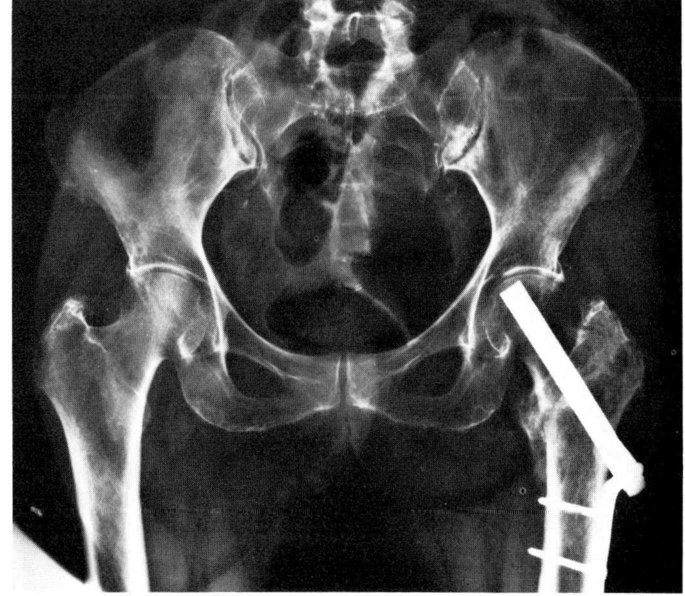

Figure 12–3. Internal fixation of the fracture of the femoral neck (AP view). A pin and plate can be seen to lie in good position, with normal alignment of the bones and correction of the deformity (see Figure 12–1).

Case E2

Amelia Bentworthy, age 68, went out shopping on an icy day. While running for the bus, she slipped and fell on her outstretched hand. What common fracture did she sustain (Fig. 12–4)?

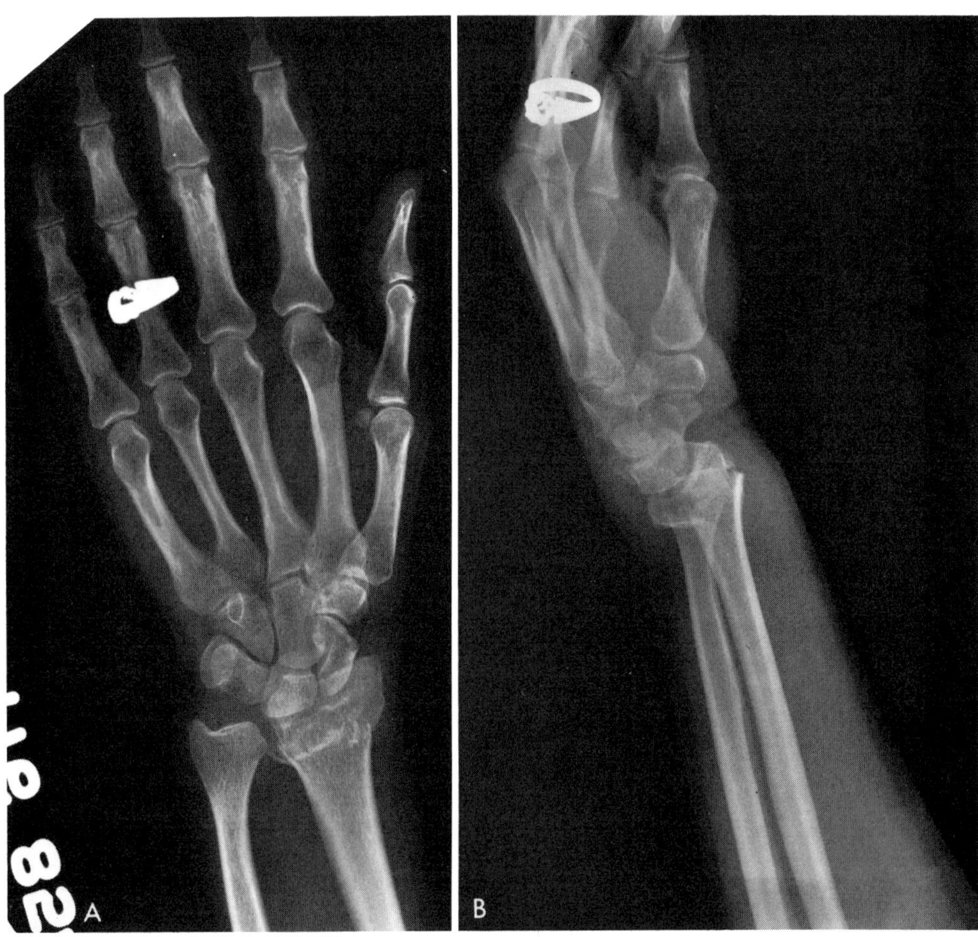

Figure 12–4. Fracture of the distal radius, AP view (*A*) and lateral view (*B*). There is a comminuted fracture of the distal radius with pronounced posterior angulation.

In most fractures, the alignment of the bones is the most important factor in prognosis. In fractures of the distal radius, alignment is especially important because of the marked dorsal (posterior) angulation that must be corrected at reduction. Radial displacement is corrected by placing the arm in an ulnar-deviated plaster cast.

The good radiologist offers the orthopedist his opinion on the alignment, presence or absence of impaction, comminution, or distraction, and position of the bones involved.

For diagnosis of any fracture, certain general principles are important to both the physician and the radiologist. The principles outlined in Chapter 1 apply to radiological diagnosis of fractures in an extremity. In almost every case, more than one view of the suspected fracture should be taken. AP and lateral views are standard, but in some areas, such as the wrist and ankle, an oblique view is helpful. The joints above and below the fracture should be included on the film, in order not to miss a second fracture. The concept of a ring of bone applies

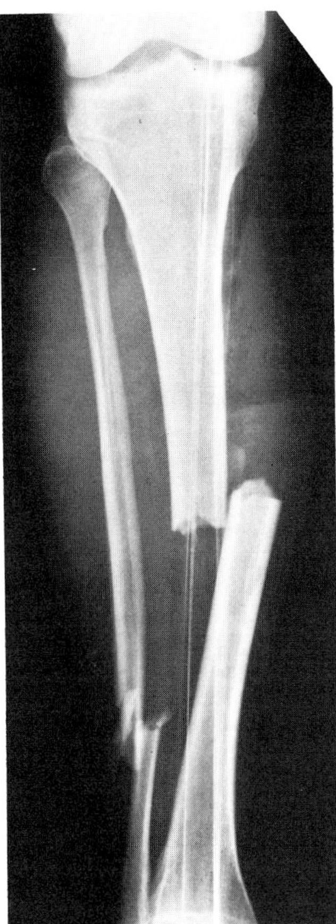

Figure 12–5. Comminuted fractures of tibia and fibula (AP view). Compound fractures of the tibia and fibula are seen in this young man who was assaulted. Note that the fractures of the two bones are at different levels; hence, it is imperative to include the whole length of both bones if a fracture is suspected.

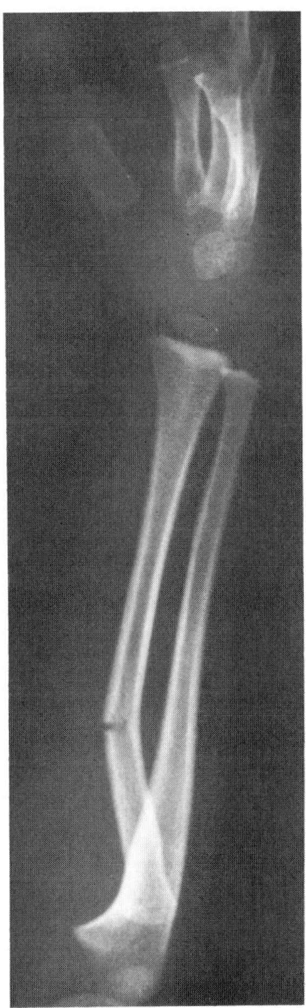

Figure 12–6. Greenstick fracture. There is a fracture through one cortex of the radius with deformity and apparent bending of the bone.

in certain areas: tibia-fibula (Fig. 12–5), radius-ulna, orbit-maxillary antrum, and pelvis. If there is any doubt or problem, x-ray the opposite side for comparison.

Children's bones are malleable and may not break completely. Thus, certain fractures occur only in children, the most common being the greenstick fracture (Fig. 12–6) and the torus fracture. In a greenstick fracture, the bone is broken on only one side and is bent on the other, which is what happens if you attempt to break a green stick. A torus fracture is an impacted fracture. The word *torus* derives from the Greek and refers to the concentric rings seen at the base of a classic column; it is also used by engineers to describe a doughnut, or concentric rings.

Case E3

Wentworth Billingsgate, age 40, fell off his motorcycle into a muddy ditch and landed on his right shoulder. He experienced some pain which was alleviated by the alcohol he had been drinking at his physician's Christmas party, and he picked himself up and went home. Three days later he presented to his local emergency room

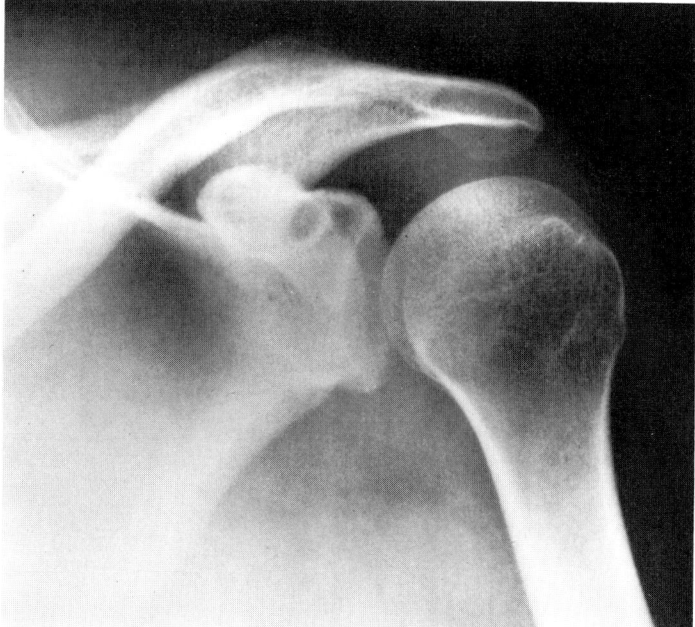

Figure 12–7. Normal shoulder. There is no apparent abnormality. (Internal and external rotation views were taken.)

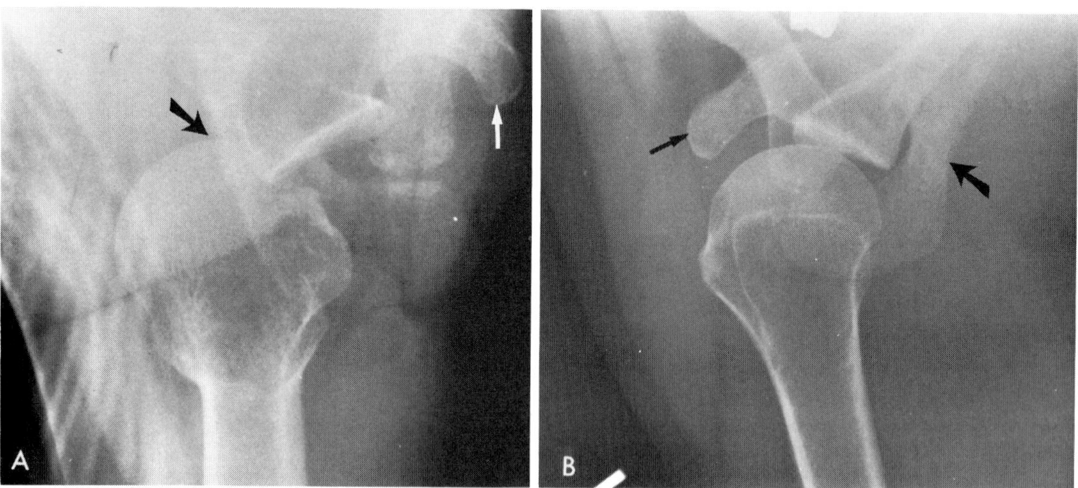

Figure 12–8. A, Posterior dislocation of the shoulder. *B*, View of a normal shoulder for comparison. Note that in the dislocated shoulder (*A*), the humeral head lies posterior to the glenoid. The orientation is worked out by finding the coracoid process anteriorly (*small arrows*) and the spine of the scapula posteriorly (*large arrows*).

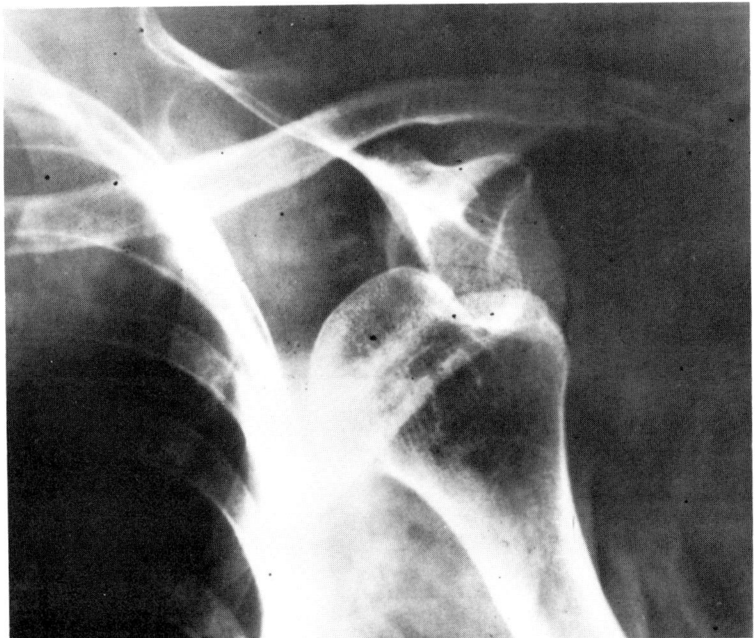

Figure 12–9. Anterior dislocation of the shoulder. The humeral head is seen to lie below and medial to the glenoid. A fracture of the humeral greater tuberosity or the labrum should be searched for on the post-reduction radiographs.

Case E3 (Continued)

with continuing pain in his shoulder associated with some difficulty in movement. Internal and external rotation views were taken and were read as normal (Fig. 12–7). Three weeks later, he came back with increasing pain, and an axial view of the shoulder showed posterior dislocation (Fig. 12–8).

Dislocations are another source of acute pain in and around a joint, but most can be diagnosed clinically even without radiography. Dislocation of the shoulder, however, is not always obvious. In injuries around the shoulder it is imperative to take a film at right angles to the normal AP view—an oblique, transthoracic lateral or true axial view is essential for the diagnosis of a posterior dislocation. Anterior dislocation (which accounts for 95 per cent of shoulder dislocations) is easy to diagnose, because the humeral head drops medially and below the glenoid (Fig. 12–9).

Dislocation of most other joints such as the elbow, knee, and ankle are easy to diagnose, but recurrent dislocation of the acromioclavicular joint may require traction views. Dislocation of the spine such as atlantoaxial subluxation often produces neurological signs and symptoms; tomography is usually needed because of confusing shadows produced on plain films by overlying bones and soft tissues.

Case E4

Prendergast Fotheringly Smythe, age 72, came in complaining of increasing pain and deformity in his left tibia. The pain appeared to be rather vague, and was associated with a throbbing sensation. The area showed an increase in temperature, and the leg was significantly bowed. The x-rays were diagnostic (Fig. 12–10).

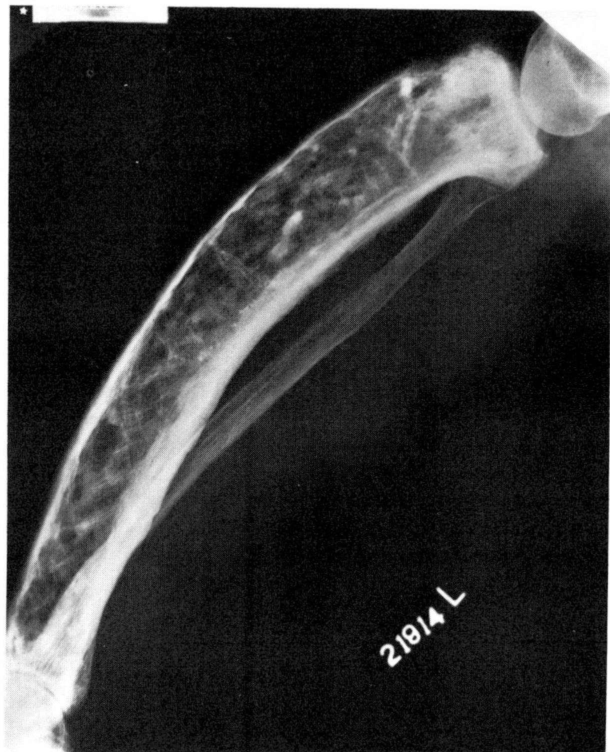

Figure 12–10. Paget's disease: tibia. Note the distortion of the normal architecture of the tibia with expansion, bowing, loss of the anterior cortex, and the presence of abnormal trabeculae throughout the bone—both cortical and intramedullary.

Paget's disease, perhaps one of the most interesting bone diseases, is also one of the most common. Its incidence is said to vary from 5 per cent up to 30 per cent in people over 60, and the incidence apparently increases the further north one lives. The condition is often diagnosed serendipitously in an elderly patient without relevant symptoms for whom a KUB has been taken (i.e., as a scout film for an IVP or upper GI study), but it can cause symptoms, particularly if it involves an extremity.

In most people, Paget's disease is polyostotic, and the bones most frequently involved are the pelvis, femurs, spine, and skull, although it can affect virtually any bone. Paget's disease is a condition afflicting the elderly and is probably never seen in patients under the age of 40 and rarely in patients under the age of 50. Paget's disease is a condition associated with reorganization of bone formation and bone resorption without any known antecedent etiological factor. Initially, excessive resorption of bone occurs, leading to a "candle flame" lucency (Fig. 12–11). This is followed by the laying down of excessive disorganized bone, usually causing thickening of the cortices and widening of the bone itself, which is characteristic and virtually pathognomonic of Paget's disease (Fig. 12–12).

There are a number of side effects of Paget's disease. Pain is often manageable with calcitonin therapy. An increase in blood flow occurs because the pagetoid bone acts like a large arteriovenous malformation, and this may lead to congestive heart failure in susceptible elderly patients. There is an increased incidence of fractures in the area of increased resorption.

Osteosarcomatous malignant degeneration occurs in some patients with Paget's disease. Malignant change is extremely rare in our opinion, and in the United States, a bone radiologist sees hundreds of cases of Paget's disease in a year but probably only one malignancy in three or four years. Since Paget's disease is often asymptomatic and found only at autopsy, its true incidence is unknown, and the risk of malignant change in Paget's disease is probably in the order of one in many thousand.

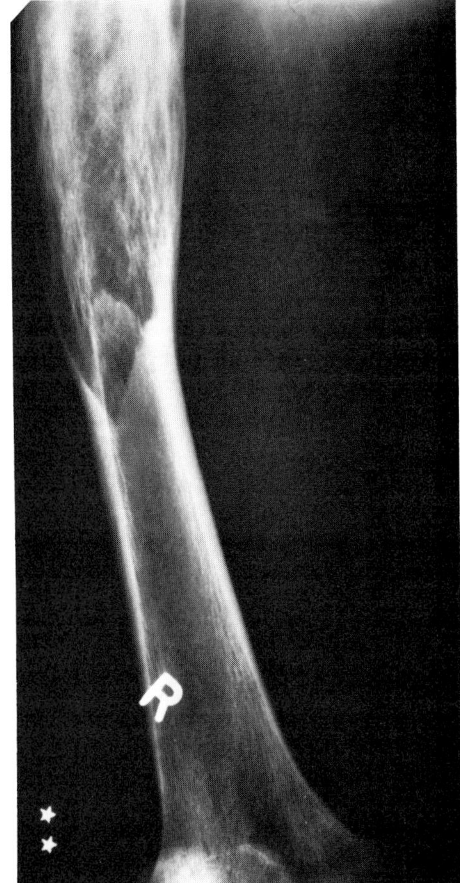

Figure 12–11. Paget's disease: femur. In long bones, the resorptive phase of Paget's disease precedes the formative osteoblastic phase. Thus a lucent expansion may be seen running down a bone, characteristically asymmetrical in that it affects only one cortex. This picture is said to resemble a "candle flame."

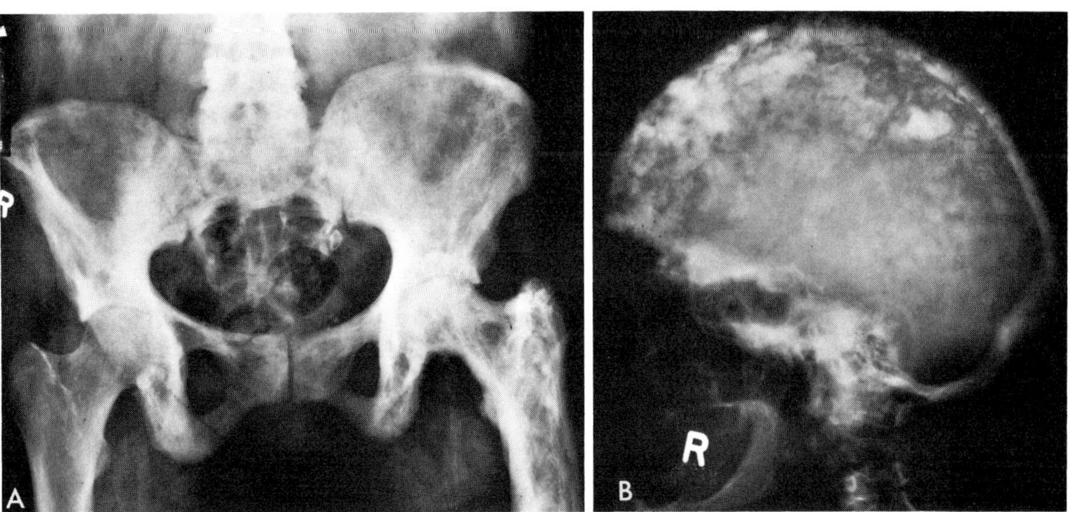

Figure 12–12. Paget's disease. *A*, In this pelvis, grossly disorganized bone can be seen in the left femur and the rami bilaterally as well as in both iliac bones. There is an irregular patchy increase in density, with thickened cortices, abnormal trabecular pattern, and expansion and deformity of the involved bones. *B*, In the skull, gross deformity can be seen, with thickening and areas of increased density as well as blurring of the normal trabecular pattern.

Case E5

Johnny Peewit, age 11, was noticed to be limping for a few days. He was brought to the emergency room and on examination was found to have a red swollen leg. An x-ray showed only soft-tissue swelling. What would you do now?

Five years ago, this situation would have presented a clinical problem, but the current procedure is to do a technetium scan, by means of which very early osteomyelitis can be detected. A gallium scan demonstrates a "hot" area, indicating infection of either soft tissue (cellulitis) or bone, but a technetium scan in suspected osteomyelitis shows a hot area only for a bone infection (Fig. 12–13).

Figure 12–14 illustrates the classic radiographic changes of a long bone infection as it progresses. Note that the initial soft-tissue swelling is followed by the loss of soft-tissue (fat) planes, followed by periosteal

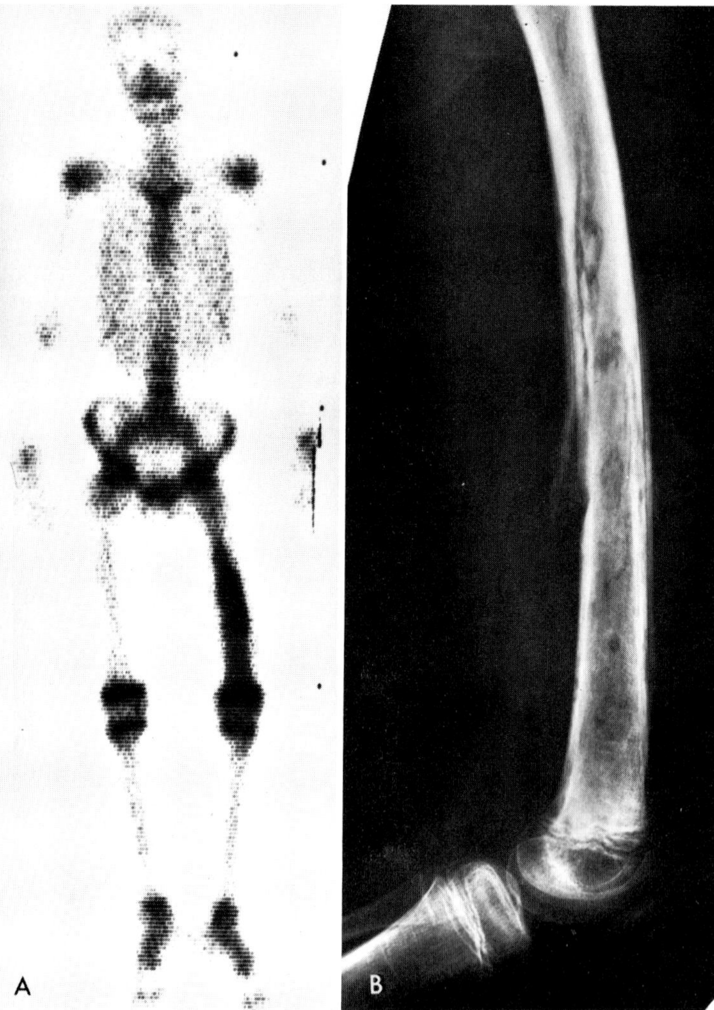

Figure 12–13. Osteomyelitis of the femur. The initial radiographs appeared to be normal. *A*, A bone scan showed the extent of the involvement of the left femur at ten days. *B*, A film taken at six weeks shows the periosteal reaction, with an "onionskin" appearance as well as the patchy resorption of bone from the diaphysis into the distal metaphysis of the femur.

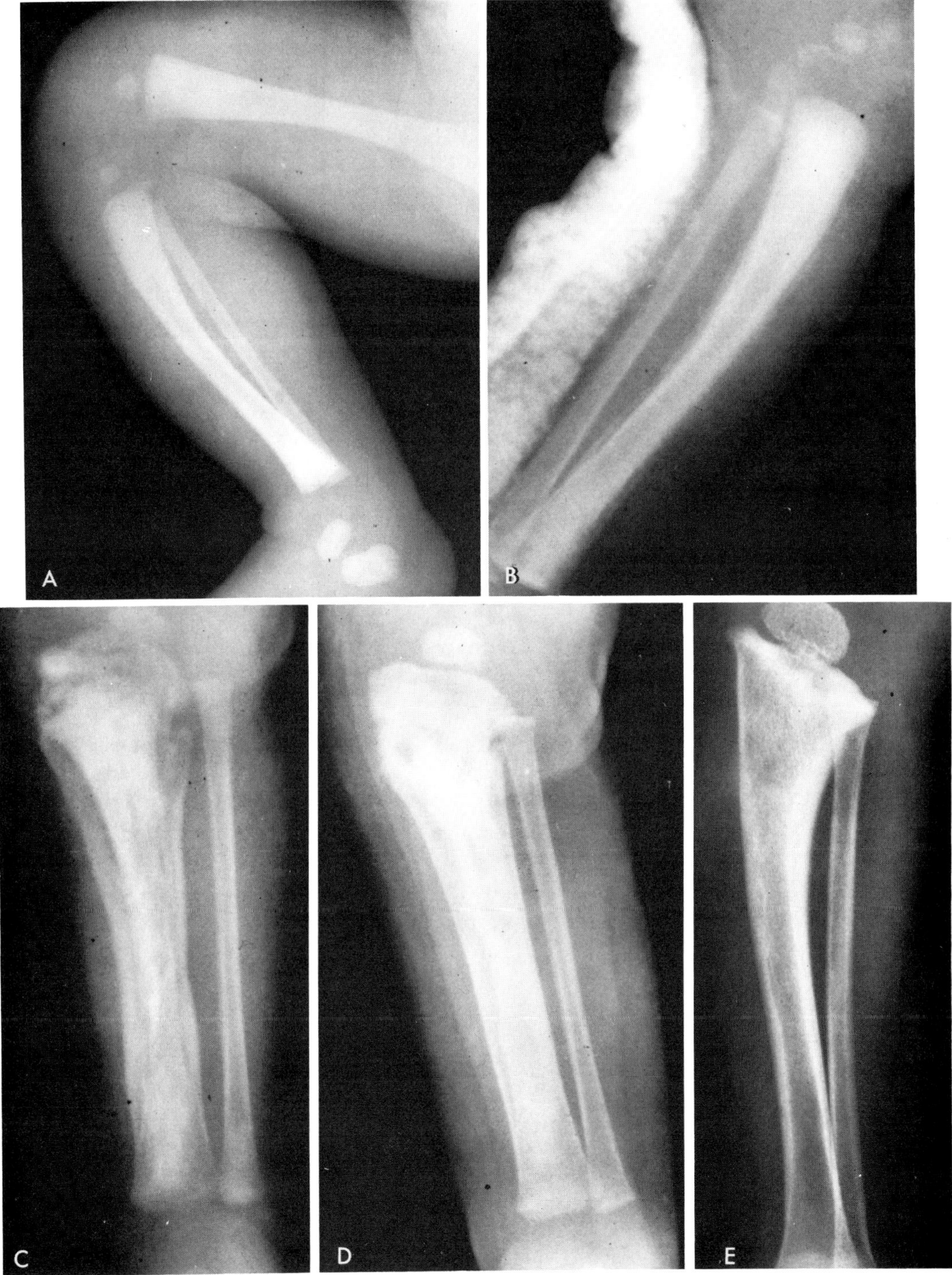

Figure 12–14. Classic osteomyelitis of a long bone. *A*, There is soft tissue swelling around the tibia with possibly some increase in the density of the bone. *B*, Two weeks later, there is an obvious periosteal reaction and increasing density in the upper tibia. *C*, After three months of antibiotic therapy, the periosteal new bone (involucrum) has surrounded the old tibia, which is now noticeably increased in density (sequestrum). *D*, One year later, the remains of the sequestrum can be seen. The involucrum has become smoother and more organized, although there is deformity of the upper metaphyseal region of the tibia. *E*, Three years later, the involucrum has now been virtually replaced by normal bone, and the sequestrum has all but disappeared. The upper tibial slant persists.

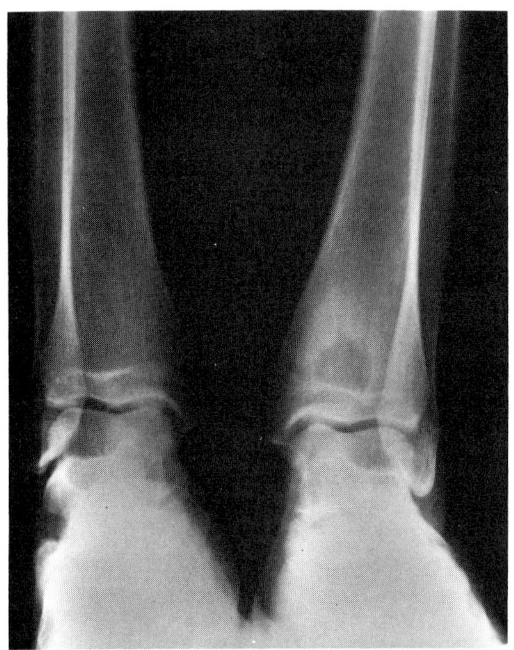

Figure 12–15. Brodie's abscess. There is a well-defined lucency in the left distal tibial metaphysis. Note that it abuts on the epiphysis and has a sharp margin with reactive new bone surrounding it. These are the characteristic appearances of a chronic abscess. The abscess was excised, and the organism responsible was found to be *Staphylococcus aureus.*

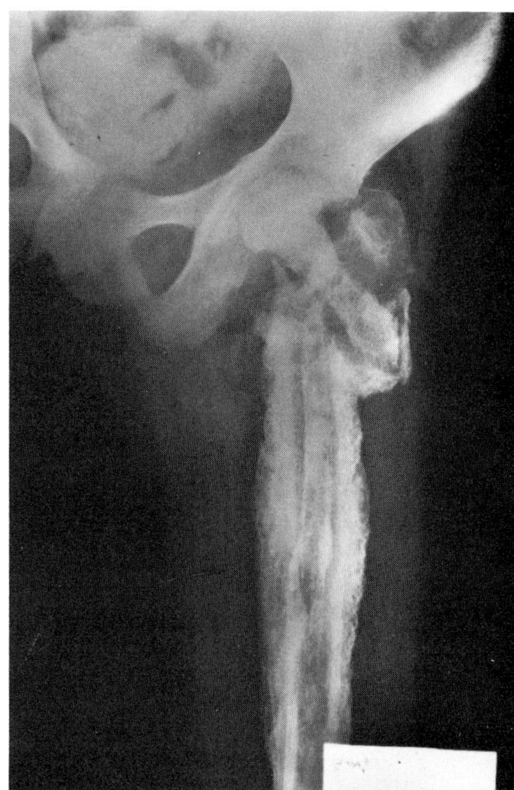

Figure 12–16. Chronic osteomyelitis. This 14-year-old girl had an immunological disease and developed staphylococcal osteomyelitis that was refractory to treatment. The sequestrum and involucrum can be easily identified. Note the pathological fracture of the femoral neck.

reaction, the first positive radiographic sign. As the infection progresses, it causes the bone to have a permeative appearance as the process invades the cortex and cancellous bone, stripping off the periosteum and provoking the formation of an intense periosteal reaction. Finally, a large intraosseous "abscess" forms, with a thick but noncontinuous margin of bone (involucrum) containing the remains of the cortex (sequestrum). It is to be hoped that this situation will not occur today because of the sensitivity of most forms of osteomyelitis to antibiotics, particularly if the disease is caught early. Some rarer organisms still cause progressive osteomyelitis. Tuberculosis, although rare in bone, occurs in underdeveloped countries and occasionally causes true osteomyelitis. More commonly, an infection caused by a weak microorganism or affecting a strong host may cause osteomyelitis with a chronic abscess as the presenting finding (Fig. 12–15). This appears to occur most often in young males; the abscess is seen close to the physeal plate (often in the lower tibia) and is known as a *Brodie's abscess.*

In many patients, chronic osteomyelitis can result from a previous penetrating wound (Fig. 12–16). These patients usually have recurrent infections and may develop a number of complications, such as amyloidosis and squamous cell carcinoma of the sinus tract.

Case E6

Siobhan MacRafferty, age 54, was in chronic renal failure and on hemodialysis. She complained of back pain over the course of three months, and x-rays of the lumbar region were taken (Fig. 12–17).

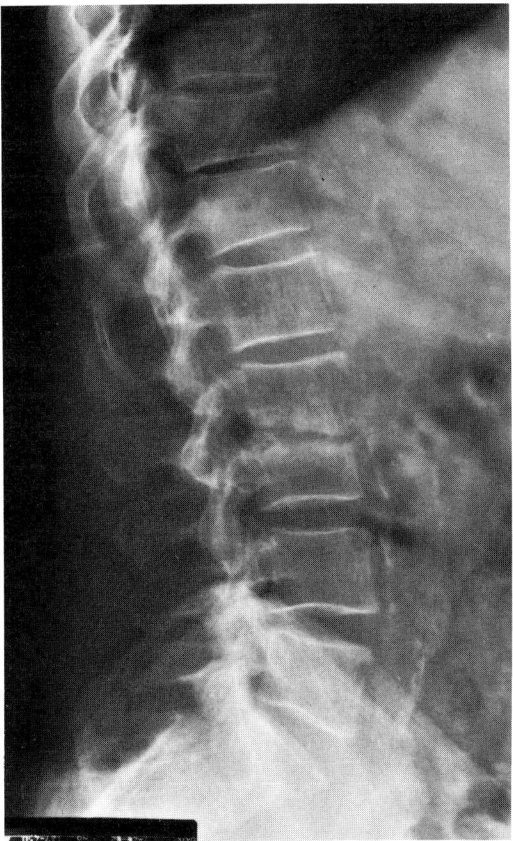

Figure 12–17. Staphylococcal osteomyelitis of the lumbar spine. This lateral view shows loss of height and destruction of the adjacent end plates of L2 and L3. Note the surrounding reactive new bone, which is more typical of bacterial infections than of tuberculosis.

Twenty years ago, it would have been correct to say that most bacterial infections of the spine involved the anterior part of the vertebral body itself with destruction and reactive sclerosis while conserving the disc space, and that most tuberculous infections destroyed the disc and the adjacent vertebral endplates without any radiographically visible new bone formation. This is, unfortunately, not true today.

In this patient, note that although the infection predominantly affects the vertebral bodies themselves, it also involves the disc space. What organism is most likely to be the culprit? In fact, it was *E. coli,* as the patient's history might suggest. Bacterial osteomyelitis of the spine has become relatively frequent, occurring in drug addicts, patients on immunosuppressive drugs, and hospital workers.

Tuberculosis of the spine is still seen in debilitated elderly patients (Fig. 12–18), and differentiating between bacterial and tuberculous infections of the spine has be-

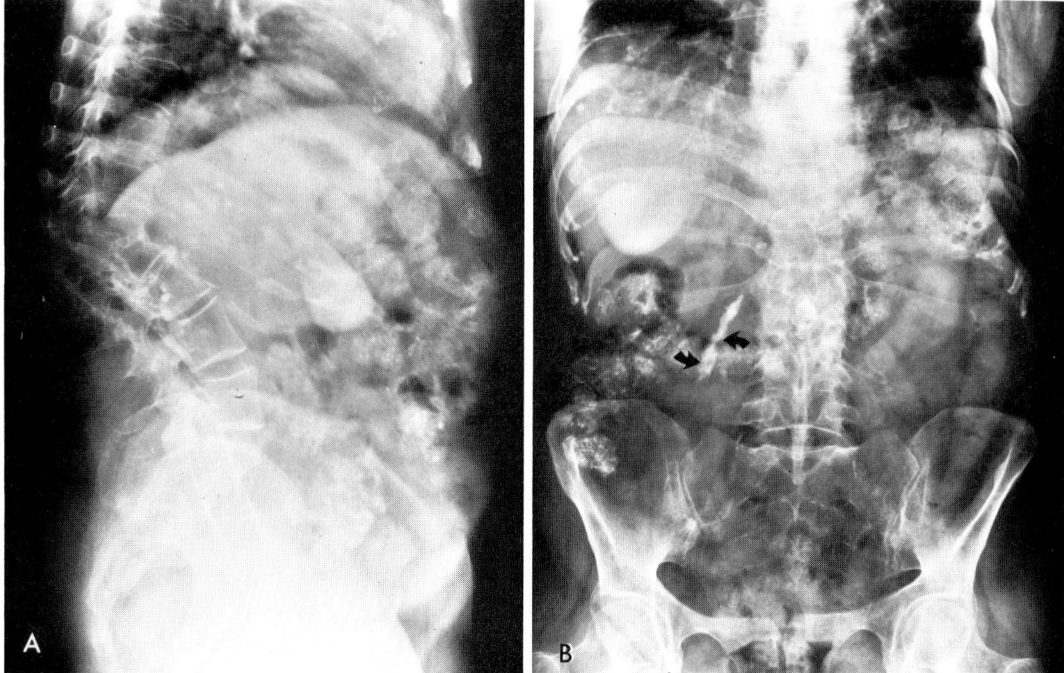

Figure 12–18. Healed tuberculosis of the spine, lateral view (*A*) and AP view (*B*). Note the fused vertebral bodies with loss of the entire disc space between T12 and L1 and partial loss of the one below. Subsequently, fusion of the bodies occurred with acute angulation (gibbus formation). Note the calcified iliopsoas abscess (*arrows*), the opacified gallbladder, and the retained barium in the colon.

come difficult radiographically. Several of the factors outlined above may be helpful. The definite diagnosis will be made today using a biopsy needle either to aspirate pus or to perform a bone biopsy in order to incubate the bony particles.

One other type of infection should be briefly mentioned: In septic arthritis, the organism, although presumably originating in the subperiosteal region of the metaphysis of a long bone, has spread rapidly into a neighboring joint. In underdeveloped countries, tuberculous arthritis of various joints is more common than pure tuberculous osteomyelitis. Elsewhere, septic arthritis is relatively rare. The characteristic radiographic appearance of rapid onset and juxta-articular osteopenia in a patient who is complaining of pain in the relevant joint should lead to the diagnosis, which is confirmed by aspiration. The most important factor in differentiating between bacterial arthritis and tuberculous arthritis is time: it takes three weeks or so for bacterial infection to affect a joint and three months to one year for tuberculous arthritis to produce the same degree of damage (Fig. 12–19).

More than one joint is usually involved in arthritis. Some aspects of arthritis have been discussed in connection with low back pain (see Table 11–2), but a more formal approach is needed. The age and sex of the patient, the joints involved (whether large or small), the clinical signs and symptoms, the symmetry or asymmetry of involvement, and the results of laboratory tests for uric acid levels and the presence of rheumatoid factor and HLA-B27 must all be taken into account by both the clinician and the radiologist.

Usually joint films are read "blindly," partly because it is more of an intellectual exercise that way and partly because radiologists are rarely given adequate clinical information. Often the diagnosis is a clinical one, and the main function of the x-rays is to document the degree of involvement and amount of damage. X-rays will also act as a baseline to observe the effects of therapy, particularly in rheumatoid arthritis. In osteoarthritis, x-rays allow a search for loose bodies, associated fractures, and narrowing of the joint space.

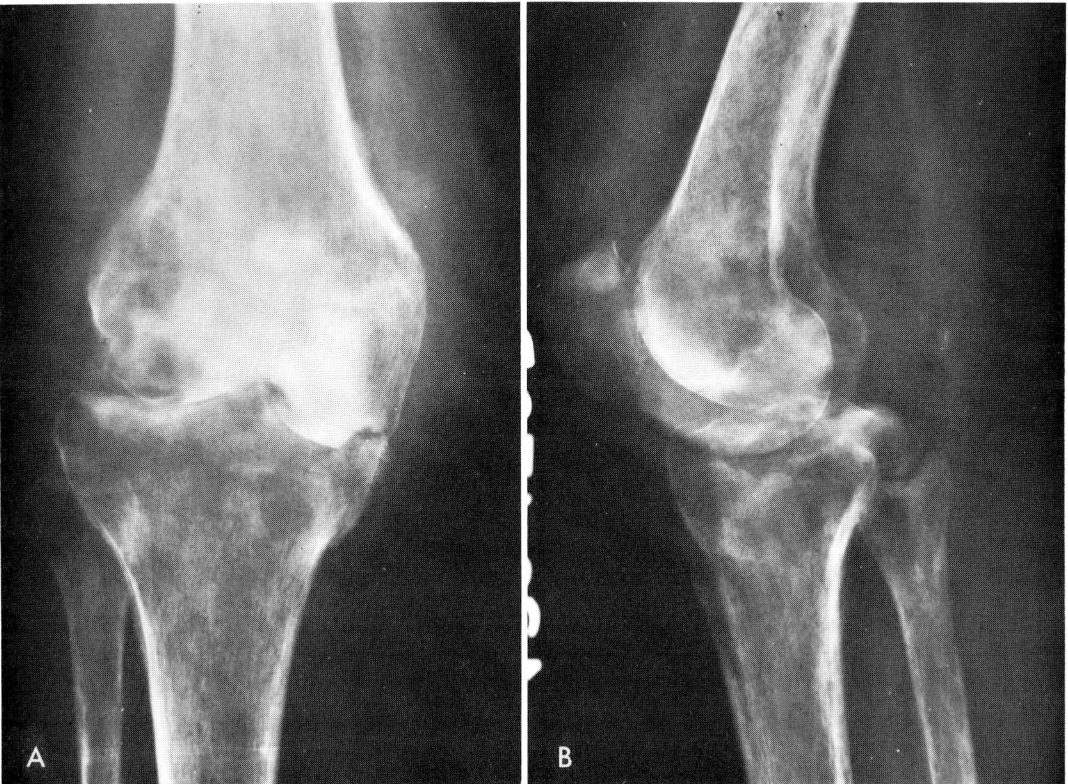

Figure 12–19. Septic arthritis. Note the soft tissue swelling, the almost total loss of cartilage, the bone destruction, and some reactive new bone formation. A periosteal reaction can be seen around the tibia and femur. This patient had a long history of systemic lupus erythematosus that was treated with steroids, and she developed a chronic staphylococcal infection in her right knee.

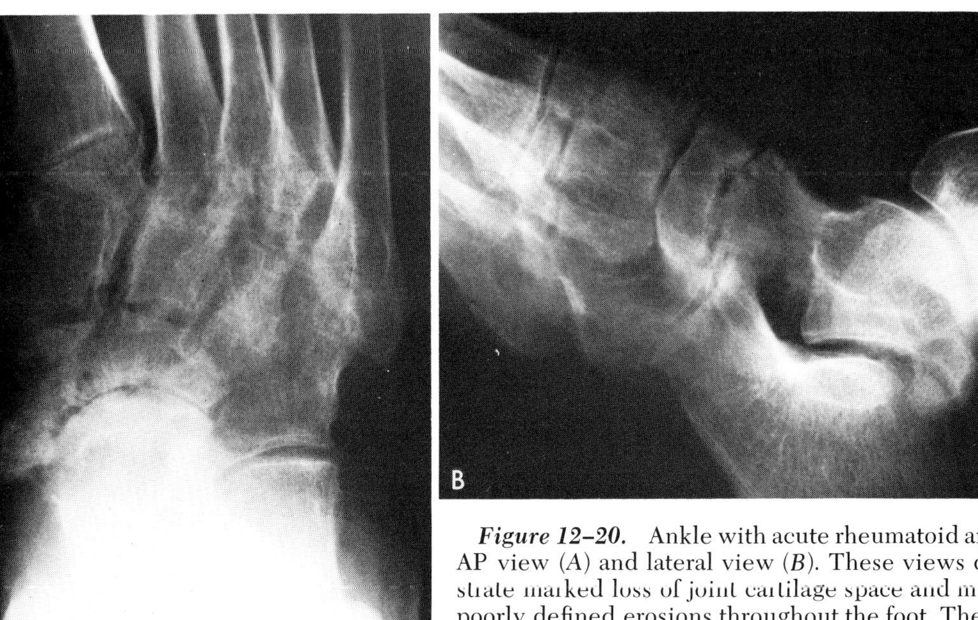

Figure 12–20. Ankle with acute rheumatoid arthritis, AP view (*A*) and lateral view (*B*). These views demonstrate marked loss of joint cartilage space and multiple, poorly defined erosions throughout the foot. The differential diagnosis would include infection (particularly tuberculosis) and hemophilia.

Case E7

Jeremiah Klunk, age 25, came in complaining of pain in his foot that had lasted for three weeks. There was no relevant information in his own or his family's medical history, and no other joints were involved. His foot and ankle appeared rather swollen and red and were tender to palpation. What do the x-rays show (Fig. 12–20)?

Not all cases of arthritis are easy to diagnose clinically. On this patient's x-ray, there are numerous poorly defined erosions of many articular surfaces in the foot. There is little osteoblastic reaction, presumably because the history of the disease is so short. What is your differential diagnosis?

A normal uric acid level makes the diagnosis of gout highly unlikely but not totally impossible. The white blood count was normal, and the erythrocyte sedimentation rate was only mildly elevated, suggesting that this is not a pure infection (tuberculosis would, however, still be a possibility if the duration of disease were longer). Synovial biopsy revealed that this patient had a very unusual manifestation of acute rheumatoid arthritis.

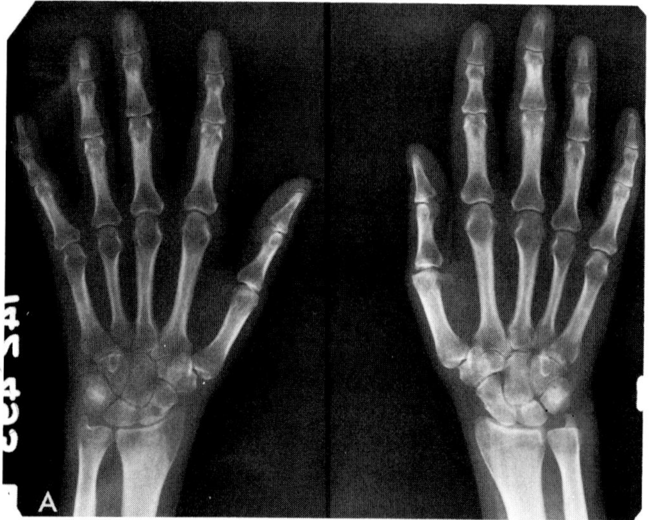

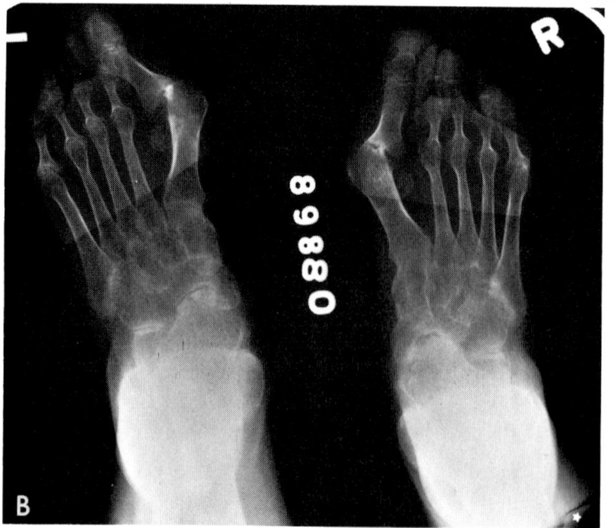

Figure 12–21. Rheumatoid arthritis. *A*, Early rheumatoid arthritis in the hands. Juxta-articular osteoporosis is seen in association with soft tissue swelling around the wrists and metacarpophalangeal joints. Very early erosions are just visible on a number of metacarpal heads and on the ulnar aspect of the proximal end of each proximal phalanx. These are the characteristic early radiographic changes of rheumatoid arthritis. *B*, Moderate rheumatoid arthritis in the feet. Generalized osteoporosis with subluxations and erosions of most of the metatarsophalangeal joints can be seen. Loss of articular cartilage space in the tarsi is also apparent.

Characteristically, rheumatoid arthritis is a symmetrical, slowly progressive process predominantly involving the small joints of the hands and feet (Fig. 12–21). Erosions occur at the points of capsular and synovial insertion into the bone (in the region of the metaphysis just below the physeal plate) and are so poorly defined that early erosions are best seen using magnification radiography (Fig. 12–21A). The first radiographically visible erosions commonly occur at the ulnar aspect of the proximal phalanx of the third and fourth digits. Various rheumatoid variants, particularly psoriatic arthritis, are asymmetrical and are not associated with juxta-articular osteopenia. Psoriatic arthritis involves the distal and middle interphalangeal joints rather than the metacarpophalangeal and proximal interphalangeal joints. Rheumatoid arthritis can produce laxity of the atlantoaxial ligaments and subluxation of the odontoid, with dire effects on the

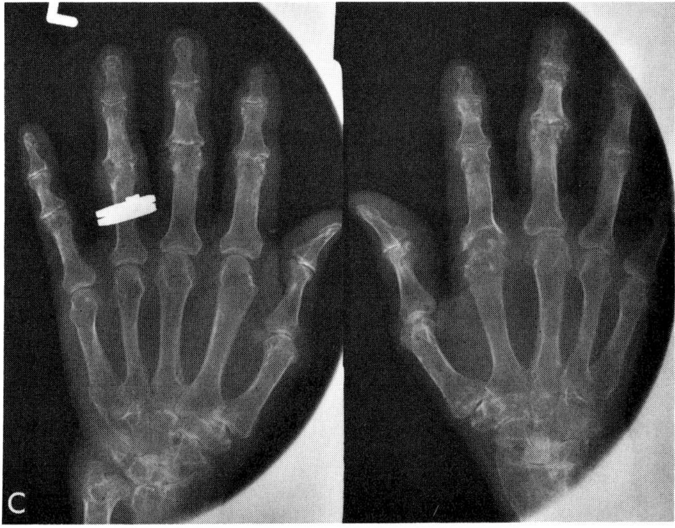

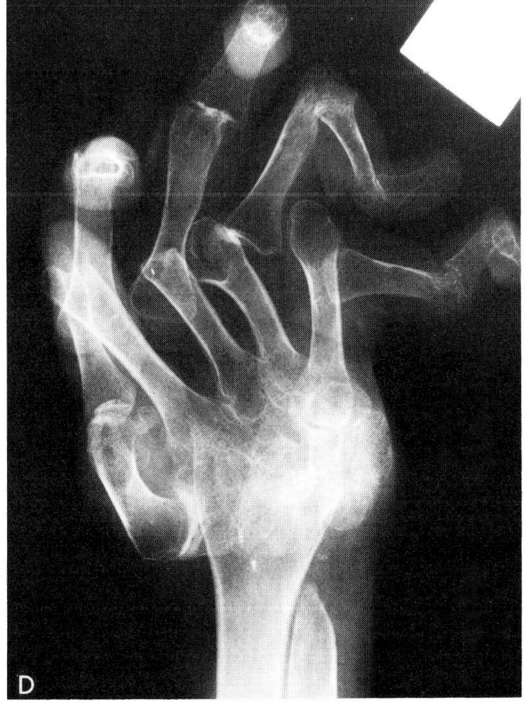

Figure 12–21. *Continued. C,* Moderate rheumatoid arthritis in the hands. In both wrists, there are large erosions associated with decreased joint cartilage space, which also involve other joints in the hand, predominantly the proximal interphalangeal joints. This 67-year-old man had long-standing rheumatoid arthritis. *D,* Severe rheumatoid arthritis in the hand. Note the destruction of the carpus as well as the ulnar deviation of the fingers, with subluxations of the metacarpophalangeal joints and severe juxta-articular osteoporosis.

patient's cervical spinal cord. Involvement of the sacroiliac joints occurs in a number of rheumatoid variants.

Although it is bilateral, osteoarthritis is rarely symmetrical and predominantly involves the larger weight-bearing joints, usually the hips and the knees (Fig. 12–22A). For some reason, osteoarthritis in the hands involves the distal interphalangeal joints, where the osteophytes are somewhat prominent and are known as *Heberden's nodes* (Fig. 12–22B). The classic radiographic features are decreased joint space, sclerosis, osteophyte formation, and large subchondral central cysts with well-defined margins. Often, bony or cartilaginous pieces break off and become loose bodies within the joint; these are known as "joint mice." To some extent, the disease process is self-limiting. Since it hurts the patient to move the involved joint too much, he often tends not to use it at all and manages for years with severe osteoarthritis.

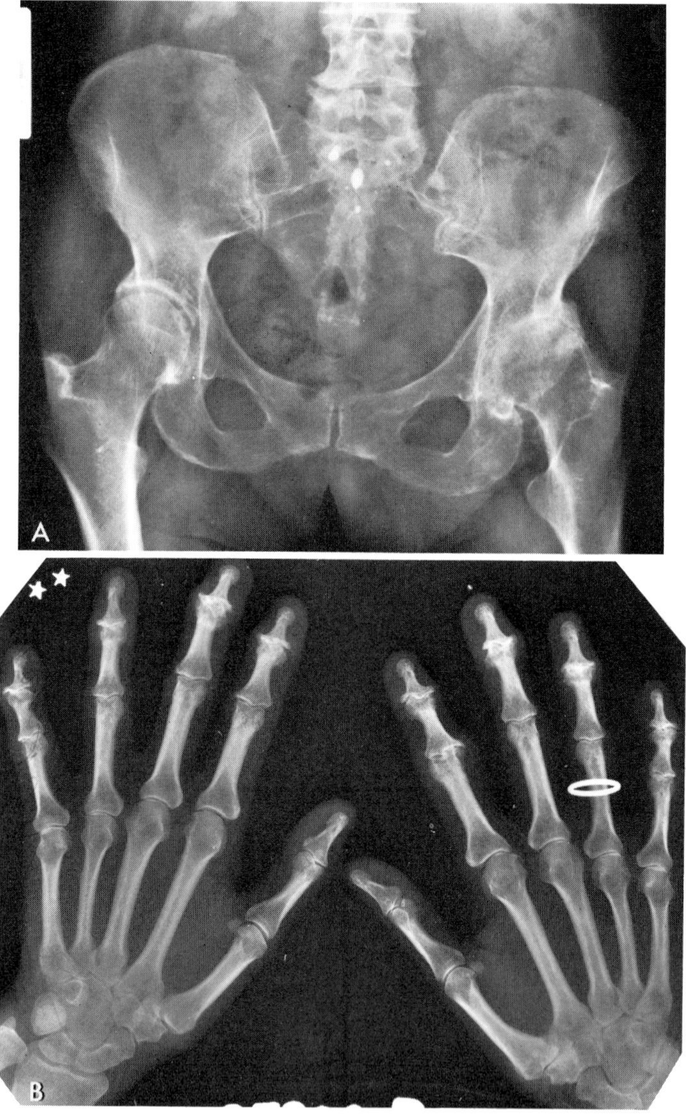

Figure 12–22. Osteoarthritis. *A*, In this view of the hips, note loss of the joint space, sclerosis, and marginal osteophyte formation mainly involving the left hip. Some small subchondral cysts (geodes) may be seen. *B*, In the hands, there is narrowing of the distal interphalangeal joints with osteophyte formation and sclerosis. These findings are typical of osteoarthritis of the hands, and the clinically apparent swellings overlying the osteophytes are known as *Heberden's nodes*.

Case E8

Dominic Doedow, age 45, had chronic renal failure and came in because his ankle "looked funny." On examination, it was certainly rather swollen, was freely mobile in all normal and some extraordinary directions, and made a curious grinding sound on movement. The x-rays were diagnostic (Fig. 12–23). What do they show?

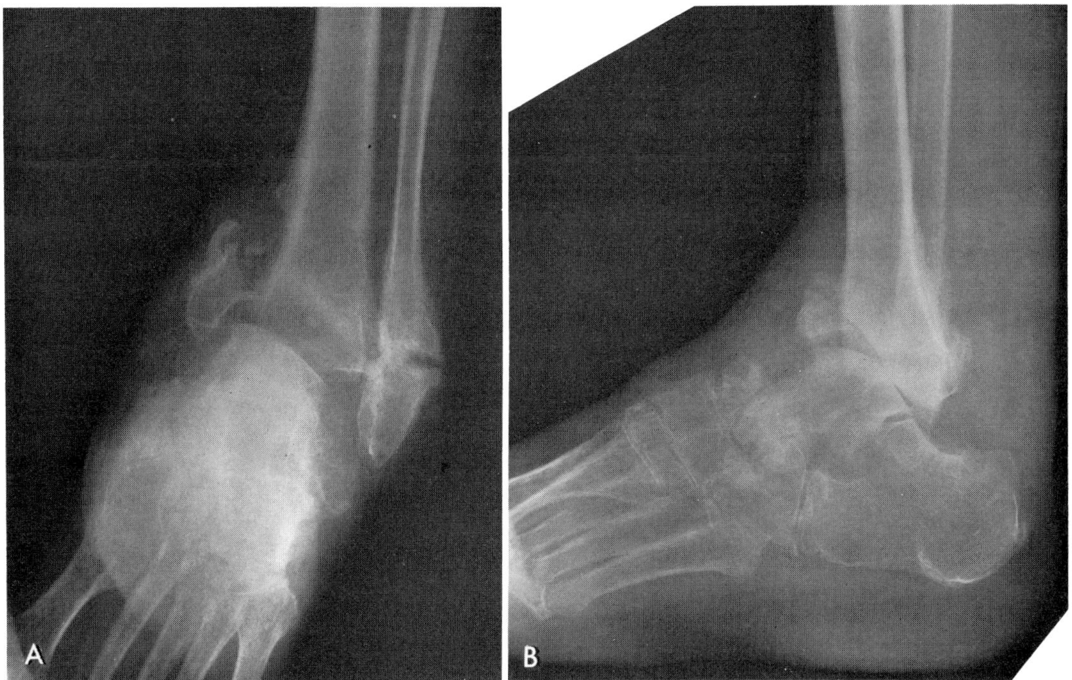

Figure 12–23. Charcot joint, AP view (*A*) and lateral view (*B*). There are fractures through the distal fibula and the medial malleolus. The tibiotalar joint is totally disorganized, and bone dust and fragments are present around the joint. Similar changes are visible in the subtalar joint. These appearances are typical of a neuropathic joint.

The fracture through the lower tibia, the total lack of alignment of the joint, the bone "dust" floating within the joint capsule, and the fact that all this is almost painless give the diagnosis away. Charcot joints were originally described in syphilis (particularly in tabes dorsalis) but now the most common cause is diabetes mellitus. This patient had diabetes, and he refused to have an operation for six months because his ankle didn't hurt. Although it is extremely exaggerated a Charcot joint is a manifestation of severe osteoarthritis, usually in a peripheral joint, just as cervical spondylosis is a manifestation of severe osteoarthritis in the neck.

Another manifestation of diabetes should be mentioned. Diabetic osteoarthropathy is a unique combination of bone destruction and bone formation occurring in the feet of a diabetic. The radiographic features are: signs of osteolysis, often with total dissolution of bone, around the metatarsophalangeal and proximal interphalangeal joints, periosteal new bone surrounding the proximal end of the metatarsals, joint-space narrowing throughout the foot and ankle, and medial wall calcification in the distal arteries (Mönckeberg's sclerosis).

Gout is another common joint disease to be discussed. The stereotype of an obese, middle-aged man who likes his port and looks like Henry VIII no longer applies; anyone can have gout. The average patient presents with an acutely tender swollen joint — often the first metatarsophalangeal joint (Fig. 12–24). Radiographically, only

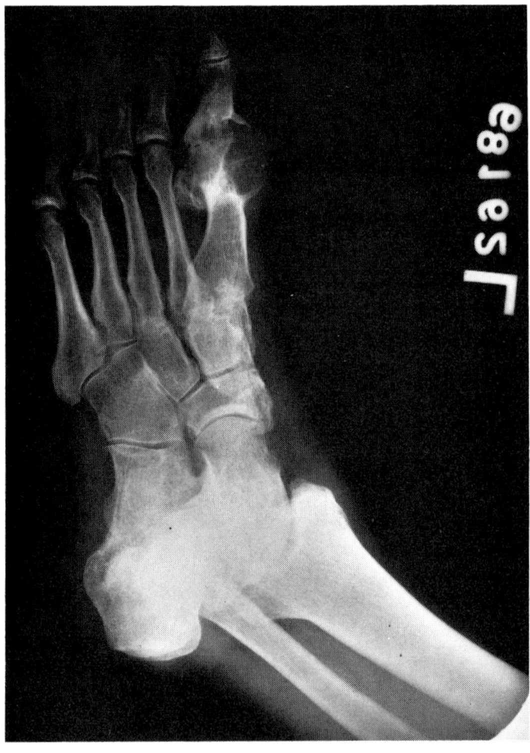

Figure 12–24. Gout. Localized destruction of the first metatarsophalangeal joint is visible, with large well-marginated erosions and destruction of the articular cartilage as well as the underlying bone. There is calcification in the soft tissues adjacent to the metatarsal head; this represents a tophus.

soft-tissue swelling may be seen early in the disease, but after six weeks or so the characteristic punched-out erosions may be clearly seen. The deposition of monosodium urate crystals may occur in places other than the joints, so that in clinical examination one may look for tophi in the earlobes or at the elbows, for example. Radiographically, a clearly marginated punched-out lesion in a bone but not near a joint is pathognomonic of gout. The diagnosis can usually be reinforced by the finding of an elevated serum uric acid level.

In a discussion of joint disease, one brief mention should be made of an arthritis that for some reason is beloved of generations of medical students. Acute gonococcal arthritis is a destructive process of the articular cartilage that has no specific radiographic features to differentiate it from other forms of septic arthritis.

Case E9

Count Trinkleheim von Dracula, age 28, presented with pain in his left elbow and both knees (Fig. 12–25). All joints were severely deformed, had limited range of motion, and were swollen. A radiological survey of all joints was performed, but only the knees and the left elbow were found to be involved. What disease does the Count have?

The severely destructive nature of this form of arthritis, with enlargement of the epiphyses and thickening of primary trabeculae, makes a diagnosis of hemophilia easy. Although a hemophiliac often bleeds into many joints, usually only one or two joints sustain recurrent serious bleeds and ultimately undergo the changes of severely destructive degenerative osteoarthritis.

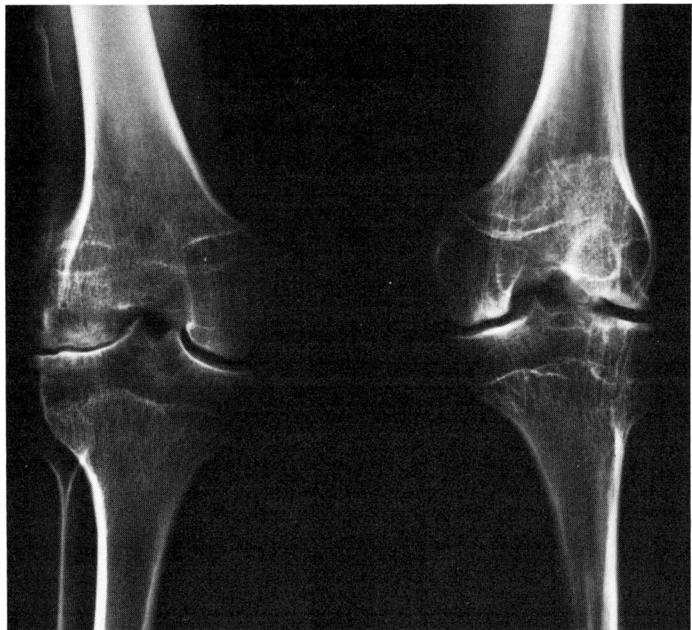

Figure 12–25. Hemophilic arthritis in the knees. Bilateral loss of articular joint space can be seen, with erosions and distortion of the articular condyles. There is also widening of the intercondylar notch and relative enlargement of the epiphyses and metaphyseal parts of the femurs and tibias. These are the typical radiographic changes seen in hemophilia of the knee.

Case E10

Roosevelt Washington, a 28-year-old black male, had recurrent bone and soft-tissue pains. His doctor finally sent him to the hospital for x-rays, which were diagnostic (Fig. 12–26).

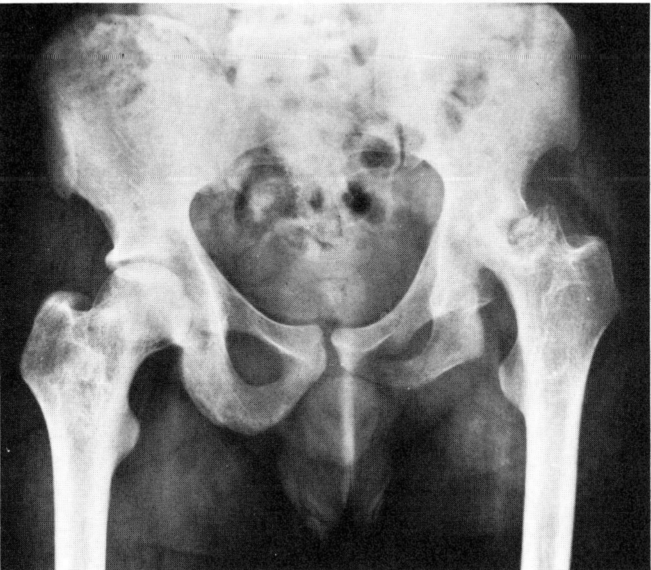

Figure 12–26. Sickle-cell anemia. There is avascular necrosis with collapse of the left femoral head. Multiple areas of increased density seen in both upper femurs as well as in the pelvis represent infarcts. There is also evidence of endosteal new bone formation with thickened cortices. Note the old fracture of the left pubic and ischial rami.

TABLE 12–1. Causes of Avascular Necrosis

Fracture (33% subcapital fractures)
Dislocation (20% of posterior hip dislocation)
Microfracture
Osteoarthritis
Steroid therapy
Cushing's syndrome
Hemoglobinopathies (e.g., sickle-cell anemia, sickle-cell thalassemia, sickle-cell trait)
Connective tissue disorders (e.g., polyarteritis nodosa, systemic lupus erythematosus, giant cell arteritis, Fabry's disease)
Pancreatitis
Alcoholism
Irradiation
Gout or hyperuricemia
Caisson disease
Multiple injuries or burns
Pregnancy
Gaucher's disease
Hyperparathyroidism
Idiopathic

The pelvis shows the classic radiographic features of osseous involvement in sickle-cell anemia, but of course the diagnosis is often made clinically years before the bones undergo such extensive changes. Sickle-cell anemia is one of the causes of avascular necrosis of an epiphysis, which characteristically affects the femoral head. Table 12–1 lists the conditions in which avascular necrosis has been described.

Case E11

Gloria Codspiece, age 55, presented with intense pain in the humerus following a very minor injury. She had never been ill before and had no other signs or symptoms. An x-ray of the arm was taken (Fig. 12–27).

This shows a destructive lesion with a pathological fracture running through it. The appearance is that of a malignant tumor. The patient's age and the appearance of this tumor make it unlikely that the lesion is benign. What would you do next?

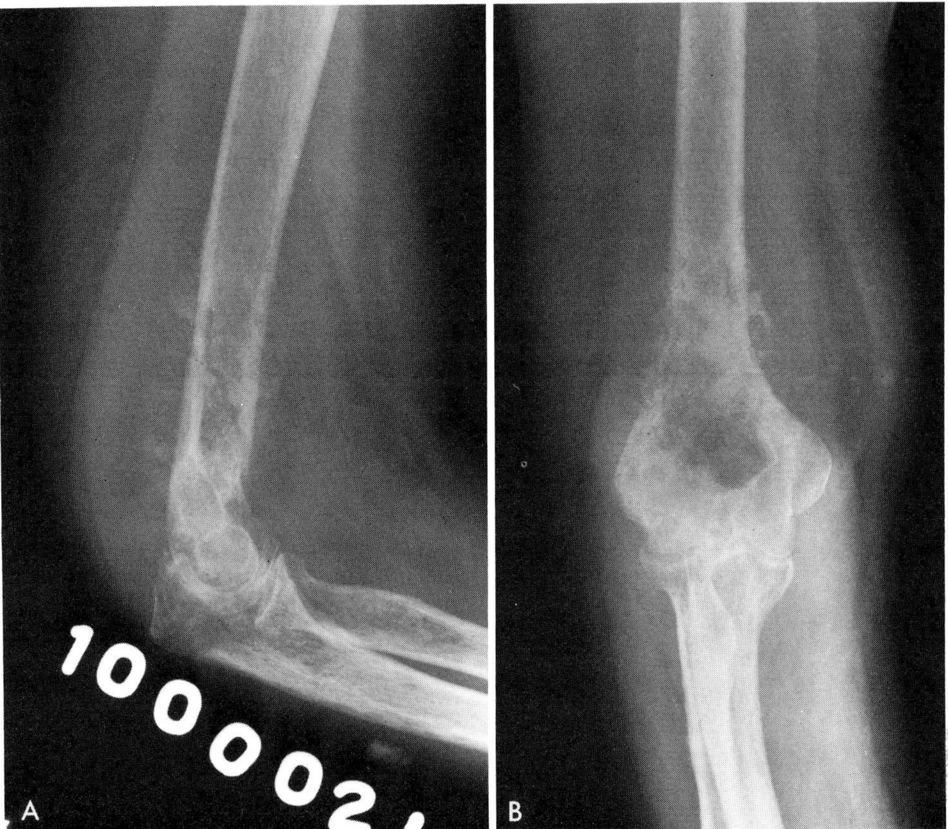

Figure 12–27. Solitary metastasis to the humerus from sigmoid colon. There is a destructive lesion of the distal humerus with a pathological fracture running through it. A periosteal reaction and a "sunburst" appearance as well as some soft tissue swelling can be seen (*A* and *B*).

A logical approach would be a bone scan or a skeletal survey to determine if there are other lesions present. The bone scan, however, is a more economically sensible approach and provides more information than radiography alone. In this patient, the lesion was found to be solitary. The differential diagnosis would include primary osseous malignancy and malignant metastasis, which is high on the list of probabilities. A solitary lesion appearing in a middle-aged patient should suggest metastasis from one of four primary sites: lung, kidney, thyroid, and (in females) breast. A chest x-ray, IVP, and thyroid scan in this patient were normal, but a barium enema study revealed a small sigmoid carcinoma which was successfully resected.

Case E12

Esmeralda Witherspoon, age 64, presented with right arm pain and a somewhat non-specific history of recurrent chest infections. An x-ray of the arm was diagnostic. Unfortunately, however, while positioning the arm for a second radiograph, the technician heard the arm crack. A pathological fracture had occurred (Fig. 12–28).

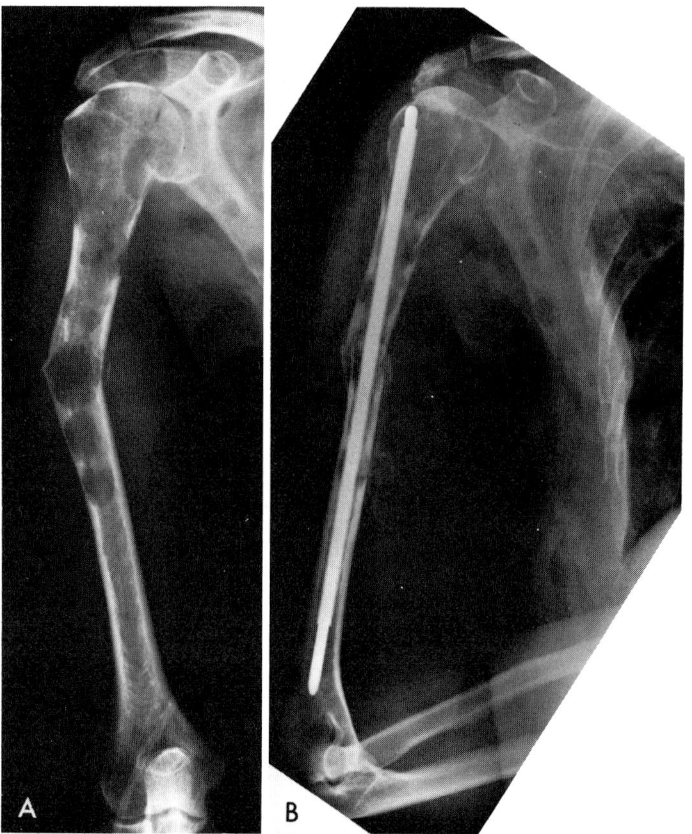

Figure 12–28. Metastases from breast cancer. *A*, Multiple lytic areas can be seen throughout all visualized bones, particularly in the humerus, where a pathological fracture has occurred. Note the extremely destructive nature of these metastases. *B*, This patient was treated using an intramedullary rod for the fracture and by local radiotherapy.

There are many destructive lesions in this humerus that are obviously not benign. For a primary tumor to occur at this site would be very unusual, so a metastasis has to be suspected. A bone scan revealed multiple metastases (Fig. 12–29). A chest x-ray showed loss of volume in the right middle lobe. A chest x-ray taken 10 years previously, however, showed an identical appearance; this was thought to be a chronic right middle lobe syndrome in a patient with chronic bronchitis. No evidence of a primary site was found in the gastrointestinal and genitourinary tracts, mammograms were considered normal, and a thorough clinical examination failed to reveal any abnormality. A biopsy of one of the lytic lesions revealed anaplastic carcinoma of unknown origin. Often we must rely on time to indicate the diagnosis. This patient developed severe osseous pain and multiple pathological fractures before she died. At autopsy, the primary site was found to be a very small breast carcinoma that presumably had been growing slowly over many years.

Perhaps we have overemphasized lytic metastases, but they are far more common than blastic metastases. Prostatic metastases also cause bone pain, but they may be found serendipitously (Fig. 12–30). They are usually multiple and may be rounded or may involve the whole width of a bone. Increase in bone density without the disordered formation of bone and thickening of cortices seen in Paget's disease is characteristic of bony metastases.

The primary site of blastic metastases in older men is almost invariably the prostate, and elevated serum acid phosphatase levels and clinical examination will usually confirm the diagnosis. Other primary sites in the male are the breast, bladder, lung, and

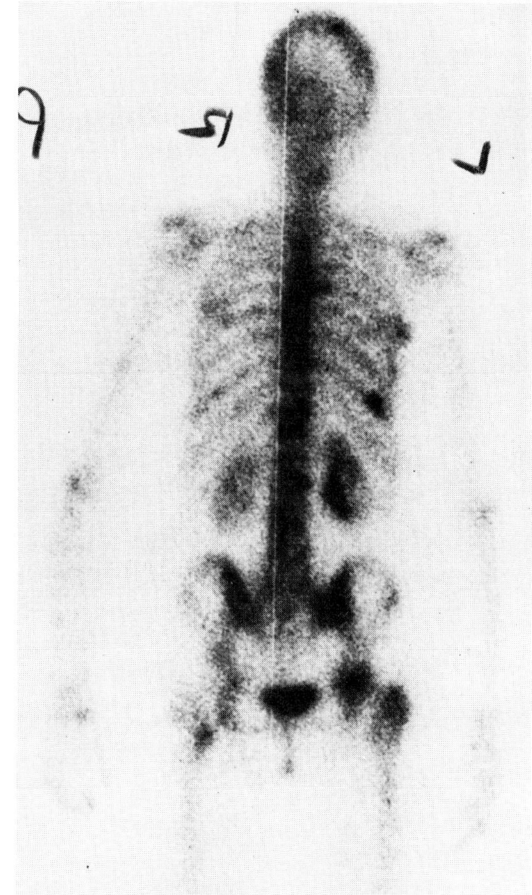

Figure 12–29. Bone scan with multiple metastases. "Hot spots," or areas of increased uptake, can be seen in the skull, ribs, spine, pelvis, and both upper femurs as well as the right humerus. These represent metastatic deposits.

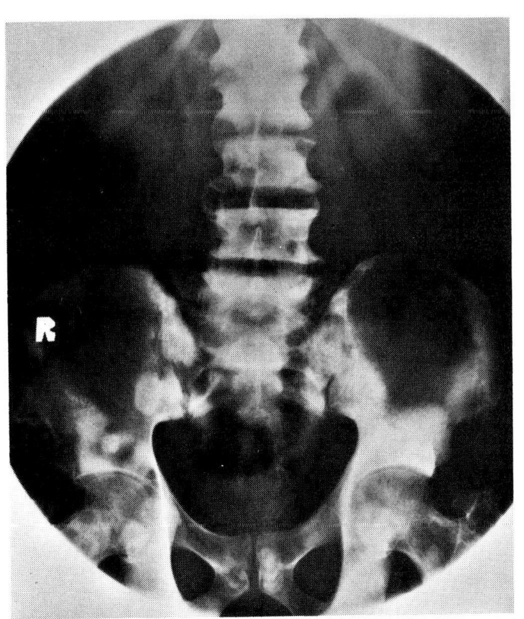

Figure 12–30. Pelvis metastases from prostatic carcinoma. Dense bony sclerosis obliterates the normal architecture throughout the pelvis, upper femurs, and spine. This patient had prostatic carcinoma, which stimulates osteoblastic activity in the skeleton and is the most common cause of sclerotic metastases.

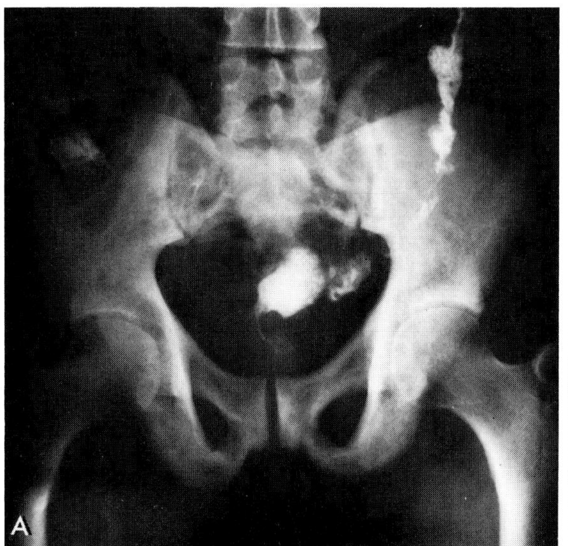

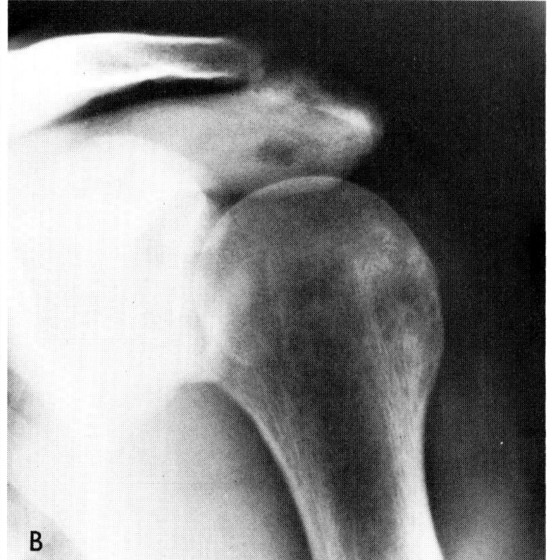

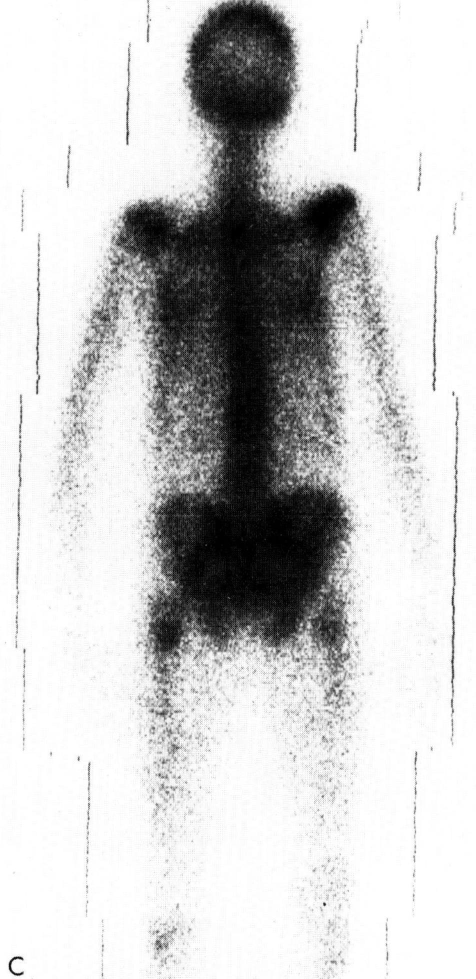

Figure 12–31. Differential diagnosis: Paget's disease versus metastases. This patient had a history of Paget's disease. *A*, This view of the pelvis shows the fairly typical areas of increased density and widened cortices of Paget's disease, although the left innominate bone is rather denser than would be expected with pure Paget's disease. *B*, In left shoulder, note the overall increased density of the scapula with a single lucency in the acromion. On biopsy, this lesion was found to be metastatic. *C*, The bone scan shows positive uptake in both shoulders, the skull, pelvis, and upper femur. Biopsy showed that although most of these areas had pagetoid bone, the left shoulder, right femoral neck, and left pelvis also showed evidence of metastases from prostatic carcinoma.

sometimes the brain (as from astrocytomas), In women, it is very rare to find sclerotic metastases as a primary manifestation of malignancy; however, after almost any form of therapy for breast cancer (mastectomy, hormonal therapy, steroids, or radiotherapy), many previously lytic metastases become blastic.

Case E13

Jonathan Painpickle, age 72, had a long history of Paget's disease, but recently he began complaining that his pain was not being controlled by calcitonin. Radiographs revealed that new sclerotic areas had developed in the skeleton (Fig. 12–31A). A new bone scan was compared with previous scans and revealed new "hot spots." Biopsy was made of the left scapula, because it had proven radiographically impossible to differentiate between Paget's disease and blastic metastasis. In fact, Mr. Painpickle had also developed prostatic carcinoma.

One point of interest: in spite of the increased blood flow that occurs in Paget's disease, metastatic involvement of pagetoid bone is extremely rare.

Case E14

Landsborough Goodenough, age 57, came into the outpatient department of the local hospital complaining of pain in his wrists and ankles. Examination revealed clubbing and extreme shortness of breath. X-rays of the chest, wrists, and other joints were pathognomic (Fig. 12–32).

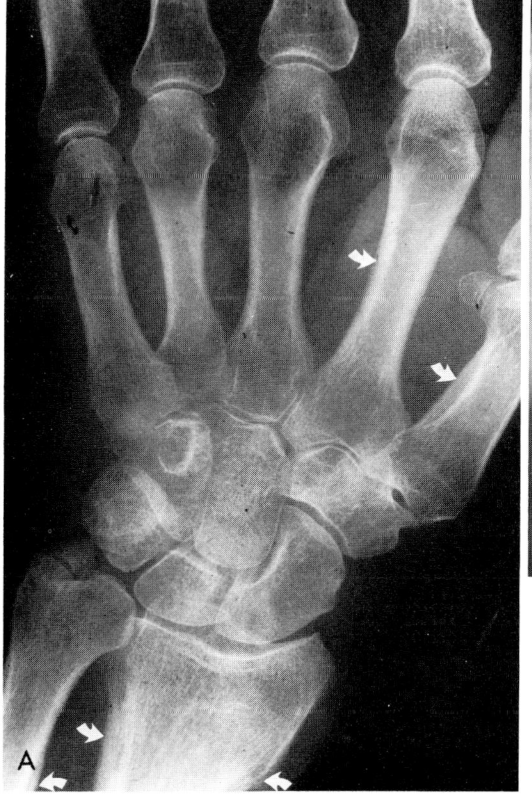

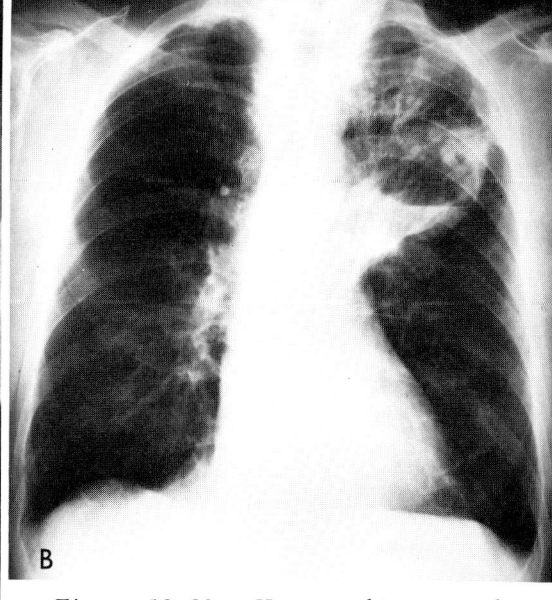

Figure 12–32. Hypertrophic osteoarthropathy. *A*, In the hands, a marked periosteal reaction can be seen on the lower radius and ulna as well as two of the metacarpals (*arrows*). *B*, In the chest, there is a mass adjacent to the upper left hilum with a peripheral cavitation and pneumonia. On bronchoscopy, the mass proved to be a bronchogenic carcinoma that was causing hypertrophic pulmonary osteoarthropathy.

TABLE 12–2. Causes of Hypertrophic (Pulmonary) Osteoarthropathy

Bronchogenic carcinoma, oat cell carcinoma, metastasis, mesothelioma, hamartoma, carcinoid
Chronic obstructive pulmonary disease, chronic bronchitis
Tuberculosis, sarcoidosis, Wegener's granulomatosis
Chronic infection, empyema, fungal infection
Chronic pericarditis
Subacute bacterial endocarditis
Congenital heart disease (including shunts)
Fibrocystic disease of the pancreas
Biliary cirrhosis, biliary atresia
Mucoid-producing gastrointestinal carcinoma, particularly of the stomach and colon
Hepatitis
Cirrhosis of the liver
Chronic pancreatitis
Chronic cholecystitis
Gallbladder carcinoma
Crohn's disease
Ulcerative colitis

There are many causes of hypertrophic pulmonary osteoarthropathy, but the best known is undoubtedly bronchogenic carcinoma (Table 12–2). The condition is probably better referred to as *hypertrophic osteoarthropathy,* since there are many nonpulmonary causes. The etiology is unknown, but the occurrence of hypertrophic osteoarthropathy in so many different conditions implies that it is caused by a humoral factor. Hypertrophic osteoarthropathy is usually associated with clubbing, and the pain may be relieved by vagotomy. The symptoms may also be relieved by thoracotomy, even without removal of the primary tumor.

For every primary bone tumor, a radiologist sees twenty or more bone metastases. Even though they are rare, malignant bone tumors are of some interest (if only as an intellectual exercise for the radiologist), because they have to be differentiated from other lesions. Most benign bone tumors fill in and heal by themselves without treatment, but malignant bone tumors are almost invariably fatal. It is possible for the well-trained eye (or even the computer) to correctly diagnose some 95 per cent of all bone tumors on the basis of a radiograph. Diagnosis depends on the age and sex of the patient, the bone involved, the position of the tumor within the bone (in the epiphysis, metaphysis, or diaphysis), the symmetry or asymmetry of the tumor, and the tumor's margin (solid, thick, thin, destructive, poorly delineated, feathery or non-existent), contents (whether trabeculae, calcifications, ossifications, fat or nothing), and periosteal reaction (present or absent, whether parallel or at an angle to the bone), the distortion or destruction of the surrounding soft tissues, and most important, the overall appearance of the tumor (does it look benign or malignant?). Since there are over 20 described types of benign bone tumor and perhaps 10 types of malignant bone tumor, a few illustrations of the more common tumors must represent the group.

Case E15

Alphonse Figpot, age 27, a circus sword-thrower, came in complaining of pain in his wrist that occurred particularly while he was working. On examination, there appeared to be some swelling over the lower radius, and the area was tender on palpation. X-rays were taken (Fig. 12–33).

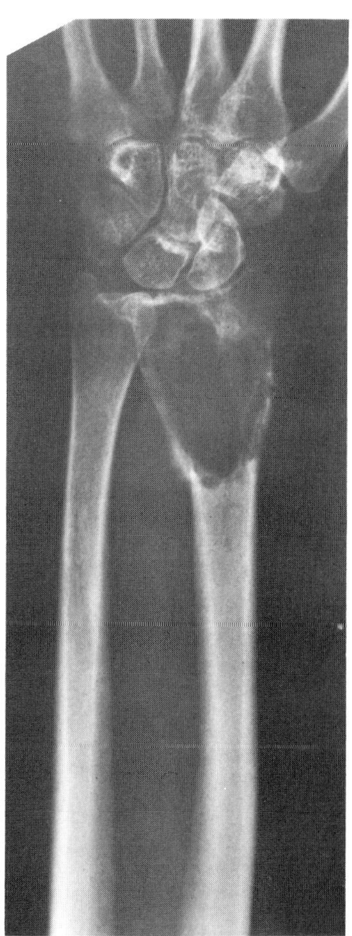

Figure 12–33. Giant cell tumor of the radius. A large asymmetrical lucent lesion involving the metaphysis and epiphysis of the distal radius has caused expansion of the bone, although there is no periosteal reaction and the cortex is largely intact. These appearances are characteristic of a giant cell tumor, which was confirmed at operation.

The x-ray showed an asymmetrical lucent tumor involving the metaphysis but spreading into the epiphysis of the radius. These findings are pathognomonic of a giant cell tumor, which although basically benign has a 1 to 4 per cent incidence of recurrence and local malignancy. Most other benign cystic tumors of bone spread from the

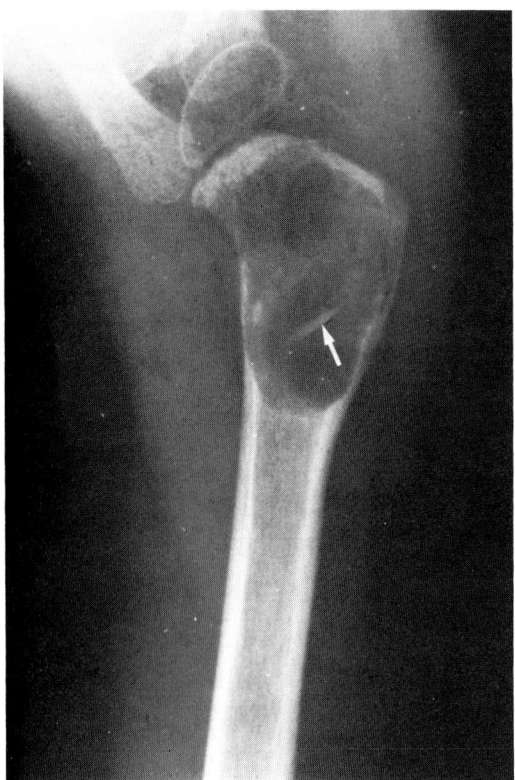

Figure 12–34. Benign cyst. There is an expansile solitary lytic lesion in the metaphyseal region of the upper humerus with a pathological fracture running through it. A "fallen fragment" (*arrow*) represents a small cortical fragment that "fell" into a hollow lesion (i.e., a cyst).

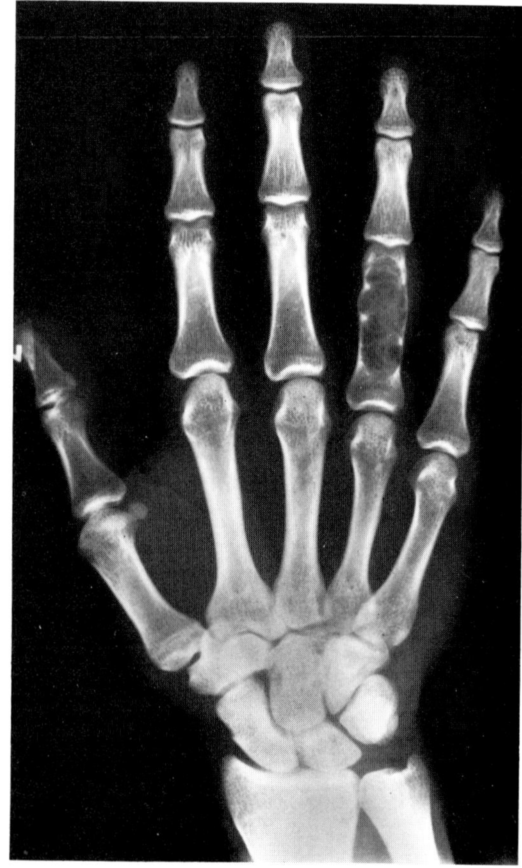

Figure 12–35. Enchondroma. There is expansion of the proximal phalanx of the fourth finger with a suggestion of calcification within the lesion. The lesion spreads from the diaphysis into the distal metaphysis and is characteristic of an enchondroma.

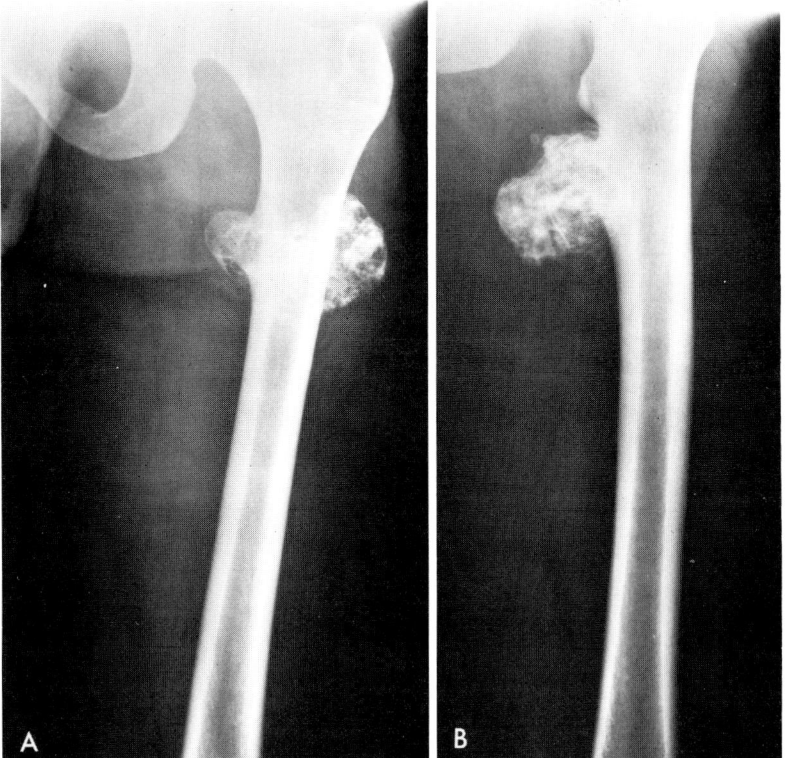

Figure 12–36. Osteochondroma, AP view (*A*) and lateral view (*B*). A large mass arising from the posterior aspect of the right femur has a solid bony base with a well-circumscribed cartilaginous cap. These findings are typical of a benign osteochondroma.

metaphysis into the diaphysis, because as the tumor is laid down in the patient's younger years, the bone grows "away" from the tumor, leaving the tumor isolated from the physeal plate in the diaphysis (Figs. 12–34 and 12–35).

One other tumor is important enough to be illustrated: the osteochondroma (Fig. 12–36). Most people will have one bony spur or exostosis on the skeleton, and Virchow postulated a theory to account for this (Fig. 12–37). Thus, many exostoses have a cartilaginous cap. If the cap can be seen radiographically as stippled calcification, there is a 5 to 8 per cent risk of malignant change into a chondrosarcoma as the patient ages.

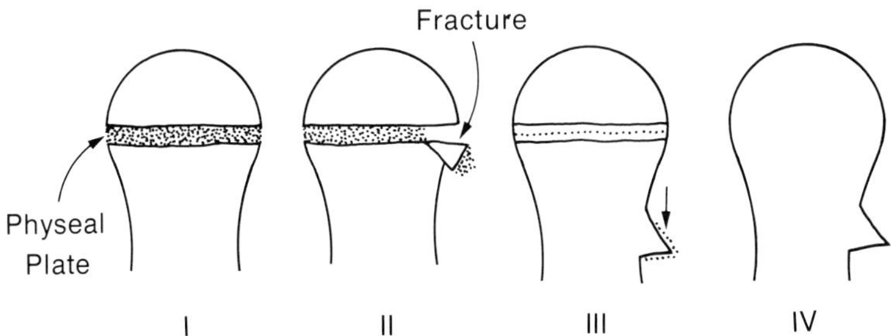

Figure 12–37. Diagram of Virchow's theory of the origin of an osteochondroma. A small fragment of metaphysis and physeal plate gets knocked off and continues to grow away from the growing end of the bone, so that as the bone grows in length, the fragment becomes isolated, with its cartilaginous cap away from the epiphysis.

Primary malignant tumors of bone also have characteristic appearances and occur particularly in certain age groups and certain bones; a competent radiologist should therefore be able to give an informed opinion on most of them.

Case E16

William Fielding, age 22, pitcher for the Snuksville baseball team, developed pain in his knee three months after having been hit in that knee by a line drive from the bat of the local Henry Aaron. On examination, there was a mass on the medial aspect of the right femur, and the x-rays were characteristic (Fig. 12–38A).

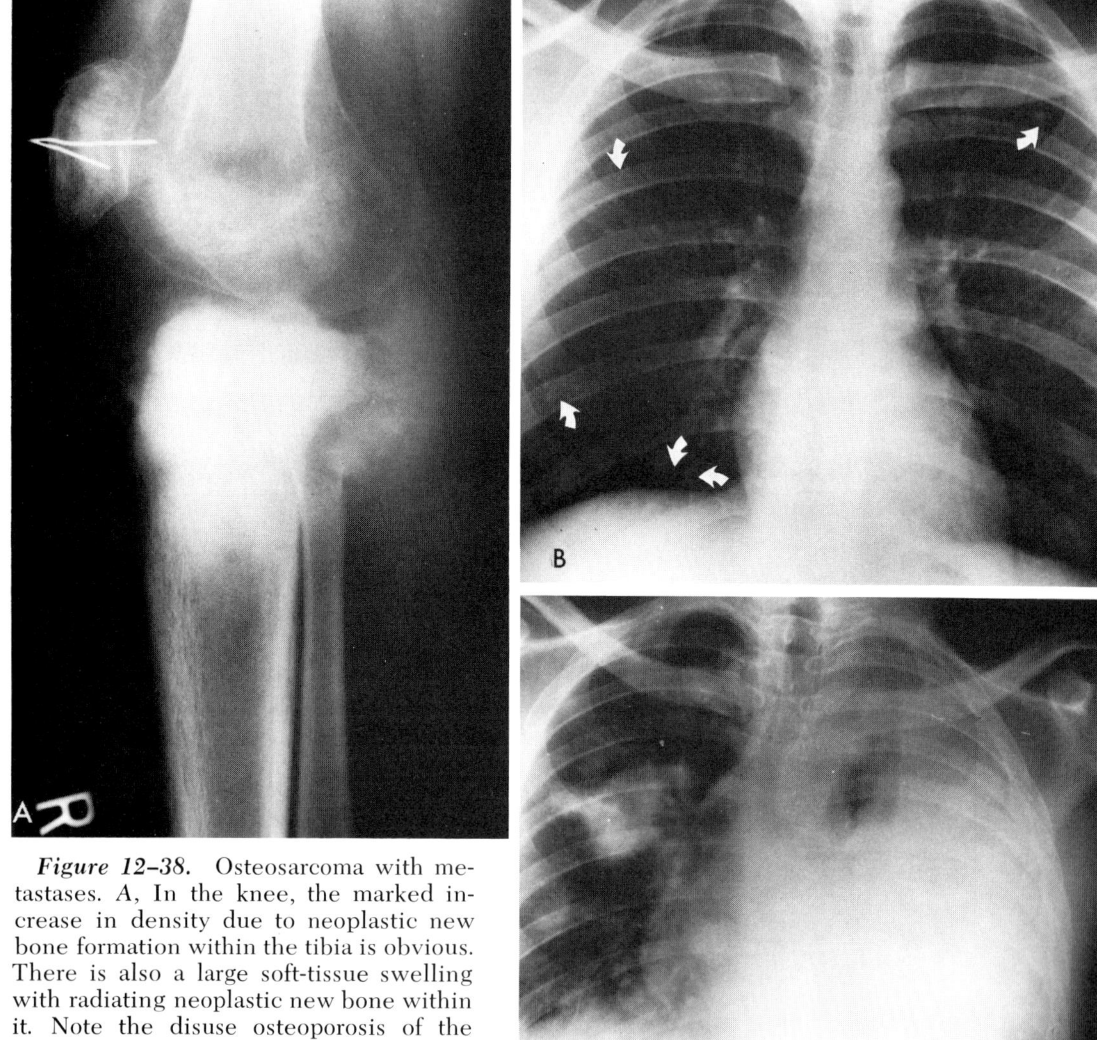

Figure 12–38. Osteosarcoma with metastases. *A*, In the knee, the marked increase in density due to neoplastic new bone formation within the tibia is obvious. There is also a large soft-tissue swelling with radiating neoplastic new bone within it. Note the disuse osteoporosis of the distal femur, which occurred because the patient refused amputation and did not use his leg because it hurt. *B*, A chest x-ray taken at three months shows a number of discrete dense ossified metastases (*arrows*). *C*, Chest x-ray taken at nine months shows marked increase in the size and number of metastases as well as a huge accumulation of fluid in the left hemithorax. The patient succumbed shortly thereafter.

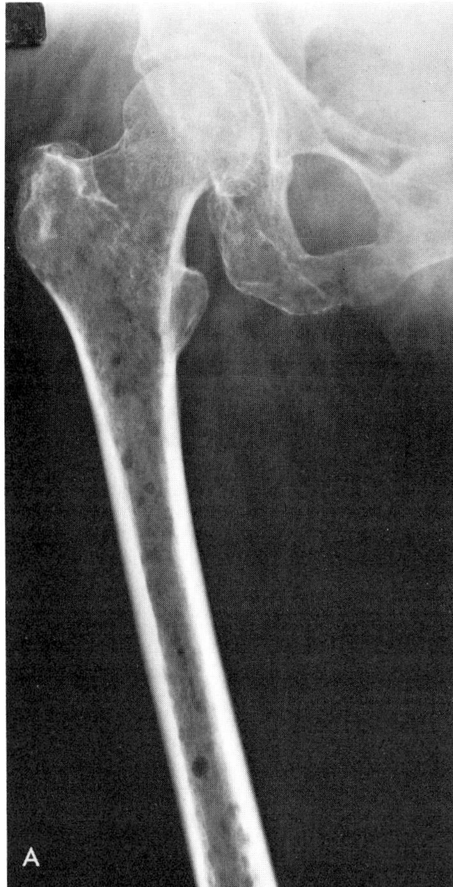

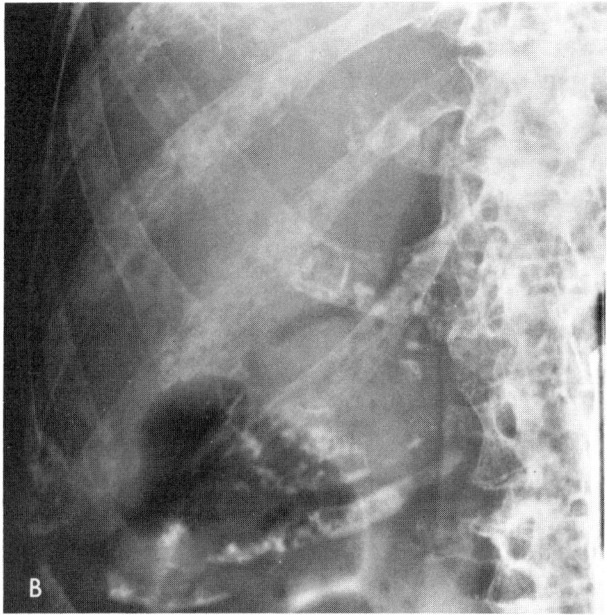

Figure 12–39. Multiple myeloma, pelvis (*A*) and ribs (*B*). Multiple well-defined "punched-out" lesions can be seen in the ribs, pelvis, and femur. The differential diagnosis between myeloma and lytic metastases may be difficult to make radiographically. Myeloma deposits, however, usually have clear-cut margins and rarely "light up" on a bone scan; lytic metastases have blurred margins because they are more infiltrative, and they always "light up" on a bone scan.

Osteogenic sarcoma occurs predominantly in patients from 15 to 30 years old and usually involves the metaphyseal regions of the major growth centers (the lower femur, upper tibia, and humeral head). Unlike the tumors shown in previous radiographs, this tumor is undoubtedly very destructive and looks malignant. The five-year survival rate, even with the modern forms of ablative surgery, radiotherapy, and chemotherapy, is still around 10 per cent. The patient died within 10 months of diagnosis from pulmonary metastases (Fig. 12–38C).

Osteogenic sarcomas generate soft-tissue metastases to lung and liver as well as osseous metastases, which are bone-forming and hence blastic. Hypertrophic osteoarthropathy may also occur. The metastases to the lungs may have one or two unusual manifestations: they may ossify or they may cavitate and lead to pneumothorax. Osteogenic sarcoma also occurs in some elderly patients with Paget's disease and in patients with chronic inflammatory conditions such as osteomyelitis.

Chondrosarcomas of bone either arise secondary to a pre-existing benign cartilaginous tumor such as an osteochondroma or exostosis or develop *de novo,* mainly in flat bones such as the rib or pelvis. They occur in the 40 to 60 year age group. Fibrosarcomas probably arise from the periosteum or fibrous tissue cells within the bone itself and occur in the 30 to 55 year age range.

Lymphoma and leukemia involving bone lie outside the scope of this book, although Hodgkin's disease is discussed earlier. Multiple myeloma has also been mentioned with osteoporosis as a primary presentation, but the patient with this disease usually presents with multiple punched-out lytic areas and appears to be severely ill, and the diagnosis is obvious (Fig. 12–39).

CHAPTER 13

THE HEAD

In a discussion of the signs and symptoms relating to the head, it is probably easier to consider the plain film findings first before discussing specific intracranial conditions and their radiological approach. For the investigation of brain lesions, a number of well-tried sophisticated techniques as well as the newly emerging science of CT scanning are available.

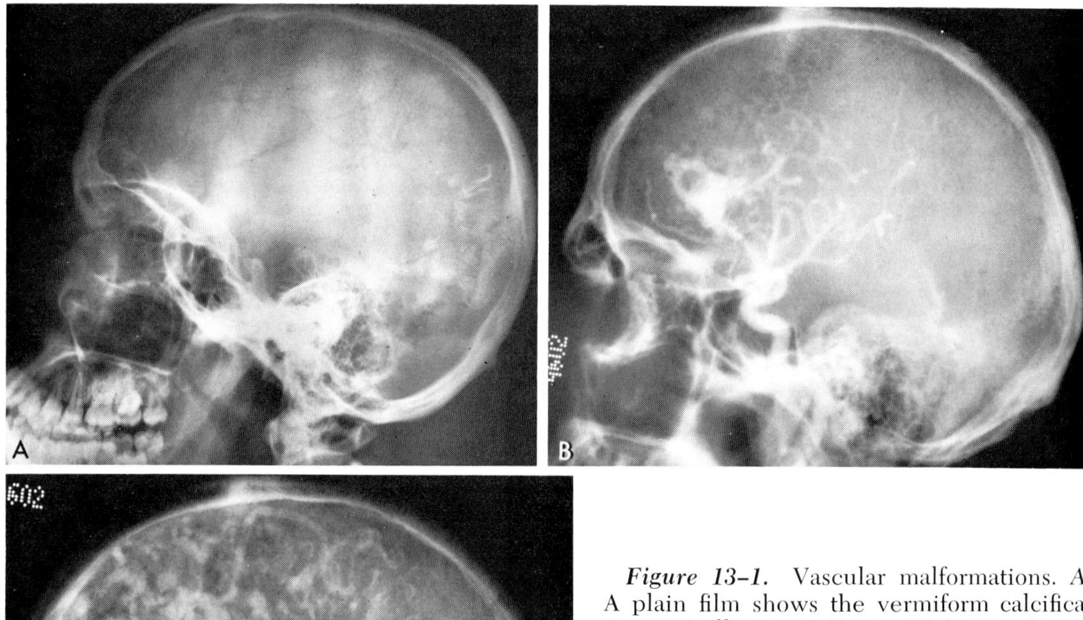

Figure 13–1. Vascular malformations. *A*, A plain film shows the vermiform calcification typically seen in Sturge-Weber syndrome (encephalotrigeminal angiomatosis). *B* and *C*, Angiograms of a different patient. The early arterial film (*B*) shows a collection of contrast agent lying anteriorly and being supplied by the anterior cerebral artery. The venous phase (*C*) shows the typical ramifications seen in a large arteriovenous malformation.

Case H1

Fern Farckle, age 78, came into the emergency room complaining of headaches that became worse when she performed headstands at the fairground where she worked. On examination, no abnormality could be found and a skull series was taken (Fig. 13–1). What do the films show?

This is one example of pathological calcification in the brain. There are some significant physiological calcifications that should not be taken for signs of disease: The pineal gland is frequently calcified, in which case it will act as a marker for the position of the midline of the brain in a PA, AP, or Townes view of the skull. The gland is calcified in some 20 per cent of people aged 20 and 80 per cent of people aged 80 (Fig. 13–2). The falx and tentorium also frequently calcify in older people, and the choroid plexuses calcify in some normal people, although this is more frequently seen in diabetic patients. (Fig. 13–2). It is not uncommon to see calcification of the parasellar portion of the internal carotid artery in arteriosclerotic and diabetic patients. Many calcifications are neither benign nor physiological and represent areas of pathological change. Many primary brain tumors calcify, including meningiomas, gliomas, and craniopharyngiomas. Some infections, such as cytomegalovirus inclusion disease and toxoplasmosis, cause intracerebral calcification (Fig. 13–3). Tuberculosis causes calcification elsewhere in the body, and meningeal calcification may develop after a bout of tuberculous meningitis. Chronic hematomas, arteriovenous malformations, and aneurysms also lead to characteristic calcifications in the head.

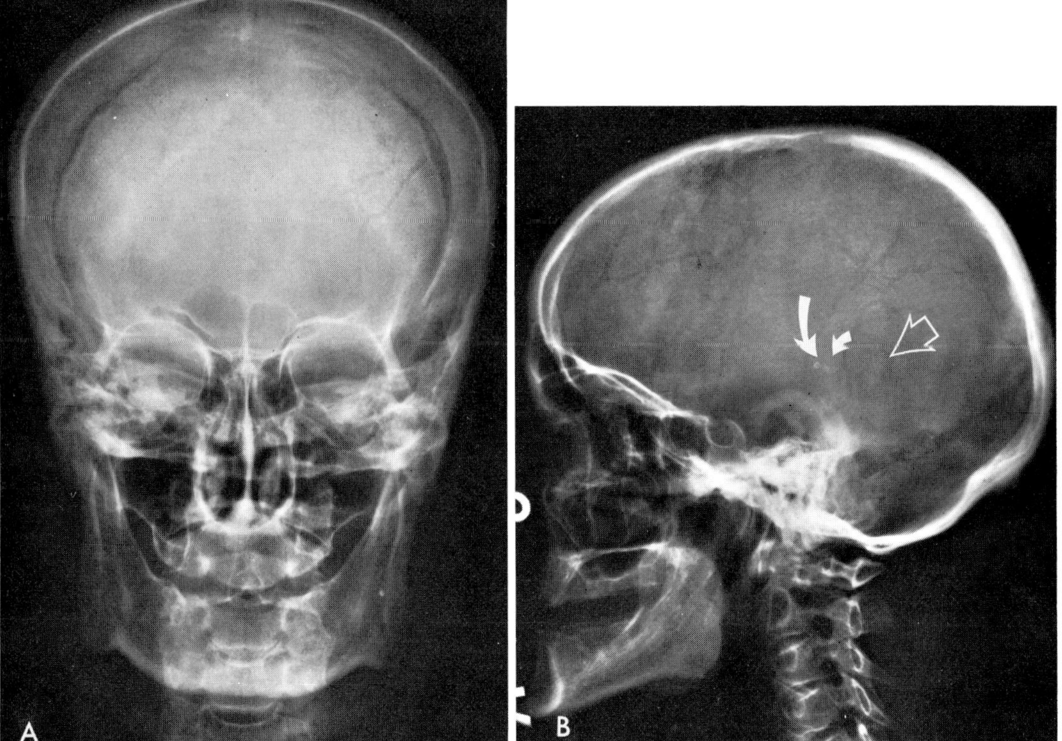

Figure 13–2. Calcified pineal gland and habenula, AP view (*A*) and lateral view (*B*). This 69-year-old man was admitted for evaluation of his arthritis. The skull x-ray shows calcification in the pineal gland (*short arrow*), habenula (*long arrow*), and choroid plexus (*hollow arrow*).

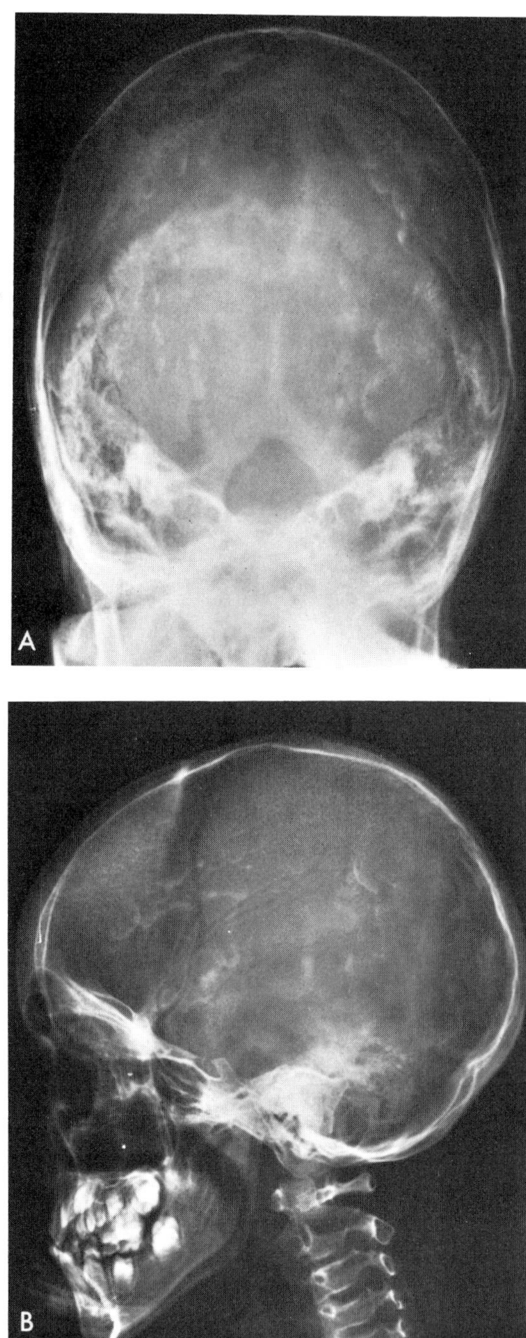

Figure 13–3. Toxoplasmosis, Townes view (*A*) and lateral view (*B*). This 10-year-old child was anemic and mentally retarded and had a cleft lip and palate. Irregular bilateral calcifications seen over the cerebral cortex were caused by toxoplasmosis.

Case H2

Pippin Quagmire, age 27, was having a quiet drink in a bar at 4:00 a.m. when he took exception to someone's laughing at his name. A fight ensued, and Pippin, who was all of 4 feet 8 inches tall, was easily subdued by his opponent, who was 6 feet 2 inches tall. Pippin was admitted to the emergency room in a semicomatose state with multiple bruises and complaining of pain around his left eye. Plain films proved not to be helpful because of the overlying edema, although there was a suggestion of a "blowout" fracture of the orbit (Fig. 13–4A). What would you do now?

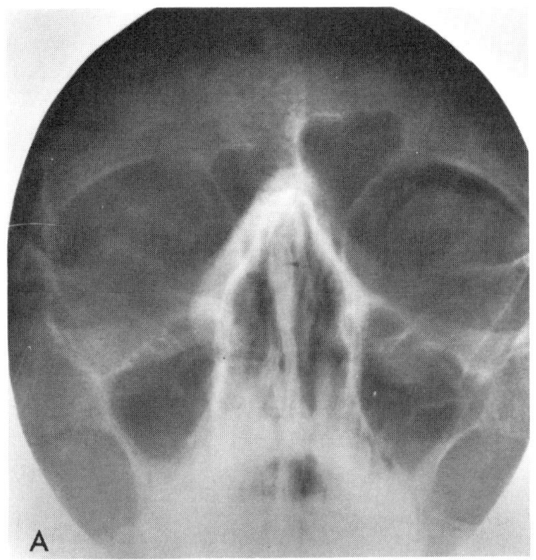

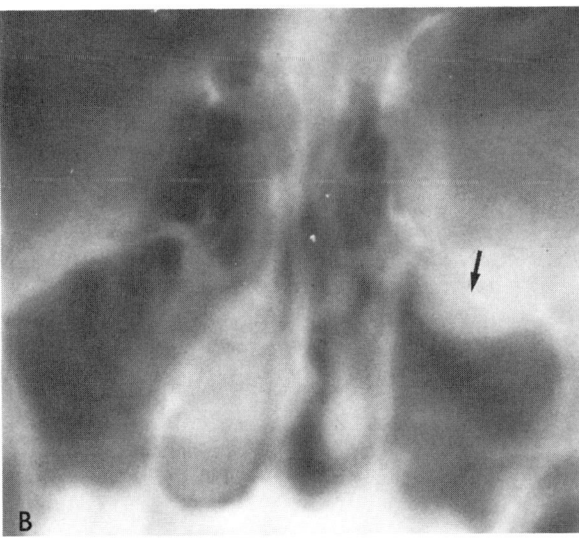

Figure 13–4. Orbital blowout fracture. *A*, The plain film shows a soft tissue density projecting from the left orbital floor into the maxillary antrum. *B*, The tomogram confirms the fracture of the orbital floor (*arrow*).

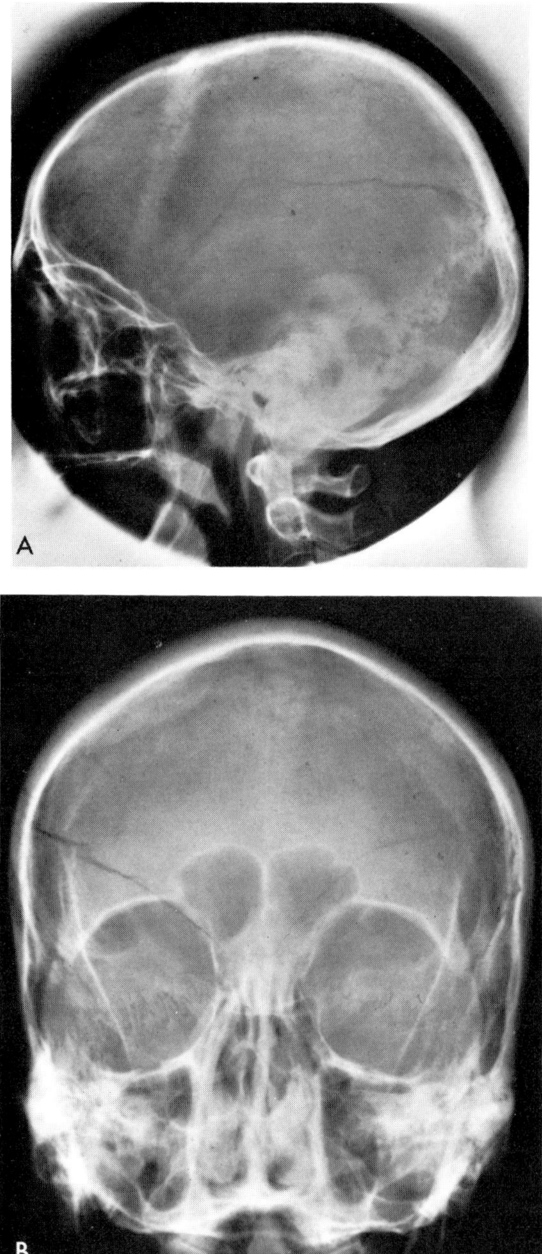

Figure 13–5. Skull fracture, lateral view (*A*) and frontal view (*B*). This 20-year-old man was punched by a bartender and fell from a barstool onto his back. He presented three days later complaining of headaches. There is a circumferential linear fracture running from one temporal bone to the other.

The swelling was allowed to recede for a day or two, and tomography was performed (Fig. 13–4B). This confirmed the diagnosis of an orbital fracture and allowed the radiologist to check for other fractures. The orbit is a "ring" of bone, and a second fracture, which usually occurs through the lateral wall of the maxillary sinus, should always be sought. A soft-tissue finding of some importance is opacification of the left maxillary antrum by blood; this usually accompanies a true fracture rather than a mere bruise or blow to this region.

Most fractures are not as spectacular as this example. The patient involved in an altercation or a road accident may present to the emergency room in an unconscious to semicomatose state, with altering states of consciousness, or fully conscious and complaining of a headache. In any case, a full skull series should be done. In the vast majority of patients with minor neurological symptoms, a lateral skull film is all that is required, but oblique views are often necessary. There are many different types of skull fracture; only one is illustrated here (Fig. 13–5).

Case H3

Elijah Crabtree, age 17, came into the emergency room complaining of frequent headaches. On examination, no abnormality could be found, and a plain lateral film of the skull was taken (Fig. 13–6). What does it show?

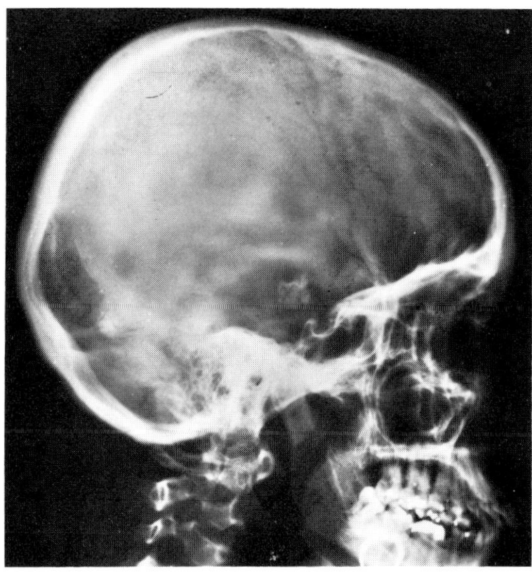

Figure 13–6. Craniopharyngioma (calcified). On this lateral skull radiograph, a calcified lesion can be seen in the suprasellar region. At operation, a craniopharyngioma with calcification was found.

There are some stippled calcifications above the sella. This appearance is characteristic of a craniopharyngioma, the most common primary tumor of the sellar region. In most cases of craniopharyngioma the sella is also enlarged, but parasellar craniopharyngiomas are not uncommon.

Case H4

Samuel Hamfist, age 45, went to his family doctor complaining that his head had grown too large for his hat. When questioned, he also revealed that his rings were too small because his hands were enlarging. There was some doubt about whether his feet had enlarged, because he didn't wear shoes. On examination, he appeared somewhat somnolent and had a jutting jaw, prominent forehead, and large tongue. His hands and feet were "spade-like." Apart from his skull (Fig. 13–7A) and extremities (Fig. 13–7C), what other part of his body should be radiographed?

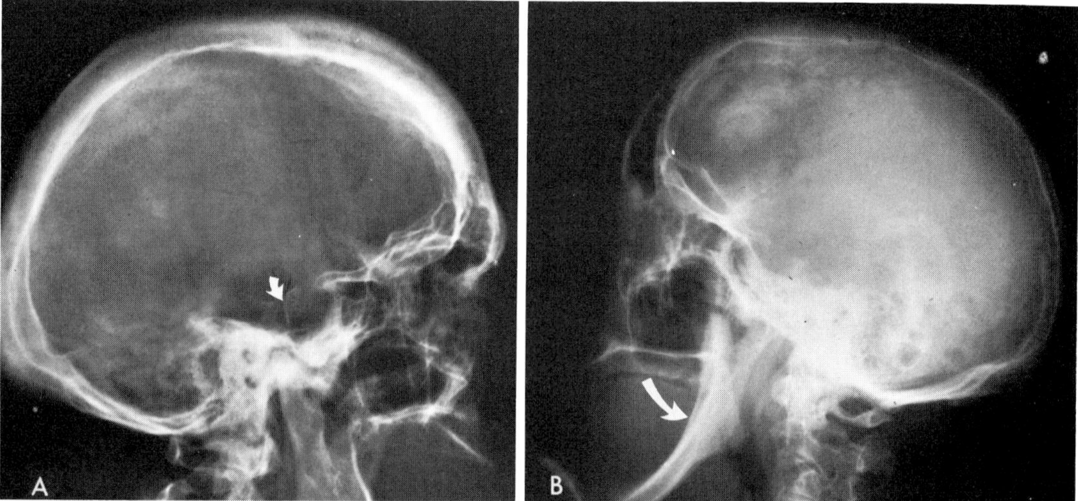

Figure 13–7. Acromegaly. *A* and *B*, Lateral views of the skulls of two different patients. In the first patient (*A*), note the thickening of the calvarium and the obvious expansion of the sella with thinning and straightening of the dorsum sella (*small arrow*). In the second patient (*B*), alteration in the angle of the jaw (*large arrow*) and enlargement of the tongue can be seen. Both patients are edentulous. The frontal sinuses are enlarged.

This patient is suffering from a classic eosinophilic pituitary adenoma, which produces acromegaly in adults and gigantism in children if it occurs before the epiphyses close. Excessive secretion of growth hormone causes the bones and soft tissues to grow where they are able. In adults, the bones are unable to grow longitudinally and so the bones appear to widen, particularly in the metaphyseal regions, the tufts of the fingers, and the calvarium. Characteristic changes are also seen in the spine (Fig. 13–7D). The soft tissue changes are often predominant, and there is marked overgrowth of the subcutaneous tissues, articular cartilage, heart, tongue, and heel pad (Fig. 13–7E).

Correct investigation of this patient includes angiography and a modified pneumoencephalogram to assess the lateral and upward extension of the pituitary tumor prior to therapy. CT scanning may be of some assistance, but the investigation of choice is still a modified pneumoencephalo-

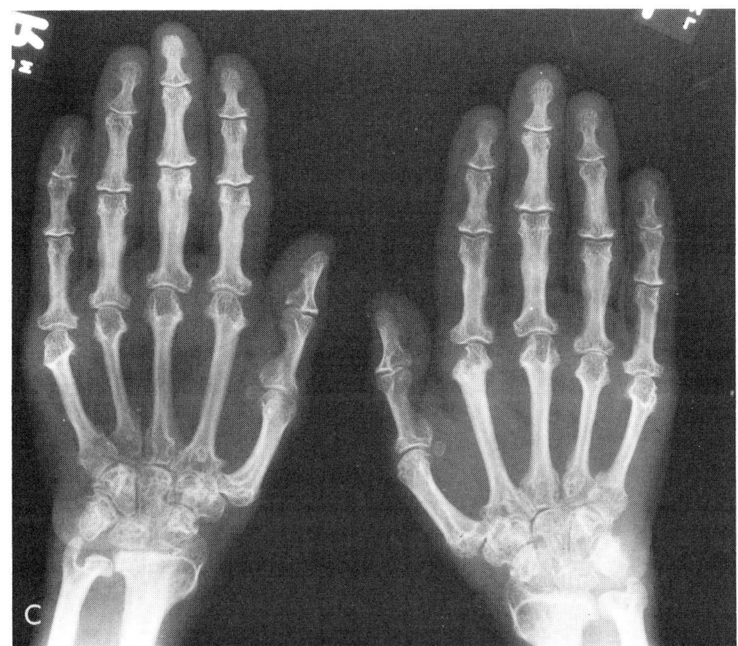

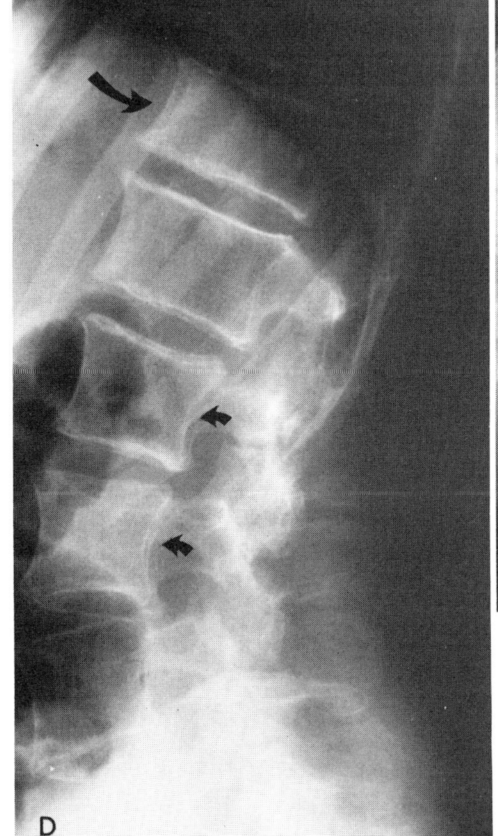

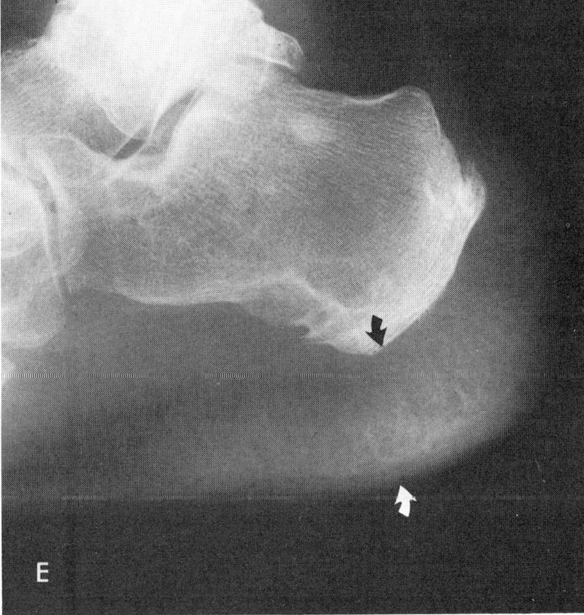

Figure 13–7. Continued. C, AP view of the hands. In acromegaly the hands take on a "spade-like" appearance, with thickening of the soft tissues, widening of the bones at their metaphyses (note particularly the distal radii), and enlargement of the tufts. Note the widening of the joint spaces due to overgrowth of the cartilage. *D,* Lateral view of the spine. Scalloping of the posterior surfaces of the lumbar vertebral bodies (*small arrows*) due to overgrowth of the soft tissues (i.e., theca, meninges) can be seen. New bone has been laid down anteriorly in the lower thoracic spine (*large arrow*). Both of these findings are characteristic of acromegaly. *E,* View of the heel pad. In acromegaly, the soft tissues enlarge all over the body, but measurement of the thickening of the heel pad (between the *arrows*) can give an indication of the degree of acromegaly. In normal people this measurement is 21 mm or less, unless they have calluses on their feet or peripheral edema; any other patient with a heel pad thickness of more than 25 mm has acromegaly.

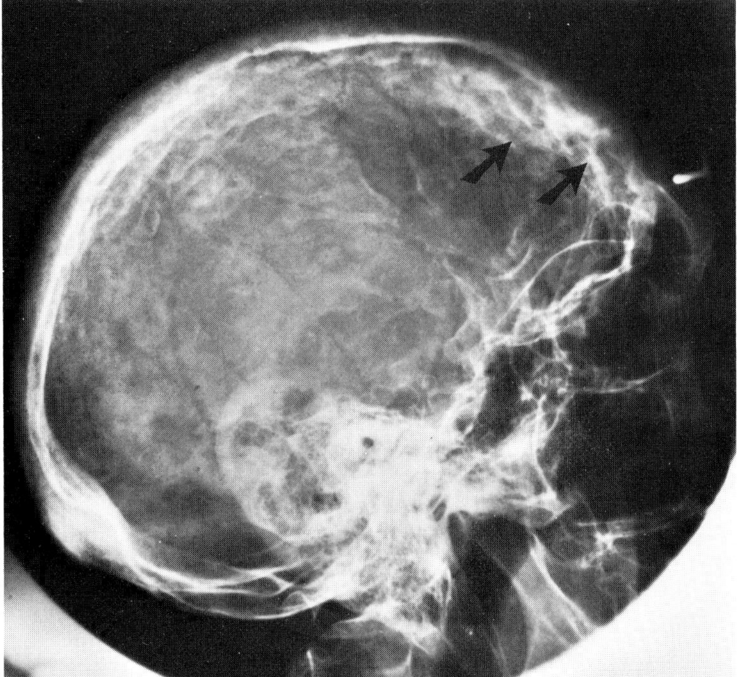

Figure 13–8. Hyperostosis frontalis interna, lateral view. This 65-year-old female patient complained of headaches. She was found to be normal apart from marked internal overgrowth of the calvarium—particularly in the frontal region (*arrows*). This condition is known as hyperostosis frontalis interna and is of no significance.

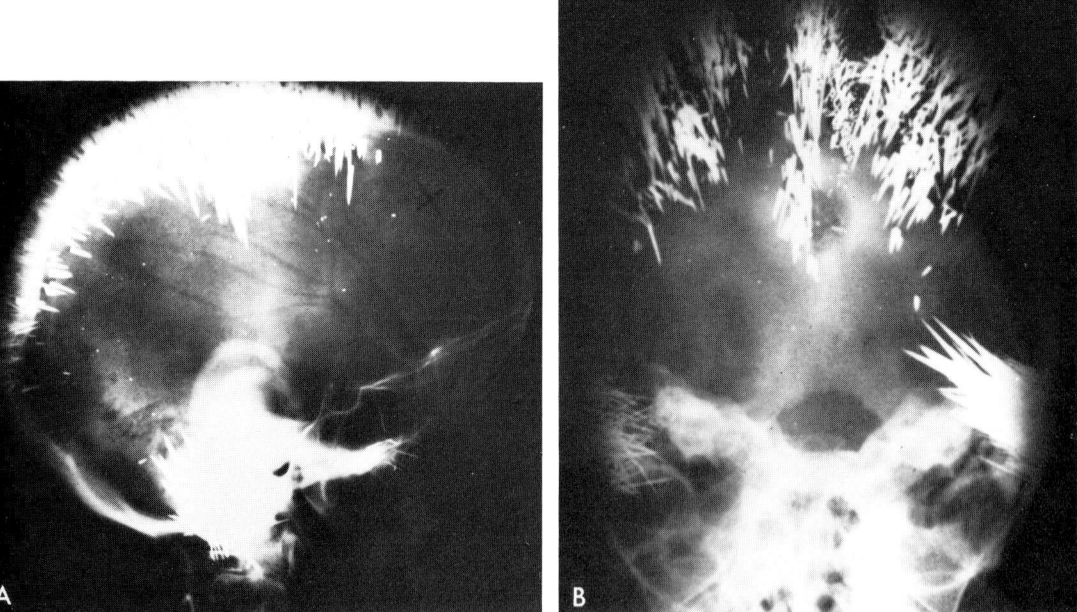

Figure 13–9. Nails in head, lateral view (*A*) and Townes view (*B*). This man was serving time in a penitentary and apparently "got his kicks" from having people hammer cobbler's nails into his skull. Note that the nails are mainly in the mastoid and posterolateral parietal regions.

gram. Other pituitary tumors are investigated in the same way, although the diagnosis is usually made on the basis of plain film findings of enlargement of the sella or a double sella floor (which can be confirmed by tomography in the AP and lateral planes).

Hyperostosis frontalis interna is a very common finding in older patients, particularly women, and is not related to any specific disorder (Fig. 13–8). On rare occasions, the etiology of recurrent headaches is not difficult to ascertain (Fig. 13–9).

Intracranial hemorrhage may have a number of different causes, and the bleeding may be intracerebral (from a ruptured aneurysm, for example) or subdural (following trauma).

Case H5

Phinias Blackberry, age 34, was scaling the Empire State Building when he slipped and fell five floors. He rapidly lost consciousness and was admitted to a local hospital. Plain films of the skull revealed no abnormality, and since the pineal was not calcified, it was not possible to obtain radiological information about possible midline shift. What investigations would you do now and in what order?

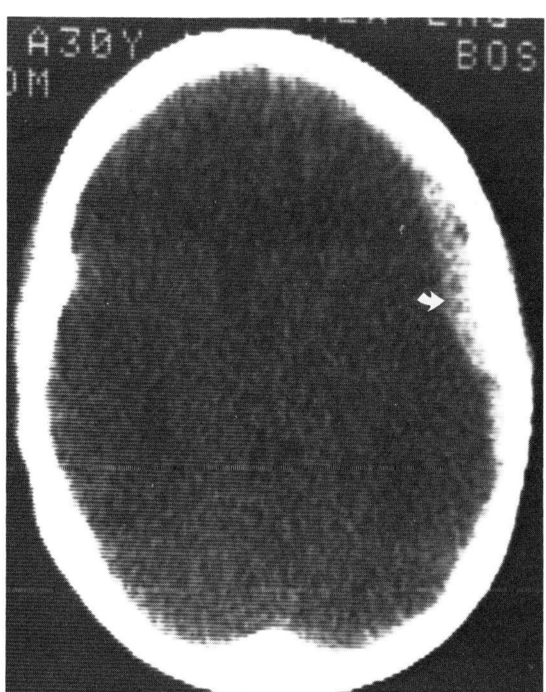

Figure 13–10. Subdural hemorrhage. A single CT scan of the cranial vault shows an area of increased attentuation value in the left frontoparietal region (*arrow*) that represents an intracranial collection of blood.

An ultrasonographic A-scan showed evidence of midline shift. If a CT scanner is available, a subdural hemorrhage is easily diagnosed (Fig. 13–10); it usually appears as a relative change in density but is sometimes suggested only by a shift in the position of the ventricles. Injection of contrast agent often enhances the outline of the hemorrhage, or appears in the blood itself. The traditional approach, however, is to perform angiography in the AP plane. An advantage of angiography is that it occasionally makes possible visualization of the bleeding site. Both a CT scan and an angio-

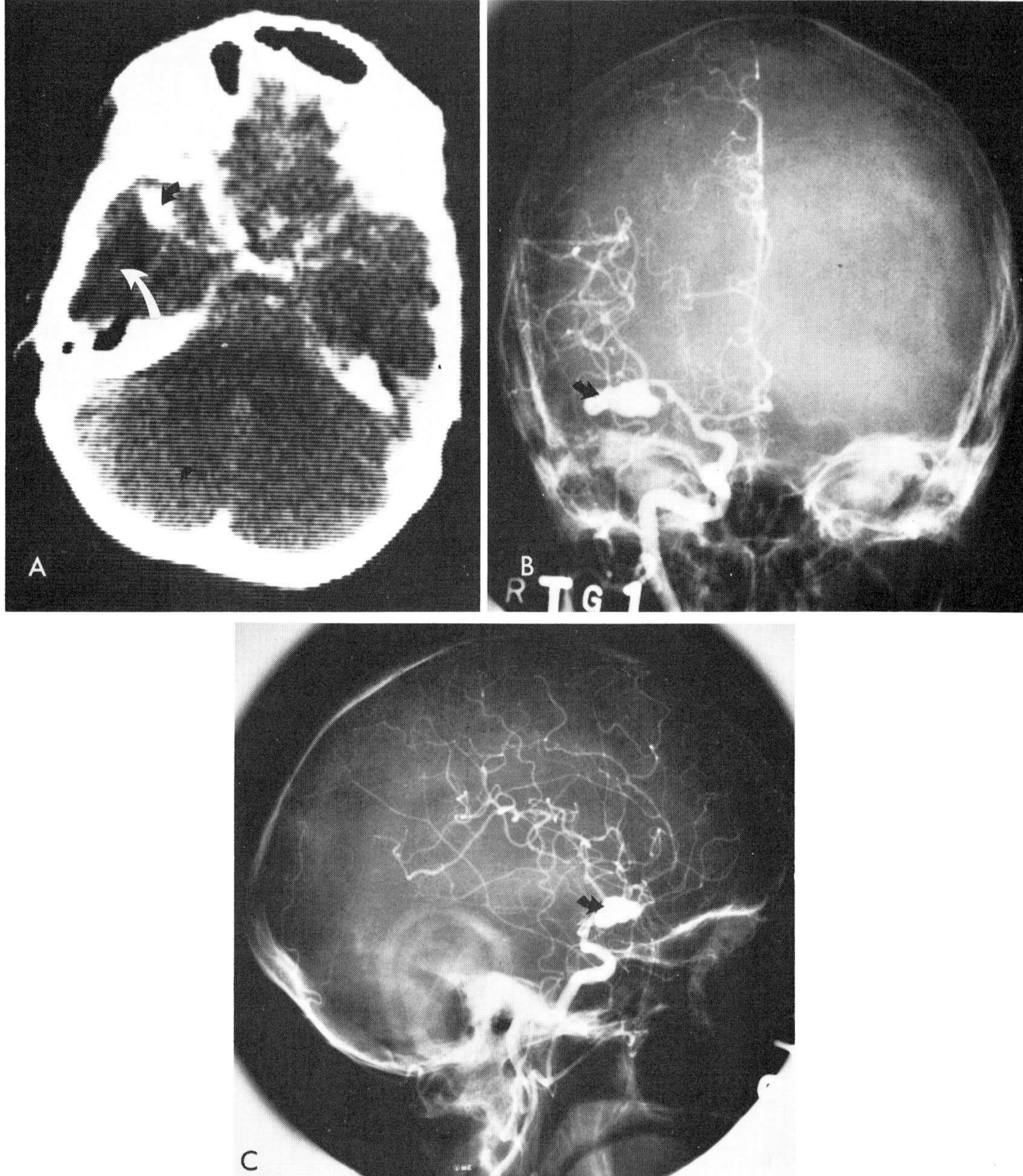

Figure 13–11. Intracranial hemorrhage. This 70-year-old patient presented with a CVA. *A*, The enhanced CT scan shows an area of increased density in the region of the right middle cerebral artery (*small black arrow*) that was surrounded by an area of edema (*large white arrow*). The area of increased density was thought to represent contrast agent in an aneurysm. *B* and *C* Frontal and lateral angiograms confirmed the suspicion of an aneurysm.

gram would reveal any associated intracerebral hemorrhage, which can be evacuated by the surgeon when he evacuates the primary subdural hemorrhage.

Many elderly patients who present with a stroke or cerebrovascular accident (CVA) have sustained a thrombosis rather than an intracranial hemorrhage. A CT scan demonstrates the hemorrhage, which usually appears as an area of increased density surrounded by an area of decreased density that represents cerebral edema (Fig. 13–11A). If the underlying cause of a CVA in a younger patient is being sought, a cerebral angiogram is essential. This procedure demonstrates the source of the bleeding to be an aneurysm or an arteriovenous malformation as well as showing the size and volume of the hemorrhage (Figs. 13–11B and 13–11C). Some long-standing intracranial hematomas calcify and thus can be seen on plain films.

Case H6

Beany Haricotvert, age 36, complained to his doctor of headaches. His wife had noted a change in his personality. Beany, who had always been very quiet and retiring, had now become noisy and demonstrative. He had also begun to exhibit himself to the 98-year-old widow who lived next door. The doctor ordered plain films of the skull, which showed bony hyperostosis, a characteristic occurrence in one third of all cases of meningioma. Angiography and CT scanning confirmed the diagnosis (Fig. 13–12).

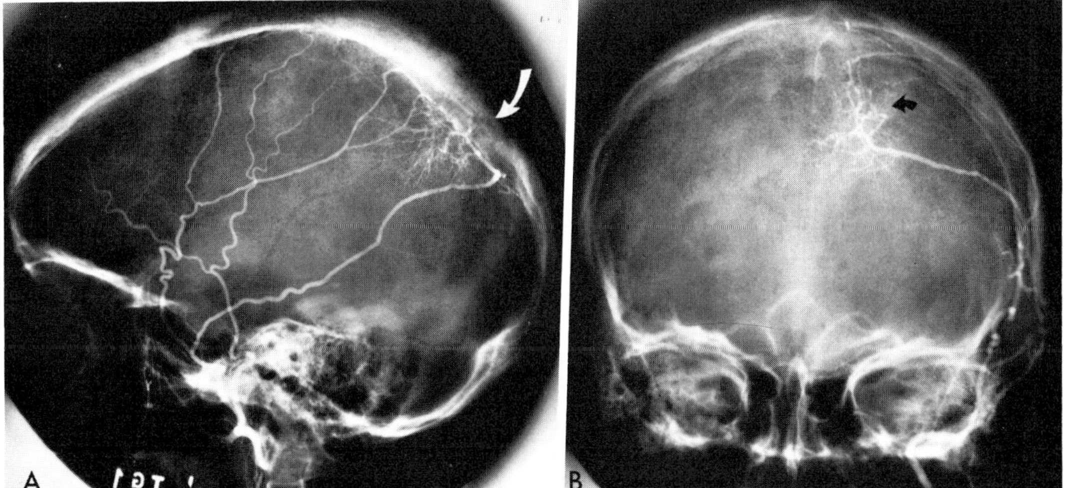

Figure 13–12. Meningioma, lateral angiogram (*A*) and frontal angiogram (*B*). Left external carotid angiograms demonstrate a large tumor blush in the region of the posterior parietal area (*arrows*). The tumor is supplied by branches of the middle meningeal artery. Note the hyperostosis and destruction of the overlying skull, best seen on the lateral view.

Approximately 75 per cent of meningiomas cause signs that can be detected on plain films: hyperostosis or local erosions with enlarged vascular channels. Psammomatous calcifications occur in 10 per cent of meningiomas, which are relatively benign, grow slowly, and represent 15 per cent of all intracranial tumors.

Case H7

Hortense Mayseed, age 52, presented with a change in personality and in a confusional state. A respectable high court judge, she had decided that she was Napoleon Bonaparte. She complained of headaches and had been known to have seizures in the courtroom. Plain films of the skull showed no abnormality apart from the shift of the pineal gland to the left. A CT scan and an angiogram were performed (Fig. 13–13). What do they show?

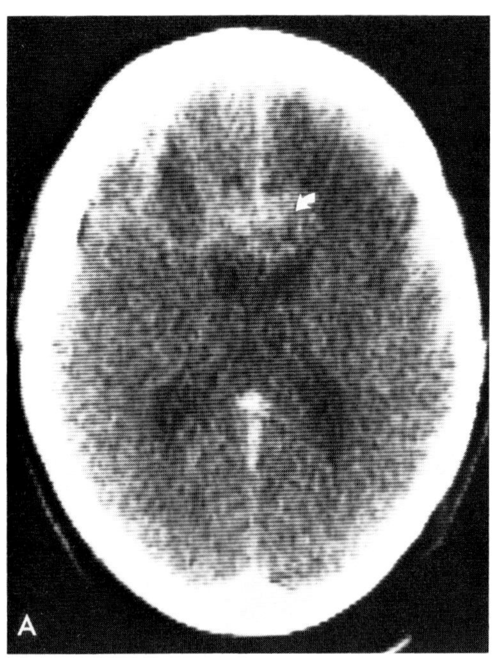

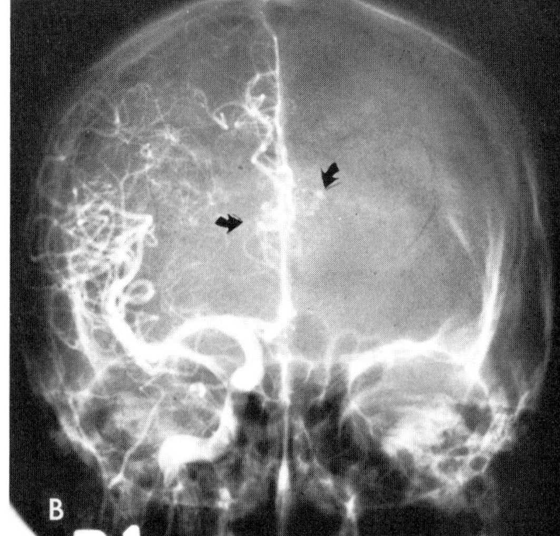

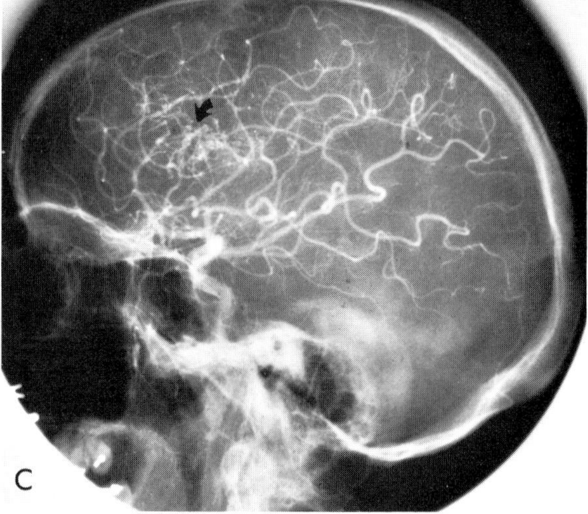

Figure 13–13. Glioma. *A*, An enhanced CT scan shows an area of increased density in the region of the left frontal lobe that extends across the midline in the region of the corpus callosum (*arrow*). *B* and *C*, Frontal and lateral angiograms show an area of neovascularity (*arrows*) in the anterior portion of the corpus callosum.

Both these studies indicate the presence of a large space-occupying lesion, and biopsy confirmed that this was a glioma. Gliomas are the largest group of intracranial tumors and are classified for diagnostic, therapeutic, and prognostic purposes according to five cell types: glioblastoma multiforme, astrocytoma, oligodendroglioma, medulloblastoma, and ependymoma. Gliomas are very malignant and generally rapidly fatal.

They may occur anywhere in the brain but are more common in the parietal and temporal lobe areas. The radiological investigation of choice is the CT scan, often followed by angiography, although CT scans are more convenient for following the effects of therapy (either surgical removal of the tumor, radiotherapy, or chemotherapy).

Case H8

Aphrodite Crapweed, age 63, experienced a gradual change in personality. Eventually she thought she was a new Messiah sent down to save physicians from themselves. Her family had her committed to a large private mental hospital, where as part of the admission procedure she had a chest radiograph and a skull series, both of which were normal. The hospital had just acquired a CT scanner, and CT scans were being performed routinely on all new admissions. The scan for this patient showed multiple areas of increased density (Fig. 13–14). What would you do now?

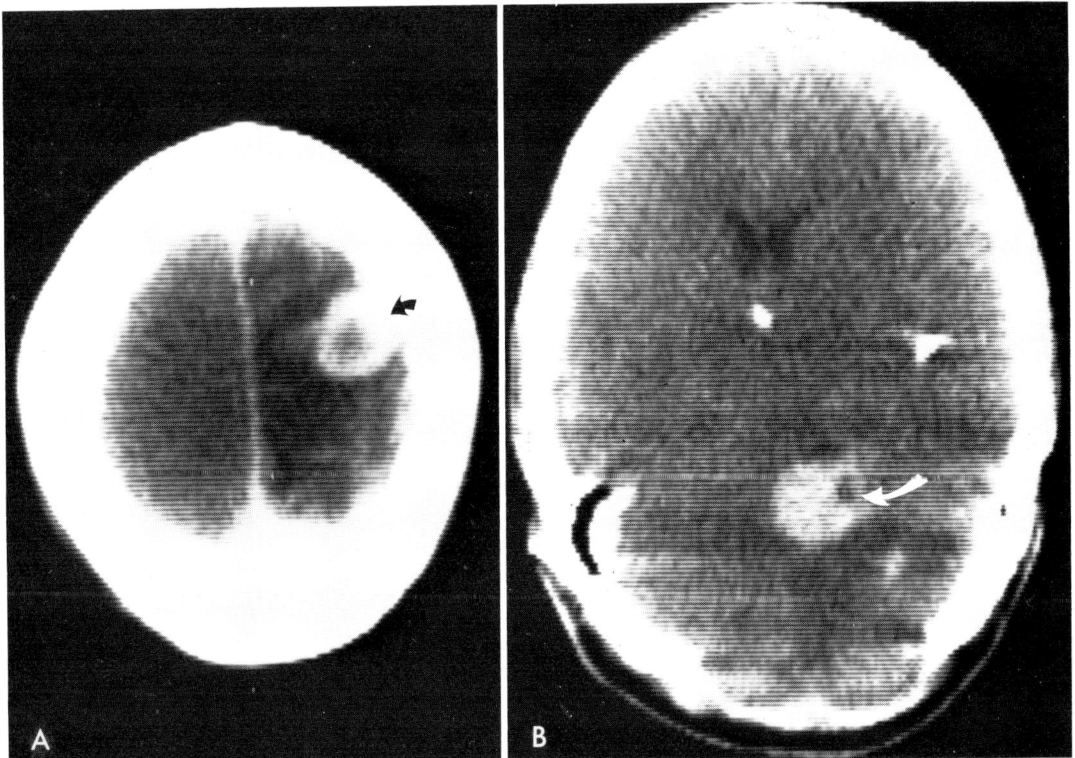

Figure 13–14. Multiple cerebral metastases. *A* and *B*, CT scans at different levels demonstrate two separate densities in the brain: one in the left parietal area (*small black arrow*) and the other in the cerebellum (*large white arrow*). Two other areas of increased density, representing a midline intraventricular shunt and some residual Pantopaque are also seen.

A diagnosis of multiple metastases from an unknown primary site can be confidently made. Metastatic tumors constitute over 20 per cent of all intracranial tumors. Usually the patient presents with evidence of a primary malignancy in another part of the body and later develops cerebral metastases. Occasionally, however, intracerebral metastases are the first manifestations of a distant malignancy. A radiographic search for the primary site should include a CXR, studies of the gastrointestinal and genitourinary tracts, mammograms (in a woman) and, of course, a careful clinical examination. This patient was found to have a breast carcinoma. Although hormonal therapy did not save her life, it was of some help in returning her personality to normal.

Case H9

Alwyn Grout, age 58, a well-known psychologist, had become extremely absent-minded. One day on the way home he lost his way. Espying a child, he asked, "Little girl, do you know where I live?" The young lady replied, "Yes, Daddy. Please follow me." His wife took him to the hospital, and CT scan revealed the cause of his problem (Fig. 13–15).

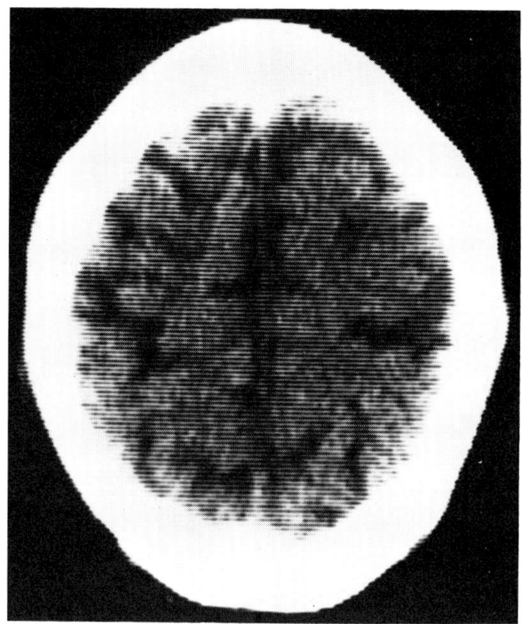

Figure 13–15. Cortical atrophy. Nonenhanced CT scan shows widening of the cortical sulci, typical of cortical atrophy.

Cortical atrophy affects every person as he ages, but premature atrophy of the cerebral cortex appears to be more common than was suspected before the advent of the CT scanner. This was a difficult diagnosis to make using traditional radiological techniques, but the diagnosis is simple with computerized tomography.

A brief discussion of raised intracranial pressure is included in this chapter, because there a few causes other than the major neurological disorders already discussed. Brain tumor, intracranial abscess, granuloma, benign intracranial hypertension, and internal hydrocephalus cause intracranial pressure to increase. On plain films, a "beaten copper" appearance is seen in the vault of the skull in children with prolonged raised intracranial pressure, whereas in adults the first radiographic sign is usually loss of the posterior clinoids.

Case H10

Rex Minimus, age 4, presented with seizures and complaining of a severe headache. Lumbar puncture revealed an elevated cerebrospinal fluid pressure. Shortly thereafter, the child suddenly went into coma. Blood tests were diagnostic, and x-rays of the wrists and knees as well as a plain film of the abdomen were taken and found to be characteristic (Fig. 13–16).

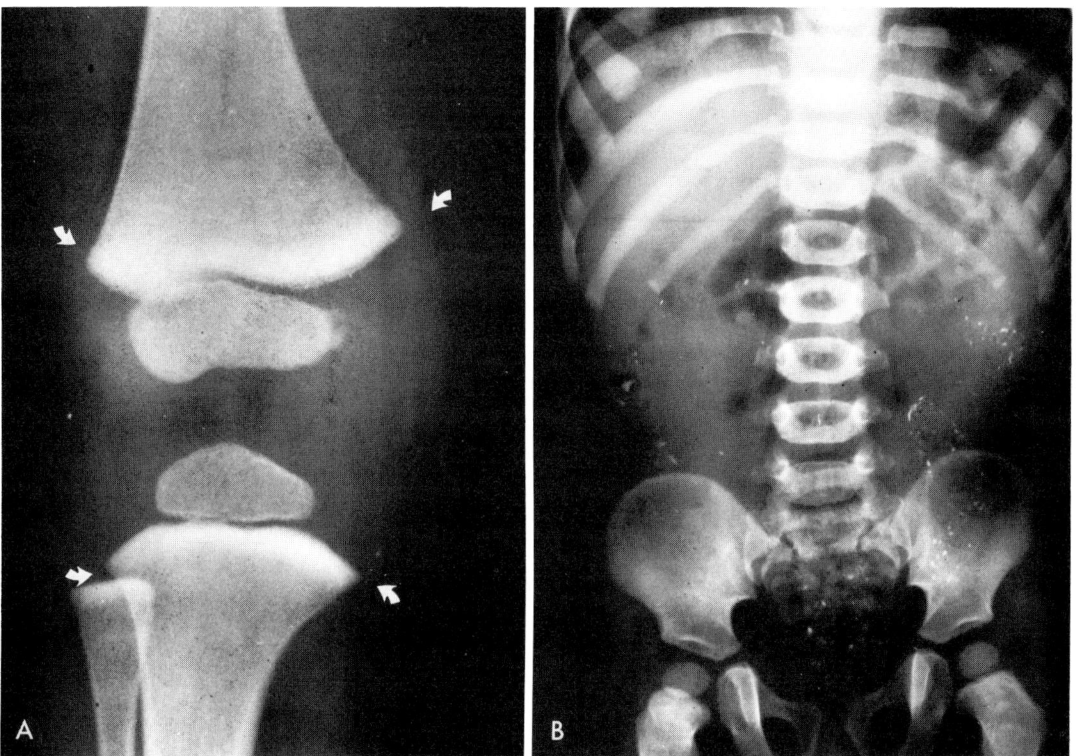

Figure 13–16. Lead poisoning. *A*, AP view of knee clearly shows an increase in density in the juxtaphyseal regions (*arrows*) that is usually due to heavy metal poisoning. *B*, KUB shows multiple speckled densities lying within the bowel that were found to represent particles of lead-containing paint.

Encephalopathies may be caused by many toxins as well as by various infections. Lead poisoning may cause encephalopathy in a child if a sufficient amount of lead has been ingested. The growing ends of the long bones show the characteristic lead lines, which are caused partially by reactive hyperplasia of the bone and partially by deposition of lead. Abdominal films occasionally demonstrate lead particles (usually from lead-based paint) throughout the alimentary tract.

EPILOGUE

"Take from the altar of knowledge the fire – and not the ashes."
–GYÖRGYI

We hope this book has stimulated you into doing some further reading about radiology or whatever branch of medicine you intend to pursue for the rest of your career. Because the book is meant to be an introduction to clinical radiology, we deliberately omitted references for specific discussions. If any reader wishes references to any of the more controversial points, we will be delighted to supply them. We have, however, cited certain texts for each area we covered. Where possible, more than one text is mentioned, and the first reference is usually the most basic.

RECOMMENDED TEXTS

General

Paul, L.W., and Juhl, J.H.: The Essentials of Roentgen Interpretation. Harper & Row, Publishers, Inc., 1972 (3rd edition).

Meschan, I.: Analysis of Roentgen Signs in General Radiology. W. B. Saunders Company, 1973 (3 volumes).

Sutton, D.: A Textbook of Radiology. Churchill Livingstone (Medical Division of Longman, Inc.), 1975 (2nd edition).

Nuclear Medicine

Gottschalk, A., et al.: Diagnostic Nuclear Medicine. The Williams & Wilkins Company, 1976 (Golden's Diagnostic Radiology Series, section 20).

Ultrasound

Gramiak, R., and Waag, R.C.: Cardiac Ultrasound. The C. V. Mosby Company, 1975.

Chest Radiology

Felson, B.: Chest Roentgenology. W. B. Saunders Company, 1973.

Fraser, R.G., and Paré, P.J.A.: Diagnosis of Diseases of the Chest. An Integrated Study Based on the Abnormal Roentgenogram. W. B. Saunders Company, 1977–78 (4 volumes).

Cardiac Radiology

Swischuk, L.E.: Plain Film Interpretation in Congenital Heart Disease. Lea & Febiger, 1970.

Gastrointestinal Radiology

Margulis, A.R., and Burhenne, H.J., eds.: Alimentary Tract Roentgenology. The C. V. Mosby Company, 1973 (2 volumes, 2nd edition).

Genitourinary Radiology

Emmett, J.L., and Witten, D.M.: Clinical Urography: An Atlas and Textbook of Roentgenographic Diagnosis. W. B. Saunders Company, 1971 (3 volumes, 3rd edition).

Witten, D.M., Meyers, G.H., and Utz, D.C.: Emmett's Clinical Urography: An Atlas and Textbook of Roentgenographic Diagnosis. W. B. Saunders Company, 1977 (3 volumes, 4th edition).

Lalli, A.: The Tailored Urogram. Year Book Medical Publishers, 1973.

Bone and Joint Radiology

Greenfield, G.B.: Radiology of Bone Diseases. J. B. Lippincott Company, 1975 (2nd edition).

Edeiken, J., and Hodes, P.J.: Roentgenologic Diagnosis of Diseases of Bone. The Williams & Wilkins Company, 1973 (Golden's Diagnostic Radiology Series, section 6, 2 volumes, 2nd edition).

Murray, R.O., and Jacobson, H.G.: The Radiology of Skeletal Disorders: Exercises in Diagnosis. Churchill Livingstone (Medical Division of Longman, Inc.), 1977 (4 volumes, 2nd edition).

Poznanski, A.K.: The Hand in Radiologic Diagnosis. W. B. Saunders Company, 1974 (Saunders Monographs in Clinical Radiology, volume 4).

Forrester, D.M., Brown, J.M., and Nesson, J.W.: The Radiology of Joint Disease. W. B. Saunders Company, 1978 (Saunders Monographs in Clinical Radiology, volume 2, 2nd edition).

Neuroradiology

Peterson, H.O., and Kieffer, S.A.: Introduction to Neuroradiology. Harper & Row, Publishers, Inc., 1972.

Taveras, J.M., and Wood, E.H.: Diagnostic Neuroradiology. The Williams & Wilkins Company, 1976 (Golden's Diagnostic Radiology Series, section 1, 2nd edition).

Pediatric Radiology

Caffey, J.P., et al.: Pediatric X-ray Diagnosis: A Textbook for Students and Practitioners of Pediatrics, Surgery and Radiology. Year Book Medical Publishers, 1972 (6th edition).

INDEX

Numbers in *italics* indicate illustrations. Numbers followed by t indicate tables.

Common Radiological Terms

AP	Anteroposterior
BE	Barium enema
CT (CAT)	Computerized (axial) tomography
CXR	Chest x-ray
IVP	Intravenous pyelogram
KUB	Plain view of abdomen (kidneys, ureters, bladder)
LAO	Left anterior oblique
LPO	Left posterior oblique
OCG	Oral cholecystogram
PA	Posteroanterior
PEG	Pneumoencephalography
RAO	Right anterior oblique
RPO	Right posterior oblique
RUQ	Right upper quadrant
SBFT	Small bowel follow-through
UGI	Upper gastrointestinal series
VCUG	Voiding cystourethrogram